HIGH-YIELD IMAGING

Chest

HIGH-YIELD IMAGING

Chest

EDITORS

Nestor L. Müller, MD, PhD
Professor and Chairman
Department of Radiology
University of British Columbia
Head and Medical Director
Department of Radiology
Vancouver General Hospital
Vancouver, British Columbia
Canada

C. Isabela S. Silva, MD, PhD
Research Associate
Department of Radiology
University of British Columbia and Vancouver
General Hospital
Vancouver, British Columbia
Canada

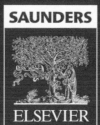

SAUNDERS

ELSEVIER

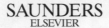

1600 John F. Kennedy Blvd.
Ste 1800
Philadelphia, PA 19103-2899

HIGH-YIELD IMAGING: CHEST

ISBN: 978-1-4160-6161-8

Library of Congress Cataloging-in-Publication Data

High-yield imaging. Chest / editors, Nestor L. Müller, C. Isabela S. Silva. — 1st ed.
   p. ; cm.
  ISBN 978-1-4160-6161-8
  1. Chest—Imaging—Handbooks, manuals, etc. 2. Respiratory organs—Imaging—Handbooks, manuals, etc. I. Müller, Nestor Luiz. II. Silva, C. Isabela S. III. Title: Chest.
  [DNLM: 1. Radiography, Thoracic. 2. Respiratory Tract Diseases—radiography. WF 975 H638 2010]
  RC941.H487 2010
  617.5′407572—dc22   2009041687

Acquisitions Editor: Rebecca Gaertner
Publishing Services Manager: Tina Rebane
Project Manager: Fran Gunning
Design Direction: Steven Stave

Printed in the United States of America

Last digit is the print number: 9 8 7 6 5 4 3 2 1

To Alison and Phillip Müller
and to Nicinha Silva

Preface

The aim of *High-Yield Imaging: Chest* is to provide an overview of the main aspects of chest imaging in a succinct and user-friendly bulleted format and with state-of-the art illustrations. It includes a review of the various radiographic and high-resolution CT patterns of disease and their differential diagnosis and a summary of the main pulmonary, mediastinal, pleural, and chest wall diseases. The text provides the essential information that the radiologist needs to know, including definition of the various abnormalities, radiologic manifestations, clinical utility of the various imaging modalities, characteristic clinical presentation, pathologic features, main diagnostic pearls, and differential diagnosis, as well as the key information that the referring physician needs to know about the condition and its imaging manifestations. The text is based on the 2-volume book *Imaging of the Chest,* published in 2008 by Elsevier, with the text updated in 2009. The figures include the most representative illustrations from that textbook plus new updated images.

The chest radiograph continues to be the most common imaging modality used in diagnostic imaging. The combination of high-quality chest radiographs and a good clinical history allows the radiologist and the respiratory physician to diagnose or to markedly narrow the differential diagnosis of many chest diseases. However, it is well recognized that the chest radiograph has important limitations. High-resolution CT and multidetector spiral CT have become the imaging modalities of choice in many chest diseases, and one or the other technique is performed almost routinely in the evaluation of patients with suspected interstitial lung disease, bronchiectasis, pulmonary embolism, abnormalities of the aorta, and pulmonary or mediastinal tumors. MR imaging has an important role in the assessment of cardiovascular, mediastinal, and chest wall abnormalities. PET imaging and integrated PET-CT have replaced CT as the imaging modalities of choice for the staging of pulmonary carcinoma and lymphoma. The main role of ultrasound in chest imaging is as a guide for aspiration and drainage of pleural fluid collections and for biopsy of pleura-based tumors.

This book is aimed at radiologists, respiratory physicians, and radiology and pulmonary medicine residents and fellows, as well as internists and family practitioners taking care of patients with chest disease. We hope that it will be of value in improving the understanding of the various chest diseases and thus be helpful in improving patient care.

Nestor L. Müller
C. Isabela S. Silva

Acknowledgments

The text of *High-Yield Imaging: Chest* is based on the 2-volume book *Imaging of the Chest,* published in 2008, with the text updated in 2009, and the figures include the most representative illustrations from that textbook plus new updated images. We wish to acknowledge all of our colleagues throughout the world listed below who contributed to *Imaging of the Chest* and without whom neither that book nor this one would have been possible. Our special thanks to the outstanding contributions by Drs. David Hansell, Kyung Soo Lee, Martine Remy-Jardin, Jacques Remy, and Kiminori Fujimoto. We wish also to thank Drs. Philippe Grenier, Catherine Beigelman-Aubry, Jim Barrie, Gustavo Meirelles, Claudia M. Figueiredo, and Marcos Manzini for the images they kindly provided.

Contributors

Masanori Akira
Galit Aviram
Anoop P. Ayyappan
Alexander A. Bankier
Phillip M. Boiselle
John F. Bruzzi
M. Kara Bucci
Susan J. Copley
Sujal R. Desai
Jeremy J. Erasmus
Anthony Febles
Joel E. Fishman
Thomas O. Flukinger
Tomás Franquet
Kiminori Fujimoto

Deepa Gopalan
Marc V. Gosselin
Ahuva Grubstein
David M. Hansell
Thomas E. Hartman
Christian J. Herold
Joshua R. Hill
Peder E. Horner
Kazuya Ichikado
Harumi Itoh,
Takeshi Johkoh
Jeffrey S. Klein
Karen S. Lee
Kyung Soo Lee
Ann Leung

Rebecca M. Lindell
Jaume Llauger
Reginald F. Munden
Clara G. Ooi
Steven L. Primack
Maureen Quigley
Jacques Remy
Martine Remy-Jardin
Nicholas J. Screaton
Jean M. Seely
Nicholas J. Statkus
Maryellen R.M. Sun
Nicola Sverzellati
William D. Travis
Charles S. White

Nestor L. Müller
C. Isabela S. Silva

Contents

SECTION XIII   Diseases of the Airways

SECTION XIV   Inhalational Diseases and Aspiration

SECTION XV   Iatrogenic Lung Disease and Trauma

Radiologic Manifestations of Lung Disease

Focal Consolidation: Acute Causes

DEFINITION: Focal consolidation is replacement of gas within airspaces by fluid, protein, cells, or other material at a single pulmonary focus.

IMAGING

Radiography
Findings
- Fairly homogeneous opacity that is associated with obscuration of the pulmonary vessels and little or no volume loss.
- Adjacent soft tissue structures are obscured: silhouette sign.
- Margins are poorly defined except where the consolidation abuts the pleura.
- Air-containing bronchi (air bronchograms) are frequently visible within areas of consolidation.
- Nonsegmental (lobar) pneumonia may be associated with increased volume and bulging of the interlobar fissure.
- Segmental consolidation may be seen in pneumonia, distal to bronchial obstruction, and in association with acute pulmonary embolism.
- Spherical (round) areas of consolidation may occur in pneumonia or occasionally in pulmonary hemorrhage.
- Lung contusion results in focal consolidation that crosses normal anatomic boundaries.
- Focal right upper lobe pulmonary edema typically occurs secondary to papillary muscle dysfunction after acute myocardial infarction.

Utility
- Silhouette sign is most useful in differentiation of middle lobe and lingular disease from lower lobe disease and may also provide precise anatomic information in other sites.
- Radiography is usually the first and often the only imaging modality used in the assessment of focal consolidation.

CT
Findings
- Consolidation: homogeneous increase in pulmonary parenchymal attenuation that obscures the margins of vessels and airway walls.
- Ground-glass opacities indicating incomplete filling of alveoli adjacent to airspace consolidation.

DIAGNOSTIC PEARLS
- Nonsegmental consolidation is associated with air bronchograms and normal or increased lung volume.
- Segmental consolidation is typically associated with atelectasis and lack of air bronchograms.
- Parenchymal consolidation may result in poorly defined 5- to 10-mm nodular opacities known as airspace nodules.

Utility
- Superior to radiography in demonstrating presence of focal consolidation or ground-glass opacity and the presence of underlying lung disease.

CLINICAL PRESENTATION
- Fever and cough are present in patients with pneumonia.
- Acute shortness of breath may occur in patients with pulmonary embolism.
- Some patients may be asymptomatic or present with nonspecific symptoms.

DIFFERENTIAL DIAGNOSIS
- Bacterial, viral, or fungal pneumonia
- Aspiration pneumonia
- Acute pulmonary embolism
- Pulmonary hemorrhage

PATHOLOGY
- Replacement of gas within the airspaces by fluid, blood, or other material.

INCIDENCE/PREVALENCE AND EPIDEMIOLOGY
- Common causes of acute focal consolidation include pneumonia (bacterial, viral, fungal), hemorrhage, and pulmonary edema.

WHAT THE REFERRING PHYSICIAN NEEDS TO KNOW
- Assessment of silhouette sign is only reliable on radiographs performed using proper technique.
- Hemorrhage should be considered particularly in patients with hemoptysis and those with blunt chest trauma.
- Focal opacities are more commonly seen on high-resolution CT than on radiography.

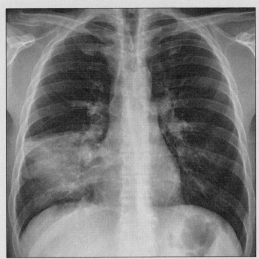

Figure 1. Parenchymal consolidation and silhouette sign. Posteroanterior chest radiograph shows consolidation in the right lower lung zone. Note obscuration of the right-sided heart border (silhouette sign) consistent with consolidation in the right middle lobe. The dome of the right hemidiaphragm is clearly seen consistent with sparing of the basal segments of the lower lobes. The patient was a 37-year-old man with right middle lobe pneumonia.

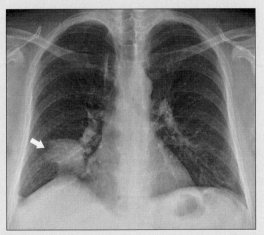

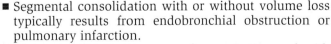

Figure 3. Round pneumonia. Posteroanterior chest radiograph shows round mass-like area of consolidation (*arrow*) in the right middle lobe. The patient was a 41-year-old man who presented with fever and cough. Incidental note is made of azygos fissure.

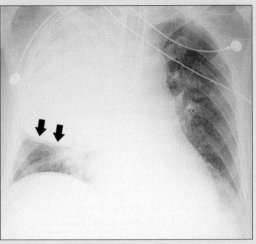

Figure 2. Bulging fissure sign. Anteroposterior chest radiograph shows dense right upper lobe consolidation with increase in volume of the right upper lobe and inferior bulging of the minor fissure (*arrows*). The patient was a 64-year-old man with *Streptococcus. pneumoniae* pneumonia.

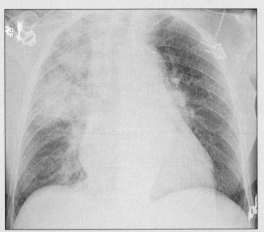

Figure 4. Right upper lobe pulmonary edema due to acute mitral regurgitation. Anteroposterior chest radiograph shows prominence and ill-definition of the pulmonary vascular markings and septal lines consistent with interstitial pulmonary edema. Also noted is extensive right upper lobe consolidation. Although the upper lobe consolidation is most suggestive of a pneumonia, it was proved to be due to airspace pulmonary edema secondary to acute mitral regurgitation after myocardial infarction. The patient was an 83-year-old woman.

- Segmental consolidation with or without volume loss typically results from endobronchial obstruction or pulmonary infarction.
- Segmental distribution seen after aspiration and with pneumonia caused by *Staphylococcus aureus*, *Streptococcus pyogenes*, or a variety of gram-negative bacteria.
- Round pneumonia occurs much more frequently in children than in adults.
- Although round pneumonia in adults may result from bacterial infection, most commonly no organism is identified.
- Focal right upper lobe pulmonary edema is seen most typically with myocardial infarction resulting in papillary muscle dysfunction or rupture and acute mitral regurgitation.

Suggested Readings

Gluecker T, Capasso P, Schnyder P, et al: Clinical and radiologic features of pulmonary edema. *RadioGraphics* 19:1507-1531, 1999.

Grenon H, Bilodeau S: Pulmonary edema of the right upper lobe associated with acute mitral regurgitation. *Can Assoc Radiol J* 45:97-100, 1994.

Wagner AL, Szabunio M, Hazlett KS, Wagner SG: Radiologic manifestations of round pneumonia in adults. *AJR Am J Roentgenol* 170:723-726, 1998.

Focal Consolidation: Chronic Causes

DEFINITION: Focal consolidation is replacement of gas within airspaces by fluid, protein, cells, or other material at a single pulmonary focus.

IMAGING

Radiography
Findings
- Fairly homogeneous opacity associated with obscuration of the pulmonary vessels and adjacent soft tissue structures is known as a silhouette sign.
- Air-containing bronchi (air bronchograms) are frequently visible within areas of consolidation.
- Consolidation in pulmonary carcinoma and lymphoma may be round or have irregular margins.
- Chronic segmental or lobar consolidation with or without associated volume loss suggests bronchial obstruction by tumor or foreign body.
- Chronic focal nonsegmental consolidation often with irregular and poorly defined margins may be seen in lipoid pneumonia.

Utility
- Silhouette sign is most useful in differentiation of middle lobe and lingular disease from lower lobe disease and it may also provide precise anatomic information in other sites.
- Chest radiograph is useful in demonstrating the presence of focal consolidation and in monitoring changes over time.

CT
Findings
- Consolidation is a homogeneous increase in pulmonary parenchymal attenuation that obscures the margins of vessels and airway walls.
- Ground-glass opacity is a homogeneous increase in attenuation that does not obscure underlying vessels.
- A small, round, focal ground-glass opacity is a common manifestation of bronchioloalveolar cell carcinoma.
- The presence of a solid component in association with the focal ground-glass opacity is suggestive of adenocarcinoma.
- Chronic focal area of consolidation with air bronchograms may represent a carcinoma or primary pulmonary lymphoma (maltoma).
- Focal consolidation with localized areas of fat density (−30 to −120 Hounsfield units) is virtually diagnostic of extrinsic lipoid pneumonia.

DIAGNOSTIC PEARLS

- Focal consolidation progressing slowly over several months is suggestive of bronchioloalveolar carcinoma or lymphoma.
- Pulmonary lymphoma may result in single or multiple mass-like areas of consolidation.
- Presence of fat attenuation in focal consolidation is characteristic of lipoid pneumonia.

Utility
- Superior to radiography in the differential diagnosis.
- Superior to radiography in demonstrating presence of bronchial obstruction.
- Frequently allows diagnosis of lipoid pneumonia by demonstrating areas of fat density.

CLINICAL PRESENTATION

- Focal ground-glass opacity or consolidation is frequently an incidental finding in asymptomatic patients.
- Symptoms when present are nonspecific, usually consisting mainly of cough and, occasionally, shortness of breath and hemoptysis.

DIFFERENTIAL DIAGNOSIS

- Organizing pneumonia
- Lipoid pneumonia
- Pulmonary Hodgkin lymphoma
- Pulmonary non-Hodgkin lymphoma
- Bronchioloalveolar cell carcinoma
- Adenocarcinoma

PATHOLOGY

- Replacement of gas within the airspaces by fluid, protein, cells, or other material
- Bronchial obstruction with distal obstructive pneumonitis and atelectasis in endobronchial lesions

WHAT THE REFERRING PHYSICIAN NEEDS TO KNOW

- Pulmonary carcinoma should be suspected in patients with ground-glass opacities or consolidation that is progressive over several months.
- Chronic segmental consolidation with or without atelectasis should suggest the presence of an endobronchial lesion with distal obstruction.
- CT commonly allows the diagnosis of lipoid pneumonia by demonstrating the presence of fat within the consolidation.

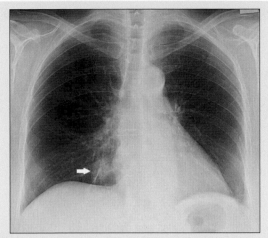

Figure 1. Primary pulmonary lymphoma. Posteroanterior chest radiograph shows focal consolidation in the right lower lung zone (*arrow*). Note focal obliteration of the right-sided heart border (silhouette sign) at the level of the consolidation. The patient was a 53-year-old man with primary lymphocytic lymphoma of the lung (maltoma).

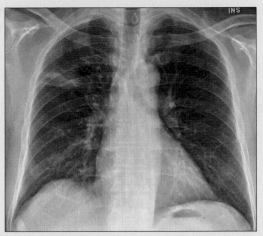

Figure 2. Lipoid pneumonia. Posteroanterior chest radiograph shows focal consolidation in the right upper lobe. The patient was a 55-year-old man with lipoid pneumonia confirmed by fine-needle biopsy and clinical history.

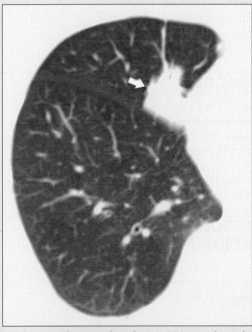

Figure 3. Primary pulmonary lymphoma. CT image shows focal consolidation (*arrow*) in the right middle lobe. The patient was a 53-year-old man with primary lymphocytic lymphoma of the lung (maltoma).

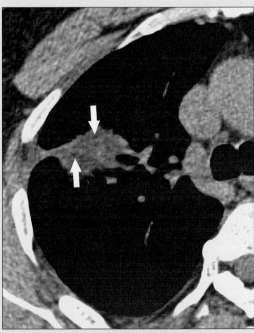

Figure 4. Lipoid pneumonia. High-resolution CT image demonstrates small foci of fat attenuation (*arrows*) within the parenchymal consolidation. The patient was a 55-year-old man with lipoid pneumonia confirmed by fine-needle biopsy and clinical history.

INCIDENCE/PREVALENCE AND EPIDEMIOLOGY

- Segmental consolidation with or without volume loss typically results from endobronchial obstruction or pulmonary infarction.
- Chronic lobar consolidation and atelectasis are usually due to an endobronchial tumor.
- Lipoid pneumonia results from aspiration of mineral, vegetable, or animal oil.
- In approximately 80% of patients with lipoid pneumonia, focal areas of fat attenuation can be seen on CT.

Suggested Readings

King LJ, Padley SP, Wotherspoon AC, et al: Pulmonary MALT lymphoma: Imaging findings in 24 cases. *Eur Radiol* 10:1932-1938, 2000.

Lee KS, Kim Y, Han J, et al: Bronchioloalveolar carcinoma: Clinical, histopathologic, and radiologic findings. *RadioGraphics* 17:1345-1357, 1997.

Lee KS, Müller NL, Hale V, et al: Lipoid pneumonia: CT findings. *J Comput Assist Tomogr* 19:48-51, 1995.

Raz DJ, Kim JY, Jablons DM: Diagnosis and treatment of bronchioloalveolar carcinoma. *Curr Opin Pulm Med* 13:290-296, 2007.

Travis WD, Garg K, Franklin WA, et al: Bronchioloalveolar carcinoma and lung adenocarcinoma: The clinical importance and research relevance of the 2004 World Health Organization pathologic criteria. *J Thorac Oncol* 1(9 Suppl):S13-S19, 2006.

Multifocal Consolidation: Acute Causes

DEFINITION: Multifocal consolidation is replacement of gas within airspaces by fluid, protein, cells, or other material in two or more areas of the lungs.

IMAGING

Radiography
Findings
- Multifocal areas of consolidation presenting acutely are commonly ill defined but may become rapidly confluent.
- Air bronchogram may be associated.
- Bronchopneumonia (bacterial, fungal, or viral) typically results in patchy unilateral or bilateral asymmetric consolidation that may have lobular, subsegmental, or segmental distribution.
- Poorly defined fluffy 5- to 10-mm nodules (airspace nodules) may be evident on the radiograph.
- Diffuse pulmonary hemorrhage (e.g., Goodpasture syndrome, microscopic polyangiitis, Wegener granulomatosis) most commonly results in symmetric, bilateral, poorly defined areas of consolidation.
- Hydrostatic pulmonary edema tends to involve mainly the central lung regions and is commonly associated with septal (Kerley B) lines.

Utility
- Usually the first imaging modality performed in the evaluation of patients with suspected acute airspace disease.
- Helpful in detecting the presence of consolidation and in monitoring disease progression.

CT
Findings
- Bronchopneumonia is characterized by multifocal lobular or confluent areas of consolidation, centrilobular nodules, and branching linear opacities ("tree-in-bud" pattern).
- Ground-glass opacities denote incomplete filling of alveoli adjacent to airspace consolidation.
- Diffuse pulmonary hemorrhage most commonly results in symmetric bilateral ground-glass opacities or poorly defined areas of consolidation that often have a lobular distribution.

Utility
- Superior to chest radiography in demonstrating presence and extent of disease, presence of underlying lung disease, and presence of complications.

CLINICAL PRESENTATION
- Acute multifocal consolidation usually results in cough and shortness of breath.

DIAGNOSTIC PEARLS
- Bronchopneumonia is characterized by multifocal lobular areas of consolidation, centrilobular nodules, and tree-in-bud pattern.
- Pulmonary edema and diffuse pulmonary hemorrhage tend to be bilateral and symmetric and to have a central predominance.

- Fever is usually present in bronchopneumonia.
- Hemoptysis occurs in patients with diffuse pulmonary hemorrhage.

DIFFERENTIAL DIAGNOSIS
- Aspiration pneumonia
- Bronchopneumonia
- Hemorrhage

PATHOLOGY
- Replacement of gas within the airspaces by fluid, protein, cells, or other material.
- Inflammatory exudate in bronchopneumonia.
- Diffuse pulmonary hemorrhage in patients with vasculitis (e.g., Goodpasture syndrome, microscopic polyangiitis, Wegener granulomatosis).

INCIDENCE/PREVALENCE AND EPIDEMIOLOGY
- Causes of acute multifocal consolidation are bronchopneumonia (bacterial, viral, fungal), hemorrhage, and pulmonary edema.

Suggested Readings

Gluecker T, Capasso P, Schnyder P, et al: Clinical and radiologic features of pulmonary edema. *RadioGraphics* 19:1507-1531, 1999.

Herold CJ, Sailer JG: Community-acquired and nosocomial pneumonia. *Eur Radiol* 14(Suppl 3):E2-20, 2004 Mar.

Hiorns MP, Screaton NJ, Muller NL: Acute lung disease in the immunocompromised host. *Radiol Clin North Am* 39:1137-1151, 2001:vi.

Kjeldsberg KM, Oh K, Murray KA, Cannon G: Radiographic approach to multifocal consolidation. *Semin Ultrasound CT MR* 23:288-301, 2002.

WHAT THE REFERRING PHYSICIAN NEEDS TO KNOW
- Hemorrhage should be considered particularly in patients with hemoptysis and in patients with blunt chest trauma.
- Nodular opacities are more commonly seen on high-resolution CT than on radiography.

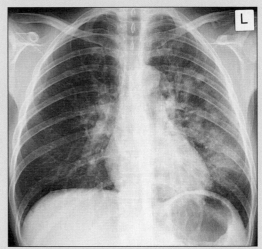

Figure 1. **Multifocal consolidation in bronchopneumonia.** Posteroanterior chest radiograph shows patchy consolidation in the left upper and lower lobes. Note inhomogeneous increased opacity of the left heart compared with the region of the right atrium consistent with consolidation in the retrocardiac region of the left lower lobe.

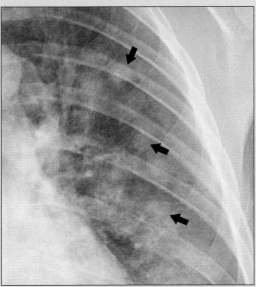

Figure 2. **Airspace nodules.** Magnified view of the left upper lobe in a patient with bronchopneumonia shows several round opacities with poorly defined margins. These represent airspace nodules and have been shown histologically to reflect the presence of peribronchiolar (centrilobular) consolidation.

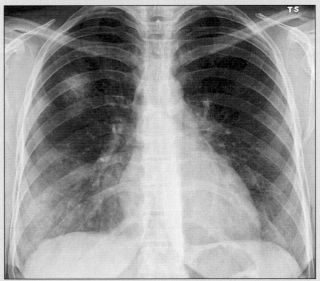

Figure 3. **Multifocal consolidation in diffuse pulmonary hemorrhage.** Posteroanterior chest radiograph shows dense consolidation in the right upper lobe and poorly defined areas of consolidation and ground-glass opacities in the lower lung zones.

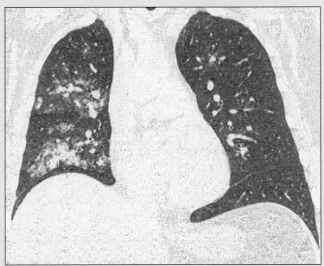

Figure 4. **Bronchopneumonia due to *Streptococcus pneumoniae*.** Coronal reformatted CT image demonstrates centrilobular nodular opacities and small foci of consolidation in the right upper and middle lobes and, to lesser extent, left upper lobe. The patient was a 29-year-old man with acute myelogenous leukemia and *S. pneumoniae* pneumonia.

Multifocal Consolidation: Chronic Causes

DEFINITION: Multifocal consolidation is replacement of gas within airspaces by fluid, protein, cells, or other material in two or more areas of the lungs.

IMAGING

Radiography
Findings
- Air-containing bronchi (air bronchograms) are frequently visible within areas of consolidation.
- Organizing pneumonia most frequently presents as patchy nonsegmental unilateral or bilateral areas of consolidation.
- Chronic eosinophilic pneumonia typically has homogeneous consolidation involving mainly peripheral lung regions of middle and upper lung zones.
- Sarcoidosis may result in peribronchial or, less commonly, peripheral areas of consolidation.
- Multifocal consolidation may be seen in pulmonary lymphoma.

Utility
- Usually the first imaging modality used in the evaluation of patients with suspected consolidation.
- Of limited value in the differential diagnosis of chronic multifocal consolidation.

CT
Findings
- Multifocal consolidation typically associated with ground-glass opacities and small nodules is an uncommon manifestation of bronchioloalveolar carcinoma.
- Organizing pneumonia most commonly results in bilateral consolidation that is often predominantly peribronchial or peripheral in distribution.
- Less common findings include ground-glass opacities, centrilobular nodules, perilobular opacities, and reverse halo sign (focal area of ground-glass opacity surrounded by crescentic or ring-shaped consolidation).
- Chronic eosinophilic pneumonia appears as peripheral and predominantly upper lobe consolidation; similar findings may be seen in Churg-Strauss syndrome.
- Localized collections of fat in patients with consolidation are characteristic of lipoid pneumonia.
- Multifocal consolidation may be seen in pulmonary lymphoma.

DIAGNOSTIC PEARLS
- Organizing pneumonia (bronchiolitis obliterans organizing pneumonia) typically has a peribronchial and peripheral distribution.
- Chronic eosinophilic pneumonia typically has upper lobe predominance and peripheral distribution.
- Pulmonary lymphoma may result in single or multiple mass-like areas of consolidation.

Utility
- CT is superior to radiography in the differential diagnosis of chronic multifocal consolidation.
- Presence of foci of fat density in areas of consolidation on CT is highly suggestive of lipoid pneumonia.

CLINICAL PRESENTATION
- Some patients may be asymptomatic or present with nonspecific symptoms.
- Patients with sarcoidosis typically have mild symptoms even in the presence of extensive bilateral consolidation.
- Patients with cryptogenic organizing pneumonia commonly present with cough, dyspnea, and low-grade fever.
- The majority of patients with chronic eosinophilic pneumonia have peripheral eosinophilia, and approximately 50% have a history of asthma or atopy.

DIFFERENTIAL DIAGNOSIS
- Organizing pneumonia of known etiology
- Lipoid pneumonia
- Pulmonary Hodgkin lymphoma
- Pulmonary non-Hodgkin lymphoma
- Chronic eosinophilic pneumonia
- Lung cancer: Bronchioloalveolar cell carcinoma
- Cryptogenic organizing pneumonia (idiopathic bronchiolitis obliterans organizing pneumonia)

WHAT THE REFERRING PHYSICIAN NEEDS TO KNOW
- In the proper clinical context, the presence of bilateral areas of consolidation that are increasing in extent over several weeks in spite of antibiotics is suggestive of organizing pneumonia.
- In chronic eosinophilic pneumonia, the characteristic pattern of bilateral consolidation involving predominantly or exclusively the peripheral regions of the upper lobes is apparent on the chest radiograph in approximately 60% of patients and on CT in 85% to 100% of cases.
- The diagnosis of lipoid pneumonia can be frequently made on CT by the presence of foci of fat density within the areas of consolidation.

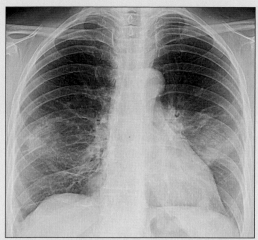

Figure 1. Cryptogenic organizing pneumonia. Posteroanterior chest radiograph shows patchy bilateral areas of consolidation and ground-glass opacities. The patient was a 50-year-old woman with cryptogenic organizing pneumonia.

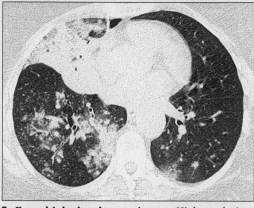

Figure 2. Bronchioloalveolar carcinoma. High-resolution CT image shows extensive consolidation and mild volume loss in the right middle lobe and patchy consolidation, ground-glass opacities, and small nodular opacities in the lower lobes. The patient was a 71-year-old woman with bronchioloalveolar carcinoma.

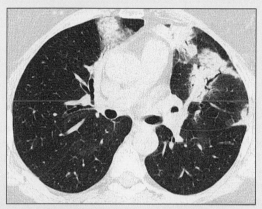

Figure 3. Cryptogenic organizing pneumonia. High-resolution CT image shows bilateral, peripheral, and peribronchial consolidation in the upper lobes. The patient was a 55-year-old woman with cryptogenic organizing pneumonia.

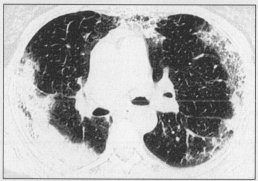

Figure 4. Chronic eosinophilic pneumonia. High-resolution CT image shows bilateral peripheral areas of consolidation. The patient was a 48-year-old woman with chronic eosinophilic pneumonia.

PATHOLOGY

- Gas within the airspaces is replaced by fluid, protein, cells, or other material.
- Organizing pneumonia is characterized by presence of buds of loose granulation tissue within alveolar ducts and air spaces.
- Chronic eosinophilic pneumonia is characterized by filling of the alveolar airspaces by an inflammatory infiltrate containing a high proportion of eosinophils.
- Numerous lipid-laden macrophages, inflammatory cellular infiltration, and a variable amount of fibrosis in lipoid pneumonia.

INCIDENCE/PREVALENCE AND EPIDEMIOLOGY

- Although most cases of organizing pneumonia are idiopathic, similar reaction pattern may also be seen in many clinical settings.

- Lipoid pneumonia results from aspiration of mineral, vegetable, or animal oil.
- Approximately 50% of patients with chronic eosinophilic pneumonia have a history of asthma or atopy.

Suggested Readings

Cordier JF: Cryptogenic organising pneumonia. *Eur Respir J* 28:422-446, 2006.

Jeong YJ, Kim KI, Seo IJ, et al: Eosinophilic lung diseases: A clinical, radiologic, and pathologic overview. *RadioGraphics* 27:617-637, 2007:discussion 637–639.

King LJ, Padley SP, Wotherspoon AC, et al: Pulmonary MALT lymphoma: Imaging findings in 24 cases. *Eur Radiol* 10:1932-1938, 2000.

Kjeldsberg KM, Oh K, Murray KA, Cannon G: Radiographic approach to multifocal consolidation. *Semin Ultrasound CT MR* 23:288-301, 2002.

Diffuse Consolidation: Acute Causes

DEFINITION: Diffuse consolidation occurs after replacement of gas within the airspaces by fluid, protein, cells, or other material throughout most of the lungs.

IMAGING

Radiography

Findings
- Hydrostatic pulmonary edema: consolidation in the perihilar regions (butterfly or bat wing distribution) associated with thickening of interlobular septa.
- Common ancillary findings: cardiomegaly and enlarged pulmonary vessels.
- Acute respiratory distress syndrome: initially patchy then becomes rapidly confluent and diffuse.
- Diffuse pulmonary hemorrhage: patchy or confluent bilateral areas of consolidation that tend to involve middle and lower lung zones.

Utility
- Usually the first and frequently the only imaging modality used in the assessment of these patients.
- Limited value in the differential diagnosis.

CT

Findings
- Hydrostatic pulmonary edema tends to have perihilar and gravitational distribution.
- Association is common with smooth interlobular septal thickening and small pleural effusions.
- Acute respiratory distress syndrome shows as bilateral consolidation and/or ground-glass opacities that may be patchy or diffuse.
- Septal thickening and smooth intralobular lines are frequently superimposed on ground-glass opacities resulting in "crazy-paving" pattern.
- Radiologic manifestations of acute interstitial pneumonia are those of acute respiratory distress syndrome.
- Diffuse pulmonary hemorrhage shows as bilateral patchy or confluent areas of consolidation and/or ground-glass opacities; poorly defined centrilobular nodules may be seen.

Utility
- High-resolution CT is superior to radiography in demonstrating the presence and extent of abnormalities and the presence of complications.
- High-resolution CT findings are relatively nonspecific.

CLINICAL PRESENTATION

- Dyspnea
- Hemoptysis in diffuse pulmonary hemorrhage

DIAGNOSTIC PEARLS

- Fairly homogeneous opacity associated with obscuration of the pulmonary vessels and little or no volume loss.
- Acute respiratory distress syndrome: initially patchy then becomes rapidly confluent and diffuse.
- Diffuse pulmonary hemorrhage: bilateral patchy or confluent areas of consolidation and/or ground-glass opacities.

DIFFERENTIAL DIAGNOSIS

- Severe pneumonia
- Pulmonary edema
- Pulmonary hemorrhage
- Acute respiratory distress syndrome
- Acute interstitial pneumonia

PATHOLOGY

- Interstitial and airspace pulmonary edema associated with thickening of interlobular septa in hydrostatic pulmonary edema.
- Diffuse alveolar damage in acute respiratory distress syndrome and acute interstitial pneumonia.
- Filling of the airspace with blood in diffuse pulmonary hemorrhage.
- Pulmonary capillaritis in patients with underlying immunologic disorders such as Goodpasture syndrome.

INCIDENCE/PREVALENCE AND EPIDEMIOLOGY

- Acute causes of diffuse consolidation are edema, pneumonia, acute respiratory distress syndrome, and hemorrhage.
- Acute interstitial pneumonia is a rare fulminant disease of unknown etiology that usually occurs in a previously healthy person and manifests as clinical, radiologic, and pathologic findings of acute respiratory distress syndrome.

Suggested Readings

Gluecker T, Capasso P, Schnyder P, et al: Clinical and radiologic features of pulmonary edema. *RadioGraphics* 19:1507-1531, 1999.

WHAT THE REFERRING PHYSICIAN NEEDS TO KNOW

- Radiologic appearance of extensive or diffuse bilateral consolidation is often similar regardless of cause.
- The differential diagnosis greatly influenced by the clinical history and immune status of the patient.

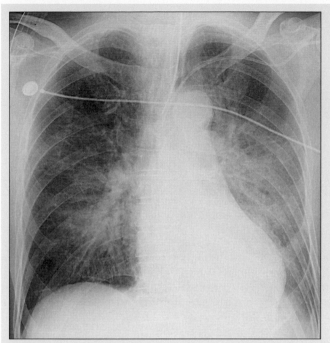

Figure 1. Hydrostatic pulmonary edema. Posteroanterior chest radiograph shows extensive consolidation with relative sparing of the subpleural regions. A permanent pacemaker and an endotracheal tube are in place. The patient was a 63-year-old man with recurrent episodes of acute left-sided heart failure.

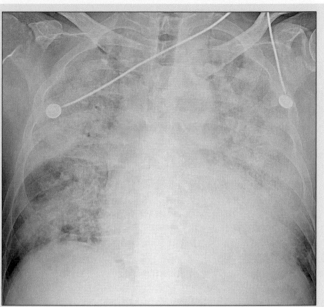

Figure 2. Acute respiratory distress syndrome. Anteroposterior chest radiograph shows extensive bilateral areas of consolidation. The patient was a 71-year-old man with acute respiratory distress syndrome. He was intubated shortly after obtaining the chest radiograph.

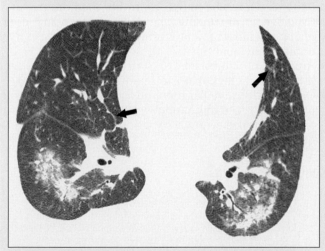

Figure 3. Perihilar distribution of pulmonary edema. High-resolution CT image shows consolidation and ground-glass opacities in the lower lobes. Also noted are mild interlobular septal thickening (*arrows*) and small pleural effusions. The patient was a 45-year-old man with acute hydrostatic pulmonary edema due to left-sided heart failure.

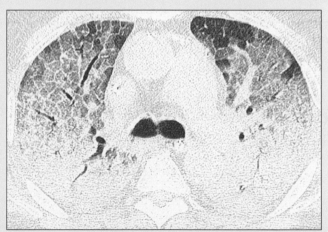

Figure 4. Acute respiratory distress syndrome. High-resolution CT image shows bilateral consolidation with air bronchograms in the dependent regions of the lungs. Also noted are extensive ground-glass opacities with superimposed smooth septal thickening ("crazy-paving" pattern). The patient was a 71-year-old man with acute respiratory distress syndrome.

Ichikado K, Suga M, Muranaka H, et al: Prediction of prognosis for acute respiratory distress syndrome with thin-section CT: Validation in 44 cases. *Radiology* 238:321-329, 2006.

Johkoh T, Müller NL, Taniguchi H, et al: Acute interstitial pneumonia: Thin-section CT findings in 36 patients. *Radiology* 211:859-863, 1999.

Primack SL, Miller RR, Müller NL: Diffuse pulmonary hemorrhage: Clinical, pathologic, and imaging features. *AJR Am J Roentgenol* 164:295-300, 1995.

Diffuse Consolidation: Chronic Causes

DEFINITION: Diffuse consolidation is replacement of gas within the airspaces by fluid, protein, cells, or other material throughout most of the lungs.

IMAGING

Radiography
Findings
- Organizing pneumonia: typically multifocal consolidation; occasionally may be diffuse.
- Chronic eosinophilic pneumonia: typically involving mainly peripheral lung and upper lobes (reverse pulmonary edema pattern).
- Alveolar proteinosis: bilateral areas of consolidation that have a vaguely nodular appearance and in up to 50% of cases is perihilar (bat wing or butterfly distribution).

Utility
- Helpful in demonstrating presence and extent of abnormalities.
- Limited value in the differential diagnosis.

CT
Findings
- Organizing pneumonia: bilateral consolidation, peripheral, perilobular, and peribronchial distribution, reversed halo sign, and ground-glass opacities.
- Chronic eosinophilic pneumonia: bilateral parenchymal consolidation mainly peripheral lung regions ("the photographic negative of pulmonary edema").

Utility
- Superior to radiography in showing distribution of disease and in the differential diagnosis.

CLINICAL PRESENTATION

- Cough and progressive shortness of breath.
- History of asthma and peripheral eosinophilia common in chronic eosinophilic pneumonia.

DIFFERENTIAL DIAGNOSIS

- Chronic eosinophilic pneumonia
- Organizing pneumonia of known etiology
- Cryptogenic organizing pneumonia
- Pulmonary alveolar proteinosis

DIAGNOSTIC PEARLS

- Chronic eosinophilic pneumonia: upper lobe predominance, peripheral distribution pattern.
- Organizing pneumonia: peribronchial and peripheral distribution, reversed halo sign.

PATHOLOGY

- Chronic eosinophilic pneumonia: abundant accumulation of eosinophils in pulmonary interstitium and airspaces.
- Organizing pneumonia: presence of buds of loose granulation tissue within alveolar ducts and air spaces.
- Alveolar proteinosis: accumulation of protein- and lipid-rich material resembling surfactant within the parenchymal airspaces.

INCIDENCE/PREVALENCE AND EPIDEMIOLOGY

- Chronic diffuse pulmonary consolidation is much less common than acute diffuse consolidation.
- Patterns tend to be multifocal rather than diffuse.
- Cryptogenic organizing pneumonia, secondary organizing pneumonia, and eosinophilic lung disease may occasionally be diffuse.
- Alveolar proteinosis is an uncommon condition of unknown etiology that is often diffuse.
- Occasionally, alveolar proteinosis may be secondary to inhalation of large quantities of silica dust (silicoproteinosis) or be seen in association with marked immunosuppression.

Suggested Readings

Chung MJ, Lee KS, Franquet T, et al: Metabolic lung disease: Imaging and histopathologic findings. *Eur J Radiol* 54:233-245, 2005.

Jeong YJ, Kim KI, Seo IJ, et al: Eosinophilic lung diseases: A clinical, radiologic, and pathologic overview. *RadioGraphics* 27:617-637, 2007.

Lee KS, Kim EA: High-resolution CT of alveolar filling disorders. *Radiol Clin North Am* 39:1211-1230, 2001.

Lee KS, Kullnig P, Hartman TE, Müller NL: Cryptogenic organizing pneumonia: CT findings in 43 patients. *AJR Am J Roentgenol* 162:543-546, 1994.

WHAT THE REFERRING PHYSICIAN NEEDS TO KNOW

- Radiologic appearance of extensive or diffuse bilateral consolidation is often similar regardless of cause.
- It is essential to know clinical history, laboratory findings, and immune status of patient.

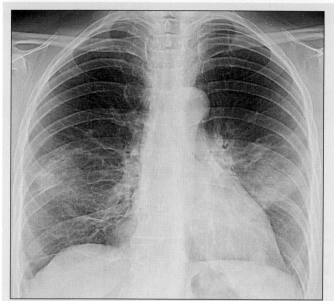

Figure 1. Cryptogenic organizing pneumonia. Posteroanterior chest radiograph shows patchy bilateral areas of consolidation and ground-glass opacities. The patient was a 50-year-old woman with cryptogenic organizing pneumonia.

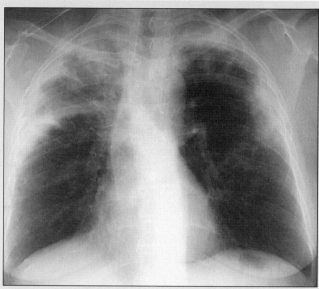

Figure 2. Chronic eosinophilic pneumonia. Posteroanterior chest radiograph shows bilateral areas of consolidation involving the peripheral regions of the upper and middle lung zones. The patient was a 48-year-old woman with chronic eosinophilic pneumonia.

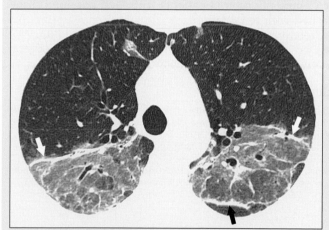

Figure 3. Cryptogenic organizing pneumonia. High-resolution CT in a 58-year-old immunocompromised woman with organizing pneumonia shows extensive bilateral ground-glass opacities, a few small nodular opacities, and bilateral crescentic and ring-like consolidation (*arrows*) surrounding areas of ground-glass opacification (reversed halo sign).

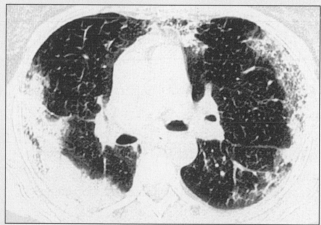

Figure 4. Chronic eosinophilic pneumonia. High-resolution CT image shows bilateral peripheral areas of consolidation. The patient was a 48-year-old woman with chronic eosinophilic pneumonia.

Central Consolidation (Butterfly or Bat Wing Distribution)

DEFINITION: Central consolidation is replacement of gas within airspaces by fluid, protein, cells, or other material with bilateral distribution mainly in the central two thirds of the lungs.

IMAGING

Radiography

Findings
- Fairly homogeneous opacity associated with obscuration of pulmonary vessels and little or no volume loss.
- Obscures adjacent soft tissue structures.

Utility
- Usually only imaging modality used in the assessment of these patients.
- High sensitivity and specificity.

CT

Findings
- Bilateral ground-glass opacities with superimposed interlobar septal thickening and intralobular lines ("crazy-paving" pattern).
- Perihilar and gravitational distribution of edema.
- Possible association with severe edema of areas of consolidation involving mainly the dependent lung regions.
- "Crazy-paving" pattern also seen in alveolar proteinosis and pulmonary hemorrhage.
- Peribronchial consolidation noted in bronchiolitis obliterans organizing pneumonia.

Utility
- Superior to radiography in showing the pattern and extent of abnormalities

CLINICAL PRESENTATION

- Dyspnea, cough
- Hemoptysis in diffuse pulmonary hemorrhage

DIFFERENTIAL DIAGNOSIS

- Hydrostatic pulmonary edema
- Diffuse pulmonary hemorrhage

DIAGNOSTIC PEARLS

- Acute causes: Hydrostatic pulmonary edema, diffuse pulmonary hemorrhage.
- Chronic causes: Organizing pneumonia, alveolar proteinosis.

- Cryptogenic organizing pneumonia
- Organizing pneumonia reaction pattern
- Bronchopneumonia
- *Pneumocystis* pneumonia
- Alveolar proteinosis

INCIDENCE/PREVALENCE AND EPIDEMIOLOGY

- Common manifestation of hydrostatic pulmonary edema.
- Commonly seen in patients with fluid overload associated with renal failure.
- Relatively common in *Pneumocystis* pneumonia.
- Occasionally seen in bronchiolitis obliterans organizing pneumonia and alveolar proteinosis.

Suggested Readings

Gluecker T, Capasso P, Schnyder P, et al: Clinical and radiologic features of pulmonary edema. *RadioGraphics* 19:1507-1531, 1999.

Primack S, Miller RR, Muller NL: Diffuse pulmonary hemorrhage: Clinical, pathologic, and imaging features. *AJR Am J Roentgenol* 164:295-300, 1995.

Storto ML, Kee ST, Golden JA: Hydrostatic pulmonary edema: High-resolution CT findings. *AJR Am Roentgenol* 165:817-820, 1995.

WHAT THE REFERRING PHYSICIAN NEEDS TO KNOW

- Radiologic appearance of extensive or diffuse bilateral consolidation is often similar regardless of cause.
- It is essential to know the clinical history (e.g., trauma, known systemic disease), presence of fever, and immune status of patient.

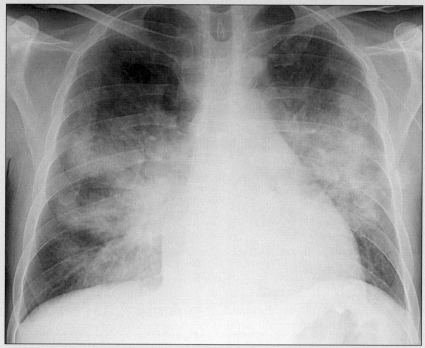

Figure 1. **Bat wing pattern of pulmonary edema.** Posteroanterior radiograph shows consolidation of the perihilar and medullary portions of both lungs, creating a bat wing or butterfly appearance; the cortex of both lungs is relatively unaffected. The consolidation is fairly homogeneous and is associated with well-defined air bronchograms on both sides. Also noted is a central venous line. The patient was a 38-year-old man with severe acute hydrostatic pulmonary edema.

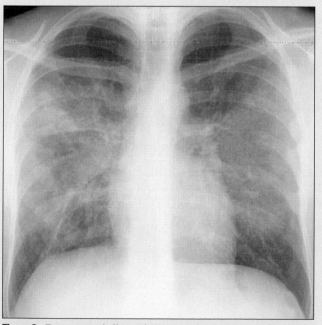

Figure 2. *Pneumocystis jiroveci* **pneumonia.** Posteroanterior chest radiograph shows bilateral areas of consolidation and ground-glass opacities in a predominantly perihilar distribution. The patient was a 32-year-old with AIDS and *P. jiroveci* pneumonia.

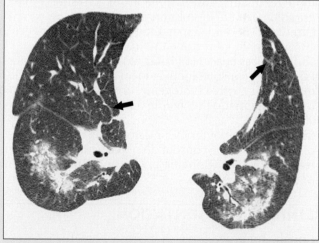

Figure 3. **Perihilar distribution of pulmonary edema.** High-resolution CT image shows consolidation and ground-glass opacities in the lower lobes. Also noted are mild interlobular septal thickening (*arrows*) and small pleural effusions. The patient was a 45-year-old man with acute hydrostatic pulmonary edema due to left-sided heart failure.

Peripheral Consolidation (Reverse Pulmonary Edema Pattern)

DEFINITION: Peripheral consolidation is replacement of gas within airspaces by fluid, protein, cells, or other material predominantly in the outer third of the lungs.

IMAGING

Radiography
Findings
- Bilateral parenchymal consolidation involves mainly the peripheral lung regions ("photographic negative of pulmonary edema").
- May be seen in chronic eosinophilic pneumonia, cryptogenic organizing pneumonia (idiopathic bronchiolitis obliterans organizing pneumonia), and, less commonly, pneumonia, acute respiratory distress syndrome, sarcoidosis, and bronchioloalveolar carcinoma.
- Peripheral distribution, involving mainly upper lobes, is apparent in approximately 60% of patients with chronic eosinophilic pneumonia.
- Peripheral consolidation is apparent on the radiograph in a small percentage of patients with cryptogenic organizing pneumonia.

Utility
- Helpful in showing presence, distribution, and extent of parenchymal abnormalities.

CT
Findings
- Bilateral parenchymal consolidation.
- Involves mainly the peripheral lung regions ("photographic negative of pulmonary edema").
- Often middle and upper lung zone predominance in chronic eosinophilic pneumonia.
- Ground-glass opacities adjacent to areas of consolidation.
- Peripheral consolidation evident on CT in 60%-80% of patients with cryptogenic organizing pneumonia, mainly involving the middle and lower lung zones.

Utility
- Superior to radiography in determining the peripheral distribution of the consolidation particularly in patients with chronic eosinophilic pneumonia and cryptogenic organizing pneumonia.

CLINICAL PRESENTATION

- Cough and progressive shortness of breath.
- Low-grade fever common in chronic eosinophilic pneumonia and cryptogenic organizing pneumonia.
- History of atopy or asthma in approximately 50% of patients with chronic eosinophilic pneumonia.

DIAGNOSTIC PEARLS

- Cryptogenic organizing pneumonia: Peribronchial and peripheral distribution, reverse halo sign.
- Chronic eosinophilic pneumonia: Upper lobe predominance.
- Uncommon causes: Sarcoidosis, bronchioloalveolar carcinoma, and Churg-Strauss syndrome.

- Peripheral eosinophilia in majority of patients with chronic eosinophilic pneumonia.

DIFFERENTIAL DIAGNOSIS

- Cryptogenic organizing pneumonia
- Organizing pneumonia of known etiology
- Chronic eosinophilic pneumonia
- Sarcoidosis
- Churg-Strauss syndrome
- Bronchioloalveolar carcinoma

PATHOLOGY

- Chronic eosinophilic pneumonia: abundant accumulation of eosinophils in the pulmonary interstitium and airspaces; may be manifestation of Churg-Strauss syndrome.
- Eosinophilic vasculitis seen almost exclusively in patients with asthma.
- Organizing pneumonia: intraluminal plugs of granulation tissue within alveolar ducts and surrounding alveoli with or without concomitant granulation tissue polyps within the respiratory bronchioles.

INCIDENCE/PREVALENCE AND EPIDEMIOLOGY

- Approximately 50% of patients with chronic eosinophilic pneumonia have history of atopy, most often asthma, and most have peripheral eosinophilia.

WHAT THE REFERRING PHYSICIAN NEEDS TO KNOW

- Radiologic appearance of bilateral consolidation is often similar regardless of cause.
- It is essential to know clinical history (e.g., known systemic disease), presence of fever, and immune status of patient.

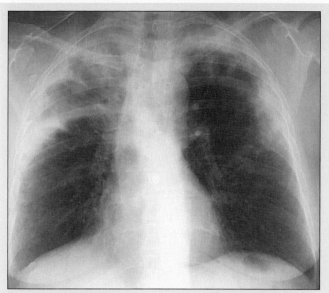

Figure 1. **Peripheral consolidation in chronic eosinophilic pneumonia.** Posteroanterior chest radiograph shows bilateral areas of consolidation involving the peripheral regions of the upper and middle lung zones. The patient was a 48-year old woman with chronic eosinophilic pneumonia.

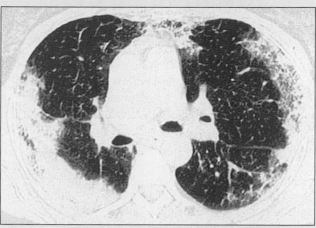

Figure 2. **Peripheral consolidation in chronic eosinophilic pneumonia.** High-resolution CT image shows bilateral peripheral areas of consolidation. The patient was a 48-year-old woman with chronic eosinophilic pneumonia.

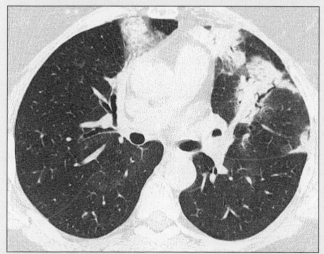

Figure 3. **Peripheral consolidation in cryptogenic organizing pneumonia.** High-resolution CT image shows bilateral peripheral and peribronchial areas of consolidation in the upper lobes. The patient was a 55-year-old woman with cryptogenic organizing pneumonia.

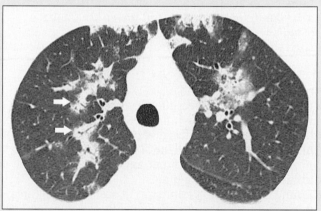

Figure 4. **Peribronchial and peripheral consolidation in cryptogenic organizing pneumonia.** High-resolution CT image shows bilateral areas of consolidation in a peribronchial (*arrows*) and subpleural distribution. The patient was a 34-year-old man with cryptogenic organizing pneumonia.

Suggested Readings

Allen JN, Davis WB: Eosinophilic lung diseases. *Am J Respir Crit Care Med* 150:1423-1438, 1994.

Cordier JF: Cryptogenic organising pneumonia. *Eur Respir J* 28:422-446, 2006.

Kim Y, Lee KS, Choi DC, et al: The spectrum of eosinophilic lung disease: Radiologic findings. *J Comput Assist Tomogr* 21:920-930, 1997.

Lynch DA, Travis WD, Müller NL, et al: Idiopathic interstitial pneumonias: CT features. *Radiology* 236:10-21, 2005.

Atelectasis

DEFINITION: Atelectasis is defined as less than normal inflation of all or part of the lung with corresponding diminution in lung volume.

IMAGING

Radiography
Findings
- Direct signs: displaced interlobar fissures, crowding of vessels and bronchi.
- Indirect signs: increased opacity; displacement of hilum, mediastinum, hemidiaphragm; tenting (juxta-phrenic peak) of hemidiaphragm; compensatory over-inflation of remaining lung.
- Silhouette sign: obliteration of right-sided heart border in right middle lobe atelectasis and left cardiac border/mediastinum in left upper lobe atelectasis.
- Luftsichel: a crescent of hyperlucency ("air crescent") adjacent to aortic arch in left upper lobe atelectasis.
- Round atelectasis: bronchi and vessels gather in curvi-linear fashion as they pass toward pleural-based nodu-lar opacity or mass (comet tail sign).
- Linear soft tissue opacities of 1-3 mm thickness and 4-10 cm in length in mid and lower lung zone.

Utility
- High sensitivity and specificity in diagnosis of atelectasis.

CT
Findings
- Direct signs: displaced interlobar fissures, crowding of vessels and bronchi within the atelectatic lobe.
- Indirect signs: increased opacity, displacement of hilum, mediastinum, hemidiaphragm; tenting (juxta-phrenic peak) of hemidiaphragm; compensatory over-inflation of remaining lung.
- Round atelectasis: peripheral "mass" abutting area of thickening pleura, associated with volume loss, and bronchi and vessels gathering in curvilinear fashion as they pass toward pleural-based nodular opacity or mass (comet tail sign).
- Dependent atelectasis: ill-defined area of increased attenuation/subpleural curvilinear opacities in dorsal

DIAGNOSTIC PEARLS

- Displacement of the fissures that form the boundary of atelectatic lobe.
- Crowding of vessels and bronchi visible within area of atelectasis.
- Increased opacity accompanied by diaphragmatic elevation, mediastinal shift, and overinflation of remainder of unaffected lung.

lung regions that typically resolves when patient is prone.
Utility
- Provides valuable additional information in obstruc-tive atelectasis with regard to location and extent.
- Distinguishes proximal obstructing tumor from col-lapsed lung/adjacent mediastinal structures with intra-venous contrast material.
- Differentiates dependent atelectasis from interstitial/airspace disease by scanning with patient in supine and prone position.

CLINICAL PRESENTATION

- Patient may be asymptomatic.
- Cough, dyspnea.

DIFFERENTIAL DIAGNOSIS

- Diffuse consolidation: Acute causes
- Diffuse consolidation: Chronic causes
- Focal consolidation: Acute causes
- Focal consolidation: Chronic causes
- Lobar pneumonia
- Acute pulmonary embolism
- Aspiration pneumonia

WHAT THE REFERRING PHYSICIAN NEEDS TO KNOW

- Lack of air bronchograms within atelectatic lung is suggestive of bronchial obstruction (resorptive atelectasis).
- CT, particularly contrast-enhanced CT, often provides valuable additional information in patients with obstructive atelectasis, particularly with regard to the precise location and extent of the obstructing process.
- Round atelectasis is seen most commonly in patients with asbestos-related pleural disease.
- The diagnosis of rounded atelectasis can often be made confidently on CT.

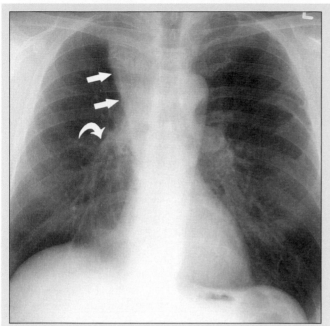

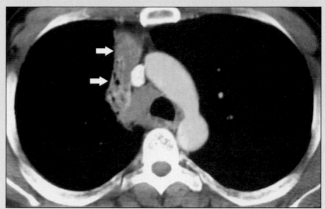

Figure 2. Direct and indirect signs of atelectasis. Contrast-enhanced CT image shows cephalad and medial displacement of the minor fissure (*arrows*). Also note presence of mediastinal lymphadenopathy. The patient was a 47-year-old man with right upper lobe atelectasis due to endobronchial pulmonary carcinoma.

Figure 1. Direct and indirect signs of atelectasis. View from a chest radiograph shows cephalad and medial displacement of the minor fissure (*straight arrows*), a direct sign of right upper lobe atelectasis. Also note several indirect signs, including increased opacity of the atelectatic lobe, superior displacement of the right hilum, lateral displacement of the right interlobar pulmonary artery (*curved arrow*), and elevation of the right hemidiaphragm. The patient was a 47-year-old man with right upper lobe atelectasis due to endobronchial pulmonary carcinoma.

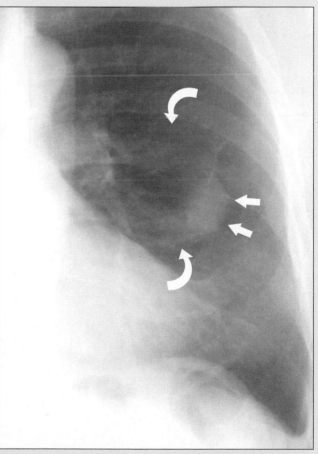

Figure 4. Round atelectasis. Magnified view of the left lung from a posteroanterior chest radiograph shows an oval opacity. The lateral margins (*straight arrows*) are well defined (where the opacity abuts the lung) and the medial margins are poorly defined (where the opacity abuts the pleura). Pulmonary vessels (*curved arrows*) can be seen to curve toward the opacity (comet tail sign). The patient was a 71-year-old man with asbestos-related pleural plaques and round atelectasis.

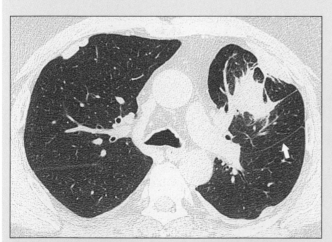

Figure 3. Round atelectasis. High-resolution CT image shows irregular mass in the left upper lobe with band-like opacities extending toward an area of pleural thickening. Also note volume loss of the left upper lobe causing curvilinear anterior displacement of the left major fissure (*straight arrow*). The patient was a 75-year-old man with a history of asbestos exposure.

PATHOLOGY

- Obstructive/resorptive atelectasis: air flow to region of lung interrupted due to airway obstruction.
- Loss of volume as lung retracts in presence of pneumothorax.
- Compression of lung by adjacent space-occupying process.
- Deficiency in surfactant increases surface tension of alveoli; increase in distending pressure.
- Retraction of fibrous tissue as it matures, resulting in volume loss of affected portion of lung.

INCIDENCE/PREVALENCE AND EPIDEMIOLOGY

- Segmental, lobar, and whole-lung atelectasis is commonly due to bronchial obstruction by secretions or tumor.
- Most cases of round atelectasis are seen in patients exposed to asbestos.
- Lower left lobe atelectasis occurs in the majority of patients after cardiac surgery.

Suggested Readings

Lee KS, Logan PM, Primack SL, Müller NL: Combined lobar atelectasis of the right lung: Imaging findings. *AJR Am J Roentgenol* 163:43-47, 1994.

Molina PL, Hiken JN, Glazer HS: Imaging evaluation of obstructive atelectasis. *J Thorac Imag* 11:176-186, 1996.

Proto AV: Lobar collapse: Basic concepts. *Eur J Radiol* 23:9-22, 1996.

Woodring JH, Reed JC: Types and mechanisms of pulmonary atelectasis. *J Thorac Imag* 11:92-108, 1996.

Woodring JH, Reed JC: Radiographic manifestations of lobar atelectasis. *J Thorac Imag* 11:109-144, 1996.

Lobar Atelectasis

DEFINITION: Lobar atelectasis is less than normal inflation of all or part of the lung with corresponding diminution in lung volume.

IMAGING

Radiography
Findings
- Direct signs: displaced interlobar fissures, crowded air bronchograms.
- Indirect signs: increased opacity; displacement of hilum, mediastinum, hemidiaphragm; tenting (juxtaphrenic peak) of hemidiaphragm; compensatory over-inflation of remaining lung.
- Left upper lobe atelectasis: left major fissure shifted cephalad and anteriorly seen on the lateral view; over-inflated superior segment often resulting in hyperlucent crescent adjacent to aortic arch ("Luftsichel" sign) on frontal view.
- Right middle lobe atelectasis: approximation of minor fissure and lower half of major fissure seen on the lateral radiograph; obscuration of right-sided heart border on frontal view.
- Combined right middle and lower lobe atelectasis: major and minor fissures displaced downward and backward so that opacity occupies posteroinferior portion of hemithorax; right hemidiaphragm obscured by atelectatic right lower lobe; right-sided heart border obscured by atelectatic right middle lobe.
- Combined right middle and upper lobe atelectasis: findings similar to those of left upper lobe atelectasis.
- Obstructive lobar atelectasis typically associated with increased opacity of atelectatic lobe and lack of air bronchograms.
- Hilar tumor with distal atelectasis typically shown by S sign of Golden, with a downward bulge in medial portion and concave appearance of lateral portion of interlobar fissure; most commonly seen in association with right upper lobe atelectasis.
Utility
- First and often only imaging modality used in assessment of patients with lobar atelectasis.

CT
Findings
- Direct signs: displaced interlobar fissures, crowded air bronchograms.
- Indirect signs: increased opacity; displacement of hilum, mediastinum, hemidiaphragm; tenting (juxtaphrenic peak) of hemidiaphragm usually related to presence of inferior

DIAGNOSTIC PEARLS
- Displacement of interlobar fissures is a direct sign of atelectasis.
- Patterns of atelectasis of right and left upper lobes differ because there is no minor fissure on the left.
- Findings of right lower lobe atelectasis are similar to those of left lower lobe atelectasis.
- Right middle lobe atelectasis is often detectable only on the lateral radiograph or CT.

accessory fissure; compensatory overinflation of remaining lung.
- Often demonstrates cause of atelectasis.
Utility
- Provides valuable additional information in patients with obstructive atelectasis, regarding precise location and extent of obstructing process.

MRI
Findings
- Decreased volume and increased signal intensity of atelectatic lobe.
Utility
- May be helpful in assessment of obstructive atelectasis due to central tumor.

CLINICAL PRESENTATION
- Patients may be asymptomatic.
- Acute symptoms are cough and shortness of breath in patients with acute atelectasis due to bronchial obstruction by mucus, aspiration, or foreign body.
- Chronic cough and, occasionally, hemoptysis occur in patients with lobar atelectasis due to bronchiectasis or endobronchial tumor.

DIFFERENTIAL DIAGNOSIS
- Lobar pneumonia
- Single and multiple pulmonary masses

WHAT THE REFERRING PHYSICIAN NEEDS TO KNOW
- Displacement of fissures that form boundaries of atelectatic lobes is a dependable and easily recognized sign of atelectasis.
- CT is commonly helpful in demonstrating cause of atelectasis.
- Contrast-enhanced CT is particularly helpful in demonstrating central obstructing tumors.

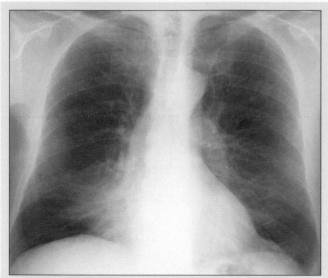

Figure 1. Right middle lobe atelectasis. Posteroanterior radiograph shows poorly defined area of increased attenuation, associated with obscuration of the right-sided heart border ("silhouette" sign).

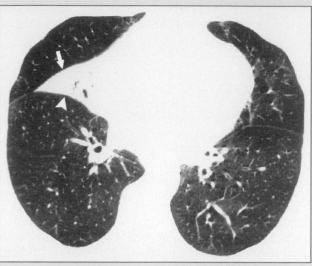

Figure 2. Right middle lobe atelectasis. High-resolution CT image shows characteristic broad triangular configuration of atelectatic right middle lobe. The anterior border of the atelectatic lobe is outlined by the minor fissure, which is displaced downward (*arrow*), and the posterior border by the major fissure, which is displaced upward and forward (*arrowhead*). The patient was a 72-year-old woman with chronic right middle lobe atelectasis secondary to bronchiectasis.

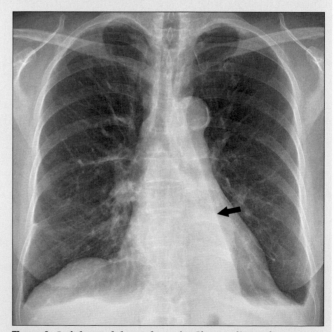

Figure 3. Right middle lobe atelectasis. Lateral view shows downward shift of the minor fissure and forward shift of the right major fissure, leading to a triangular area of increased opacity (*arrow*) characteristic of right middle lobe atelectasis.

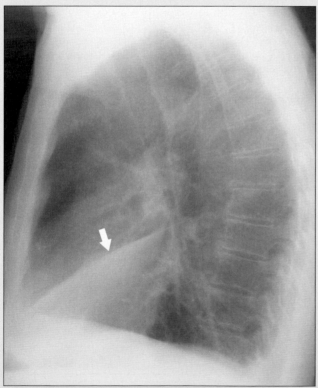

Figure 4. Left lower lobe atelectasis. Chest radiograph shows inferior and medial displacement of the left major fissure resulting in a well-defined interface (*arrow*) extending obliquely downward and laterally from the region of the hilum, characteristic of left lower lobe atelectasis. The atelectatic left lower lobe obscures the silhouette of the left descending pulmonary artery and the left hemidiaphragm. The patient was a 69-year-old woman with asthma.

INCIDENCE/PREVALENCE AND EPIDEMIOLOGY

- Hilar displacement occurs more commonly in atelectasis of upper than lower lobes.
- Downward displacement of right hilum in cases of lower lobe atelectasis is seldom clearly appreciated.
- Downward displacement of only the left hilum is seen in only 3% of normal individuals.
- Combined right upper and middle lobe atelectasis occurs most commonly with mucus plugs and pulmonary carcinoma.
- Less commonly, right upper and middle lobe collapse occur with carcinoid tumors, metastatic tumors, and inflammatory processes.
- Combined right upper and lower lobe atelectasis is rare.
- Atelectasis is seen in a majority of patients after cardiac surgery.

Suggested Readings

Davis SD, Yankelevitz DF, Wand A, Chiarella DA: Juxtaphrenic peak in upper and middle lobe volume loss: Assessment with CT. *Radiology* 198:143-149, 1996.

Lee KS, Logan PM, Primack SL, Müller NL: Combined lobar atelectasis of the right lung: Imaging findings. *AJR Am J Roentgenol* 163:43-47, 1994.

Naidich DP, McCauley DI, Khouri NF, et al: Computed tomography of lobar collapse: 1. Endobronchial obstruction. *J Comput Assist Tomogr* 7:745-757, 1983.

Proto AV: Lobar collapse: Basic concepts. *Eur J Radiol* 23:9-22, 1996.

Woodring JH, Reed JC: Types and mechanisms of pulmonary atelectasis. *J Thorac Imag* 11:92-108, 1996.

Woodring JH, Reed JC: Radiographic manifestations of lobar atelectasis. *J Thorac Imag* 11:109-144, 1996.

Round Atelectasis

DEFINITION: Round atelectasis is a distinct form of atelectasis characteristically associated with focal pleural thickening.

IMAGING

Radiography
Findings
- Fairly homogeneous round, oval, wedge-shaped, or irregularly shaped mass in peripheral lung adjacent to thickened pleura.
- Comet tail sign.
- Usually Measures 3.0-6.0 cm in greatest diameter.

Utility
- Helpful in demonstrating presence of abnormality but of limited value in specific diagnosis.

CT
Findings
- Comet tail sign occurs when vessels and bronchi curve into periphery of mass.
- Bronchi and vessels curve and converge toward a round/oval mass that abuts an area of pleural thickening.
- Evidence of volume loss occurs in affected lobe.
- Subpleural fat may be identified within the mass, a feature that reflects chronicity.
- Lung parenchyma adjacent to round atelectasis shows compensatory hyperinflation.

Utility
- CT diagnostic in most cases.
- Diagnosis requires that round atelectasis be adjacent to thickened pleura, with vessels and bronchi curving into the periphery of the "mass"; lung volume loss is proportional to the size of "mass."
- Multiplanar reconstructed images are helpful in better determining the course of blood vessels and bronchi in these cases.

MRI
Findings
- Signal intensity is higher than that of muscle and lower than that of fat on T1-weighted images and similar to or lower than that of fat on T2-weighted images.
- Atelectatic mass enhances homogeneously after administration of gadopentetate dimeglumine.

DIAGNOSTIC PEARLS

- Homogeneous round, oval, wedge-shaped, or irregularly shaped mass in the peripheral lung adjacent to thickened pleura.
- Comet tail sign.
- Atelectasis proportional to the size of the mass.
- Mass represents atelectatic lung.

- Pulmonary vessels and bronchi converge toward area of atelectasis (comet tail sign), which is often best seen on sagittal/oblique sagittal images.

Utility
- Of limited value in assessment of round atelectasis.

Positron Emission Tomography
Findings
- Little or no uptake

Utility
- Helpful in distinguishing round atelectasis from carcinoma.

CLINICAL PRESENTATION

- Usually asymptomatic

DIFFERENTIAL DIAGNOSIS

- Pulmonary carcinoma
- Granuloma
- Inflammatory pseudo-tumor

PATHOLOGY

- Pleural-based mass that consists of atelectasis associated with pleural fibrosis.
- Seen most commonly in patients exposed to asbestos.
- Other causes: pleural effusion from tuberculosis, infections other than tuberculosis, pulmonary infarction, left-sided heart failure, surgery (mainly cardiac), malignant tumor.

WHAT THE REFERRING PHYSICIAN NEEDS TO KNOW

- CT findings are often sufficiently characteristic that neither biopsy nor further investigative procedures are necessary to exclude more ominous disease.
- PET typically shows no uptake.
- Needle biopsy may occasionally be required to rule out carcinoma.
- Follow-up of patients who have round atelectasis has shown that the majority of lesions are stable for many years.
- Occasionally, a lesion decreases in size, resolves within a few weeks to several years, or enlarges.

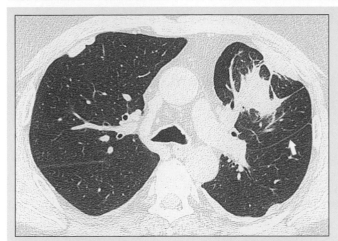

Figure 1. Round atelectasis. A high-resolution CT scan shows an irregular mass in the left upper lobe with band-like opacities extending toward an area of pleural thickening. Also note the volume loss in the left upper lobe causing curvilinear anterior displacement of the left major fissure (*arrow*). The patient was a 75-year-old man with a history of asbestos exposure.

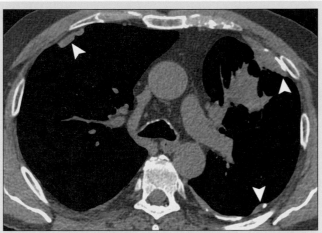

Figure 2. Round atelectasis. Soft tissue windows demonstrate bilateral calcified pleural plaques (*arrowheads*). The patient was a 75-year-old man with a history of asbestos exposure.

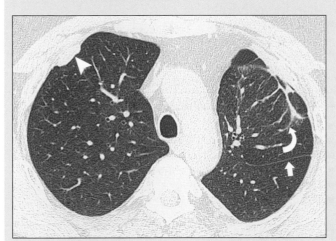

Figure 3. Round atelectasis. A high-resolution CT scan at a more cephalad level than in Figures 1 and 2 shows pulmonary vessels (*curved arrow*) curving toward the area of pleural thickening. Also noted are superior and anterior displacement of the left major fissure (*straight arrow*) and a right pleural plaque (*arrowhead*). The patient was a 75-year-old man with a history of asbestos exposure.

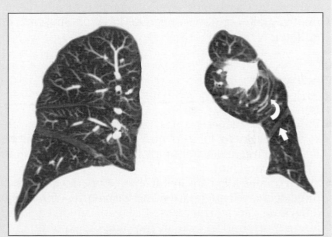

Figure 4. Round atelectasis. A coronal maximum intensity projection reformatted image shows the pulmonary vessels curving toward the left upper lobe mass and superior displacement of the left major fissure. The patient was a 75-year-old man with a history of asbestos exposure.

INCIDENCE/PREVALENCE AND EPIDEMIOLOGY

- Seen most commonly in patients with asbestos-related pleural plaques or diffuse pleural thickening.

Suggested Readings

Batra P, Brown K, Hayashi K, Mori M: Rounded atelectasis. *J Thorac Imaging* 11:187-197, 1996.

Hillerdal G: Rounded atelectasis: Clinical experience with 74 patients. *Chest* 95:836-941, 1989.

Ludeman N, Elicker BM, Reddy GP, et al: Atypical rounded atelectasis: Diagnosis and management based on results of F-18 FDG positron emission tomography. *Clin Nucl Med* 30:734-735, 2005.

McHugh K, Blaquiere RM: CT features of rounded atelectasis. *AJR Am J Roentgenol* 153:257-260, 1989.

Yamaguchi T, Hayashi K, Ashizawa K, et al: Magnetic resonance imaging of rounded atelectasis. *J Thorac Imaging* 12:188-194, 1997.

Mediastinal Shift

DEFINITION: Mediastinal shift is deviation of the mediastinum and its contents away from its normal midline location.

IMAGING

Radiography
Findings
- Atelectasis of lung or lobe: ipsilateral shift of mediastinum and trachea.
- Pulmonary agenesis/aplasia/severe hypoplasia: absence of aerated lung in one hemothorax; ipsilateral hemidiaphragm elevation; ipsilateral mediastinal shift; rib approximation.
- Swyer-James-McLeod syndrome: hyperlucent lobe/lung, decreased vascularity of involved lobe/lung, normal/decreased size of involved lobe/lung, and decreased size of ipsilateral hilum.
- Pectus excavatum: obscuration of right-sided heart border; displacement of heart to left hemithorax.
- Contralateral shift of mediastinum in large pneumothorax, pleural effusion, or pleural malignancy.
- Contralateral shift in large pulmonary space-occupying lesion, such as tumor, cyst, congenital cystic adenomatoid malformation, congenital lobar emphysema, or bulla(e).

CT
Findings
- Atelectasis of lung or lobe: ipsilateral shift of mediastinum and trachea.
- Pulmonary agenesis/aplasia/severe hypoplasia: absence of aerated lung in one hemothorax; ipsilateral hemidiaphragm elevation; ipsilateral mediastinal shift; rib approximation.
- Swyer-James-McLeod syndrome: hyperlucent lobe/lung, decreased attenuation and vascularity of involved lobe/lung, normal/decreased size of involved lobe/lung on inspiration, and air trapping on expiration.
- Contralateral shift of mediastinum in large pneumothorax, pleural effusion, pleural malignancy.
- Contralateral shift in large pulmonary space-occupying lesion such as tumor, cyst, congenital cystic adenomatoid malformation, congenital lobar emphysema, or bulla(e).
- Congenital cystic adenomatoid malformation: unilocular/multiloculated cyst or complex soft tissue and cystic mass ranging from 4-12 cm in diameter.

DIAGNOSTIC PEARLS

- Ipsilateral shift: Atelectasis, fibrothorax, mesothelioma
- Contralateral shift: Pleural effusion, pneumothorax, large tumor, mesothelioma

Utility
- Allows diagnosis of pulmonary agenesis, aplasia, and hypoplasia.

CLINICAL PRESENTATION

- Patients may be asymptomatic or have nonspecific symptoms of cough and shortness of breath.
- Swyer-James-McLeod syndrome: majority of patients are asymptomatic; occasionally they may present with a history of recurrent respiratory tract infections or shortness of breath.
- Acute shortness of breath and pleuritic chest pain occur in pneumothorax.
- Weight loss and progressive shortness of breath occur in pulmonary or pleural malignancy.

DIFFERENTIAL DIAGNOSIS

- Atelectasis of lobe or lung
- Fibrothorax
- Lobectomy or pneumonectomy
- Pleural effusion
- Pneumothorax
- Mesothelioma

PATHOLOGY

- Mediastinal shift is away from space-occupying abnormalities such as large pleural effusion, pleural malignancy, large lung tumor, or mass.
- Mediastinal shift is toward hemithorax with decreased volume due to atelectasis, fibrothorax, or mesothelioma.
- Anterior and middle mediastinal compartments are more mobile than posterior compartment, with shift to greater extent in patients with atelectasis.

WHAT THE REFERRING PHYSICIAN NEEDS TO KNOW

- Mediastinal shift is often helpful in recognizing presence of pulmonary or pleural abnormality.
- Mediastinal shift is most commonly due to atelectasis.
- Contralateral mediastinal shift is most commonly due to pneumothorax or large pleural effusion.
- Pleural malignancy, including mesothelioma and metastasis, may result in ipsilateral or contralateral mediastinal shift.
- Large pleural effusions associated with mediastinal shift are most commonly due to infection or neoplasm.

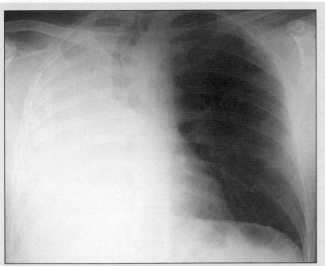

Figure 1. Obstructive atelectasis of right lung. Chest radiograph shows opacification and decreased volume of the right hemithorax. The trachea and mediastinum are shifted to the right and the left lung shows compensatory overinflation. The lack of air bronchograms within the opacified atelectatic right lung is consistent with obstructive atelectasis. The patient was a 44-year-old man with squamous cell carcinoma.

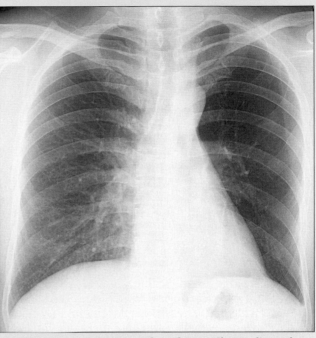

Figure 2. Swyer-James-McLeod syndrome. Chest radiograph shows hyperlucency and decreased vascularity of the left lung. The mediastinum is shifted to the left consistent with decreased left lung volume. The patient was a 40-year-old man with Swyer-James-McLeod syndrome.

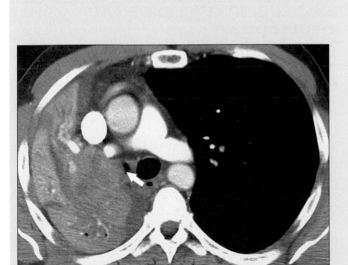

Figure 3. Obstructive atelectasis of right lung. Contrast-enhanced CT demonstrates complete obstruction of the right main bronchus by tumor (*arrow*) and distal atelectasis and obstructive pneumonitis. Note that the descending aorta is essentially in its normal position while the anterior and middle mediastinum are markedly displaced to the right. The patient was a 44-year-old man with squamous cell carcinoma.

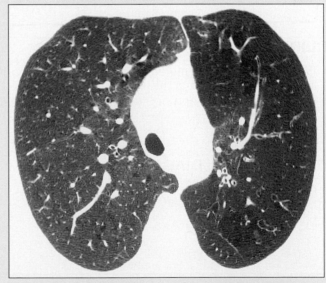

Figure 4. Swyer-James-McLeod syndrome. High-resolution CT shows decreased attenuation and vascularity of the left lung with associated bronchiectasis and mild volume loss leading to ipsilateral shift of the mediastinum and anterior junction line. The patient was a 61-year-old woman with Swyer-James-McLeod syndrome.

INCIDENCE/PREVALENCE AND EPIDEMIOLOGY

- Mediastinal shift is most commonly due to atelectasis.
- Contralateral mediastinal shift is most commonly due to pneumothorax or large pleural effusion.

Suggested Readings

Moore ADA, Godwin JD, Dietrich PA, et al: Swyer-James syndrome: CT findings in eight patients. *AJR Am J Roentgenol* 158:1211-1215, 1992.

Qureshi NR, Gleeson FV: Imaging of pleural disease. *Clin Chest Med* 27(2):193-213, 2006.

Woodring JH, Reed JC: Types and mechanisms of pulmonary atelectasis. *J Thorac Imag* 11:92-108, 1996.

Unilateral Hilar Displacement

DEFINITION: Unilateral hilar displacement is upward or downward displacement of the hilum while the medial aspect of the lung usually remains fixed.

IMAGING

Radiography
Findings
- Elevation of hilum in upper lobe atelectasis, scarring, or upper lobectomy.
- Downward displacement of hilum in lower lobe atelectasis, scarring, or lower lobectomy and in combined middle and lower lobe atelectasis.

Utility
- Often first and only imaging modality used in assessment of patient.

CT
Findings
- Elevation and forward displacement of hilum in upper lobe atelectasis, scarring, or upper lobectomy.
- Downward and posterior displacement of hilum in lower lobe atelectasis, scarring, or lower lobectomy and in combined middle and lower lobe atelectasis.
- Atelectatic lobe tapers smoothly toward hilum.
- Obstructive tumor or mass.

Utility
- Helpful in demonstrating underlying cause of volume loss.

CLINICAL PRESENTATION

- Patients may be asymptomatic or have nonspecific symptoms of cough and dyspnea.
- Occasionally, hemoptysis due to endobronchial lesion.

DIFFERENTIAL DIAGNOSIS

- Postprimary tuberculosis
- Lobar atelectasis
- Lobectomy

DIAGNOSTIC PEARLS

- Loss of lung volume.
- Upward displacement in upper lobe atelectasis, scarring or lobectomy.
- Downward displacement in lower lobe atelectasis, scarring or lobectomy.

PATHOLOGY

- Because medial aspect of lung is fixed at hilum, atelectatic forms are affected by relatively rigid lung components (bronchi, arteries, veins).
- As lobe loses volume, two surfaces approximate, with the end result of total atelectasis being a flattened triangle instead of a normal pyramid.
- Signs related to shift of other structures to compensate for loss of volume include unilateral hilar displacement.

INCIDENCE/PREVALENCE AND EPIDEMIOLOGY

- Occurs more commonly in atelectasis of upper and lower lobes.
- Becomes more marked as atelectasis becomes chronic.

Suggested Readings

Lee KS, Logan PM, Primack SL, Müller NL: Combined lobar atelectasis of the right lung: Imaging findings. *AJR Am J Roentgenol* 163:43-47, 1994.
Molina PL, Hiken JN, Glazer HS: Imaging evaluation of obstructive atelectasis. *J Thorac Imag* 11:176-186, 1996.
Proto AV: Lobar collapse: Basic concepts. *Eur J Radiol* 23:9-22, 1996.
Woodring JH, Reed JC: Radiographic manifestations of lobar atelectasis. *J Thorac Imag* 11:109-144, 1996.
Woodring JH, Reed JC: Types and mechanisms of pulmonary atelectasis. *J Thorac Imag* 11:92-108, 1996.

WHAT THE REFERRING PHYSICIAN NEEDS TO KNOW

- Unilateral cephalad or caudal displacement of hila is common manifestation of atelectasis.
- Hilar displacement becomes more marked as atelectasis becomes chronic.

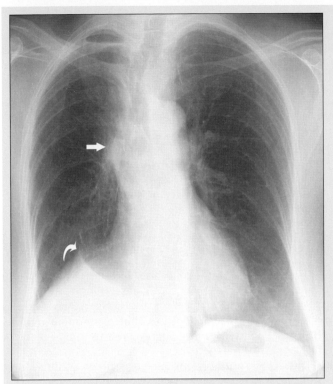

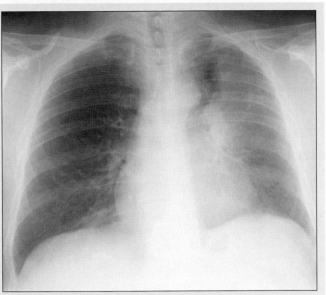

Figure 1. Elevation of hilum due to previous lobectomy. Chest radiograph shows decrease in size of the right hemithorax, elevation of the right hilum (*straight arrow*), lateral displacement of the right interlobar pulmonary artery, and tenting of the right hemidiaphragm (*curved arrow*). The patient was a 73-year-old woman with previous right upper lobectomy.

Figure 2. Elevation of hilum due to atelectasis. Posteroanterior chest radiograph shows poorly defined increased opacity of the left hemithorax associated with obliteration of the left-sided heart border (silhouette sign), volume loss of the left hemithorax, elevation of the left hemidiaphragm, and superior displacement of the left hilum characteristic of left upper lobe atelectasis. Note crescent-shaped lucency between the apex of the atelectatic left upper lobe and the aortic arch (Luftsichel sign).

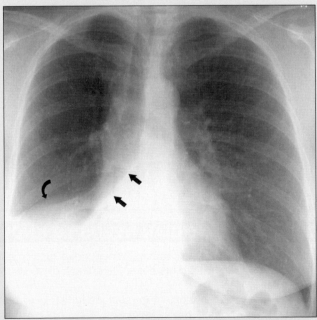

Figure 3. Combined right middle lobe and lower lobe atelectasis. Posteroanterior chest radiograph shows caudad displacement of the right major (*straight arrows*) and minor (*curved arrow*) fissures. Caudal displacement of the right hilum and overinflation of the right upper lobe are also evident. The silhouette of the right atrium is obscured by the atelectatic middle lobe.

Part 3

NODULES AND MASSES

Solitary Lung Nodule

DEFINITION: A pulmonary nodule is any pulmonary lesion characterized by a well-defined, discrete, approximately circular opacity ≤3 cm in diameter.

IMAGING

Radiography
Findings
- Intrapulmonary nodule forming an acute angle with contiguous pleura and well-defined margins seen en face.
- Pleural or extrapleural nodule that tends to have tapered margins, is poorly defined en face, and forms an obtuse angle with chest wall.
- Diffuse or central (target) calcification in a benign nodule.

Utility
- Calcification within pulmonary nodule is more readily seen on low-kilovoltage than high-kilovoltage radiographs.
- Presence of diffuse or central calcification in a smoothly marginated nodule is virtually diagnostic of a granuloma (tuberculoma, histoplasmoma).

CT
Findings
- Fat-attenuation value on thin-section CT within smoothly marginated lung nodule is virtually diagnostic of hamartoma.
- Fat within spiculated lesion is most suggestive of focal lipoid pneumonia.
- Water density and thin or invisible wall are diagnostic of cystic lesion (bronchogenic cyst, congenital cystic adenomatoid malformation, hydatid cyst, fluid-filled bulla).
- Air bronchograms and air bronchiolograms are seen more commonly with pulmonary carcinomas than with benign nodules.
- Bubble lucencies within nodule are often seen in bronchioalveolar carcinomas, acinar adenocarcinomas, and other malignancies and are uncommon in benign tumors.
- Nodule with ground-glass opacity surrounding solid component or with a mixed ground-glass and solid component is more likely to be malignant.

DIAGNOSTIC PEARLS

- Main diagnostic radiologic criteria to differentiate benign from malignant nodules: size, change in size over time, calcification, fat, margins.
- Calcification within solitary pulmonary nodule most reliable sign that lesion is benign.
- Likelihood for malignancy: 0.5- to 1.0-cm diameter, 35%; 2-cm diameter, 50%; 2- to 3-cm diameter, 80%; 3-cm diameter, 95%.

- Nodules with predominantly solid component tend to be associated with more aggressive tumors.

Utility
- CT is used routinely for assessment of solitary lung nodule.
- CT is superior to chest radiography in detection and characterization of nodules.
- CT can show if nodule is clearly benign, as determined by rigidly defined radiologic signs, or of indeterminate nature
- Nodule detection is optimized by thinner sections, multiplanar and maximum intensity projection reconstructions, and dynamic viewing on workstation.
- Optimal assessment of lung nodules for presence of calcification by CT requires thin sections (1- to 3-mm collimation).

Positron Emission Tomography
Findings
- Enhancement seen in malignant and inflammatory lesion.

Utility
- FDG-PET has sensitivity of 97% and specificity of 78% for diagnosis of malignancy in nodules ≥10 mm.

WHAT THE REFERRING PHYSICIAN NEEDS TO KNOW

- Clinical findings to consider include age, risk factors, recent travel history, and symptoms.
- Likelihood for malignancy is: 0.5- to 1.0-cm diameter, 35%; 2-cm diameter, 50%; 2- to 3-cm diameter, 80%; 3-cm diameter, 95%.
- Only two findings are considered to be sufficient to preclude further evaluation: benign pattern of calcification and stability in size for more than 2 years.
- Fleischner Society recommends schedule of follow-up studies classified by nodule size and presence of risk factor.
- Transthoracic needle aspiration or biopsy is indicated in patients with solitary lung nodules who cannot/would not undergo surgery.

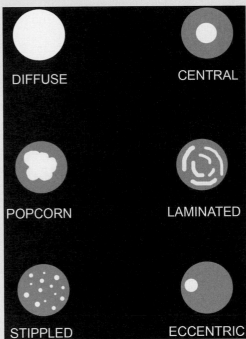

Figure 1. Patterns of calcification. A schematic drawing shows the characteristic patterns of pulmonary nodule calcification. Diffuse calcification, central calcification in nodules ≤2.0 cm in diameter, popcorn calcification, and laminated calcification are virtually diagnostic of a benign nodule. Diffuse, central, and laminated types of calcification are seen most commonly in calcified granulomas as a result of previous tuberculosis or histoplasmosis, and popcorn calcification, albeit rare, is virtually diagnostic of hamartoma. Stippled calcification, particularly when seen in large masses, and eccentric calcification are worrisome for malignancy. They occur most commonly in pulmonary carcinoma.

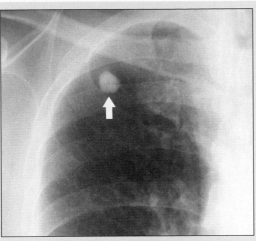

Figure 2. Calcified granuloma with diffuse calcification. A magnified view of the right upper lobe from a frontal chest radiograph shows a diffusely calcified nodule (*arrow*). The patient was a 70-year-old man with previous tuberculosis.

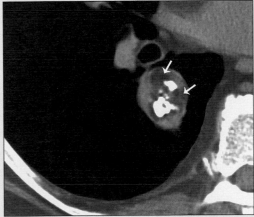

Figure 3. Popcorn calcification in pulmonary hamartoma. A magnified view of the right lower lobe from a CT scan shows a smoothly marginated nodule with several coarse foci of calcification (popcorn calcification). Also note the presence of foci of fat attenuation (*arrows*). The findings are virtually pathognomonic of hamartoma.

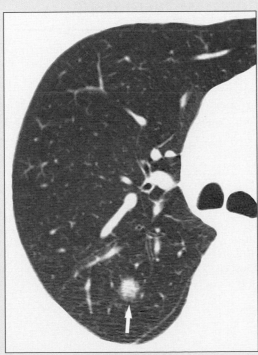

Figure 4. Nodule with mixed attenuation. A magnified view of the right lung from a high-resolution CT scan shows a nodule with a predominantly solid component and a halo of ground-glass attenuation (CT halo sign) (*arrow*) in a patient with invasive pulmonary adenocarcinoma.

- False-negative FDG-PET studies can be seen with carcinoid tumor, bronchioloalveolar carcinoma, and pulmonary carcinoma <10 mm in diameter.
- False-positive scans can occur with inflammatory conditions such as tuberculosis, histoplasmosis, and rheumatoid nodules.
- Role of PET has increased with integration of PET and multidetector CT technology in hybrid PET/CT scanners.

MRI
Findings
- Bronchogenic cyst: virtually all have characteristic high signal intensity similar to that of cerebrospinal fluid on T2-weighted images.
Utility
- MRI has very limited role in evaluation of solitary lung nodule and is not indicated in the routine workup.
- MRI is superior to CT in the diagnosis of bronchogenic cysts and foregut duplication cysts.

CLINICAL PRESENTATION

- History of smoking common in carcinoma
- Cough
- Fever usually associated with infectious cause

DIFFERENTIAL DIAGNOSES

- Tuberculosis
- Histoplasmosis
- Coccidioidomycosis
- Pulmonary carcinoma
- Pulmonary carcinoid tumor
- Hamartoma
- Bronchogenic cyst
- Metastasis

PATHOLOGY

- Malignant neoplasm may be primary carcinoma or metastasis (sarcoma, testicular tumor).
- Infectious causes include tuberculous granuloma, histoplasmosis, coccidioidomycosis, round pneumonia, *Echinococcus* infection, abscess, and conglomerate fibrosis in talcosis.

- Inflammatory causes include lipoid pneumonia, Wegener granulomatosis, sarcoidosis, and rheumatoid nodules.
- Benign tumors are either neoplastic or hamartomatous.
- Congenital causes include bronchogenic cyst and pulmonary arteriovenous malformation.
- Silicosis and hematoma may also manifest as solitary lung nodule.
- Calcification in malignancies may be evident in primary carcinoma engulfing calcified granuloma, metastatic osteogenic sarcoma or chondrosarcoma, carcinoid tumors with stromal ossification, and calcified carcinomas.

INCIDENCE/PREVALENCE AND EPIDEMIOLOGY

- In the United States, solitary pulmonary nodule is seen on chest radiography or CT in more than 150,000 patients/year.
- More than 95% fall into one of three groups: malignancy, infectious granulomas, or, less commonly, benign tumors.
- Approximately 40% of solitary lung nodules detected on chest radiograph represent primary lung cancer.
- More than 50% of smokers subjected to thin-section CT have small lung nodules measuring <7 mm diameter.

Suggested Readings

Erasmus JJ, Connolly JE, McAdams HP, Roggli VL: Solitary pulmonary nodules: I. Morphologic evaluation for differentiation of benign and malignant lesions. *RadioGraphics* 20:43-58, 2000.

Erasmus JJ, McAdams HP, Connolly JE: Solitary pulmonary nodules: II. Evaluation of the indeterminate nodule. *RadioGraphics* 20:59-66, 2000.

Khan A: ACR Appropriateness Criteria on solitary pulmonary nodule. *J Am Coll Radiol* 4:152-155, 2007.

Kim SK, Allen-Auerbach M, Goldin J, et al: Accuracy of PET/CT in characterization of solitary pulmonary lesions. *J Nucl Med* 48: 214-220, 2007.

Ko JP: Lung nodule detection and characterization with multi-slice CT. *J Thorac Imaging* 20:196-209, 2005.

MacMahon H, Austin JH, Gamsu G, et al: Guidelines for management of small pulmonary nodules detected on CT scans: A statement from the Fleischner Society. *Radiology* 237:395-400, 2005.

Tan BB, Flaherty KR, Kazerooni EA, et al: The solitary pulmonary nodule. *Chest* 123(1 Suppl):89S-96S, 2003.

Multiple Lung Nodules

DEFINITION: Presence of multiple nodules ≥1 cm in diameter.

IMAGING

Radiography
Findings
- Pulmonary metastases: multiple nodules tend to be most numerous in the basal portions of the lungs, range in size from barely visible to large masses, and may be solid or cavitated.
- Tuberculosis: nodules in endobronchial spread tend to measure 4-10 mm in diameter and to have a patchy distribution, whereas those of miliary tuberculosis measure 1-3 mm in diameter and are diffuse.
- Histoplasmosis and coccidioidomycosis usually present as a single nodule measuring up to 3 cm in diameter or as multiple nodules <1 cm in diameter.
- In the immunocompromised host, multiple nodules most commonly result from invasive aspergillosis, candidiasis, cytomegalovirus pneumonia, or septic embolism.
- Angioinvasive aspergillosis: multiple nodules with ill-defined margins range from a few millimeters to approximately 3 cm in diameter.
- Septic embolism: multiple nodules 0.5 to 3.0 cm in diameter occur mainly in lower lobes and are frequently cavitated.
- Arteriovenous malformations: well-defined, lobulated, round or oval opacities range from a few millimeters to several centimeters in diameter.

Utility
- Often the first and only imaging modality used in the assessment of multiple nodules.

CT
Findings
- Pulmonary metastases range from diffuse micronodular pattern to large, well-defined masses; cavitation may occur particularly in metastatic squamous cell carcinoma.
- Septic embolism: multiple nodules measuring 1-3 cm in diameter are frequently cavitated.
- Arteriovenous malformations appear as characteristic large feeding arteries and draining veins.
- Halo of ground-glass attenuation surrounding nodules (CT halo sign) is commonly seen in angioinvasive

DIAGNOSTIC PEARLS
- Pulmonary metastases are evident as numerous bilateral nodules and masses of various sizes.
- Halo of ground-glass attenuation surrounding nodules (CT halo sign) is commonly seen in highly vascular or hemorrhagic tumors (angiosarcoma) and also in metastatic mucinous colon carcinoma, angioinvasive aspergillosis, and Wegener granulomatosis.
- Wegener granulomatosis typically presents as multiple nodules and masses ranging from few mm up to 10 cm in diameter that often cavitate and have no lung zone predilection.

aspergillosis, candidiasis, cytomegalovirus pneumonia, Kaposi sarcoma, Wegener granulomatosis, and metastases (angiosarcoma, choriocarcinoma, melanoma).
- Wegener granulomatosis typically presents as multiple nodules and masses ranging from few mm up to 10 cm in diameter that often cavitate and have no lung zone predilection.
- Endobronchial spread of tuberculosis is shown by centrilobular nodules and "tree-in-bud" pattern.
- Miliary tuberculosis has a random distribution of numerous 1-3 mm diameter nodules.

Utility
- Superior to radiography in demonstrating presence of nodules and cavitation.

CLINICAL PRESENTATION
- Patients may be asymptomatic.
- Majority of patients with multiple pulmonary metastases have previously diagnosed extrathoracic neoplasm or clinical findings directly referable to synchronous primary tumor.
- Fever is commonly associated with infection (e.g., septic embolism, tuberculosis, and fungal infection).
- Severely neutropenic patient with fever and lung nodules is highly suggestive of angioinvasive aspergillosis.

WHAT THE REFERRING PHYSICIAN NEEDS TO KNOW
- Most pulmonary metastases presenting as single or multiple nodules are asymptomatic.
- Causes of multiple nodules with CT halo sign include angioinvasive aspergillosis, candidiasis, cytomegalovirus pneumonia, Kaposi sarcoma, Wegener granulomatosis, and metastases from angiosarcoma, mucinous adenocarcinoma, and melanoma.
- Common causes of multiple nodules are pulmonary infection (septic embolism, tuberculosis, histoplasmosis, coccidioidomycosis, and cryptococcosis) and metastases.
- CT, particularly volumetric thin-section CT, is superior to radiography in the detection of pulmonary nodules.

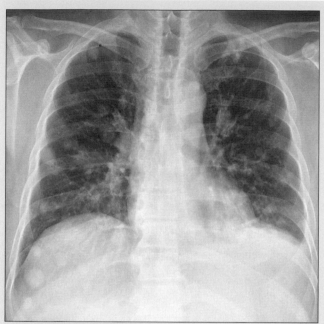

Figure 1. Pulmonary metastases: radiographic findings. Chest radiograph demonstrates multiple bilateral pulmonary nodules ranging from a few millimeters to 2 cm in diameter. The nodules have smooth margins and involve mainly the lower lung zones. Small left pleural effusion is also present. The patient was a 53-year-old man with metastatic sarcoma.

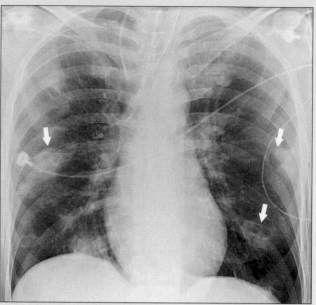

Figure 2. Septic embolism. A chest radiograph shows several bilateral nodules, some of which are cavitated (*arrows*). Also noted is a right pneumothorax. The patient was a 41-year-old male intravenous drug user with septic emboli caused by *Staphylococcus aureus*.

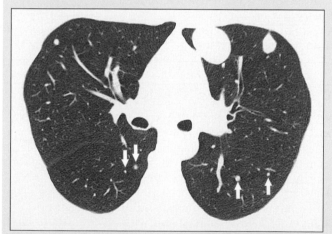

Figure 3. CT scan showing several large nodules in the anterior aspects of the right and left lungs and several small nodules (*arrows*) in the lower lobes. The nodules have well-defined smooth margins and range from 2 to 35 mm in diameter. The patient was a 40-year-old man with lung metastases from synovial sarcoma.

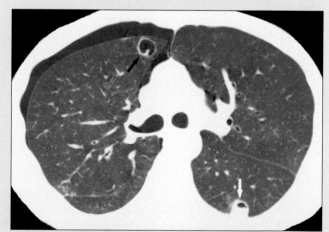

Figure 4. Septic embolism. CT scan at the level of the right upper lobe bronchus shows a thin-walled cavity in the right upper lobe and one in the left lower lobe (*arrows*). Also noted is a right pneumothorax. The patient was a 41-year-old male intravenous drug user with septic emboli caused by *Staphylococcus aureus*.

DIFFERENTIAL DIAGNOSIS

- Metastases
- Septic embolism
- Lung cancer: Adenocarcinoma
- Pulmonary lymphoma
- Wegener granulomatosis

PATHOLOGY

- Common causes of multiple nodules are pulmonary infection (septic embolism, tuberculosis, histoplasmosis, coccidioidomycosis, and cryptococcosis) and metastases.
- Pulmonary metastases are commonly seen in outer third of lungs, particularly the subpleural regions of lower zones.
- Cavitation occurs most commonly in metastases from squamous cell carcinoma of the head and cervix.

INCIDENCE/PREVALENCE AND EPIDEMIOLOGY

- Septic embolism occurs commonly in intravenous drug abusers and immunocompromised patients with central venous lines.
- Most common vascular abnormalities in multiple nodules are congenital arteriovenous malformations, often in patients with Osler-Weber-Rendu syndrome.

- More than 95% of multiple nodule cases represent pulmonary metastases or infection.
- Approximately 80% to 90% of patients with multiple pulmonary metastases have previously diagnosed extrathoracic neoplasm or clinical findings directly referable to a synchronous primary tumor.
- Cavitation occurs in approximately 4% of pulmonary metastases and is seen mostly in squamous cell carcinoma primary sites such as head and neck in men and cervix in women.
- Calcification of metastatic lesions is rare and almost invariably indicates that primary neoplasm is osteogenic sarcoma, chondrosarcoma, or synovial sarcoma.

Suggested Readings

Dodd J, Souza CA, Müller NL: High-resolution MDCT of pulmonary septic embolism: Evaluation of the feeding vessel sign. *AJR Am J Roentgenol* 187:623-629, 2006.

Franquet T, Müller NL, Gimenez A, et al: Infectious pulmonary nodules in immunocompromised patients: Usefulness of computed tomography in predicting their etiology. *J Comput Assist Tomogr* 27:446-461, 2003.

Gruden JF, Ouanounou S, Tigges S, et al: Incremental benefit of maximum-intensity-projection images on observer detection of small pulmonary nodules revealed by multidetector CT. *AJR Am J Roentgenol* 179:149-157, 2002.

Hirakata K, Nakata H, Nakagawa T: CT of pulmonary metastases with pathological correlation. *Semin Ultrasound CT MR* 16:379-394, 1995.

Primack SL, Hartman TE, Lee KS, Müller NL: Pulmonary nodules and the CT halo sign. *Radiology* 190:513-515, 1994.

Seo JB, Im JG, Goo JM, et al: Atypical pulmonary metastases: Spectrum of radiologic findings. *RadioGraphics* 21:403-417, 2001.

Solitary Cavitary Lung Nodule

DEFINITION: A solitary cavitary nodule is a gas-containing space within lung surrounded by a wall, with thickness >1 mm, formed by necrosis of the central portion of a lesion and drainage of resultant partially liquefied material via communicating airways.

IMAGING

Radiography
Findings
- Cavitary lung nodule or mass
- Well-defined or poorly defined outer margins
- Thin-walled (<4 mm) or thick-walled
- Smooth, irregular, or nodular inner lining
- Thin-walled lesions with smooth inner lining usually benign.
- Thick-walled lesions (>15 mm) usually malignant
- May contain fluid level

Utility
- Usually first imaging modality used in the assessment of these patients.

CT
Findings
- Cavitary lung nodule or mass
- Well-defined or poorly defined outer margins
- Thin-walled (<4 mm) or thick-walled
- Smooth, irregular, or nodular inner lining
- Nodular inner lining: favors carcinoma
- Enhancement of wall usually after intravenous administration of a contrast agent
- May contain fluid level

Utility
- Superior to radiography in demonstrating presence of cavitation.

CLINICAL PRESENTATION
- Cough and fever in lung abscess and fungal infection.
- Cough, hemoptysis, weight loss in pulmonary carcinoma or metastasis.

DIFFERENTIAL DIAGNOSIS
- Pulmonary carcinoma
- Tuberculosis
- Coccidioidomycosis
- Lung abscess
- Bronchogenic cyst

DIAGNOSTIC PEARLS
- Cavitation in lung carcinoma usually occurs in mass >3 cm in diameter and may be central or eccentric and 1-10 cm in diameter.
- Cavity wall is usually thick in acute lung abscess, primary and metastatic carcinoma, and Wegener granulomatosis.
- Cavity wall is usually thin in coccidioidomycosis, bronchogenic cyst, and traumatic pneumatocele.

- Wegener granulomatosis
- Rheumatoid nodule
- Traumatic pneumatocele

PATHOLOGY
- Most common histologic type of cavitating malignancy is squamous cell carcinoma.
- Cavities in neoplastic lesion are formed by necrosis of central portion of lesion and drainage of resultant partially liquefied material.
- Lung abscess is focus of suppuration surrounded by wall composed of fibrous and granulation tissue.
- Common causes of lung abscess include *Staphylococcus aureus, Pseudomonas aeruginosa, Klebsiella pneumoniae,* and anaerobes.

INCIDENCE/PREVALENCE AND EPIDEMIOLOGY
- Incidence of cavitation in pulmonary carcinoma is about 10%.
- Cavitation is a complication that occurs in tumors of any size, especially those >3 cm in diameter.
- Cavitation is seen in squamous cell carcinomas, large cell carcinomas, and adenocarcinomas, but not in small cell carcinomas.
- Common predisposing factors for lung abscess are alcoholism, anesthesia, trauma, and drug abuse.

WHAT THE REFERRING PHYSICIAN NEEDS TO KNOW
- In majority of cases a cavity is evident on the radiograph.
- CT is superior to radiography in demonstrating presence of cavitation and associated findings.
- Needle aspiration or biopsy is often helpful in establishing tissue diagnosis.

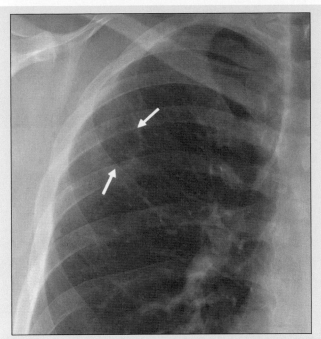

Figure 1. Chronic coccidioidomycosis. A 33-year-old man with a chronic productive cough developed acute chest pain while on vacation in Arizona. Chest radiograph showed a 3.3-cm subtle thin-walled cavity (*arrows*) in the right upper lobe. Cultures from sputum and bronchial washings grew *Coccidioides immitis.*

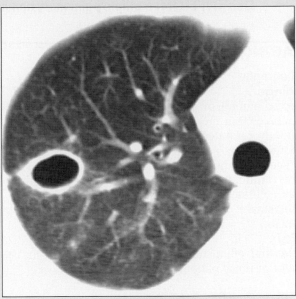

Figure 2. Chronic coccidioidomycosis. A 33-year-old man with chronic productive cough developed acute chest pain while on vacation in Arizona. CT scan confirmed a 3.3-cm thin-walled cavity in the right upper lobe. Cultures from sputum and bronchial washings grew *Coccidioides immitis.*

Suggested Readings

Chong S, Lee KS, Yi CA, et al: Pulmonary fungal infection: Imaging findings in immunocompetent and immunocompromised patients. *Eur J Radiol* 59:371-383, 2006.

Franquet T, Müller NL, Giménez A, et al: Spectrum of pulmonary aspergillosis: Histologic, clinical, and radiologic findings. *Radio-Graphics* 21:825-837, 2001.

Mueller PR, Berlin L: Complications of lung abscess aspiration and drainage. *AJR Am J Roentgenol* 178:1083-1086, 2002.

Ryu JH, Swensen SJ: Cystic and cavitary lung diseases: Focal and diffuse. *Mayo Clin Proc* 78:744-752, 2003.

Seo JB, Im JG, Goo JM, et al: Atypical pulmonary metastases: Spectrum of radiologic findings. *RadioGraphics* 21:403-417, 2001.

Woodring JH, Fried AM, Chuang VP: Solitary cavities of the lung: Diagnostic implications of cavity wall thickness. *AJR Am J Roentgenol* 135:1269-1271, 1980.

Multiple Cavitary Lung Nodules

DEFINITION: Multiple pulmonary nodules containing gas-filled space (cavity).

IMAGING

Radiography
Findings
- Septic embolism: round or wedge-shaped peripheral opacities that measure 1-3 cm in diameter and are frequently cavitated with well-defined or poorly defined margins.
- Wegener granulomatosis: usually <10 nodules from a few millimeters up to 10 cm in diameter, with about half cavitated.
- Metastases: nodules of various sizes mainly in lower lobes.

Utility
- First and often only imaging modality used in assessment of these patients.

CT
Findings
- Septic embolism: round or wedge-shaped peripheral opacities that measure 1-3 cm in diameter, frequently cavitated.
- Wegener granulomatosis: more nodules seen than with radiography without predilection for any lung zone; nodules >2 cm in diameter frequently cavitated.
- Pulmonary metastases: cavitations in bilateral nodules of various sizes.

Utility
- Superior to the radiograph in demonstrating presence of cavitation.

CLINICAL PRESENTATION

- Fever and cough in pulmonary infection.
- Weight loss and malaise in pulmonary metastases.

PATHOLOGY

- Multiple lung cavitations are found in cases of infections (septic emboli, fungal infection, *Pneumocystis jiroveci* infection, tuberculosis, nontuberculous mycobacterial infection, paragonimiasis).
- Multiple lung cavitations also seen in pulmonary metastases, cystic adenomatoid malformation, lymphoma, laryngotracheal papillomatosis, Wegener granulomatosis, rheumatoid nodules, and traumatic pneumatoceles.

DIAGNOSTIC PEARLS

- Septic emboli tend to be most numerous in peripheral lung regions and lower lobes.
- Wegener granulomatosis is characterized by <10 nodules from a few millimeters up to 10 cm in diameter.
- Most cavitating pulmonary metastases are from squamous carcinoma, with primary site at head and neck in men and at cervix in women.

INCIDENCE/PREVALENCE AND EPIDEMIOLOGY

- Septic embolism occurs most commonly in intravenous drug abusers and in immunocompromised patients with central venous lines.
- Cavitation occurs in approximately 4% of pulmonary metastases, most often in squamous cell carcinoma.
- Cavitation also occurs in metastatic adenocarcinoma and metastatic sarcoma, although it is uncommon.

Suggested Readings

Dodd JD, Souza CA, Müller NL: High-resolution MDCT of pulmonary septic embolism: Evaluation of the feeding vessel ssign. *AJR Am J Roentgenol* 187:623-629, 2006.

Franquet T, Müller NL, Giménez A, et al: Spectrum of pulmonary aspergillosis: Histologic, clinical, and radiologic findings. *RadioGraphics* 21:825-837, 2001.

Huang RM, Naidich DP, Lubat E, et al: Septic pulmonary emboli: CT-radiographic correlation. *AJR Am J Roentgenol* 153:41-45, 1989.

Kuhlman JE, Fishman EK, Teigen C: Pulmonary septic emboli: Diagnosis with CT. *Radiology* 174:211-213, 1990.

Ryu JH, Swensen SJ: Cystic and cavitary lung diseases: Focal and diffuse. *Mayo Clin Proc* 78:744-752, 2003.

Seo JB, Im JG, Goo JM, et al: Atypical pulmonary metastases: Spectrum of radiologic findings. *RadioGraphics* 21:403-417, 2001.

Sheehan RE, Flint JD, Müller NL: Computed tomography features of the thoracic manifestations of Wegener granulomatosis. *J Thorac Imaging* 18:34-41, 2003.

WHAT THE REFERRING PHYSICIAN NEEDS TO KNOW

- Primary site of squamous carcinoma resulting in cavitating lung metastases is usually in head and neck for men and cervix for women.

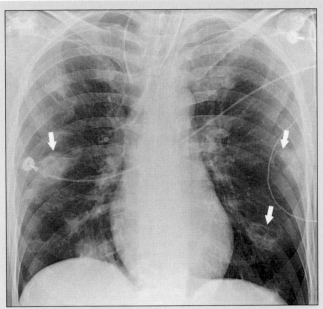

Figure 1. Septic embolism. Chest radiograph shows several bilateral nodules, some of which are cavitated (*arrows*).

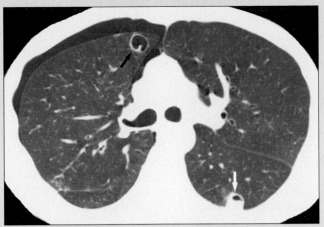

Figure 2. Septic embolism. CT image at the level of the right upper lobe bronchus shows a thin-walled cavity in the right upper lobe and one in the left lower lobe (*arrows*). Also noted is a right pneumothorax. The patient was a 41-year-old male intravenous drug user with septic emboli caused by *Staphylococcus aureus*.

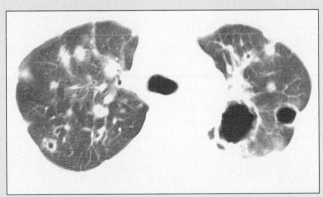

Figure 3. Cavitating metastases. CT image shows numerous bilateral nodules and masses of various sizes, most of them solid and with irregular or ill-defined margins. Two of the lesions in the left upper lobe and a smaller one in the right upper lobe are cavitated. The patient was a 21-year-old man with pulmonary metastases from carcinoma of the tongue.

CT Halo Sign

DEFINITION: CT halo sign refers to ground-glass attenuation surrounding a pulmonary nodule on a CT image.

IMAGING

CT

Findings

- Angioinvasive aspergillosis typically presents as one or multiple nodules ranging from a few millimeters to approximately 3.0 cm in diameter, frequently with a halo of ground-glass attenuation.
- Similar findings may be seen in candidiasis.
- Nodules in cytomegalovirus and herpesvirus pneumonia usually measure <1.0 cm in diameter.
- In a smoker the presence of a nodule with ground-glass opacity surrounding a solid component is suggestive of bronchogenic carcinoma, most commonly adenocarcinoma.

Utility

- Differential diagnosis is influenced by clinical history (e.g., multiple lung nodules): CT halo sign in patient with severe neutropenia is most suggestive of invasive aspergillosis; similar finding in patient with mucinous carcinoma of colon is most suggestive of metastases).

CLINICAL PRESENTATION

- Symptoms depend on underlying cause.
- Patients with CT halo sign due to pulmonary adenocarcinoma are usually asymptomatic smokers.
- Opportunistic infections associated with CT halo sign (invasive aspergillosis, candidiasis, mucormycosis, cytomegalovirus) frequently manifest as fever and cough.

DIFFERENTIAL DIAGNOSIS

- Angioinvasive aspergillosis
- Pneumonia (cytomegalovirus)
- Septic embolism
- Pulmonary manifestations of Wegener granulomatosis
- Cryptogenic organizing pneumonia (idiopathic bronchiolitis obliterans organizing pneumonia)

DIAGNOSTIC PEARLS

- Nodule with ground-glass opacity surrounds a solid component.
- This rim is due to pulmonary hemorrhage, infiltration by inflammatory process or tumor, or lepidic growth of bronchioalveolar carcinoma.
- CT finding must be interpreted in proper clinical context to arrive at most likely diagnosis.

- Pulmonary metastases: Angiosarcoma and mucinous carcinoma of the colon
- Lung cancer: Bronchioloalveolar cell carcinoma and adenocarcinoma

PATHOLOGY

- Hemorrhage surrounding nodule (e.g., invasive aspergillosis, candidiasis, Kaposi sarcoma).
- Less dense infiltration by inflammatory process (e.g., organizing pneumonia) or tumor (e.g., pulmonary adenocarcinoma, lymphoma).

INCIDENCE/PREVALENCE AND EPIDEMIOLOGY

- Invasive aspergillosis is typically seen in patients with severe neutropenia.
- Kaposi sarcoma is typically seen in homosexual males with AIDS.
- Infections commonly causing CT halo sign include invasive aspergillosis, candidiasis, and cytomegaloviral pneumonia.
- Neoplasms commonly causing CT halo sign include pulmonary adenocarcinoma, Kaposi sarcoma, lymphoma, metastatic angiosarcoma, metastatic choriocarcinoma, and metastatic mucinous carcinoma of colon.

WHAT THE REFERRING PHYSICIAN NEEDS TO KNOW

- CT halo sign: can be highly suggestive of diagnosis given proper clinical context.
- Common differential diagnosis: invasive aspergillosis (neutropenic), candidiasis (immunocompromised with other findings of Candida infection), cytomegalovirus infection (≥1 month post transplantation), adenocarcinoma (≥ age 50, smoker, not immunocompromised).
- Less common differential diagnosis (infection): herpesvirus infection (immunocompromised), septic embolism (central venous line, intravenous drug user).
- Less common differential diagnosis (malignancy): metastatic hemorrhagic (angiosarcoma) or mucus-producing tumor (adenocarcinoma of colon), Kaposi sarcoma (male AIDS patient).
- Uncommon differential diagnosis: Wegener granulomatosis (sinusitis), pulmonary infarction.

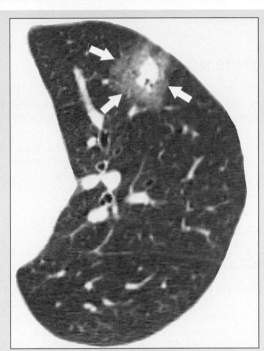

Figure 1. CT halo sign in invasive pulmonary aspergillosis.
Magnified view of the left lung from a high-resolution CT shows nodule with surrounding ground-glass attenuation (CT halo sign). The patient was a 33-year-old man with acute leukemia, severe neutropenia, and angioinvasive pulmonary aspergillosis.

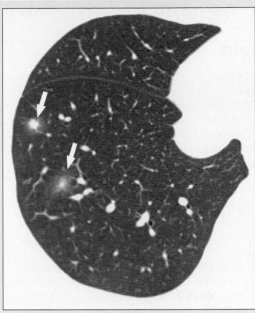

Figure 2. Angioinvasive aspergillosis. View of the right lung from a high-resolution CT shows two small nodules (*arrows*) in the right lower lobe surrounded by a rim of ground-glass attenuation (CT halo sign). The patient was a 28-year-old woman with acute leukemia and severe neutropenia following chemotherapy in whom angioinvasive aspergillosis developed.

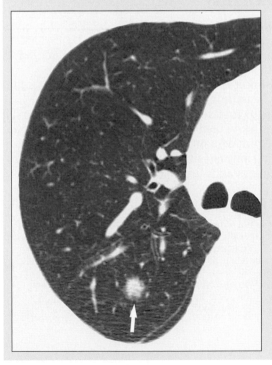

Figure 3. CT halo sign in pulmonary adenocarcinoma. Magnified view of the right lung from a high-resolution CT shows nodule with predominantly solid component and with halo of ground-glass attenuation (CT halo sign) (*arrow*) in a patient with invasive pulmonary adenocarcinoma.

Suggested Readings

Franquet T, Müller NL, Giménez A, et al: Infectious pulmonary nodules in immunocompromised patients: Usefulness of computed tomography in predicting their etiology. *J Comput Assist Tomogr* 27(4):461-468, 2003.

Greene RE, Schlamm HT, Oestmann JW, et al: Imaging findings in acute invasive pulmonary aspergillosis: Clinical significance of the halo sign. *Clin Infect Dis* 44(3):373-379, 2007.

Kim Y, Lee KS, Jung KJ, et al: Halo sign on high resolution CT: Findings in spectrum of pulmonary diseases with pathologic correlation. *J Comput Assist Tomogr* 23(4):622-626, 1999.

Lee YR, Choi YW, Lee KJ, et al: CT halo sign: The spectrum of pulmonary diseases. *Br J Radiol* 78(933):862-865, 2005.

Lindell RM, Hartman TE, Swensen SJ, et al: Five-year lung cancer screening experience: CT appearance, growth rate, location, and histologic features of 61 lung cancers. *Radiology* 242(2):555-562, 2007.

Single and Multiple Pulmonary Masses

DEFINITION: Pulmonary masses are lesions >3 cm in diameter.

IMAGING

Radiography
Findings
- Single or multiple lesions >3 cm in diameter.
- Solitary masses: most commonly pulmonary carcinoma, lung abscess, post-traumatic lung cyst/hematoma.
- Multiple masses: most commonly metastases or Wegener granulomatosis.
- Mass may contain foci of calcification or cavity.

Utility
- Usually first imaging modality used

CT
Findings
- Single or multiple lesions >3 cm in diameter.
- Solitary masses: most commonly due to pulmonary carcinoma, lung abscess, post-traumatic lung cyst/hematoma.
- Large pulmonary carcinomas that may cavitate or contain foci of calcification.
- Homogeneous water density in hydatid cyst and 50% of bronchogenic cysts.
- If located within a cavity, most commonly an aspergilloma.
- Multiple masses: most commonly metastases or Wegener granulomatosis.
- Cavitating metastases: most commonly due to squamous cell carcinoma but may also be seen in other tumors.

Utility
- Superior to the radiograph in demonstrating the presence of calcification and cavitation and associated findings such as lymphadenopathy.

MRI
Findings
- Bronchogenic cyst: almost all have homogeneous high signal intensity on T2-weighted images.

Utility
- Helpful in distinction of cystic from solid masses

DIFFERENTIAL DIAGNOSIS

- Pulmonary carcinoma
- Pulmonary metastases
- Wegener granulomatosis
- Lung abscess

DIAGNOSTIC PEARLS

- Masses are more likely than nodules to be malignant.
- Some diseases are characteristically solitary (e.g., primary pulmonary carcinoma, acute lung abscess, post-traumatic lung cyst).
- Other diseases are characteristically multiple (e.g., metastatic carcinoma, Wegener granulomatosis, septic emboli, Churg-Strauss syndrome)

- Hydatid cyst
- Bronchogenic cyst

PATHOLOGY

- Calcifications are related to psammoma bodies, dystrophic calcification of necrotic carcinoma, incorporation of focus of previous granulomatous inflammation, or calcified bronchial cartilage within tumor.
- Cavities are formed by necrosis of central portion of lesion and drainage of resultant partially liquefied material via communicating airways.

INCIDENCE/PREVALENCE AND EPIDEMIOLOGY

- Pulmonary mass has approximately 95% likelihood of being malignant.
- Incidence of cavitation in pulmonary carcinoma is about 10%.
- Most common histologic type with cavitation is squamous cell carcinoma (22%).
- Thin-walled cavitated lesions are more likely to be benign; thick-walled (>15 mm) cavitated lesions are more likely malignant.
- Single lung metastases may occur particularly in testicular tumors and sarcomas.

Suggested Readings

Aquino SL: Imaging of metastatic disease to the thorax. *Radiol Clin North Am* 43(3):481-495, 2005:vii.

Lee KS, Kim TS, Fujimoto K, et al: Thoracic manifestation of Wegener's granulomatosis: CT findings in 30 patients. *Eur Radiol* 13(1):43-51, 2003.

Zylak CJ, Eyler WR, Spizarny DL, Stone CH: Developmental lung anomalies in the adult: Radiologic-pathologic correlation. *RadioGraphics* 22:S25-S43, 2002.

WHAT THE REFERRING PHYSICIAN NEEDS TO KNOW

- Masses are more likely than nodules to be malignant.
- Majority of differential diagnosis falls into any one of the following groups: malignant neoplasm, infectious granulomas, benign tumors.
- Calcification in mass does not exclude malignancy.

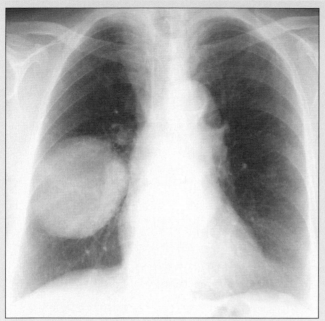

Figure 1. Pulmonary carcinoma. Posteroanterior chest radiograph shows large mass in the right lower lobe. The patient was a 73-year-old woman with pulmonary carcinoma.

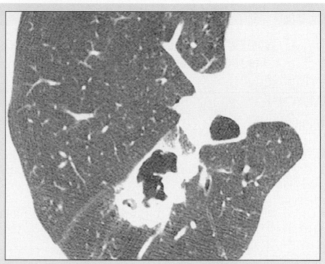

Figure 2. Cavitation in pulmonary carcinoma. View of the right lung from a high-resolution CT shows right lower lobe mass with cavitation. The wall of the cavity is thick and has a nodular appearance. The patient was a 73-year-old man with pulmonary squamous cell carcinoma.

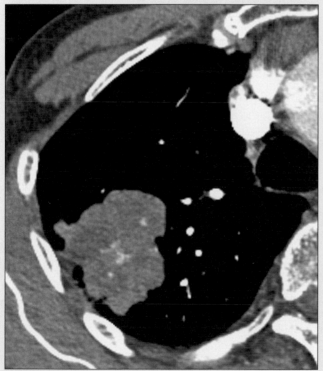

Figure 3. Calcification in carcinoma. CT image demonstrates foci of amorphous calcification within lobulated mass in a patient with metastatic adenocarcinoma of the colon.

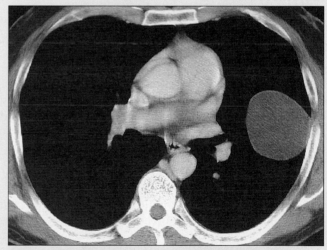

Figure 4. Hydatid cyst. CT image shows homogeneous, water-density, thin-walled cyst in the left lung. The patient was a 51-year-old man with hydatid cyst due to *Echinococcus granulosus*.

Intracavitary Mass (Meniscus or Air Crescent Sign)

DEFINITION: A crescent-shaped area of air surrounding round or oval opacity within a cavity on CT and radiography.

IMAGING

Radiography
Findings
- Crescent-shaped area of lucency within a cavity, nodule, mass, or consolidation (air crescent sign or meniscus sign).

Utility
- Often first and only imaging modality used to make diagnosis.

CT
Findings
- Crescent-shaped area of air density surrounding round or oval opacity within cavity (air crescent sign or meniscus sign).

Utility
- Superior to radiography in demonstrating cavitation and air crescent sign.

CLINICAL PRESENTATION

- Hemoptysis, fever, cough

PATHOLOGY

- Aspergilloma (fungus ball) is a conglomeration of intertwined fungal hyphae admixed with mucus and cellular debris within a pulmonary cavity or ectatic bronchus.
- Cavitating nodule, mass, or consolidation may be seen after angioinvasive fungal infection (*Aspergillus, Mucor*).
- Angioinvasion leads to infarction; retraction of infarcted center and reabsorption of peripheral necrotic tissue results in air crescent between devitalized tissue and surrounding parenchyma.

DIAGNOSTIC PEARLS

- Meniscus or air crescent sign surrounds an intracavitary mass.
- This sign is commonly seen in aspergilloma and angioinvasive aspergillosis and also may be occasionally seen in necrotizing pneumonia and ruptured hydatid cyst.

- Occasionally this sign may be seen in necrotizing pneumonia and after rupture of hydatid cyst.

INCIDENCE/PREVALENCE AND EPIDEMIOLOGY

- Vast majority of cases are related to *Aspergillus fumigatus*.
- Aspergilloma (fungus ball) with air crescent sign is seen most commonly in patients with upper lobe bronchiectasis or cavitation due to previous tuberculosis or long-standing sarcoidosis.
- Angioinvasive aspergillosis is seen most commonly in immunocompromised patients with severe neutropenia.
- Necrotizing pneumonia and ruptured hydatid cyst are uncommon causes of air crescent sign.

Suggested Readings

Abramson S: The air crescent sign. *Radiology* 218:230-232, 2001.
Franquet T, Müller NL, Giménez A, et al: Spectrum of pulmonary aspergillosis: Histologic, clinical, and radiologic findings. *RadioGraphics* 21:825-837, 2001.
Jamadar DA, Kazerooni EA, Daly BD, et al: Pulmonary zygomycosis: CT appearance. *J Comput Assist Tomogr* 19:733-738, 1995.
Koul PA, Koul AN, Wahid A, Mir FA: CT in pulmonary hydatid disease: Unusual appearances. *Chest* 118:1645-1647, 2000.

WHAT THE REFERRING PHYSICIAN NEEDS TO KNOW

- Air crescent sign results most commonly from aspergilloma (fungus ball) within pulmonary cavity or ectatic bronchus or from angioinvasive aspergillosis in patients with severe neutropenia.
- CT is imaging modality of choice in diagnosis of aspergilloma and angioinvasive aspergillosis.

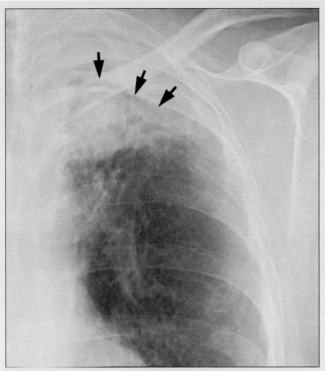

Figure 1. **Aspergilloma in tuberculous cavity.** Magnified view of the left upper lobe from a frontal chest radiograph shows air crescent (*arrows*) surrounding an intracavitary mass. Also noted is bronchiectasis.

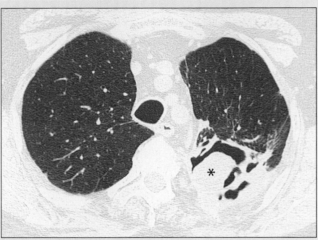

Figure 2. **Aspergilloma in tuberculous cavity.** High-resolution CT image demonstrates large cavity in the left upper lobe containing homogeneous soft tissue mass (*asterisk*). The mass lies in the dependent portion of the cavity, suggesting that it is mobile. The findings are characteristic of intracavitary fungus ball. Note bilateral centrilobular emphysema and areas of scarring and bronchiectasis in the left upper lobe and extensive pleural thickening adjacent to the cavity.

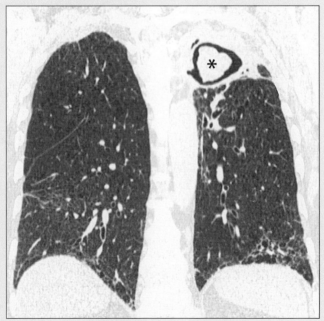

Figure 3. **Aspergilloma in tuberculous cavity.** Coronal reformatted image better shows the intracavitary aspergilloma (*asterisk*) in the left upper lobe. Also noted is subpleural honeycombing in the lower lobes consistent with idiopathic pulmonary fibrosis. The patient was a 58-year-old man with previous tuberculosis and intracavitary aspergilloma.

Small Nodular Pattern

DEFINITION: A small nodular pattern occurs with evidence of numerous round opacities <1 cm in diameter.

IMAGING

Radiography
Findings
- Small nodular opacities.
- Sarcoidosis: nodular or reticulonodular pattern in upper to middle lung with bilateral symmetric hilar lymphadenopathy.
- Silicosis and coal worker's pneumoconiosis: diffuse nodules with middle and upper lung predominance.
- Hypersensitivity pneumonitis: diffuse poorly defined nodular opacities with ground-glass opacities.
- Hematogenous processes (miliary tuberculosis, miliary fungal infection, metastatic carcinoma): diffuse nodules with lower lung predominance.
- Endobronchial spread of tuberculosis: patchy unilateral or bilateral small nodules commonly in association with cavity.

Utility
- Initial modality for suspected cases
- Used in follow-up
- Overall distribution of nodules on radiograph helps to narrow differential diagnosis

CT
Findings
- Several patterns on high-resolution CT: perilymphatic, centrilobular, and random.
- Perilymphatic distribution on CT: typical of sarcoidosis and less common in lymphatic spread of carcinoma, lymphoma, lymphoid hyperplasia, and lymphoid interstitial pneumonia.
- Centrilobular nodules on CT: infectious bronchiolitis, cellular bronchiolitis, hypersensitivity pneumonitis, and endobronchial spread of tuberculosis.
- Random nodules on CT: hematogenous infection (miliary tuberculosis, miliary fungal infection, septic embolism) and metastases.

Utility
- High-resolution CT gives more accurate assessment of presence, pattern, and extent of disease.
- High-resolution CT is superior to radiography in differential diagnosis.

DIAGNOSTIC PEARLS
- Diffuse: Miliary tuberculosis, miliary fungal infection, miliary metastases
- Upper lobe predominance: Silicosis, coal worker's pneumoconiosis, sarcoidosis

CLINICAL PRESENTATION
- Febrile patient with acute disease suggestive of hematogenous infection (e.g., miliary tuberculosis, miliary fungal infection, septic embolism).
- Chronic symptoms suggestive of various pneumoconioses or neoplasm.
- Pneumoconioses: history of exposure.
- Hypersensitivity pneumonitis: commonly a history of exposure to inciting antigen.

PATHOLOGY
- Expansion of parenchymal interstitium by spherical cellular infiltrate, fibrous tissue, or both
- Infection: viral, bacterial, and fungal infection; tuberculosis
- Inhalational diseases: silicosis, coal worker's pneumoconiosis, hypersensitivity pneumonitis
- Pulmonary metastases
- Miscellaneous: sarcoidosis, intravenous talcosis

INCIDENCE/PREVALENCE AND EPIDEMIOLOGY
- Chest radiograph normal in 10% of patients with interstitial lung disease
- Nodular pattern common manifestation of infection: tuberculosis; bacterial and fungal infection
- Inhalational diseases: silicosis, coal worker's pneumoconiosis, hypersensitivity pneumonitis
- Sarcoidosis
- Pulmonary metastases

WHAT THE REFERRING PHYSICIAN NEEDS TO KNOW
- Chest radiograph normal in 10% of patients with interstitial lung disease.
- Small nodular pattern in patient with fever: mainly miliary tuberculosis or fungal infection.
- Small nodular pattern in afebrile patient: inhalational process (e.g., silicosis, coal worker's pneumoconiosis, hypersensitivity pneumonitis); sarcoidosis; pulmonary metastases.

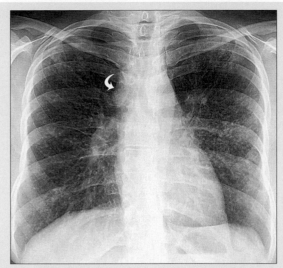

Figure 1. Nodular pattern in sarcoidosis. Posteroanterior chest radiograph shows numerous bilateral nodules involving mainly the upper and middle lung zones. Also note evidence of right paratracheal lymph node enlargement (*arrow*). The patient was a 37-year-old woman with sarcoidosis.

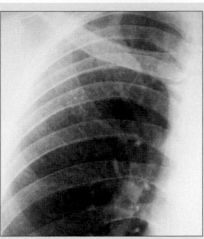

Figure 2. Silicosis. View of the right upper lobe from a posteroanterior chest radiograph shows small nodules. *(Case courtesy of Dr. Ericson Bagatin, Area of Occupational Health, State University of Campinas [UNICAMP], Campinas, São Paulo, Brazil.)*

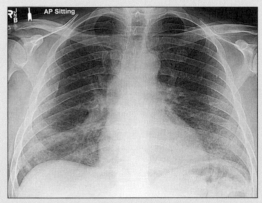

Figure 3. Hypersensitivity pneumonitis. Chest radiograph shows hazy increased opacity (ground-glass opacity) in the middle and lower lung zones and poorly defined nodular opacities. The patient was a 42-year-old man with hypersensitivity pneumonitis.

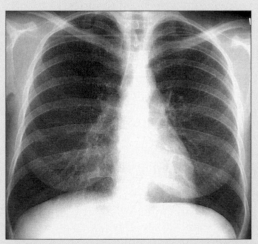

Figure 4. Miliary tuberculosis. Chest radiograph shows numerous 1- to 2-mm diameter nodules throughout both lungs (miliary pattern). The patient was a 27-year-old woman with miliary tuberculosis.

Suggested Readings

Chong S, Lee KS, Chung MJ, et al: Pneumoconiosis: Comparison of imaging and pathologic findings. *RadioGraphics* 26:59-77, 2006.

Collins J: CT signs and patterns of lung disease. *Radiol Clin North Am* 39(6):1115-1135, 2001.

McGuinness G, Naidich DP, Jagirdar J, et al: High resolution CT findings in miliary lung disease. *J Comput Assist Tomogr* 16:384-390, 1992.

Miller WT Jr: Chest radiographic evaluation of diffuse infiltrative lung disease: Review of a dying art. *Eur J Radiol* 44(3):182-197, 2002.

Perilymphatic Nodules

DEFINITION: Perilymphatic nodules are nodules along the bronchovascular interstitium, interlobular septa, and subpleural lung regions.

IMAGING

CT
Findings
- Sarcoidosis: symmetric bilateral hilar and mediastinal lymph node enlargement with/without associated parenchymal abnormalities.
- Sarcoidosis: nodules along bronchovascular and pleural interstitium and adjacent to interlobar fissures mainly in upper to middle lung zones.
- Lymphangitic carcinomatosis: occasional peribronchovascular and subpleural nodules but predominantly septal pattern.
- Silicosis and other pneumoconioses: nodules in subpleural regions and along interlobar fissures, but predominantly centrilobular, mostly in dorsal upper lobes.

Utility
- High-resolution CT gives more accurate assessment of presence, pattern, and extent of disease.
- Diagnosis can usually be made based on pattern of involvement and associated findings.

CLINICAL PRESENTATION

- Pneumoconioses: history of exposure.
- Sarcoidosis: asymptomatic, dry cough, dyspnea.
- Lymphangitic carcinomatosis: history of primary tumor, dyspnea, weight loss, malaise.

DIFFERENTIAL DIAGNOSIS

- Sarcoidosis
- Lymphangitic carcinomatosis
- Silicosis
- Coal worker's pneumoconiosis
- Lymphoma
- Lymphoid hyperplasia

DIAGNOSTIC PEARLS

- Well-defined, 2- to 5-mm nodular opacities are seen along bronchovascular interstitium and in interlobular septa and subpleural areas.
- Most common cause: sarcoidosis.

PATHOLOGY

- Nodular expansion of perilymphatic interstitium by cellular infiltrate, fibrous tissue, or tumor.
- Common causes: sarcoidosis, lymphangitic carcinomatosis, lymphoma, lymphoid hyperplasia.

INCIDENCE/PREVALENCE AND EPIDEMIOLOGY

- Present in 90%-100% of sarcoidosis patients with abnormal parenchyma.
- Commonly present in patients with lymphatic spread of cancer.
- Less common causes: lymphoma, lymphoid interstitial pneumonia, lymphoid hyperplasia, amyloidosis.

Suggested Readings

Chong S, Lee KS, Chung MJ, et al: Pneumoconiosis: Comparison of imaging and pathologic findings. *RadioGraphics* 26(1):59-77, 2006.

Gruden JF, Webb WR, Naidich DP, McGuinness G: Multinodular disease: Anatomic localization at thin-section CT—multireader evaluation of a simple algorithm. *Radiology* 210(3):711-720, 1999.

Honda O, Johkoh T, Ichikado K, et al: Comparison of high resolution CT findings of sarcoidosis, lymphoma, and lymphangitic carcinoma: Is there any difference of involved interstitium? *J Comput Assist Tomogr* 23:374-379, 1999.

Lee KS, Kim TS, Han J, et al: Diffuse micronodular lung disease: HRCT and pathologic findings. *J Comput Assist Tomogr* 23(1):99-106, 1999.

Nunes H, Brillet PY, Valeyre D, et al: Imaging in sarcoidosis. *Semin Respir Crit Care Med* 28(1):102-120, 2007.

WHAT THE REFERRING PHYSICIAN NEEDS TO KNOW

- Chest radiograph is normal in 10% of patients with interstitial lung disease.
- Perilymphatic distribution of nodules and upper and middle lung predominance are characteristic features of sarcoidosis.
- Main differential diagnosis of nodular perilymphatic pattern includes sarcoidosis and lymphangitic carcinomatosis.
- Both diagnoses can usually be confirmed by transbronchial biopsy.

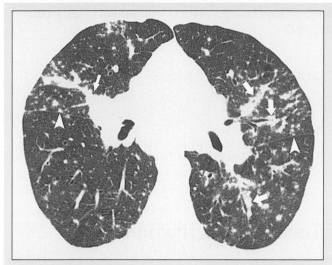

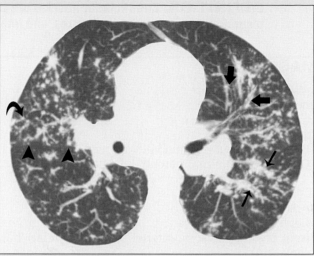

Figure 1. Perilymphatic nodules in sarcoidosis. High-resolution CT scan at the level of the middle lobe bronchus shows numerous small nodules located mainly along the bronchi (*broad straight arrows*), vessels (*narrow straight arrow*), and interlobar fissures (*arrowheads*). Also noted is lymph node enlargement in the subcarinal region. The patient was a 28-year-old man with sarcoidosis.

Figure 2. Perilymphatic nodules in sarcoidosis. Maximum intensity projection image demonstrates peribronchial (*broad straight arrows*) and perivascular (*narrow straight arrows*) predominance of nodules. Also note presence of subpleural nodules and nodules along interlobular septa (*curved arrow*) and interlobar fissures (*arrowheads*). The patient was a 28-year-old man with sarcoidosis.

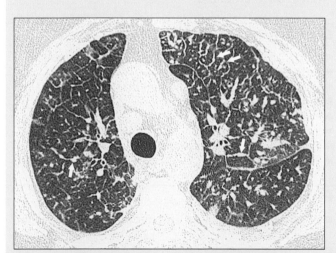

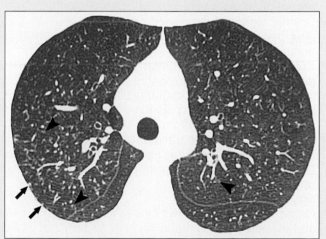

Figure 3. Nodular septal thickening in lymphangitic carcinomatosis. High-resolution CT image shows extensive bilateral septal thickening and small left pleural effusion. Several of the thickened septa have a beaded nodular appearance (*arrows*). The patient was an 80-year-old man with lymphangitic carcinomatosis. Also evident are enlarged mediastinal lymph nodes.

Figure 4. Silicosis. High-resolution CT image shows small well-defined nodules mainly in the dorsal half of the upper lobes. Some of the nodules can be seen to be in a subpleural (*arrows*) and centrilobular (*arrowheads*) distribution. *(Case courtesy of Dr. Ericson Bagatin, Area of Occupational Health, State University of Campinas [UNICAMP], Campinas, São Paulo, Brazil.)*

Centrilobular Nodules

DEFINITION: Centrilobular nodules are pulmonary nodules located several millimeters away from pleural surfaces, interlobar fissures, and interlobular septa.

IMAGING

Radiography
Findings
- Small nodular pattern

Utility
- Usually first imaging modality utilized
- Of limited value in differential diagnosis

CT
Findings
- Centrilobular nodules are several millimeters away from pleural surfaces, interlobar fissures, interlobular septa.
- No nodules are along pleura or interlobular septa.
- Bilateral, symmetric, poorly defined nodules are most commonly seen in hypersensitivity pneumonitis, respiratory bronchiolitis, and respiratory bronchiolitis/interstitial lung disease.
- Patchy, unilateral or bilateral, asymmetric well-defined nodules are most commonly seen in infectious bronchiolitis and endobronchial spread of tuberculosis or nontuberculous mycobacteria.
- Lobular areas of decreased attenuation and air trapping usually present in patients with hypersensitivity pneumonitis.
- Branching linear and nodular opacities ("tree-in-bud") pattern is commonly present in infectious bronchiolitis and endobronchial spread of tuberculosis or nontuberculous mycobacteria; a similar pattern is a rare manifestation of pulmonary arterial disease.
- In silicosis and other pneumoconioses there are nodules in subpleural regions and along interlobar fissures but predominantly centrilobular, mostly in dorsal upper lobes.

Utility
- High-resolution CT allows best assessment of presence and extent of centrilobular nodular pattern and associated parenchymal or airway abnormalities.

DIAGNOSTIC PEARLS

- Centrilobular nodules usually reflect bronchiolocentric process.
- Acute causes: usually infection, typically infectious bronchiolitis or bronchopneumonia.
- Chronic causes: most commonly inhalation of organic dusts (hypersensitivity pneumonitis) and inorganic dusts (silicosis and coalworker's pneumoconiosis).

CLINICAL PRESENTATION

- Fever and cough occur in patients with infectious bronchiolitis and with endobronchial spread of tuberculosis.
- Chronic cough and progressive dyspnea are noted in hypersensitivity pneumonitis.
- Respiratory bronchiolitis occurs in smokers and has no associated symptoms.
- Respiratory bronchiolitis/interstitial lung disease usually occurs in smokers and results in cough and progressive dyspnea.

DIFFERENTIAL DIAGNOSIS

- Acute and subacute hypersensitivity pneumonitis
- Respiratory bronchiolitis
- Respiratory bronchiolitis/interstitial lung disease
- Infectious bronchiolitis
- Tuberculosis
- Panbronchiolitis
- Coalworker's pneumoconiosis
- Silicosis

PATHOLOGY

- Infectious bronchiolitis due to viral, bacterial, or fungal infection
- Early bronchopneumonia

WHAT THE REFERRING PHYSICIAN NEEDS TO KNOW

- Chest radiograph is normal in 10% of patients with interstitial lung disease.
- Centrilobular nodules on high-resolution CT usually reflect the presence of bronchiolitis or peribronchiolar inflammation.
- Main differential diagnosis in patients presenting with acute symptoms includes viral, bacterial, or fungal bronchiolitis and endobronchial spread of tuberculosis.
- Main differential diagnosis in patients with chronic symptoms includes hypersensitivity pneumonitis, respiratory bronchiolitis, respiratory bronchiolitis/interstitial lung disease, *Mycobacterium avium-intracellulare* infection, and pneumoconiosis.
- Main differential diagnosis in patients with pulmonary arterial hypertension includes pulmonary capillary hemangiomatosis, pulmonary veno-occlusive disease, and idiopathic pulmonary arterial hypertension.

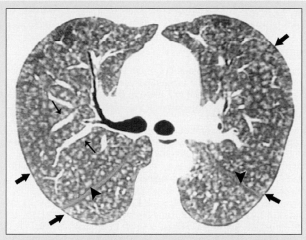

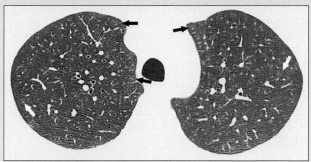

Figure 2. **Respiratory bronchiolitis.** High-resolution CT image shows poorly defined centrilobular nodules (*arrows*) in the upper lobes. The patient was a 33-year-old man with a 20-pack-year smoking history.

Figure 1. **Hypersensitivity pneumonitis.** High-resolution CT image shows diffuse parenchymal abnormalities consisting of poorly defined centrilobular nodular opacities. The centrilobular opacities typically are a few millimeters away from the pleura (*thick arrows*), interlobular septa (*arrowheads*), and large vessels (*thin arrows*) and bronchi. The patient was a bird breeder with subacute hypersensitivity pneumonitis.

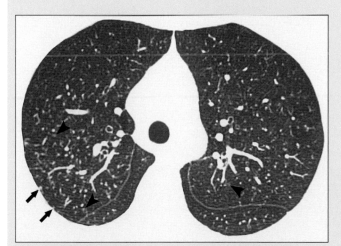

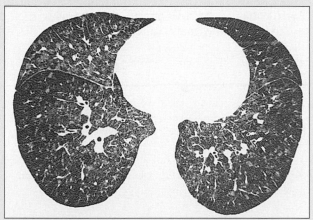

Figure 3. **Silicosis.** High-resolution CT image shows small well-defined nodules mainly in the dorsal half of the upper lobes. Some of the nodules can be seen to be in a subpleural (*straight arrows*) and centrilobular (*arrowheads*) distribution. (*Case courtesy of Dr. Ericson Bagatin, Area of Occupational Health, State University of Campinas [UNICAMP], Campinas, São Paulo, Brazil.*)

Figure 4. **Pulmonary veno-occlusive disease.** High-resolution CT image in patient with pulmonary hypertension shows widespread ground-glass opacities with centrilobular nodules and smooth interlobular septal thickening in a patient with histologically proven pulmonary veno-occlusive disease.

- Endobronchial spread of tuberculosis or nontuberculous mycobacteria
- Bronchiolitis and bronchiolocentric inflammation in hypersensitivity pneumonitis, respiratory bronchiolitis, and respiratory bronchiolitis/interstitial lung disease

INCIDENCE/PREVALENCE AND EPIDEMIOLOGY

- Respiratory bronchiolitis and respiratory bronchiolitis/interstitial lung disease are seen almost exclusively in cigarette smokers.
- Hypersensitivity pneumonitis occurs most commonly in susceptible individuals exposed to birds (bird fancier's lung) or various molds.
- Viral, bacterial, and fungal bronchiolitis often progresses to bronchopneumonia.
- Endobronchial spread is evident on CT in majority of patients with tuberculosis.
- Panbronchiolitis is seen most commonly in East Asia, particularly Japan, and is uncommon in North America.
- Bronchiolitis and peribronchial inflammation and fibrosis may occur in inhalational diseases such as smoke inhalation, coal worker's pneumoconiosis, and silicosis.

- Occasionally centrilobular nodules may result from vascular abnormality such as intravascular metastases.

Suggested Readings

Heyneman LE, Ward S, Lynch DA, et al: Respiratory bronchiolitis, respiratory bronchiolitis-associated interstitial lung disease, and desquamative interstitial pneumonia: Different entities or part of the spectrum of the same disease process? *AJR Am J Roentgenol* 173:1617-1622, 1999.

Kanne JP, Godwin JD, Franquet T, et al: Viral pneumonia after hematopoietic stem cell transplantation: High-resolution CT findings. *J Thorac Imaging* 22(3):292-299, 2007.

Okada F, Ando Y, Yoshitake S, et al: Clinical/pathologic correlations in 553 patients with primary centrilobular findings on high-resolution CT scan of the thorax. *Chest* 132(6):1939-1948, 2007.

Pipavath SJ, Lynch DA, Cool C, et al: Radiologic and pathologic features of bronchiolitis. *AJR Am J Roentgenol* 185(2):354-363, 2005.

Remy-Jardin M, Remy J, Gosselin B, et al: Lung parenchymal changes secondary to cigarette smoking: Pathologic-CT correlations. *Radiology* 186:643-651, 1993.

Rossi SE, Franquet T, Volpacchio M, et al: Tree-in-bud pattern at thin-section CT of the lungs: Radiologic-pathologic overview. *RadioGraphics* 25(3):789-801, 2005.

Silva CIS, Müller NL, Churg A: Hypersensitivity pneumonitis: Spectrum of high-resolution CT and pathologic findings. *AJR Am J Roentgenol* 188:334-344, 2007.

"Tree-in-Bud" Pattern

DEFINITION: The "tree-in-bud" pattern is one of well-defined pulmonary nodules and branching opacities that resemble a budding tree.

IMAGING

CT
Findings
- Well-defined nodular and branching opacities ("tree-in-bud" pattern)
- Infectious bronchiolitis or endobronchial spread of tuberculosis: findings mostly in the mid to lower lobes
- Panbronchiolitis: diffuse throughout both lungs but often lower lobe predominance; commonly associated air trapping and bronchiectasis
- Mucoid impaction distal to bronchiectasis or bronchial obstruction or in association with allergic bronchopulmonary aspergillosis
- Aspiration bronchiolitis: mainly dependent lung regions
- Intravascular metastases: mainly lower lung zones and peripheral distribution

Utility
- "Tree-in-bud" pattern is a characteristic pattern seen on high-resolution CT.

CLINICAL PRESENTATION

- Fever and cough in infectious bronchiolitis and endobronchial spread of tuberculosis
- Chronic cough in patient with mucoid impaction associated with bronchiectasis
- Worsening of symptoms of asthma in patients with allergic bronchopulmonary aspergillosis
- History of impaired consciousness or esophageal motility disorder in aspiration bronchiolitis
- Dyspnea and weight loss in intravascular metastases

DIFFERENTIAL DIAGNOSIS

- Infectious bronchiolitis
- Postprimary tuberculosis
- Bronchiectasis
- Allergic bronchopulmonary aspergillosis
- Bronchopneumonia
- Aspiration bronchiolitis

DIAGNOSTIC PEARLS

- Acute causes: infectious bronchiolitis, bronchopneumonia
- Chronic causes: tuberculosis, *Mycobacterium avium-intracellulare*, mucoid impaction, aspiration bronchiolitis, panbronchiolitis
- Usually due to bronchiolar abnormality
- Occasionally may reflect vascular disease such as intravascular metastases

- Panbronchiolitis
- Intravascular pulmonary metastases
- *Mycobacterium avium-intracellulare*

PATHOLOGY

- Associated with infection of small airways (e.g., infectious bronchiolitis, bronchopneumonia, endobronchial spread of tuberculosis or *Mycobacterium avium-intracellulare*)
- Impaction of bronchiolar lumens with mucus, fluid, or pus resulting from infection
- Dilated centrilobular bronchioles
- May also be caused by abnormality in centrilobular pulmonary arteries

INCIDENCE/PREVALENCE AND EPIDEMIOLOGY

- "Tree-in-bud" pattern is a common and characteristic manifestation of infectious bronchiolitis and endobronchial spread of tuberculosis.
- Aspiration bronchiolitis is seen mainly in the elderly and in patients with history of impaired consciousness (trauma, anesthesia, drugs), hiatal hernia, or esophageal dysmotility.
- Panbronchiolitis is seen almost exclusively in Asia, particularly Japan.
- "Tree-in-bud" pattern is an uncommon manifestation of pulmonary metastases.

WHAT THE REFERRING PHYSICIAN NEEDS TO KNOW

- "Tree-in-bud" pattern is a common and characteristic manifestation of infectious bronchiolitis and endobronchial spread of tuberculosis.
- "Tree-in-bud" pattern may result from viral, bacterial, and fungal infection.
- The differential diagnosis is based on clinical and high-resolution CT findings, but definitive diagnosis requires confirmation by culture, serology, and, occasionally, transbronchial or surgical lung biopsy.

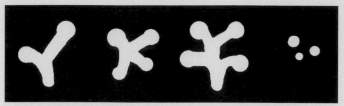

Figure 1. Schematic drawing of "tree-in-bud" pattern. A "tree-in-bud" pattern is characterized by centrilobular branching linear and nodular opacities. It is most suggestive of infectious bronchiolitis.

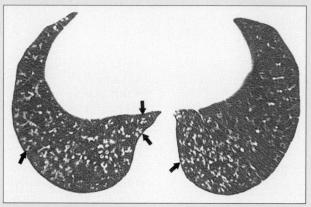

Figure 2. "Tree-in-bud" pattern in infectious bronchiolitis. High-resolution CT image shows centrilobular branching nodular and linear opacities resulting in a "tree-in-bud" appearance (*arrows*). The patient was a 20-year-old woman with recurrent respiratory infections.

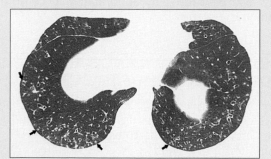

Figure 3. Diffuse panbronchiolitis: high-resolution CT findings. High-resolution CT at presentation in a 47-year-old man with panbronchiolitis shows centrilobular nodules and branching opacities resulting in a "tree-in-bud" pattern (*straight arrows*), extensive bronchiectasis, and localized areas of decreased attenuation and perfusion.

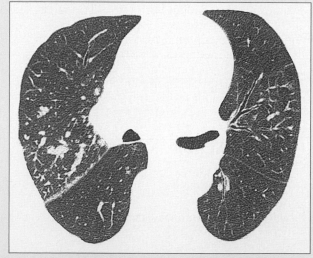

Figure 4. Tree-in-bud pattern due to intravascular metastases. High-resolution CT shows centrilobular nodular and branching opacities ("tree-in-bud" pattern) in the periphery of the right upper lobe. Also noted is nodular thickening of the pulmonary vessels. The patient was a 78-year-old man with intravascular metastatic renal cell carcinoma.

Suggested Readings

Aquino SL, Gamsu G, Webb WR, Kee SL: Tree-in-bud pattern: Frequency and significance on thin section CT. *J Comput Assist Tomogr* 20:594-599, 1996.

Collins J, Blankenbaker D, Stern EJ: CT patterns of bronchiolar disease: What is "tree-in-bud"? *AJR Am J Roentgenol* 171:365-370, 1998.

Franquet T, Müller NL: Disorders of the small airways: High-resolution computed tomographic features. *Semin Respir Crit Care Med* 24(4):437-444, 2003.

Gruden JF, Webb WR, Naidich DP, McGuinness G: Multinodular disease: Anatomic localization at thin-section CT—multireader evaluation of a simple algorithm. *Radiology* 210:711-720, 1999.

Rossi SE, Franquet T, Volpacchio M, et al: Tree-in-bud pattern at thin-section CT of the lungs: Radiologic-pathologic overview. *Radio-Graphics* 25(3):789-801, 2005.

Randomly Distributed Nodules

DEFINITION: Pulmonary nodules that have random distribution in relation to the lobular structures.

IMAGING

CT

Findings
- Multiple nodular opacities are randomly distributed in relation to the secondary pulmonary lobules.
- Mainly the lower lung zones and peripheral lung regions are involved.
- Miliary pattern (diffuse randomly distributed 1- to 3-mm nodules) is typically seen in hematogenous dissemination of infection (tuberculosis, histoplasmosis, coccidioidomycosis) or tumor metastases.
- Larger randomly distributed nodules occur most commonly in septic embolism, angioinvasive aspergillosis, and hematogenous metastases.

Utility
- High-resolution CT gives more accurate assessment of presence, pattern, and extent of disease.
- Maximum intensity projection reconstructions may demonstrate pattern and distribution better.

CLINICAL PRESENTATION

- Acute presentation with fever and shortness of breath in miliary infection (tuberculosis, histoplasmosis, coccidioidomycosis).
- Progressive shortness of breath in hematogenous spread of metastases.

DIFFERENTIAL DIAGNOSIS

- Miliary tuberculosis
- Miliary histoplasmosis
- Miliary coccidioidomycosis
- Pulmonary metastases

DIAGNOSTIC PEARLS

- Nodular opacities
- Bilateral, symmetric, random distribution
- Mostly in periphery and lung bases
- Usually results from hematogenous dissemination of infection or metastases

PATHOLOGY

- Pulmonary nodules with diffuse, random distribution
- May represent small granulomas (miliary infection) or tumors

INCIDENCE/PREVALENCE AND EPIDEMIOLOGY

- The most common causes of randomly distributed nodules are miliary tuberculosis, miliary fungal infection, and hematogenous metastases.
- Miliary tuberculosis may occur in primary or reactivation tuberculosis.
- Miliary tuberculosis, histoplasmosis, and coccidioidomycosis occur more commonly in immunocompromised patients.
- Lungs are the most common site of hematogenous metastases.

Suggested Readings

Lee KS, Kim TS, Han J, et al: Diffuse micronodular lung disease: HRCT and pathologic findings. *J Comput Assist Tomogr* 23(1): 99-106, 1999.

McGuinness G, Naidich DP, Jagirdar J, et al: High resolution CT findings in miliary lung disease. *J Comput Assist Tomogr* 16:384-390, 1992.

Murata K, Takahashi M, Mori M, et al: Pulmonary metastatic nodules: CT-pathologic correlation. *Radiology* 182:331-335, 1992.

WHAT THE REFERRING PHYSICIAN NEEDS TO KNOW

- The most common causes of randomly distributed nodules are miliary tuberculosis, miliary fungal infection, and hematogenous metastases.
- In patients with acute onset of fever and shortness of breath the main consideration is miliary tuberculosis.
- Hematogenous metastases most commonly result in various-sized nodules in random distribution in relation to secondary lobule but usually involving mainly lower lung zones and subpleural regions.

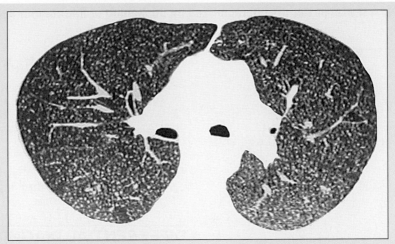

Figure 1. Miliary tuberculosis. High-resolution CT demonstrates random distribution of numerous nodules. The patient was a 27-year-old woman with miliary tuberculosis.

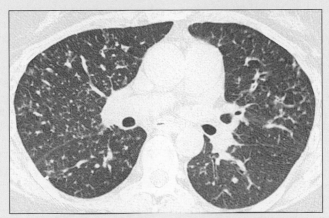

Figure 2. Pulmonary metastases: miliary pattern. CT image demonstrates multiple small nodules that have a random distribution in relation to the secondary pulmonary lobules. Also noted are a few septal lines. The patient was a 48-year-old woman with miliary pattern and biopsy-proven lymphangitic carcinomatosis due to metastatic adenocarcinoma of the colon.

Septal Pattern

DEFINITION: A septal pattern is characterized by thickening of interlobular septa.

IMAGING

Radiography
Findings
- Linear opacities
- Kerley A: 2- to 6-cm lines oriented toward hila
- Kerley B: 1- to 2-cm lines perpendicular to and continuous with pleura

Utility
- Initial modality for suspected cases
- Used in follow-up

CT
Findings
- Septal lines: short lines 0.5-2.0 cm apart extending to pleura; polygonal arcades
- Hydrostatic pulmonary edema: symmetric bilateral smooth septal thickening involving mainly dependent regions
- Lymphangitic carcinomatosis: smooth or nodular septal thickening; may have associated lymphadenopathy and pleural effusion
- Lymphoma: bilateral smooth or nodular septal thickening with associated mediastinal mass
- Churg-Strauss syndrome: bilateral smooth septal thickening due to heart failure or eosinophilic infiltration
- Niemann-Pick syndrome: bilateral smooth septal thickening associated with hepatosplenomegaly
- Acute lung rejection and pleural inflammation: smooth septal thickening in transplanted lung or adjacent to pleura
- Sarcoidosis: nodular septal thickening; other findings of nodular peribronchial thickening and nodules along pleura
- Idiopathic pulmonary fibrosis: irregular septal thickening; other findings of intralobular reticulation, architectural distortion, and honeycombing

Utility
- High-resolution CT gives more accurate assessment of presence, pattern, and extent of disease.

CLINICAL PRESENTATION

- Shortness of breath
- Acute (e.g., hydrostatic pulmonary edema) or chronic (e.g., lymphangitic carcinomatosis) symptoms

DIAGNOSTIC PEARLS

- Smooth: hydrostatic pulmonary edema, lymphangitic carcinomatosis, acute lung transplant rejection
- Nodular: lymphangitic carcinomatosis, sarcoidosis
- Irregular: pulmonary fibrosis

- Systemic symptoms related to underlying condition such as lymphoma, lymphangitic carcinomatosis, and Churg-Strauss syndrome

DIFFERENTIAL DIAGNOSIS

- Hydrostatic pulmonary edema
- Lymphangitic carcinomatosis
- Leukemia
- Churg-Strauss syndrome
- Pulmonary Hodgkin lymphoma
- Pulmonary non-Hodgkin lymphoma
- Niemann-Pick disease
- Erdheim-Chester disease
- Lymphoid interstitial pneumonia
- Acute respiratory distress syndrome
- Idiopathic pulmonary fibrosis
- Asbestos-related parenchymal disease
- Sarcoidosis
- Acute lung transplant rejection
- Diffuse pulmonary hemorrhage
- Pulmonary amyloidosis

PATHOLOGY

- Thickened septa are caused by edema, cellular infiltration, or fibrosis.
- Diseases with a septal pattern include hydrostatic pulmonary edema, lymphatic spread of carcinoma, lymphoma, leukemia, Churg-Strauss syndrome, acute lung rejection, congenital lymphangiectasia, and Niemann-Pick syndrome.
- Irregular septal thickening occurs in interstitial fibrosis, particularly idiopathic pulmonary fibrosis, asbestosis, and sarcoidosis.

WHAT THE REFERRING PHYSICIAN NEEDS TO KNOW

- Chest radiograph is normal in 10% of patients with interstitial lung disease.
- High-resolution CT is the imaging modality of choice for diagnosis of interstitial lung disease.
- The two most common causes of a diffuse septal pattern on high-resolution CT are interstitial pulmonary edema and lymphangitic carcinomatosis.
- With the exception of pulmonary edema, the definitive diagnosis of the cause of a septal pattern often requires transbronchial or, less commonly, surgical biopsy.

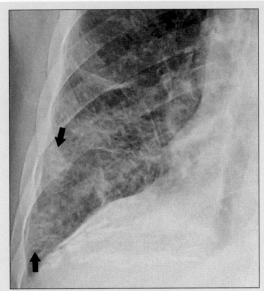

Figure 1. Septal pattern in a patient with lymphangitic carcinomatosis. Magnified view of right lower lung zone shows linear opacities (*arrows*) measuring 1 to 2 cm in length and perpendicular to the pleura. These represent septal lines (Kerley B lines). The patient was an 80-year-old man with lymphangitic carcinomatosis.

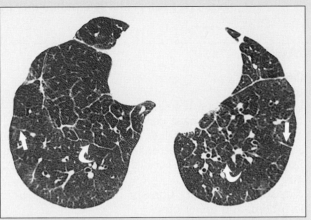

Figure 2. Smooth septal thickening in a patient with interstitial pulmonary edema. High-resolution CT at the level of the lower lung zones shows smooth septal lines perpendicular to the pleura (*straight arrows*) and more centrally as polygonal arcades (*curved arrows*). The patient was an 84-year-old woman with left-sided heart failure and interstitial pulmonary edema.

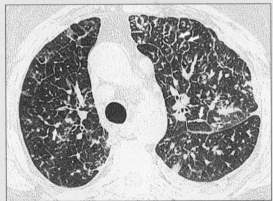

Figure 3. Nodular septal thickening in lymphangitic carcinomatosis. High-resolution CT image shows extensive bilateral septal thickening and small left pleural effusion. Several of the thickened septa have a beaded nodular appearance (*arrows*). The patient was an 80-year-old man with lymphangitic carcinomatosis. Also evident are enlarged mediastinal lymph nodes.

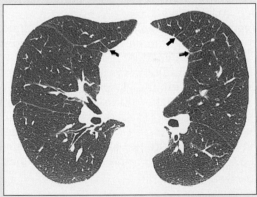

Figure 4. Smooth septal thickening in Churg-Strauss syndrome. High-resolution CT image shows mild bilateral smooth thickening of several interlobular septa (*arrows*). The patient was a 41-year-old man with Churg-Strauss syndrome. The patient had normal cardiac function; the interlobular septal thickening was due to eosinophilic infiltration.

INCIDENCE/PREVALENCE AND EPIDEMIOLOGY

- Most common cause is hydrostatic pulmonary edema.
- Nodular septal thickening occurs most commonly in lymphangitic carcinomatosis.
- Irregular septal thickening is seen most commonly in interstitial fibrosis.

Suggested Readings

Bessis L, Callard P, Gotheil C, et al: High-resolution CT of parenchymal lung disease: Precise correlation with histologic findings. *RadioGraphics* 12(1):45-58, 1992.

Kang EY, Grenier P, Laurent F, Müller NL: Interlobular septal thickening: Patterns at high-resolution computed tomography. *J Thorac Imaging* 11(4):260-264, 1996.

Müller NL, Miller RR: Computed tomography of chronic diffuse infiltrative lung disease: I. *Am Rev Respir Dis* 142:1206-1215, 1990.

Webb WR: Thin-section CT of the secondary pulmonary lobule: Anatomy and the image—the 2004 Fleischner lecture. *Radiology* 239:322-338, 2006.

Cystic Pattern

DEFINITION: Multiple pulmonary cysts result in a cystic pattern on high-resolution CT.

IMAGING

Radiography

Findings

- Reticular pattern due to superimposed cyst walls
- Pulmonary Langerhans cell histiocytosis: diffuse bilateral reticulation with relative lower lung sparing
- Lymphangioleiomyomatosis: diffuse bilateral reticulation, sometimes with visible cysts and signs of pulmonary hyperinflation
- Idiopathic pulmonary fibrosis: bilateral reticulation in peripheral and lower lung

Utility

- Initial modality for suspected cases
- Used in follow-up
- Limited value in diagnosis of cystic pattern

CT

Findings

- Pulmonary Langerhans cell histiocytosis: numerous bilateral cysts of various sizes and shapes and subcentimeter nodules with relative sparing of lung bases.
- Lymphangioleiomyomatosis: diffuse numerous 0.2- to 2.0-cm thin-walled cysts with normal surrounding parenchyma.
- *Pneumocystis* pneumonia: single or multiple cysts superimposed on ground-glass opacities in upper lobes.
- Lymphoid interstitial pneumonia and hypersensitivity pneumonitis: multiple cysts mainly in lower lobes superimposed on ground-glass opacities.
- Idiopathic pulmonary fibrosis: honeycombing in peripheral and lower lung associated with other findings of fibrosis.
- Birt-Hogg-Dubé syndrome: multiple thin-walled cysts of 1.0-6.0 cm in diameter mainly in lower lobes.

Utility

- High-resolution CT gives more accurate assessment of presence, pattern, and extent of disease.
- Confident diagnosis often can be made based on high-resolution CT findings.

CLINICAL PRESENTATION

- Progressive shortness of breath and dry cough
- Birt-Hogg-Dubé syndrome: patients typically have facial papules that represent fibrofolliculomas

DIAGNOSTIC PEARLS

- Diffuse: Lymphangioleiomyomatosis
- Upper and middle lung zones and basal sparing: Langerhans cell histiocytosis
- Variable size, basal predominance: Birt-Hogg-Dubé syndrome
- Superimposed on ground-glass opacities: *Pneumocystis* pneumonia, lymphoid interstitial pneumonia, hypersensitivity pneumonitis

DIFFERENTIAL DIAGNOSIS

- Lymphangioleiomyomatosis
- *Pneumocystis* pneumonia
- Lymphoid interstitial pneumonia
- Idiopathic pulmonary fibrosis
- Hypersensitivity pneumonitis
- Pulmonary Langerhans histiocytosis
- Birt-Hogg-Dubé

PATHOLOGY

- Round circumscribed space that is surrounded by an epithelial or fibrous wall of variable thickness
- Usually contains air; may contain fluid
- Pulmonary Langerhans cell histiocytosis: infiltration of the lung by Langerhans cells
- Lymphangioleiomyomatosis: interstitial proliferation of smooth muscle–like cells
- Honeycombing as result of advanced pulmonary fibrosis of any cause; lined by metaplastic bronchiolar epithelium

INCIDENCE/PREVALENCE AND EPIDEMIOLOGY

- Pulmonary Langerhans cell histiocytosis is seen most commonly in young adult smokers.
- Lymphangioleiomyomatosis is a rare disease, limited to women usually of childbearing age.
- Cystic spaces are seen in approximately 30% of patients with *Pneumocystis* pneumonia.

WHAT THE REFERRING PHYSICIAN NEEDS TO KNOW

- Chest radiograph is normal in 10% of patients with interstitial lung disease.
- High-resolution CT is imaging modality of choice in the diagnosis of cystic lung disease.
- Combination of clinical history, laboratory data, and high-resolution CT allows confident diagnosis in majority of cases.
- Some patients may require lung biopsy for definitive diagnosis.

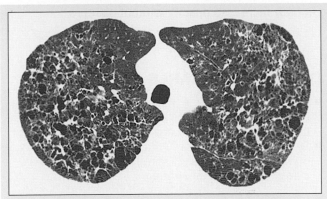

Figure 1. Pulmonary Langerhans cell histiocytosis. High-resolution CT slightly above the level of the aortic arch shows numerous bilateral cysts, a few small nodules, and ground-glass opacities. The patient was a 52-year-old man who was a smoker and developed pulmonary Langerhans cell histiocytosis. The ground-glass opacities reflect the presence of respiratory bronchiolitis ("smoker's bronchiolitis").

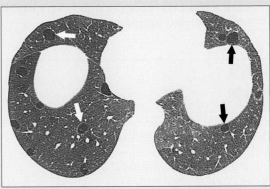

Figure 2. Lymphoid interstitial pneumonia. High-resolution CT image shows patchy bilateral ground-glass opacities and several thin-walled cysts (*arrows*). The patient was a 44-year-old woman with lymphoid interstitial pneumonia who was a life-long nonsmoker.

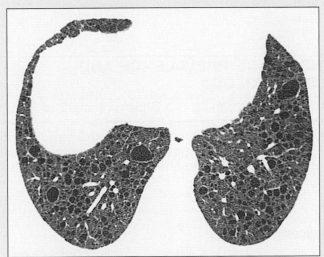

Figure 3. Lymphangioleiomyomatosis. High-resolution CT at the level of the lung bases shows diffuse involvement by thin-walled cysts. The patient was a 75-year-old woman with long-standing lymphangioleiomyomatosis.

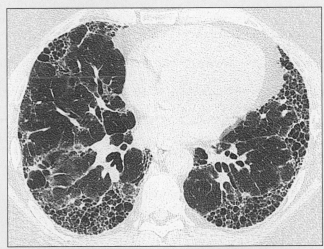

Figure 4. Honeycombing in end-stage idiopathic pulmonary fibrosis. High-resolution CT image obtained on a multidetector scanner shows extensive subpleural honeycombing. The patient was a 59-year-old man with idiopathic pulmonary fibrosis.

- Cysts are seen in 60% to 80% of lymphoid interstitial pneumonia, 30% of *Pneumocystis* pneumonia, 13% of subacute hypersensitivity pneumonitis, and 40% of chronic hypersensitivity pneumonitis.
- Honeycombing is seen most commonly in idiopathic pulmonary fibrosis.

Suggested Readings

Abbott GF, Rosado-de-Christenson ML, Franks TJ, et al: From the archives of the AFIP: Pulmonary Langerhans cell histiocytosis. *RadioGraphics* 24(3):821-841, 2004.

Bonelli FS, Hartman TE, Swensen SJ, Sherrick A: Accuracy of high-resolution CT in diagnosing lung diseases. *AJR Am J Roentgenol* 170(6):1507-1512, 1998.

Hartman TE: CT of cystic diseases of the lung. *Radiol Clin North Am* 39(6):1231-1244, 2001.

Koyama M, Johkoh T, Honda O, et al: Chronic cystic lung disease: Diagnostic accuracy of high-resolution CT in 92 patients. *AJR Am J Roentgenol* 180:827-835, 2003.

Niku S, Stark P, Levin DL, Friedman PJ: Lymphangioleiomyomatosis: Clinical, pathologic, and radiologic manifestations. *J Thorac Imaging* 20(2):98-102, 2005.

Primack SL, Hartman TE, Hansell DM, Müller NL: End-stage lung disease: CT findings in 61 patients. *Radiology* 189:681-686, 1993.

Ground-Glass Pattern: Acute Lung Disease

DEFINITION: Acute pulmonary disease resulting in hazy increased opacity without obscuration of underlying vascular markings.

IMAGING

Radiography
Findings
- Granular or hazy opacity with underlying vascular markings unobscured (ground-glass pattern)
Utility
- Initial modality for suspected cases
- Findings commonly normal
- Useful in follow-up

CT
Findings
- Hazy increased opacity is evident without obscuration of underlying vascular markings.
- Ground-glass pattern may be the only pattern on CT or may be associated with other parenchymal abnormalities.
- Ground-glass opacities surrounding nodules result in CT halo sign, which is commonly seen in invasive aspergillosis, candidiasis, and cytomegaloviral pneumonia.
- Ground-glass attenuation superimposed with smooth interlobular septal thickening and intralobular lines ("crazy-paving" pattern) is seen most commonly in acute respiratory distress syndrome, pulmonary hemorrhage, and *Pneumocystis* pneumonia.

Utility
- Represent abnormalities below resolution limit of high-resolution CT
- Relatively nonspecific finding
- Diagnosis made by correlation with associated findings and clinical data

CLINICAL PRESENTATION

- Cough and dyspnea
- Pulmonary hemorrhage: hemoptysis

DIFFERENTIAL DIAGNOSIS

- *Pneumocystis* pneumonia
- Diffuse pulmonary hemorrhage

DIAGNOSTIC PEARLS

- Diffuse: *Pneumocystis* pneumonia, cytomegalovirus pneumonia, acute respiratory distress syndrome, diffuse pulmonary hemorrhage
- Surrounding nodules (CT halo sign): invasive pulmonary aspergillosis, candidiasis, cytomegalovirus pneumonia.

- Cytomegalovirus pneumonia
- Acute respiratory distress syndrome

PATHOLOGY

- Interstitial thickening by inflammation or fibrosis
- Partial filling of the airspaces by edema, blood, or exudate

INCIDENCE/PREVALENCE AND EPIDEMIOLOGY

- Ground-glass pattern is a common pattern of abnormality on high-resolution CT.
- Common acute conditions with ground-glass pattern include pneumonia (particularly *Pneumocystis* and cytomegalovirus), hemorrhage, and acute respiratory distress syndrome.

Suggested Readings

Boiselle PM, Crans CA Jr, Kaplan MA: The changing face of *Pneumocystis carinii* pneumonia in AIDS patients. *AJR Am J Roentgenol* 172(5):1301-1309, 1999.

Collins J, Stern EJ: Ground-glass opacity at CT: The ABCs. *AJR Am J Roentgenol* 169(2):355-367, 1997.

Nowers K, Rasband JD, Berges G, Gosselin M: Approach to ground-glass opacification of the lung. *Semin Ultrasound CT MR* 23(4):302-323, 2002.

Primack SL, Miller RR, Müller NL: Diffuse pulmonary hemorrhage: Clinical, pathologic, and imaging features. *AJR Am J Roentgenol* 164:295-300, 1995.

WHAT THE REFERRING PHYSICIAN NEEDS TO KNOW

- Ground-glass pattern is a common pattern of abnormality seen on high-resolution CT.
- The chest radiograph is often normal or shows nonspecific findings.
- Ground-glass pattern is a nonspecific pattern seen in a variety of acute or chronic interstitial and airspace diseases.
- Common acute conditions with ground-glass pattern include pneumonia (particularly *Pneumocystis* and cytomegalovirus), hemorrhage, and acute respiratory distress syndrome.

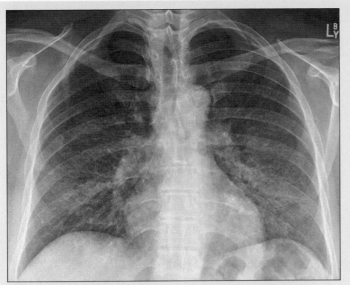

Figure 1. *Pneumocystis jiroveci* **pneumonia.** Chest radiograph shows symmetric bilateral hazy increased opacity (ground-glass opacity). The patient was a 42-year-old woman with newly diagnosed AIDS and *Pneumocystis jiroveci* pneumonia.

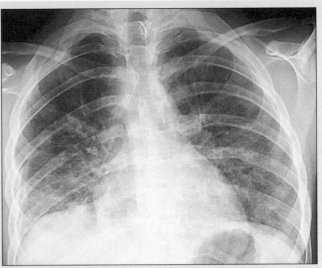

Figure 2. **Diffuse pulmonary hemorrhage.** Chest radiograph shows ground-glass opacities involving mainly the lower lung zones. The patient was an 18-year-old woman with diffuse pulmonary hemorrhage due to vasculitis.

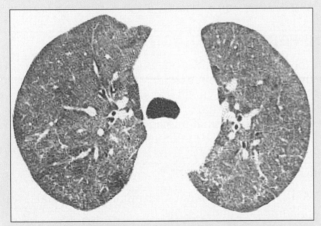

Figure 3. *Pneumocystis jiroveci* **pneumonia.** High-resolution CT at the level of the upper lobes shows extensive bilateral ground-glass opacities. The patient was a 42-year-old woman with newly diagnosed AIDS and *Pneumocystis jiroveci* pneumonia.

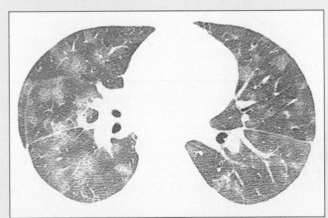

Figure 4. **Diffuse pulmonary hemorrhage.** High-resolution CT image shows patchy bilateral ground-glass opacities. The patient was an 18-year-old woman with diffuse pulmonary hemorrhage due to vasculitis.

Ground-Glass Pattern: Chronic Lung Disease

DEFINITION: Chronic pulmonary disease associated with hazy increased opacity without obscuration of underlying vascular markings.

IMAGING

Radiography
Findings
- Granular or hazy opacity with underlying vascular markings unobscured (ground-glass pattern).

Utility
- Initial modality for suspected cases
- Normal findings in approximately 10% of cases
- Useful in follow-up

CT
Findings
- Hazy increased opacity without obscuration of underlying vascular markings.
- Ground-glass pattern may be the only pattern on CT or may be associated with other parenchymal abnormalities.
- Poorly defined centrilobular nodules are commonly seen in patients with hypersensitivity pneumonitis and respiratory bronchiolitis/interstitial lung disease.
- Cysts superimposed on ground-glass opacities may be seen in lymphoid interstitial pneumonia and hypersensitivity pneumonitis.
- Reticulation and evidence of fibrosis (traction bronchiectasis and bronchiolectasis) are commonly seen in nonspecific interstitial pneumonia, usual interstitial pneumonia, and chronic hypersensitivity pneumonitis.
- Ground-glass attenuation with superimposed smooth interlobular septal thickening and intralobular lines results in pattern known as "crazy-paving," a finding seen in a number of diseases including alveolar proteinosis, lipoid pneumonia, and bronchioloalveolar carcinoma.

Utility
- Represent abnormalities below resolution limit of high-resolution CT
- Relatively nonspecific finding
- Diagnosis made by correlation with associated findings and clinical data

DIAGNOSTIC PEARLS

- Associated with centrilobular nodules: hypersensitivity pneumonitis, respiratory bronchiolitis/interstitial lung disease
- Associated with lobular air trapping: hypersensitivity pneumonitis
- Associated with reticulation: chronic hypersensitivity pneumonitis, nonspecific interstitial pneumonia, desquamative interstitial pneumonia
- Associated with cysts: lymphoid interstitial pneumonia, hypersensitivity pneumonitis

CLINICAL PRESENTATION

- Chronic symptoms: most commonly dry cough and progressive dyspnea
- Respiratory bronchiolitis/interstitial lung disease: history of smoking >30 pack-years

DIFFERENTIAL DIAGNOSIS

- Nonspecific interstitial pneumonia
- Hypersensitivity pneumonitis
- Respiratory bronchiolitis/interstitial lung disease
- Desquamative interstitial pneumonia
- Lymphoid interstitial pneumonia
- Bronchioloalveolar carcinoma

PATHOLOGY

- Nonspecific interstitial pneumonia: alveolar wall inflammation and fibrosis
- Nonspecific interstitial pneumonia: idiopathic or secondary to collagen vascular disease, drug reaction, or hypersensitivity pneumonitis
- Desquamative interstitial pneumonia: filling of alveolar airspaces with macrophages, mild alveolar wall inflammation, and mild fibrosis

WHAT THE REFERRING PHYSICIAN NEEDS TO KNOW

- Ground-glass pattern is a common pattern of abnormality seen on high-resolution CT.
- Common chronic conditions associated with a ground-glass pattern include hypersensitivity pneumonitis and nonspecific interstitial pneumonia.
- Chest radiograph is normal in 10% of patients with interstitial lung disease.

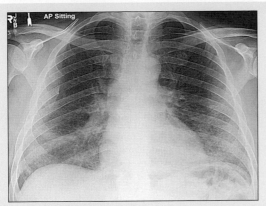

Figure 1. Hypersensitivity pneumonitis. Chest radiograph shows hazy increased opacity (ground-glass opacity) in the middle and lower lung zones and poorly defined nodular opacities. The patient was a 42-year-old man with hypersensitivity pneumonitis.

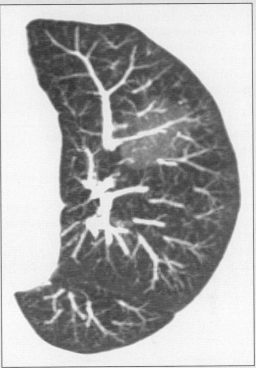

Figure 2. Ground-glass pattern. Maximum intensity projection image of the left lung illustrates characteristic appearance of ground-glass opacity with homogeneous increase in attenuation that does not result in obscuration of underlying vessels.

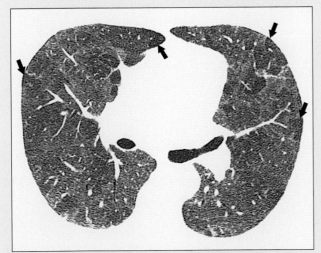

Figure 3. Hypersensitivity pneumonitis. High-resolution CT image shows extensive bilateral ground-glass opacities, a few centrilobular nodules, and lobular areas of decreased attenuation and vascularity (*arrows*). The patient was a 65-year-old woman with subacute hypersensitivity pneumonitis.

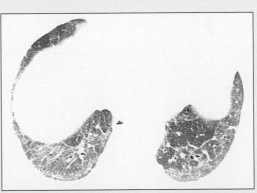

Figure 4. Nonspecific interstitial pneumonia. High-resolution CT at the level of the lung bases shows extensive bilateral ground-glass opacities. The patient was a 62-year-old man with nonspecific interstitial pneumonia.

- Respiratory bronchiolitis/interstitial lung disease: smoking-related interstitial lung disease
- Lymphoid interstitial pneumonia: benign lymphoproliferative disorder in immunologic disorders (Sjögren syndrome)
- Hypersensitivity pneumonitis: alveolitis, bronchiolitis, ill-defined granulomas

INCIDENCE/PREVALENCE AND EPIDEMIOLOGY

- Hypersensitivity pneumonitis is most common cause in normal hosts.
- Respiratory bronchiolitis/interstitial lung disease and desquamative interstitial pneumonia usually occur in smokers.
- Desquamative interstitial pneumonia and lymphoid interstitial pneumonia are uncommon conditions.

Suggested Readings

Collins J, Stern EJ: Ground-glass opacity at CT: The ABCs. *AJR Am J Roentgenol* 169(2):355-367, 1997.

Leung AN, Miller RR, Müller NL: Parenchymal opacification in chronic infiltrative lung diseases: CT-pathologic correlation. *Radiology* 188:209-214, 1993.

Lynch DA, Travis WD, Müller NL, et al: Idiopathic interstitial pneumonias: CT features. *Radiology* 236(1):10-21, 2005.

Nowers K, Rasband JD, Berges G, Gosselin M: Approach to ground-glass opacification of the lung. *Semin Ultrasound CT MR* 23(4):302-323, 2002.

Park CM, Goo JM, Lee HJ, et al: Nodular ground-glass opacity at thin-section CT: Histologic correlation and evaluation of change at follow-up. *RadioGraphics* 27(2):391-408, 2007.

Silva CIS, Müller NL, Churg A: Hypersensitivity pneumonitis: Spectrum of high-resolution CT and pathologic findings. *AJR Am J Roentgenol* 188:334-344, 2007.

Reticular Pattern

DEFINITION: A reticular pattern is one of innumerable, interlacing line shadows that suggest a mesh.

IMAGING

Radiography
Findings
- Reticulation: mesh-like shadows resulting from summation of linear opacities and/or cystic spaces.
- Idiopathic pulmonary fibrosis: diffuse, symmetric, bilateral reticulation with peripheral and lower lobe predominance.
- Nonspecific interstitial pneumonia: predominant ground-glass opacities with fine reticulation mostly in lower lungs.
- Chronic hypersensitivity pneumonitis: reticulation with middle lung predominance and ground-glass opacities.
- Sarcoidosis: upper and middle lung zone reticulation with traction and overinflation of lower lobes.
- Asbestosis: mild lower lobe reticulation with pleural plaques or thickening.
- Scleroderma: fibrosis associated with esophageal dilatation.
- Rheumatoid arthritis: fibrosis usually resembling that of idiopathic pulmonary fibrosis.

Utility
- Initial modality for suspected cases
- Used in follow-up

CT
Findings
- Small irregular intralobular linear opacities separated by only a few millimeters.
- Idiopathic pulmonary fibrosis: patchy diffuse reticulation, worse in subpleural area and lung bases associated with architectural distortion, traction bronchiectasis, traction bronchiolectasis, and honeycombing.
- Nonspecific interstitial pneumonia: predominant ground-glass opacities, mild reticulation, no or only mild honeycombing, and relative subpleural sparing.
- Hypersensitivity pneumonitis: reticulation predominantly subpleural or peribronchovascular with ground-glass opacities, centrilobular nodules, and lobular air trapping.
- Sarcoidosis: extensive upper lobe reticulation and architectural distortion with nodular opacities.
- Asbestosis: subpleural reticulation with curvilinear opacities and nodular branching; subpleural opacities mainly in dorsal regions; pleural thickening.

DIAGNOSTIC PEARLS
- Predominant ground-glass favors nonspecific interstitial pneumonia
- Lobular air trapping favors hypersensitivity pneumonitis
- Peripheral and basal honeycombing favors idiopathic pulmonary fibrosis

- Scleroderma: fibrosis usually with a pattern of nonspecific interstitial pneumonia.
- Rheumatoid arthritis: fibrosis usually resembling idiopathic pulmonary fibrosis.

Utility
- High-resolution CT gives more accurate assessment of presence, pattern, and extent of disease.

CLINICAL PRESENTATION
- Majority of patients present with history of dry cough and progressive shortness of breath.
- Nonspecific interstitial pneumonia resembles idiopathic pulmonary fibrosis clinically.
- In chronic hypersensitivity pneumonitis there is commonly a history of exposure to inciting antigens.

DIFFERENTIAL DIAGNOSIS
- Idiopathic pulmonary fibrosis
- Nonspecific interstitial pneumonia
- Chronic hypersensitivity pneumonitis
- Sarcoidosis
- Asbestosis
- Rheumatoid arthritis
- Scleroderma

PATHOLOGY
- Intralobular linear opacities reflect thickening of interstitium within secondary pulmonary lobule and are commonly caused by fibrosis.
- Causes include idiopathic interstitial fibrosis and fibrosis associated with collagen vascular disease, hypersensitivity pneumonitis, sarcoidosis, and asbestosis.

WHAT THE REFERRING PHYSICIAN NEEDS TO KNOW
- Chest radiograph is normal in 10% of patients with interstitial lung disease.
- Chest radiograph is of limited value in the differential diagnosis of interstitial lung diseases.
- High-resolution CT is imaging modality of choice for assessment of patients with interstitial lung disease.
- Definitive diagnosis requires integration of clinical and CT findings and, commonly, lung biopsy.

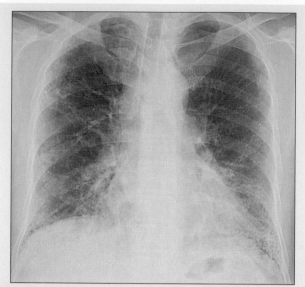

Figure 1. Reticular pattern on the chest radiograph.
Posteroanterior chest radiograph shows extensive bilateral
reticular pattern worse in the lower lung zones. The patient
was a 58-year-old man with idiopathic pulmonary fibrosis. The
reticular pattern in this patient was caused by summation of
irregular linear opacities and honeycombing.

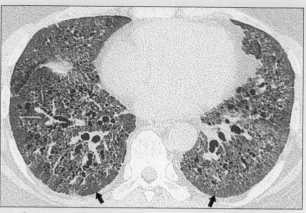

**Figure 2. Nonspecific interstitial pneumonia: relative
subpleural sparing.** High-resolution CT in a 60-year-old man
shows extensive bilateral ground-glass opacities, traction
bronchiectasis, and reticulation. The reticulation is less severe in
the lung immediately adjacent to the pleura (*arrows*) than in the
lung 1 cm away from the pleura (relative subpleural sparing), a
characteristic finding seen in approximately 50% of patients with
fibrotic nonspecific interstitial pneumonia.

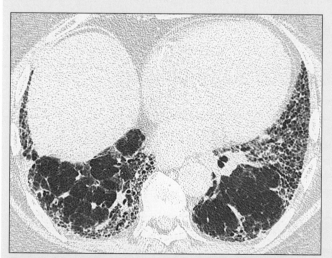

Figure 3. Idiopathic pulmonary fibrosis. High-resolution CT
at the level of the lung bases shows extensive reticulation and
subpleural honeycombing. The patient was a 70-year-old man
with idiopathic pulmonary fibrosis.

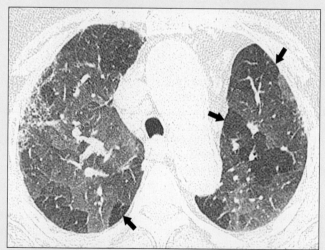

Figure 4. Chronic hypersensitivity pneumonitis. High-
resolution CT performed after maximal expiration shows
peripheral reticulation, ground-glass opacities, and extensive
areas of air trapping (*arrows*). The patient was a 78-year-old
woman with chronic hypersensitivity pneumonitis.

- Idiopathic pulmonary fibrosis: idiopathic chronic interstitial fibrosis is limited to the lung and associated with histologic appearance of usual interstitial pneumonia.
- Nonspecific interstitial pneumonia: chronic interstitial lung disease is characterized histologically by combination of interstitial fibrosis and inflammation.

INCIDENCE/PREVALENCE AND EPIDEMIOLOGY

- Usual interstitial pneumonia is the most common histologic pattern in chronic interstitial pneumonia. Majority of cases are idiopathic. Idiopathic usual interstitial pneumonia is synonymous with idiopathic pulmonary fibrosis.
- Nonspecific interstitial pneumonia may be idiopathic but is also commonly seen in patients with connective tissue disease (scleroderma) and drug reaction.
- Most common collagen vascular diseases associated with a reticular pattern on a chest radiograph and high-resolution CT are scleroderma and rheumatoid arthritis.
- Reticular pattern is seen in 15%-20% of patients who have sarcoidosis.

Suggested Readings

Aziz ZA, Wells AU, Bateman ED, et al: Interstitial lung disease: Effects of thin-section CT on clinical decision making. *Radiology* 238(2):725-733, 2006.

Devaraj A, Wells AU, Hansell DM: Computed tomographic imaging in connective tissue diseases. *Semin Respir Crit Care Med* 28(4): 389-397, 2007.

Lynch DA, Travis WD, Müller NL, et al: Idiopathic interstitial pneumonias: CT features. *Radiology* 236(1):10-21, 2005.

Miller WT Jr: Chest radiographic evaluation of diffuse infiltrative lung disease: Review of a dying art. *Eur J Radiol* 44:182-197, 2002.

Silva CI, Churg A, Müller NL: Hypersensitivity pneumonitis: Spectrum of high-resolution CT and pathologic findings. *AJR Am J Roentgenol* 188(2):334-344, 2007.

Silva CI, Müller NL, Lynch DA, et al: Chronic hypersensitivity pneumonitis: Differentiation from idiopathic pulmonary fibrosis and nonspecific interstitial pneumonia by using thin-section CT. *Radiology* 246(1):288-297, 2008.

Webb WR: Thin-section CT of the secondary pulmonary lobule: Anatomy and the image—the 2004 Fleischner lecture. *Radiology* 239:322-338, 2006.

"Crazy-Paving" Pattern

DEFINITION: Ground-glass opacities with superimposed septal lines and intralobular lines comprise the "crazy-paving" pattern.

IMAGING

CT

Findings
- Bilateral ground-glass opacities with superimposed smooth septal lines and intralobular lines

Utility
- Nonspecific high-resolution CT pattern seen in a number of acute and chronic interstitial and airspace lung diseases

CLINICAL PRESENTATION

- Cough, dyspnea
- Hemoptysis in patients with "crazy-paving" pattern due to pulmonary hemorrhage
- Symptoms either acute or chronic depending on cause of "crazy-paving" pattern

DIFFERENTIAL DIAGNOSIS

- Pulmonary alveolar proteinosis
- Acute interstitial pneumonia
- Acute respiratory distress syndrome
- *Pneumocystis* pneumonia
- Lipoid pneumonia
- Bronchioloalveolar cell carcinoma
- Hydrostatic pulmonary edema
- Radiation-induced lung disease
- Churg-Strauss syndrome
- Diffuse pulmonary hemorrhage

PATHOLOGY

- Acute conditions: acute respiratory distress syndrome, acute interstitial pneumonia, pulmonary edema, pulmonary hemorrhage, bacterial pneumonia, *Pneumocystis*

DIAGNOSTIC PEARLS

- Acute: *Pneumocystis* pneumonia, acute respiratory distress syndrome, pulmonary hemorrhage
- Chronic: Pulmonary alveolar proteinosis, lipoid pneumonia, Churg-Strauss syndrome, bronchioloalveolar cell carcinoma

pneumonia, *Mycoplasma* pneumonia, acute eosinophilic pneumonia
- Subacute and chronic conditions: radiation pneumonitis, lipoid pneumonia, alveolar proteinosis, Churg-Strauss syndrome, bronchioloalveolar cell carcinoma

INCIDENCE/PREVALENCE AND EPIDEMIOLOGY

- "Crazy-paving": common pattern seen on high-resolution CT
- Acute causes: acute respiratory distress syndrome, acute interstitial pneumonia, pulmonary edema, pulmonary hemorrhage, bacterial pneumonia, *Pneumocystis* pneumonia, *Mycoplasma* pneumonia, acute eosinophilic pneumonia
- Subacute or chronic causes: radiation pneumonitis, lipoid pneumonia, alveolar proteinosis, Churg-Strauss syndrome, bronchioloalveolar carcinoma

Suggested Readings

Chung MJ, Lee KS, Franquet T, et al: Metabolic lung disease: Imaging and histopathologic findings. *Eur J Radiol* 54(2):233-245, 2005.
Franquet T, Giménez A, Bordes R, et al: The crazy-paving pattern in exogenous lipoid pneumonia: CT-pathologic correlation. *AJR Am J Roentgenol* 170:315-317, 1998.
Johkoh T, Itoh H, Müller NL, et al: Crazy-paving appearance at thin-section CT: Spectrum of disease and pathologic findings. *Radiology* 211:155-160, 1999.
Murayama S, Murakami J, Yabuuchi H, et al: Crazy paving appearance" on high resolution CT in various diseases. *J Comput Assist Tomogr* 23:749-752, 1999.

WHAT THE REFERRING PHYSICIAN NEEDS TO KNOW

- "Crazy-paving" is a high-resolution CT pattern characterized by smooth interlobular septal thickening and intralobular lines superimposed on ground-glass opacities.
- Many common acute and chronic interstitial and airspace diseases may result in a "crazy-paving" pattern.
- Differential diagnosis is based on presence of associated findings and clinical history.
- Definitive diagnosis often requires lung biopsy.

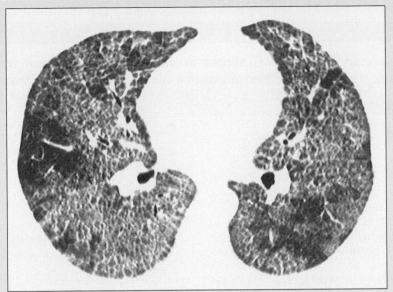

Figure 1. **"Crazy-paving" pattern in alveolar proteinosis.** High-resolution CT image demonstrates bilateral ground-glass opacities with superimposed smooth septal lines and intralobular lines resulting in a pattern known as "crazy-paving." The patient was a 45-year-old man with alveolar proteinosis.

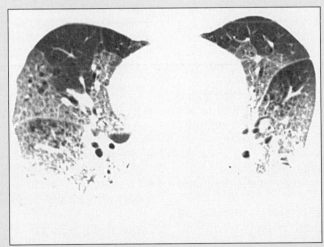

Figure 2. **"Crazy-paving" pattern acute respiratory distress syndrome.** High-resolution CT image shows bilateral ground-glass opacities and areas of consolidation involving mainly the dependent lung regions. Smooth septal lines and intralobular lines are present in the areas of ground-glass opacity ("crazy-paving" pattern). The patient was a 70-year-old man with acute respiratory distress syndrome.

Mosaic Perfusion Pattern

DEFINITION: Areas with decreased attenuation and vascularity with blood flow redistribution to normal lung result in areas of increased attenuation and vascularity called a mosaic perfusion pattern.

IMAGING

CT
Findings
- Areas of decreased attenuation and vascularity with blood flow redistribution to normal lung results in the so-called mosaic perfusion pattern on inspiratory CT.
- Mosaic perfusion pattern is seen most commonly in patients with obliterative bronchiolitis and asthma or chronic thromboembolic pulmonary arterial hypertension.
- High-resolution CT findings of asthma include thickening and narrowing of bronchi, bronchial dilatation, patchy areas of decreased attenuation and vascularity on inspiratory images, and air trapping on expiratory CT.
- Obliterative bronchiolitis (bronchiolitis obliterans) is shown by areas of decreased attenuation and vascularity on inspiratory CT scans and air trapping on expiratory scans; bronchiectasis is commonly present.
- Chronic pulmonary thromboembolic pulmonary arterial hypertension results in a mosaic perfusion pattern and increased diameter of the main, lobar, and segmental pulmonary arteries.
- Contrast-enhanced CT shows eccentric flattened mural thrombi that may be occlusive or have areas of recanalization; chronically occluded vessels are typically smaller than expected.

Utility
- CT is seldom indicated in patients with asthma.
- CT is the imaging modality of choice in the diagnosis of obliterative bronchiolitis.
- Contrast-enhanced CT is the imaging modality of choice in the diagnosis of chronic pulmonary thromboembolism.

CLINICAL PRESENTATION

- Progressive shortness of breath and cough
- Wheezing in asthma
- Pulmonary arterial hypertension in chronic pulmonary embolism

DIAGNOSTIC PEARLS

- Mosaic attenuation pattern may be due to mosaic perfusion or patchy ground-glass opacities
- Mosaic attenuation due to patchy ground-glass typically has similar size vessels in the areas of ground-glass as in the adjacent uninvolved parenchyma
- Pulmonary vessels in areas of apparent ground-glass opacity due to mosaic perfusion are typically larger and more numerous than in the adjacent parenchyma

PATHOLOGY

- Oligemia secondary to decreased vascularity may result from partial airway obstruction (asthma, obliterative bronchiolitis) or obliteration of small peripheral vessels (emphysema) and vascular obstruction (pulmonary thromboembolism).
- Blood flow redistribution to normal lung results in areas of increased attenuation and vascularity.

INCIDENCE/PREVALENCE AND EPIDEMIOLOGY

- Mosaic perfusion pattern is a common manifestation of obliterative bronchiolitis
- Commonly seen in chronic thromboembolic pulmonary arterial hypertension

Suggested Readings

King MA, Ysrael M, Bergin CJ: Chronic thromboembolic pulmonary hypertension: CT findings. *AJR Am J Roentgenol* 170:955-960, 1998.

Oikonomou A, Dennie CJ, Muller NL, et al: Chronic thromboembolic pulmonary arterial hypertension: Correlation of postoperative results of thromboendarterectomy with preoperative helical contrast-enhanced computed tomography. *J Thorac Imaging* 19:67-73, 2004.

Pipavath SJ, Lynch DA, Cool C, et al: Radiologic and pathologic features of bronchiolitis. *AJR Am J Roentgenol* 185:354-363, 2005.

WHAT THE REFERRING PHYSICIAN NEEDS TO KNOW

- Mosaic perfusion pattern is a common manifestation of obliterative bronchiolitis.
- In patients with pulmonary hypertension, presence of mosaic perfusion pattern on CT is highly suggestive of chronic pulmonary thromboembolism.

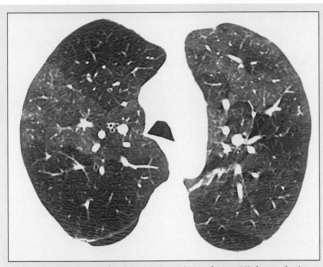

Figure 1. Mosaic perfusion pattern in asthma. High-resolution CT performed at end inspiration shows extensive bilateral areas of decreased attenuation and vascularity with blood flow redistribution to normal lung resulting in a mosaic perfusion pattern. The patient was a 54-year-old woman with severe chronic asthma.

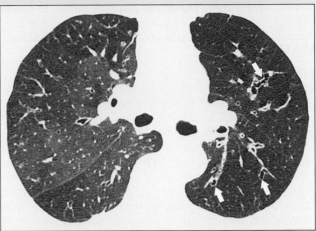

Figure 2. Obliterative bronchiolitis. High-resolution CT images shows decreased attenuation and vascularity in most of the left lung, anterior aspect of the right upper lobe, and superior segment of the right lower lobe. Also noted is bronchiectasis (*arrows*). The findings are characteristic of bronchiolitis obliterans. The uninvolved portions of the right upper lobe have increased vascularity and attenuation due to blood flow redistribution. The patient was a 69-year-old woman with obliterative bronchiolitis associated with rheumatoid arthritis.

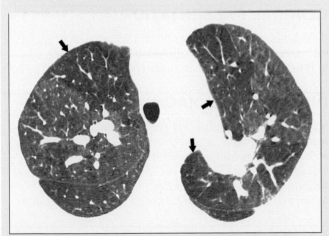

Figure 3. Mosaic perfusion in chronic thromboembolic pulmonary hypertension. High-resolution CT image at the level of the upper lobes shows areas with decreased attenuation and vascularity (*straight arrows*) and areas with increased attenuation and vascularity (mosaic perfusion pattern). Note the marked enlargement of the pulmonary arteries as compared with the normal-sized bronchi. The patient was a 57-year-old woman with chronic thromboembolic pulmonary hypertension.

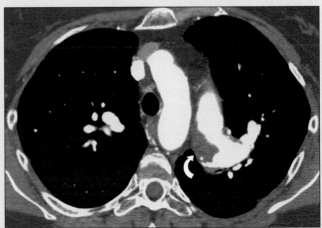

Figure 4. Mosaic perfusion in chronic thromboembolic pulmonary hypertension. CT pulmonary angiogram demonstrates eccentric filling defect in the left pulmonary artery (*curved arrow*) and irregular arterial lumen consistent with chronic pulmonary thromboembolism. The patient was a 57-year-old woman.

Silva CI, Colby TV, Müller NL: Asthma and associated conditions: High-resolution CT and pathologic findings. *AJR Am J Roentgenol* 183:817-824, 2004.

Visscher DW, Myers JL: Bronchiolitis: The pathologist's perspective. *Proc Am Thorac Soc* 3:41-47, 2006.

Worthy SA, Müller NL, Hartman TE, et al: Mosaic attenuation pattern on thin-section CT scans of the lung: Differentiation among infiltrative lung, airway, and vascular diseases as a cause. *Radiology* 205:465-470, 2005.

Air Trapping

DEFINITION: Air trapping refers to obstruction of the egress of air from affected lung parenchyma.

IMAGING

Radiography

Findings

- Inspiratory radiograph is frequently normal or may show increased radiolucency and decreased vascularity; hyperinflation may be seen in severe cases.
- Most common radiographic abnormalities in patients who have asthma are hyperinflation and bronchial wall thickening.
- Obliterative bronchiolitis (bronchiolitis obliterans) may be associated with increased lung volumes and peripheral attenuation of vascular markings.
- Unilateral or lobar air trapping on expiratory radiograph and normal or decreased ipsilateral lung volume on inspiratory radiograph may be seen in Swyer-James-McLeod syndrome and endobronchial tumor.
- Focal hyperlucency on inspiratory radiograph and air trapping on expiratory radiograph are typical findings of congenital lobar emphysema and bronchial atresia.

Utility

- Inspiratory radiograph is frequently normal.
- Expiratory radiograph is required to demonstrate air trapping.

CT

Findings

- Normal subjects: mild air trapping common, typically limited to dependent lung regions and the tip of the middle lobe and lingula area, and involves less than 25% of lung parenchyma.
- Asthma: thickening and narrowing of bronchi, bronchial dilatation, patchy areas of decreased attenuation, and vascularity (mosaic perfusion pattern) on inspiratory images and air trapping on expiratory CT.
- Obliterative bronchiolitis (bronchiolitis obliterans): areas of decreased attenuation and vascularity (mosaic perfusion pattern) on inspiratory CT scans and air trapping on expiratory scans; bronchiectasis commonly present.
- Endobronchial tumor and Swyer-James-McLeod syndrome: decreased attenuation and vascularity of affected lung on inspiration and air trapping on expiration; normal or decreased volume of affected lobe or lung in adults.
- Congenital lobar emphysema: increased volume, decreased attenuation and vascularity of involved lobe

DIAGNOSTIC PEARLS

- Unilateral: endobronchial tumor, foreign body, Swyer-James-McLeod syndrome, bronchial atresia, congenital lobar emphysema
- Bilateral: bronchiolitis obliterans, asthma, normal

(most commonly left upper lobe), and air trapping on expiratory scans.

- Bronchial atresia: increased volume, decreased attenuation and vascularity of involved pulmonary segment, and air trapping on expiratory scans.
- Bronchial atresia: bronchial dilatation immediately distal to atresia, mucoid impaction within ectatic bronchus (bronchocele), and occlusion of bronchus central to bronchocele.

Utility

- Expiratory high-resolution CT is superior to radiography in demonstrating focal and diffuse areas of air trapping.
- CT findings are usually diagnostic in patients with endobronchial tumors, Swyer-James-McLeod syndrome, congenital lobar emphysema, and bronchial atresia.

CLINICAL PRESENTATION

- Patients commonly asymptomatic
- Progressive shortness of breath and cough
- Wheezing in asthma and central endobronchial tumors

DIFFERENTIAL DIAGNOSIS

- Obliterative bronchiolitis (bronchiolitis obliterans)
- Asthma
- Swyer-James-McLeod syndrome
- Endobronchial tumor
- Endobronchial foreign body
- Normal (when mild and limited to certain regions)

PATHOLOGY

- Air trapping results from obstruction of egress of air from affected lung parenchyma.
- Volume of lung behind a partly obstructing endobronchial lesion is almost invariably reduced at total lung capacity.

WHAT THE REFERRING PHYSICIAN NEEDS TO KNOW

- Wheezing may result from asthma or partial central bronchial obstruction by tumor or foreign body.
- Inspiratory and expiratory high-resolution CT is the imaging modality of choice in the diagnosis of air trapping in patients with suspected obliterative bronchiolitis.
- CT is seldom indicated in patients with asthma.
- CT findings are usually diagnostic in patients with endobronchial tumors, Swyer-James-McLeod syndrome, congenital lobar emphysema, and bronchial atresia.

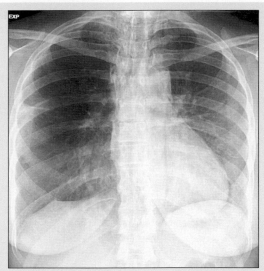

Figure 1. Air trapping due to endobronchial tumor. Expiratory chest radiograph shows air trapping of the right lung with contralateral shift of the mediastinum. The patient was a 31-year-old woman with partial obstruction of the right main-stem bronchus by an endobronchial carcinoid.

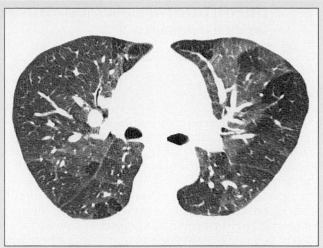

Figure 2. Air trapping in obliterative bronchiolitis. Expiratory high-resolution CT demonstrates extensive bilateral air trapping. The patient was a 54-year-old woman with obliterative bronchiolitis after stem cell transplantation for multiple myeloma.

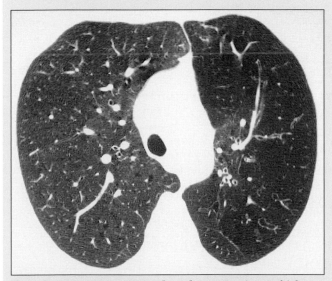

Figure 3. Swyer-James-McLeod syndrome. Inspiratory high-resolution CT image shows decreased attenuation and vascularity of the left lung with associated bronchiectasis and mild volume loss leading to ipsilateral shift of the mediastinum and anterior junction line. The patient was a 61-year-old woman with Swyer-James-McLeod syndrome.

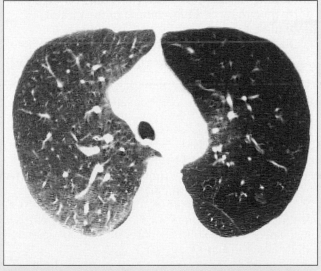

Figure 4. Swyer-James-McLeod syndrome. Expiratory high-resolution CT image shows air trapping in the left lung. The mediastinum and anterior junction line are in the midline. The patient was a 61-year-old woman with Swyer-James-McLeod syndrome.

- Density of affected parenchyma is less than that of opposite lung from decreased perfusion (oligemia) secondary to hypoventilation-mediated hypoxic vasoconstriction.

INCIDENCE/PREVALENCE AND EPIDEMIOLOGY

- Air trapping is a characteristic feature of asthma, obliterative bronchiolitis (bronchiolitis obliterans), partial bronchial obstruction by foreign body or tumor, bronchial atresia, and congenital lobar emphysema.

Suggested Readings

Matsushima H, Takayanagi N, Satoh M, et al: Congenital bronchial atresia: Radiologic findings in nine patients. *J Comput Assist Tomogr* 26:860-864, 2002.

Pipavath SJ, Lynch DA, Cool C, et al: Radiologic and pathologic features of bronchiolitis. *AJR Am J Roentgenol* 185:354-363, 2005.

Silva CI, Colby TV, Müller NL: Asthma and associated conditions: High-resolution CT and pathologic findings. *AJR Am J Roentgenol* 183:817-824, 2004.

Visscher DW, Myers JL: Bronchiolitis: The pathologist's perspective. *Proc Am Thorac Soc* 3:41-47, 2006.

Unilateral Hyperlucent Lung

DEFINITION: A hyperlucent lung is a lung that has increased lucency compared to the other lung on the chest radiograph or CT.

IMAGING

Radiography
Findings
- Swyer-James-McLeod syndrome: hyperlucent lung or lobe, decreased vascularity, normal or reduced volume during inspiration, and air trapping during expiration.
- Partial bronchial obstruction (endobronchial tumor, bronchial stenosis).
- Nonpulmonary causes of hyperlucent "lung" on chest radiograph: faulty technique (patient rotation), chest wall abnormalities (mastectomy, congenital absence of the pectoralis muscle (Poland syndrome), and pneumothorax.

Utility
- Diagnosis of Swyer-James-McLeod syndrome often first suspected on chest radiograph in asymptomatic patient

CT
Findings
- Swyer-James-McLeod syndrome: decreased attenuation and vascularity of affected lung on inspiration, normal or reduced lung volume on inspiratory CT, air trapping on expiration, bronchiectasis.
- Partial bronchial obstruction (endobronchial tumor, bronchial stenosis).
- Asymmetric emphysema.
- Extensive unilateral or asymmetric pulmonary embolism.
- Lobar collapse with compensatory overinflation of remaining lung.
- Previous lobectomy or bilobectomy.
- Unilateral lung transplant for emphysema.

Utility
- CT is superior to radiography in diagnosis of unilateral hyperlucent lung and underlying cause.
- Inspiratory and expiratory high-resolution CT is the best imaging technique for assessment of patients with suspected bronchiolitis obliterans or Swyer-James-McLeod syndrome.

CLINICAL PRESENTATION

- Patients are often asymptomatic.
- Cough, dyspnea

DIAGNOSTIC PEARLS

- Air trapping on expiratory radiograph or CT: Swyer-James-McLeod syndrome, partial bronchial obstruction
- No air trapping: proximal interruption or narrowing of the pulmonary artery
- Nonpulmonary causes: mastectomy, absence of pectoralis muscles (Poland syndrome), patient rotation
- Typically left upper lobe: congenital lobar emphysema, bronchial atresia

DIFFERENTIAL DIAGNOSIS

- Swyer-James-McLeod syndrome
- Endobronchial tumor
- Foreign body
- Atelectasis
- Pneumothorax
- Mastectomy
- Poland syndrome
- Patient rotation

PATHOLOGY

- Swyer-James-McLeod syndrome: decreased lung density results from reduction in quantity of blood due to bronchiolitis obliterans in absence of pulmonary overinflation; it most commonly results as a sequela of childhood respiratory infections, most often viral.
- Other causes of unilateral hyperlucent lung include partial endobronchial obstruction, asymmetric emphysema, and unilateral or asymmetric pulmonary embolism.

INCIDENCE/PREVALENCE AND EPIDEMIOLOGY

- Common cause of hyperlucent lung is partial endobronchial obstruction by tumor or foreign body.
- Swyer-James-McLeod or unilateral hyperlucent lung syndrome is an uncommon condition that typically is a sequela of childhood viral or *Mycoplasma* infection.

WHAT THE REFERRING PHYSICIAN NEEDS TO KNOW

- Unilateral hyperlucency on the radiograph may also result from pneumothorax and congenital and acquired abnormalities of the chest wall.
- Chest wall abnormalities, in particular mastectomy, are the most common cause of unilateral hyperlucent "lung" on radiography.
- Common cause of hyperlucent lung is partial endobronchial obstruction by tumor or foreign body.
- CT is superior to radiography in diagnosis of unilateral hyperlucent lung and the underlying cause.

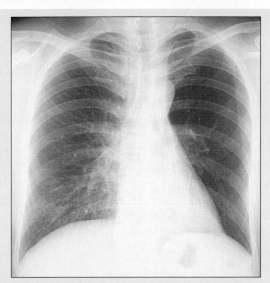

Figure 1. Swyer-James-McLeod syndrome. Chest radiograph shows hyperlucency and decreased vascularity of the left lung. The mediastinum is shifted to the left consistent with decreased left lung volume. The patient was a 40-year-old man.

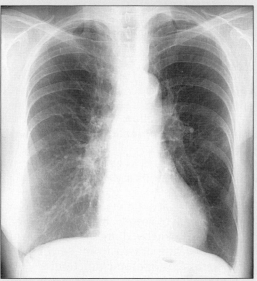

Figure 2. Unilateral hyperlucency secondary to left mastectomy. Posteroanterior chest radiograph shows increased lucency of the left hemithorax. The patient was a 74-year-old woman.

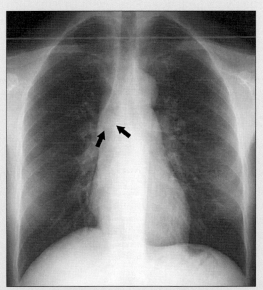

Figure 3. Unilateral hyperlucent lung due to central carcinoid tumor. Posteroanterior chest radiograph demonstrates a tumor in the right main bronchus (*arrows*). The right lung is slightly smaller than the left and shows decreased vascularity. The patient was a 48-year-old woman with a diagnosis of typical carcinoid tumor made at bronchoscopy and confirmed at surgery.

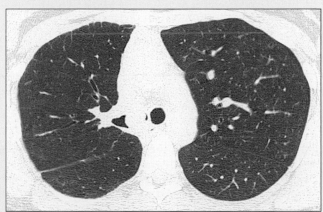

Figure 4. Unilateral hyperlucent lung. Inspiratory high-resolution CT image shows endoluminal tumor in right main bronchus. Note decreased size of right lung and diffuse decrease in attenuation and vascularity as compared with the left lung. The patient was a 31-year-old woman with a typical carcinoid tumor. She presented with recurrent episodes of shortness of breath and tightness in the chest and had a clinical diagnosis of asthma.

Suggested Readings

Jeung MY, Gasser B, Gangi A, et al: Bronchial carcinoid tumors of the thorax: Spectrum of radiologic findings. *RadioGraphics* 22:351-365, 2002.

Lucaya J, Gartner S, Garcia-Pena P, et al: Spectrum of manifestations of Swyer-James-MacLeod syndrome. *J Comput Assist Tomogr* 22:592-597, 1998.

Moore ADA, Godwin JD, Dietrich PA, et al: Swyer-James syndrome: CT findings in eight patients. *AJR Am J Roentgenol* 158:1211-1215, 1992.

Bilateral Hyperlucent Lungs

DEFINITION: Increased lucency of both lungs results from generalized excess air or alteration in pulmonary vasculature.

IMAGING

Radiography
Findings
- Emphysema: overinflation with diaphragm depressed often to level of 7th rib anteriorly, 11th interspace, or 12th rib posteriorly.
- Distance >2.5 cm between posterior sternum and most anterior margin of ascending aorta indicative of overinflation.
- Emphysema: irregular areas of radiolucency, local avascular areas, distortion of vessels, bullae, and hyperinflation.
- Overinflation shown by dome of diaphragm located <2.6 cm above line drawn from sternophrenic junction to posterior costophrenic junction.
- Asthma: bronchial wall thickening and hyperinflation.
- Bronchiolitis obliterans: hyperinflation and decrease in peripheral vascular markings.

Utility
- Chest radiograph is often normal in patients with mild to moderate emphysema.
- In majority of cases, obliterative bronchiolitis results in no definite abnormality on chest radiograph.

CT
Findings
- Emphysema: presence of areas of abnormally low attenuation without visible walls or, occasionally, walls ≤1 mm are seen.
- Thin walls may be seen particularly in patients with paraseptal emphysema and bulla formation.
- On high-resolution CT, vessels can often be seen within areas of low attenuation.
- In bronchiolitis obliterans there is decreased attenuation and vascularity on inspiration and air trapping on expiration.
- Redistribution of blood flow to uninvolved lung results in a heterogeneous pattern of attenuation and vascularity (mosaic attenuation/perfusion).

Utility
- Parenchymal abnormalities are usually readily seen on CT, particularly high-resolution CT.

CLINICAL PRESENTATION
- Dyspnea, cough

DIAGNOSTIC PEARLS
- Emphysema: flattening of the diaphragm and increased retrosternal space on the radiograph
- Emphysema: areas of abnormally low attenuation on CT
- Bronchiolitis obliterans: air trapping on expiratory CT

DIFFERENTIAL DIAGNOSIS
- Emphysema
- Bronchiolitis obliterans
- Asthma
- Lymphangioleiomyomatosis

PATHOLOGY
- Decreased lung density may result from obstructive overinflation with lung destruction (emphysema) or without lung destruction (asthma, bronchiolitis obliterans).
- Altered pulmonary vasculature in primary pulmonary hypertension results in oligemia.

INCIDENCE/PREVALENCE AND EPIDEMIOLOGY
- Most common cause of generalized overinflation of both lungs is emphysema.
- Less common causes include asthma, bronchiolitis obliterans, Langerhans cell pulmonary histiocytosis, and lymphangioleiomyomatosis.
- Hyperinflation in asthma is more common in children than in adults.

Suggested Readings
Bankier AA, Van Muylem A, Knoop C, et al: Bronchiolitis obliterans syndrome in heart-lung transplant recipients: Diagnosis with expiratory CT. *Radiology* 218:533-539, 2001.
Bankier AA, Madani A, Gevenois PA: CT quantification of pulmonary emphysema: Assessment of lung structure and function. *Crit Rev Comput Tomogr* 43:399-417, 2002.

WHAT THE REFERRING PHYSICIAN NEEDS TO KNOW
- Mild to moderate emphysema is often missed on the chest radiograph.
- High-resolution CT is superior to radiography in the detection and quantification of emphysema.
- Inspiratory and expiratory high-resolution CT is the best imaging technique for assessment of bronchiolitis obliterans.

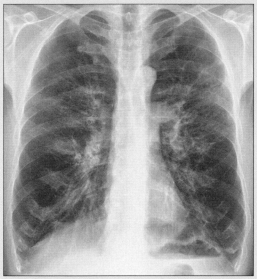

Figure 1. Hyperinflation due to panacinar emphysema.
Posteroanterior chest radiograph shows that the dome of the right
hemidiaphragm is below the level of the anterior right 7th rib,
consistent with increased lung volumes. Also noted is a decrease
in the peripheral vascular markings. The patient was a 52-year-
old man with severe panacinar emphysema due to α1-antitrypsin
deficiency.

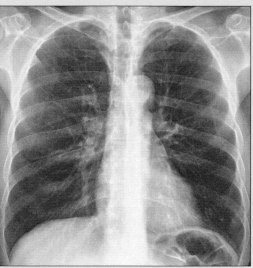

Figure 2. Centrilobular and paraseptal emphysema.
Posteroanterior chest radiograph shows increased lung volumes,
slight distortion of the upper lobe vessels, and focal areas of
lucency in the upper lobes. The patient was a 53-year-old
smoker.

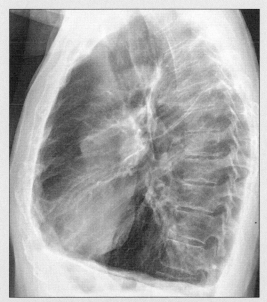

Figure 3. Hyperinflation due to panacinar emphysema. Lateral
view shows increased retrosternal airspace (> 2.5 cm distance
between the posterior sternum and the most anterior margin of
the ascending aorta) and flattening of the diaphragm. The patient
was a 52-year-old man with severe panacinar emphysema due to
α1-antitrypsin deficiency.

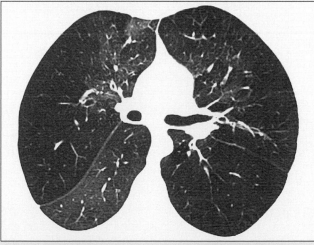

Figure 4. Postinfectious obliterative bronchiolitis. High-
resolution CT image at the level of left main bronchus
shows extensive bilateral areas of decreased attenuation and
vascularity with blood flow redistribution (mosaic perfusion
pattern). The patient was a 24-year-old woman with obliterative
bronchiolitis following severe viral infection when the patient
was 9 months old.

Hoffman EA, Simon BA, McLennan G: State of the art: A structural
    and functional assessment of the lung via multidetector-row
    computed tomography: Phenotyping chronic obstructive pulmo-
    nary disease. *Proc Am Thorac Soc* 3:519-532, 2006.
Kilburn KH, Warshaw RH, Thornton JC: Do radiographic criteria for
    emphysema predict physiologic impairment? *Chest* 107:1225-1231,
    1995.

Pratt PC: Role of conventional chest radiography in diagnosis and
    exclusion of emphysema. *Am J Med* 82:998-1006, 1987.
Silva CI, Colby TV, Muller NL: Asthma and associated conditions:
    High-resolution CT and pathologic findings. *AJR Am J Roentgenol*
    183:817-824, 2004.
Thurlbeck WM, Müller NL: Emphysema: Definition, imaging, and
    quantification. *AJR Am J Roentgenol* 163:1017-1025, 1994.

Developmental Lung Disease

Part 6

AIRWAY AND PARENCHYMAL ANOMALIES

Bronchial Atresia

DEFINITION: Bronchial atresia is a rare congenital anomaly characterized by short-segment obliteration of a lobar, segmental, or subsegmental bronchus at or near its origin.

IMAGING

Radiography
Findings
- Area of pulmonary hyperlucency (90% of cases)
- Hilar nodule or mass (80%)
- Adjacent normal lung compressed and displaced
- Mediastinal displacement: may or may not be evident
- Decreased vascularity of affected segment
- Ovoid, round, or branching opacities near hilum due to accumulation of secretions and mucoid impaction distal to bronchial atresia
- Air trapping evident on expiratory chest radiographs

Utility
- Radiographic findings usually characteristic

CT
Findings
- Mucoid impaction seen as presence of branching soft tissue densities in bronchial distribution, usually associated with bronchial dilatation.
- Bronchial occlusion and mucoid impaction with bronchial dilatation (bronchocele) immediately distal to atretic bronchus.
- Decreased vascularity and attenuation and increased volume of affected segment.

Utility
- Most sensitive imaging technique for confirming diagnosis
- Imaging modality of choice
- Disorder best appreciated on multiplanar and volumetric reconstructions
- Excellent visualization of mucoid impaction and segmental overinflation and hypovascularity

MRI
Findings
- Mucoid impaction shown as variable signal intensity on T1-weighted images and typically very high signal intensity on T2-weighted images.

DIAGNOSTIC PEARLS
- Mucoid impaction, segmental hyperlucency, and decreased vascularity
- Air trapping of affected segment and presence of hilar nodule or mass
- Most commonly apico-posterior segment of left upper lobe but may affect any pulmonary segment

Utility
- Of limited value in diagnosis

CLINICAL PRESENTATION
- Majority of cases are asymptomatic.
- Some patients present with recurrent pneumonia.

DIFFERENTIAL DIAGNOSIS
- Aspiration of foreign body
- Endobronchial tumor

PATHOLOGY
- Short-segment obliteration of lobar, segmental, or subsegmental bronchus occurs at or near its origin.
- Pathogenesis of airway interruption is unknown; airway and airspaces distal to obstruction develop normally.
- Patent bronchial tree peripheral to point of obliteration results in accumulation of mucus and mucocele distal to atresia.
- Alveoli supplied by atretic bronchus are ventilated by collateral pathways, showing air trapping and resulting in hyperinflation.
- Hyperlucency results from combination of oligemia and increase in the volume of air within the affected parenchyma.

WHAT THE REFERRING PHYSICIAN NEEDS TO KNOW
- Seldom associated with significant complications and thus rarely requires surgical resection of affected segment or lobe.
- CT findings are usually diagnostic.

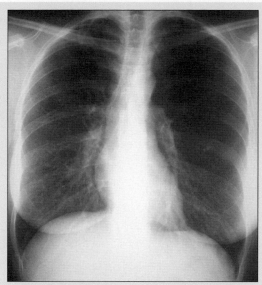

Figure 1. Bronchial atresia. Chest radiograph shows increased lucency in the left middle and upper lung zones. (*Courtesy of Dr. Jim Barrie, University of Alberta Medical Center, Edmonton, Canada.*)

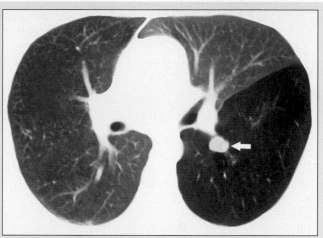

Figure 2. Bronchial atresia. CT scan demonstrates marked decrease in attenuation and vascularity of the superior segment of the left lower lobe. Also noted is anterior displacement of the left major fissure due to hyperinflation of the superior segment. An oval opacity is present posterior to the left hilum (*arrow*). This represents a bronchocele distal to the atretic superior segmental bronchus of the left lower lobe. (*Courtesy of Dr. Jim Barrie, University of Alberta Medical Center, Edmonton, Canada.*)

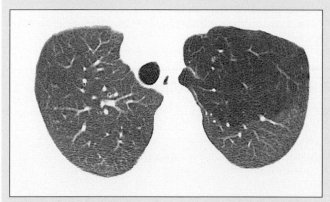

Figure 3. Bronchial atresia. High-resolution CT image at the level of the thoracic inlet demonstrates decrease in attenuation and vascularity of the anterior segment of the left upper lobe. The patient was a 19-year-old woman.

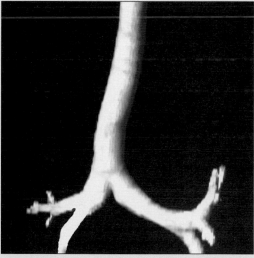

Figure 4. Bronchial atresia. 3D external volume rendering image of central airways viewed from an anterior perspective shows atresia of right upper lobe bronchus. Also noted is abnormal branching pattern of the right middle lobe bronchus.

INCIDENCE/PREVALENCE AND EPIDEMIOLOGY

- Rare congenital anomaly
- More common in men
- Estimated prevalence: approximately 1 case per 100,000 population

Suggested Readings

Berrocal T, Madrid C, Novo S, et al: Congenital anomalies of the tracheobronchial tree, lung, and mediastinum: Embryology, radiology, and pathology. *RadioGraphics* 24:17, 2004.

Ghaye B, Szapiro D, Fanchamps JM, Dondelinger RF: Congenital bronchial abnormalities revisited. *RadioGraphics* 21:105-119, 2001.

Jederlinic PJ, Sicilian LS, Baigelman W, Gaensler EA: Congenital bronchial atresia: A report of 4 cases and a review of the literature. *Medicine (Baltimore)* 66:73-83, 1987.

Kinsella D, Sissons G, Williams MP: The radiological imaging of bronchial atresia. *Br J Radiol* 65:681-685, 1992.

Bronchogenic Cyst

DEFINITION: Bronchogenic cysts are congenital cysts lined with bronchial epithelium that arise from abnormal separation of localized portions of the tracheobronchial tree from the adjacent airways.

IMAGING

Radiography
Findings
- Mediastinal cysts: round, oval masses usually in right paratracheal or subcarinal region.
- Pulmonary cysts: sharply circumscribed, solitary, round or oval mass usually involving the medial third of lower lobe.
- Air-containing cysts, with or without fluid when communication is established.

Utility
- Serial radiographs: show little change in size and shape with time.
- Chest radiograph: initial imaging modality but does not allow confident diagnosis.

CT
Findings
- Homogeneous cystic mass with thin smooth wall.
- Mediastinal cysts tend to mold to adjacent airway or vessel.
- Pulmonary cysts displace adjacent parenchyma.
- Homogeneous attenuation is at or near water density (-10 to $+10$ Hounsfield units in 50% of cases).
- Cysts are indistinguishable from soft tissue lesions in the other 50% of cases.
- Infected cysts have inhomogeneous enhancement and resemble abscess.
- Lung adjacent to cyst is frequently abnormal and shows areas of decreased attenuation and scarring.

Utility
- Confident diagnosis can be made in approximately 50% of cases; remaining cysts have soft tissue attenuation due to protein content.

MRI
Findings
- Cyst filled predominantly with water or serous fluid: low signal intensity on T1-weighted images.
- Cyst with high protein content: high signal intensity.
- Homogeneous high-signal intensity on T2-weighted spin-echo images.
- Infected or hemorrhagic cyst: inhomogeneous and variable intensity on both T1- and T2-weighted images.

DIAGNOSTIC PEARLS
- Water density on CT in approximately 50%
- Homogeneous high signal intensity on T2-weighted images
- Lack of enhancement after intravenous administration of contrast material on CT and MRI

Utility
- Superior to CT in evaluation for suspected bronchogenic cysts; allows confident diagnosis in virtually 100% of cases.
- Lack of radiation exposure and higher specificity.

CLINICAL PRESENTATION
- No symptoms evident in majority of cases
- Cough, wheezing, stridor, and pneumonia due to compression of trachea or bronchi
- Dysphagia due to compression of esophagus
- Localized pulmonary edema due to compression of adjacent pulmonary vein
- Infection in approximately 20% of patients with intraparenchymal cysts
- Hemoptysis and pneumothorax less common

DIFFERENTIAL DIAGNOSIS
- Congenital cystic adenomatoid malformation (congenital pulmonary airway malformation)
- Hydatid cyst
- Benign or malignant neoplasm
- Granuloma

PATHOLOGY
- Abnormal separation of localized portions of tracheobronchial tree from adjacent airways occurs between 3rd and 24th weeks of gestation.
- Bronchogenic cysts are thin-walled, unilocular, spherical, and either mucoid or serous filled.
- Cyst wall is lined by respiratory epithelium and contains smooth muscle and commonly cartilage.
- Established communication with tracheobronchial tree is due to infection or instrumentation.

WHAT THE REFERRING PHYSICIAN NEEDS TO KNOW
- CT allows confident diagnosis in 50% of cases.
- MRI allows confident diagnosis in virtually 100% of cases.
- CT-guided needle aspiration of cyst contents is confirmatory after inconclusive CT and MR diagnosis of cystic content.

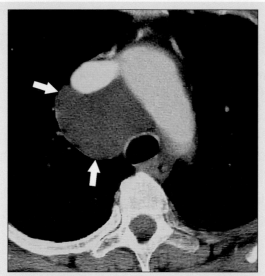

Figure 1. Bronchogenic cyst. Magnified view from contrast-enhanced CT scan shows a paratracheal mass (*arrows*) with homogeneous water density. The attenuation value of the mass was 9 Hounsfield units. The patient was a 58-year-old woman with a bronchogenic cyst.

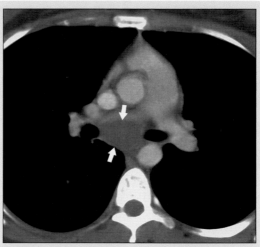

Figure 2. Mediastinal bronchogenic cyst. Contrast medium-enhanced CT demonstrates a cystic mass in the subcarinal region (*arrows*). The patient was a 32-year-old woman with a bronchogenic cyst.

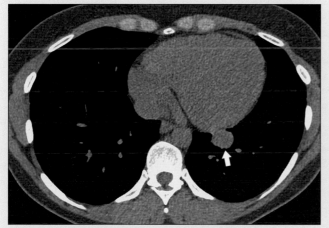
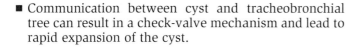

Figure 3. Pulmonary bronchogenic cyst. CT image photographed at mediastinal window setting shows that the nodule has soft tissue attenuation (*arrow*). The patient was a 41-year-old woman with a presumptive diagnosis of pulmonary bronchogenic cyst.

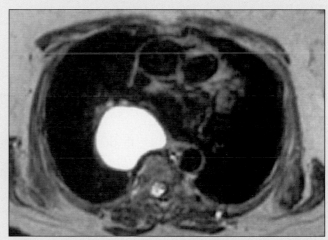

Figure 4. Bronchogenic cyst. T2-weighted MR image demonstrates homogeneous high signal intensity similar to that of cerebrospinal fluid. The findings are characteristic of a bronchogenic cyst. The patient was a 72-year-old woman.

■ Communication between cyst and tracheobronchial tree can result in a check-valve mechanism and lead to rapid expansion of the cyst.

INCIDENCE/PREVALENCE AND EPIDEMIOLOGY

■ Bronchogenic cysts are uncommon and usually isolated.
■ Approximately 75% of cysts are located in the mediastinum and 25% in the lung.
■ Infection occurs in approximately 20% of patients with intraparenchymal cysts.

Suggested Readings

Berrocal T, Madrid C, Novo S, et al: Congenital anomalies of the tracheobronchial tree, lung, and mediastinum: Embryology, radiology, and pathology. *RadioGraphics* 24:e17, 2004.

Mendelson DS, Rose JS, Efremidis SC, et al: Bronchogenic cysts with high CT numbers. *AJR Am J Roentgenol* 140:463-465, 1983.

Naidich DP, Rumancik WM, Ettenger NA, et al: Congenital anomalies of the lungs in adults: MR diagnosis. *AJR Am J Roentgenol* 151:13-19, 1988.

Nakata H, Egashira K, Watanabe H, et al: MRI of bronchogenic cysts. *J Comput Assist Tomogr* 17:267-270, 1993.

Suen HC, Mathisen DJ, Grillo HC, et al: Surgical management and radiological characteristics of bronchogenic cysts. *Ann Thorac Surg* 55:476-481, 1993.

Yoon YC, Lee KS, Kim TS, et al: Intrapulmonary bronchogenic cyst: CT and pathologic findings in five adult patients. *AJR Am J Roentgenol* 179:167-170, 2002.

Congenital Cystic Adenomatoid Malformation (Congenital Pulmonary Airway Malformation)

DEFINITION: Congenital cystic adenomatoid malformation is an abnormality characterized by a multicystic mass of pulmonary tissue with an abnormal proliferation of bronchial structures.

IMAGING

Radiography
Findings
- Unilocular or multiloculated cyst
- Complex soft tissue and cystic mass ranging from 4-12 cm in diameter
- Occasional preferential expansion of one cyst, creating a single lucent area
- Space-occupying lesion

Utility
- Pneumonia in surrounding parenchyma results in obscuration of malformation or development of fluid levels.
- Radiographic findings are suggestive of the diagnosis.

CT
Findings
- Unilocular or multiloculated cyst
- Complex soft tissue and cystic mass ranging from 4-12 cm in diameter
- Type I: at least one cyst >2 cm in diameter
- Type II: multiple thin-walled cysts ranging from 2-20 mm in diameter

Utility
- Superior to chest radiography in demonstrating both cystic and solid components.
- Performed almost routinely in adults with cystic lung lesions.

CLINICAL PRESENTATION

- Increasing respiratory distress in neonatal period
- In adults, incidental finding or accompanied by symptoms of recurrent respiratory infections (cough and fever)
- Pneumothorax (occasionally)

DIFFERENTIAL DIAGNOSIS

- Bronchogenic cyst
- Lung abscess

DIAGNOSTIC PEARLS

- Radiographs usually show cystic mass most commonly in lower lobes.
- CT finding in adults typically consists of multiple thin-walled, complex cystic masses ranging from 4-12 cm in diameter.

- Lung tumor
- Lobar sequestration

PATHOLOGY

- Heterogeneous, complex congenital malformation, typically cystic, containing smooth muscle but generally no cartilage
- Type I: large, often multiloculated cysts of >2 cm in diameter
- Type II: uniform small cysts of <2 cm in diameter
- Type III: solid-appearing lesions that microscopically demonstrate tiny cysts
- Cyst wall: contains smooth muscle, no cartilage, and a lining of bronchiolar-type epithelium; may contain fluid and/or air
- Results from localized arrest in development of fetal bronchial tree or a hamartomatous lesion of the bronchial tree

INCIDENCE/PREVALENCE AND EPIDEMIOLOGY

- Majority of these malformations are diagnosed in the first 5 years of life.
- They have been detected in adults up to 64 years of age.
- Incidence is estimated at 1:25,000 to 1:35,000 pregnancies.
- Majority seen in adults are type I (cystic form).
- Any lobe may be involved but more commonly the lower lobes are affected.

WHAT THE REFERRING PHYSICIAN NEEDS TO KNOW

- Surgical removal is necessary because the majority of cases are associated with recurrent infection and slightly increased risk for development of carcinoma.
- Lobectomy is required.
- Vast majority of these lesions are diagnosed in early childhood, and only occasionally are they seen in adults.

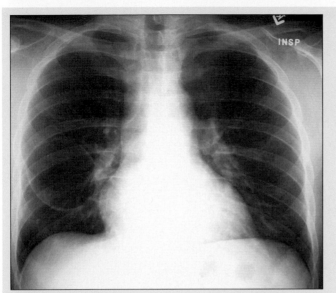

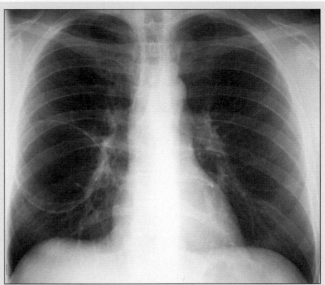

Figure 1. **Congenital cystic adenomatoid malformation.** Posteroanterior chest radiograph shows large cystic lesion in the right lower lobe. The patient was a 31-year-old man with type I cystic adenomatoid malformation.

Figure 2. **Congenital cystic adenomatoid malformation.** Chest radiograph 3 years later (see Fig. 1) demonstrates increase in the size of the cystic lesion. The patient was a 31-year-old man with type I cystic adenomatoid malformation.

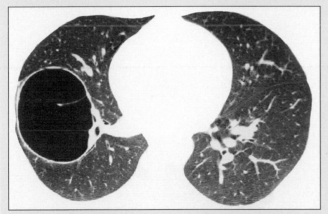

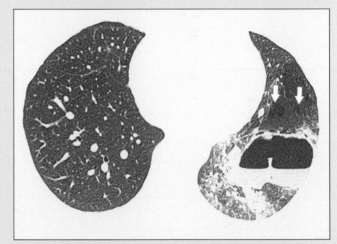

Figure 3. **Congenital cystic adenomatoid malformation.** CT image shows thin-walled cyst with septation. The patient was a 31-year-old man with type I cystic adenomatoid malformation.

Figure 4. **Congenital cystic adenomatoid malformation.** CT demonstrates a cystic mass with internal septation and a fluid level in the left lower lobe, as well as adjacent focal emphysematous changes (*arrows*). Consolidation is present in the left lower lobe secondary to pneumonia. The patient was a 33-year-old woman with infected congenital cystic adenomatoid malformation.

Suggested Readings

Ioachimescu OC, Mehta AC: From cystic pulmonary airway malformation, to bronchioloalveolar carcinoma and adenocarcinoma of the lung. *Eur Respir J* 26:1181-1187, 2005.

Oh BJ, Lee JS, Kim JS, et al: Congenital cystic adenomatoid malformation of the lung in adults: Clinical and CT evaluation of seven patients. *Respirology* 11:496-501, 2006.

Patz EF Jr, Müller NL, Swensen SJ, Dodd LG: Congenital cystic adenomatoid malformation in adults: CT findings. *J Comput Assist Tomogr* 19:361-364, 1995.

Pulmonary Sequestration

DEFINITION: Pulmonary sequestration refers to when a portion of lung is detached from the remaining normal lung.

IMAGING

Radiography
Findings
- Intralobar homogeneous opacity in posterior basal segment of lower lobe that is almost invariably contiguous with hemidiaphragm.
- Focal area of lucency, cystic mass (single or multiple, of variable sizes), prominent vessels in the lower lobe.
- Infection: air-containing cystic mass, with or without fluid levels.
- Extralobar sequestration: sharply defined, triangular opacity in posterior costophrenic angle, adjacent to left hemidiaphragm.
- Small bump on the left hemidiaphragm.

Utility
- Often first modality used in assessment of patients.
- Of limited value in diagnosis.

CT
Findings
- Intralobar sequestration: focal consolidation or areas of lucency or irregular cystic spaces with/without fluid.
- Less common: cysts and nodules, multiple dilated vessels, soft tissue mass, mucoid impaction, foci of calcification.
- Extralobar sequestration: homogeneous opacity or well-circumscribed mass.
- Focal areas of emphysema and air trapping.
- CT angiography allows accurate assessment of the systemic arterial supply in majority of cases.

Utility
- Contrast-enhanced CT using multidetector scanner, thin sections, and multiplanar reformatted images is imaging modality of choice for diagnosis.
- The sequestration, anomalous vessels, and abnormalities in the adjacent parenchyma can be seen.

MRI
Findings
- Soft tissue signal intensity.
- MR angiography helpful in showing abnormal vessel(s) supplying the intralobar sequestration.

DIAGNOSTIC PEARLS
- Homogeneous opacity, hyperlucent area, or cystic masses.
- Typically adjacent to diaphragm, most commonly on left side.
- Arterial supply from aorta or one of its branches.

Utility
- Comparable to CT in demonstrating systemic arterial supply.
- Inferior to CT in demonstrating parenchymal findings.

Interventional Radiology
Findings
- Aortography demonstrates abnormal vessel(s) supplying the intralobar sequestration.

Utility
- Aortography and selective catheterization of feeding vessels may be required to demonstrate venous drainage.

CLINICAL PRESENTATION
- Often asymptomatic
- Signs and symptoms, when present, usually those of acute or recurrent lower lobe pneumonia
- Intralobar sequestration: suspected in young adults with nonresolving or recurrent lower lobe pneumonia

DIFFERENTIAL DIAGNOSIS
- Recurrent pneumonia
- Bronchial obstruction
- Congenital cystic adenomatoid malformation (congenital pulmonary airway malformation)
- Bronchogenic cyst
- Atelectasis
- Aspiration of foreign body

WHAT THE REFERRING PHYSICIAN NEEDS TO KNOW
- Confident diagnosis can be made by demonstrating systemic arterial supply on contrast-enhanced CT or MRI.
- Surgical resection is treatment of choice for patients with infection or symptoms resulting from compression of normal lung tissue.
- Lobectomy is procedure of choice.

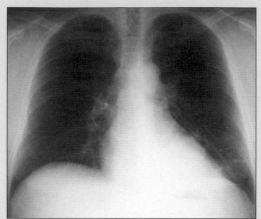

Figure 1. Intralobar pulmonary sequestration. Radiographic manifestations. Posteroanterior chest radiograph demonstrates an area of homogeneous increased opacity in the posterior basal region of the lower lobe. Note that the opacity abuts the diaphragm. The patient was a 33-year-old man with a history of recurrent pneumonia.

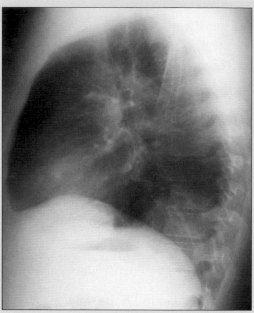

Figure 2. Intralobar pulmonary sequestration. Radiographic manifestations. Lateral chest radiograph demonstrates an area of homogeneous increased opacity in the posterior basal region of the lower lobe. Note that the opacity abuts the diaphragm. The patient was a 33-year-old man with a history of recurrent pneumonia.

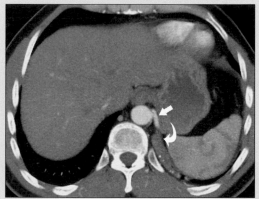

Figure 3. Intralobar pulmonary sequestration. Contrast medium—enhanced CT performed on a multidetector CT scanner demonstrates an anomalous vessel (*straight arrow*) originating from the aorta and coursing toward an area of consolidation (*curved arrow*) in the left lung base. The patient was a 44-year-old man with intralobar pulmonary sequestration.

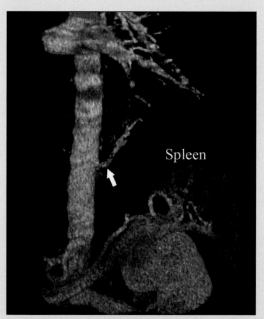

Figure 4. Intralobar pulmonary sequestration. A volume-rendered image better demonstrates the course of the anomalous vessel (*arrow*) originating from the upper abdominal aorta and extending into the sequestered lung. The patient was a 44-year-old man with intralobar pulmonary sequestration.

PATHOLOGY

- Intralobar sequestration: located within normal lung but generally demarcated from surrounding parenchyma; does not communicate with the normal bronchi.
- Intralobar sequestration: consists of one or more cystic spaces with a variable amount of intervening, more solid, tissue.
- Extralobar sequestration: completely enclosed in a pleural membrane; related to the left hemidiaphragm.
- Extralobar sequestration: contains immature lung tissue and few airways.
- Arterial supply: from aorta or one of its branches.
- Venous drainage: pulmonary venous system in intralobar sequestration; systemic veins in extralobar sequestration.

INCIDENCE/PREVALENCE AND EPIDEMIOLOGY

- Pulmonary sequestration is rare.
- Majority of intralobular sequestrations are acquired secondary to chronic bronchial obstruction and chronic infections.
- Extralobular sequestrations are always congenital and frequently associated with congenital abnormalities; they are usually diagnosed in the neonatal period.
- Pulmonary sequestration accounts for 0.15%-6% of pulmonary malformations.
- Intralobular sequestrations account for about 80% of cases; they are usually first recognized in adolescents and young adults and seldom associated with other congenital anomalies.

Suggested Readings

Ahmed M, Jacobi V, Vogl TJ: Multislice CT and CT angiography for non-invasive evaluation of bronchopulmonary sequestration. *Eur Radiol* 14:2141-2143, 2004.

Berrocal T, Madrid C, Novo S, et al: Congenital anomalies of the tracheobronchial tree, lung, and mediastinum: Embryology, radiology, and pathology. *RadioGraphics* 24:e17, 2004.

Frazier AA, Rosado-de-Christenson ML, Stocker JT, Templeton PA: Intralobar sequestration: Radiologic-pathologic correlation. *RadioGraphics* 17:725-745, 1997.

Lehnhardt S, Winterer JT, Uhrmeister P, et al: Pulmonary sequestration: Demonstration of blood supply with 2D and 3D MR angiography. *Eur J Radiol* 44:28-32, 2002.

Rosado de Christenson ML, Frazier AA, Stocker JT, Templeton PA: From the Archives of the AFIP: Extralobar sequestration: Radiologic-pathologic correlation. *RadioGraphics* 13:425-441, 1993.

Zylak CJ, Eyler WR, Spizarny DL, Stone CH: Developmental lung anomalies in the adult: Radiologic-pathologic correlation. *RadioGraphics* 22:S25-S43, 2002.

Part 7

CONGENITAL MALFORMATIONS OF THE PULMONARY VESSELS IN THE ADULT

Isolated Systemic Arterial Supply of the Lung

DEFINITION: Isolated systemic arterial supply of the lung refers to systemic arterial supply to normal lung.

IMAGING

Radiography
Findings
- Parenchymal opacification secondary to bleeding.
- Abnormal vascular opacity in paravertebral regions of lung bases.

Utility
- Chest radiographs frequently normal except with very large or aneurysmal anomalous artery.
- Abnormal vascular opacity detected more easily by postprocessing of digital images.

CT
Findings
- Parenchyma and pleura are normal
- There is moderate dilatation of bronchi to posterior basal segments not accompanied by homonymous pulmonary arteries.
- Systemic artery is abnormal.
- Parenchyma supplied by systemic artery may exhibit ground-glass opacification.

Utility
- Optimally analyzes bronchi and pulmonary and systemic vessels supplying affected lobe.
- More anatomically precise.
- Performed with electrocardiographic gating to evaluate morphologic and functional effects on the heart.

MRI
Findings
- Parenchyma and pleura are normal.
- Moderate dilatation of bronchi to posterior basal segments is not accompanied by homonymous pulmonary arteries.
- Systemic artery is abnormal.
- Parenchyma supplied by systemic artery may exhibit increased signal intensity.

DIAGNOSTIC PEARLS
- Posterobasal tubular shadow on radiograph.
- Abnormal systemic arterial supply to the lung arising from thoracic or abdominal aorta.
- Normal lung parenchyma, bronchi, and pleura.

Utility
- Less precise
- Main advantage: no radiation exposure

CLINICAL PRESENTATION
- Often asymptomatic
- Hemoptysis with no previous history of respiratory disease

DIFFERENTIAL DIAGNOSIS
- Pulmonary sequestration
- Systemic arterial supply in bronchiectasis

PATHOLOGY
- Abnormal systemic artery from aorta often follows sigmoid course toward left side and divides into branches in lower basal segments.
- Moderate dilatation of bronchi to posterior basal segments is not accompanied by homonymous pulmonary arteries.
- Increased vascular perfusion in conjunction with pulmonary artery perfusion results in morphologic and functional effects on the heart.

WHAT THE REFERRING PHYSICIAN NEEDS TO KNOW
- Chest radiographs are frequently normal.
- Contrast-enhanced spiral CT is usually diagnostic.

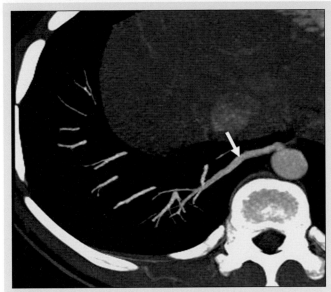

Figure 1. Isolated systemic arterial supply of the lung. Maximum intensity projection image from CT angiogram shows abnormal systemic artery (*arrow*) and its origin from the descending thoracic aorta. The patient was a young adult woman in whom isolated systemic arterial supply to the posterior basal segment of the right lower lobe was detected during workup for hemoptysis. (*Reprinted with permission of Grenier P: Imagerie Thoracique de l'Adulte. Paris, Flammarion, 2006.*)

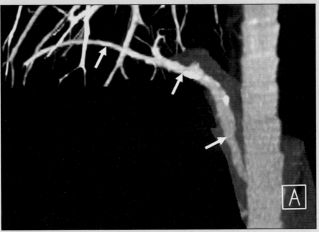

Figure 2. Systemic arterial supply of the lung. Volumetric reformatted image from a CT scan shows abnormal isolated systemic artery (*arrows*) coursing in the region of the right inferior phrenic artery. There is decreased pulmonary arterial vascularization of the medial basal segment of the right lower lobe. (*Reprinted with permission of Grenier P: Imagerie Thoracique de l'Adulte. Paris, Flammarion, 2006.*)

INCIDENCE/PREVALENCE AND EPIDEMIOLOGY

- Uncommon congenital anomaly
- More commonly involves basal segments of lower lobes
- Left lung more commonly affected than right

Suggested Readings

Albertini A, Dell'amore A, Tripodi A, et al: Anomalous systemic arterial supply to the left lung base without sequestration. *Heart Lung Circ* 17:505-507, 2008.

Do KH, Goo JM, Im JG, et al: Systemic arterial supply to the lung in adults: Spiral CT findings. *RadioGraphics* 21:387-402, 2001.

Zylak CJ, Eyler WR, Spizarny DL, Stone CH: Developmental lung anomalies in the adult: Radiologic-pathologic correlation. *RadioGraphics* 22:S25-S43, 2002.

Pulmonary Arteriovenous Malformations

DEFINITION: Pulmonary arteriovenous malformations (PAVMs) are abnormal communications between pulmonary arteries and pulmonary veins.

IMAGING

Radiography
Findings
- Aneurysmal sac
- Virtually diagnostic "comet tail" appearance (feeding and draining vessels)
- Limited value in detecting small- to moderate-sized pulmonary arteriovenous malformations

CT Angiography
Findings
- Aneurysmal sac
- Single or multiple feeding pulmonary arteries and single or multiple draining veins

Utility
- Most diagnostically accurate and least invasive examination for detection of PAVMs.
- Indications: screening (noncontrast), pretherapeutic evaluation of PAVM angioarchitecture (CT angiography), and post-treatment follow-up.

MR Angiography
Findings
- Malformations with feeding and draining vessels that are well seen if large.

Utility
- Of limited sensitivity in the detection of small PAVMs.

CLINICAL PRESENTATION

- Orthopnea, hypoxia, and cyanosis
- Paradoxical septic or thrombotic emboli
- May be asymptomatic

DIFFERENTIAL DIAGNOSIS

- Lung nodule(s)
- Pulmonary vein varix

PATHOLOGY

- PAVMs may be simple or complex.
- A simple PAVM is supplied by single feeding artery and has a single draining vein.

DIAGNOSTIC PEARLS

- Single or multiple
- Majority of cases seen in patients with hereditary hemorrhagic telangiectasia (Rendu-Osler-Weber syndrome)
- Identification of feeding and draining vessels diagnostic on CT
- Screening for PAVMs in patients with hereditary hemorrhagic telangiectasia can be done with CT without intravenous contrast.

- A complex PAVM has two or more feeding arteries or draining veins.
- Approximately 80%-90% of PAVMs are simple.
- The majority of PAVMs are seen in the context of hereditary hemorrhagic telangiectasia (Rendu-Osler-Weber) syndrome, where they are often multiple.

INCIDENCE/PREVALENCE AND EPIDEMIOLOGY

- Majority of malformations are associated with Rendu-Osler-Weber syndrome.
- Most frequently they are found in the lower lobes of the lung.

Suggested Readings

Cottin V, Dupuis-Girod S, Lesca G, Cordier JF: Pulmonary vascular manifestations of hereditary hemorrhagic telangiectasia (Rendu-Osler disease). *Respiration* 74:361-378, 2007.

Gossage JR, Kanj G: Pulmonary arteriovenous malformations: A state of the art review. *Am J Respir Crit Care Med* 158:643-661, 1998.

Remy-Jardin M, Dumont P, Brillet PY, et al: Pulmonary arteriovenous malformations treated with embolotherapy: Helical CT evaluation of long-term effectiveness after 2- to 21-year follow-up. *Radiology* 239:576-585, 2006.

Remy-Jardin M, Remy J: Spiral CT angiography of the pulmonary circulation. *Radiology* 212:615-636, 1999.

WHAT THE REFERRING PHYSICIAN NEEDS TO KNOW

- In Rendu-Osler-Weber syndrome, evaluation of liver should be performed before undertaking treatment of PAVMs.
- Pulmonary arterial hypertension should be treated before embolotherapy of pulmonary arteriovenous malformations.
- Embolotherapy is contraindicated if pulmonary arterial hypertension cannot be adequately treated.

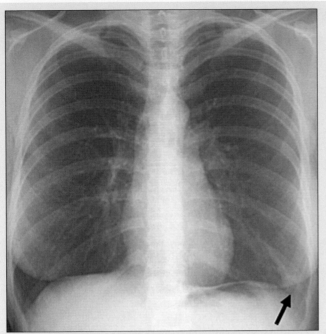

Figure 1. Pulmonary arteriovenous malformation. Frontal radiograph in a young adult woman who presented with a transient ischemic attack 10 years earlier shows a nodular opacity in the region of the left lateral costodiaphragmatic recess (*arrow*). The opacity of the aneurysmal sac was probably initially mistaken for the left breast shadow. The radiographic appearance simulates a comet tail because of a dilated pulmonary vessel connecting the inferior portion of the left hilum to the aneurysmal sac. *(Courtesy of Dr. Jacques Remy, Lille, France)*

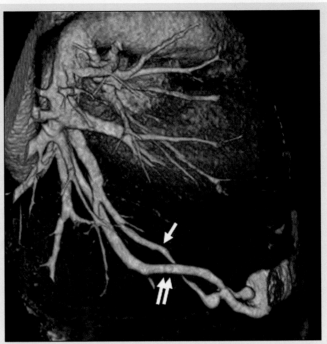

Figure 2. Pulmonary arteriovenous malformation. Volumetric reconstruction from a CT angiographic study shows the aneurysmal sac contacting the anterior arc of a rib. A single arterial pedicle arises from a branch of the left lower lobe pulmonary artery (*single arrow*). The venous pedicle is more dilated than the arterial pedicle (*double arrow*). There is no systemic arterial supply evident by CT angiography. *(Courtesy of Dr. Jacques Remy, Lille, France)*

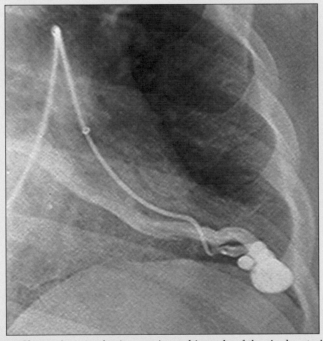

Figure 3. Pulmonary arteriovenous malformation. A selective arteriographic study of the single arterial pedicle identified on Figure 2. The tip of the catheter is located very close to the aneurysmal sac. Metal coils are about to be deployed from the tip of the catheter. This example shows the perfect correlation that exists between CT angiography and conventional selective arteriography in depicting the angioarchitecture of the malformation. *(Courtesy of Dr. Jacques Remy, Lille, France)*

Partial Anomalous Pulmonary Venous Return: Scimitar Syndrome (Hypogenetic Lung Syndrome)

DEFINITION: Scimitar syndrome is malformation of the right lung and anomalous right pulmonary vein, which resembles a scimitar on a chest radiograph.

IMAGING

Radiology
Findings
- Scimitar vein is hallmark of anomaly that often can be easily visualized and diagnosed on plain radiography, particularly if the right lung is not too underdeveloped and abnormal venous drainage is significant.
- Classic appearance is of a vertically oriented curvilinear vein that is convex inferolaterally, increasing in diameter from superior to inferior.
- Radiopaque stripe is often observed in a retrosternal region on lateral chest radiographs because the anterior aspect of right lung is situated more posteriorly than the left lung.

Utility
- Diagnosis of congenital hypogenetic lung syndrome can often be made radiographically.
- Dextrocardia resulting from small right lung can obscure scimitar vein.
- "Horseshoe lung" must be searched for routinely, even though it is very rare in adults.

CT
Findings
- Scimitar vein with approximately 50% left-to-right shunt
- Associated anomalies

Utility
- Multiplanar and 3D image reconstructions required for optimal depiction of findings.
- Has replaced aortography, pulmonary angiography, and bronchography as primary imaging modality for this malformation.

CLINICAL PRESENTATION

- Symptoms are related to associated congenital pulmonary or cardiac malformations or pulmonary arterial hypertension.
- In order of decreasing frequency, clinical symptoms include recurrent respiratory tract infections, dyspnea on effort, chronic cough, chest pain, wheezing, and recurrent hemoptysis.

DIAGNOSTIC PEARLS

- Scimitar vein with approximately 50% left-to-right shunt
- Small right lung and decreased volume of right upper lobe

- In 10% of cases, there are no symptoms and anomaly is discovered incidentally on routine chest radiograph.
- Symptoms depend on the magnitude of the left-to-right shunt associated with the anomaly.

DIFFERENTIAL DIAGNOSIS

- Aberrant pulmonary veins

PATHOLOGY

- Total or partial anomalous pulmonary venous return from right lung, most often to inferior vena cava
- Hypoplasia of right lung
- No known embryologic explanation that takes into account all of the malformations common to congenital hypogenetic lung syndrome

INCIDENCE/PREVALENCE AND EPIDEMIOLOGY

- Most common form of partial anomalous pulmonary venous return detected by radiography.
- Usually sporadic but familial cases have been reported.
- Age at detection dependent on associated malformations and may vary from neonatal period to adulthood.
- Very frequently associated with malformations of right lung.
- Associated anomalies: bronchopulmonary malformation, cardiac malformation, vascular anomalies, systemic arterialization of lung, malformations of hemidiaphragm, absence of pleura, horseshoe lung.

WHAT THE REFERRING PHYSICIAN NEEDS TO KNOW

- Diagnosis can often be made based on findings on chest radiograph or CT.
- Preoperative hemodynamic assessment of contributions from the heart and from pulmonary and systemic vascular systems can be performed by CT, MRI, and echocardiography.

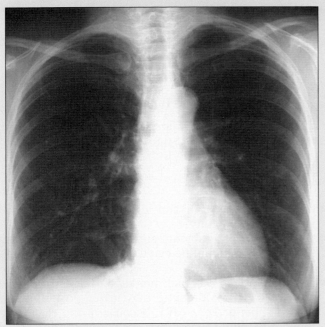

Figure 1. Scimitar syndrome. Routine chest radiograph shows large tubular opacity coursing toward the right cardiophrenic angle. The cardiac silhouette is normal. There are no obvious anomalies of the pulmonary vascular supply or of the right lung. This appearance is immediately suggestive of a scimitar syndrome. It must nevertheless be confirmed by a CT examination to exclude other diagnostic possibilities for the tubular opacity, such as bronchocele, systemic artery, and pseudo-scimitar syndrome. (*Reprinted with permission of Grenier P: Imagerie Thoracique de l'Adulte. Paris, Flammarion, 2006.*)

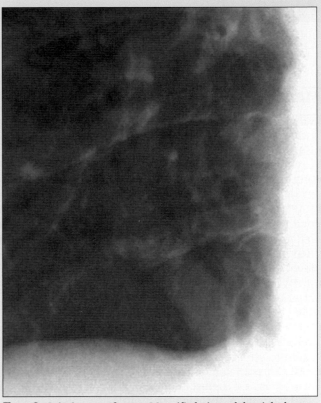

Figure 2. Scimitar syndrome. Magnified view of the right lower lung region shows large tubular opacity coursing toward the right cardiophrenic angle. The cardiac silhouette is normal. There are no obvious anomalies of the pulmonary vascular supply or of the right lung. This appearance is immediately suggestive of a scimitar syndrome. It must nevertheless be confirmed by a CT examination to exclude other diagnostic possibilities for the tubular opacity such as bronchocele, systemic artery, and pseudo-scimitar syndrome. (*Reprinted with permission of Grenier P. Imagerie Thoracique de l'Adulte. Paris, Flammarion, 2006.*)

Suggested Readings

Konen E, Raviv-Zilka L, Cohen RA, et al: Congenital pulmonary venolobar syndrome: Spectrum of helical CT findings with emphasis on computed reformatting. *RadioGraphics* 23:1175-1184, 2003.

Zylak CJ, Eyler WR, Spizarny DL, Stone CH: Developmental lung anomalies in the adult: Radiologic-pathologic correlation. *RadioGraphics* 22:S25-S43, 2002.

Partial Anomalous Pulmonary Venous Return: Other Forms

DEFINITION: Partial anomalous pulmonary venous return refers to venous drainage of one lung or part of one lung into the systemic vein or right atrium.

IMAGING

Radiography

Findings

- PAPVR draining into caudal portion of superior vena cava: this may be suspected by presence of one or several tubular opacities in right upper lobe or by opacity in right tracheobronchial angle.
- PAPVR of left upper lobe draining into vertical vein: one or two dilated tubular opacities may be visible in left upper lobe; vertical vein can at times be identified on chest radiograph as left mediastinal interface at level of aortopulmonary window and aortic arch.
- PAPVR draining into right atrium: signs of pulmonary arterial hypertension are evident.

Utility

- PAPVR draining into the caudal portion of the superior vena cava anomaly frequently goes unrecognized with radiography.
- PAPVR associated with veins that are neither ectopic nor dilated is not detectable radiographically; left-to-right shunt is not of sufficient magnitude to cause dilatation of pulmonary vessels nor alteration in cardiac silhouette.

CT

Findings

- PAPVR draining into superior vena cava: it is easy to identify abnormal tubular structures as dilated pulmonary veins.
- PAPVR draining into right atrium: abnormalities occur in alignment of interatrial septum and drainage of right pulmonary veins into right atrium.
- Associated heterotaxic syndrome will reveal levo-isomerism, left superior vena cava, polysplenia, or, more rarely, asplenia or normal spleen.

Utility

- PAPVR is more often detected on CT than on chest radiography.

DIAGNOSTIC PEARLS

- Diagnosis usually readily made on CT
- Left-to-right shunt is usually < 25% of cardiac output, except in PAPVR draining into right atrium.

- Contrast-enhanced CT can identify venous dilatation without any difficulty.
- Once PAPVR draining into superior vena cava is identified, patient should be evaluated for interatrial communication.
- The only diagnosis that remains difficult to make on CT is PAPVR draining into lower posterior portion of superior vena cava, because of the close anatomic proximity of these two structures in the normal situation.

MRI

Utility

- MRI is usually only performed when there is associated congenital cardiac disease, during the evaluation of which the PAPVR may be incidentally detected.

CLINICAL PRESENTATION

- Isolated PAPVR in adulthood is nearly always asymptomatic.
- Signs of pulmonary hypertension are evident when left-to-right shunt is >25%.

DIFFERENTIAL DIAGNOSIS

- Stenosis and atresia of pulmonary veins
- Aberrant pulmonary veins

WHAT THE REFERRING PHYSICIAN NEEDS TO KNOW

- Risk of cardiac failure occurs after lobectomy or pneumonectomy; surgery unmasks and increases magnitude of previously silent left-to-right shunt.
- Prior to surgery, interpretation of preoperative CT scan of thorax should include assessment of possible hemodynamic consequences of PAPVR that might result from planned resection.
- If vein terminates in ipsilateral pulmonary vein or in left atrium, this represents an aberrant intrapulmonary venous pathway.
- It is necessary to exclude the possibility that an ectopic vein is not a dilated collateral vein resulting from atresia of a normal pulmonary vein.
- Venous drainage into systemic vein or into right atrium should be easily identifiable on unenhanced CT images or on enhanced images where there is little or no streak artifact from central venous structures.

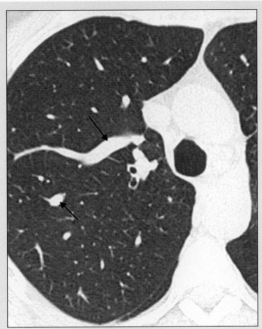

Figure 1. Partial anomalous pulmonary venous return. Magnified view of the right upper lobe from a CT scan shows tubular structures that can be identified as veins because they are not associated with accompanying bronchi *(arrows)*. *(Courtesy of Dr. Jacques Remy, Lille, France)*

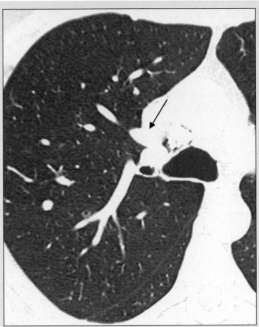

Figure 2. Partial anomalous pulmonary venous return. These venous structures (see Fig. 1) form a confluence at the posterior aspect of the superior vena cava *(arrow)*. CT was performed without intravenous administration of a contrast agent to avoid streak artifacts from the superior vena cava. *(Courtesy of Dr. Jacques Remy, Lille, France)*

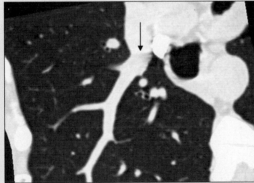

Figure 3. Partial anomalous pulmonary venous return. Multiplanar reformatted image in an axial oblique plane shows the most important features of the abnormal venous return. This image shows termination of the abnormal vein *(arrow)* in the lower posterior portion of the superior vena cava, immediately adjacent to a calcified lymph node in the lower right paratracheal region. *(Courtesy of Dr. Jacques Remy, Lille, France)*

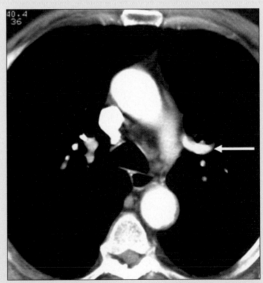

Figure 4. Partial anomalous pulmonary venous return from the left upper lobe into a vertical vein. A tributary of the left upper lobe pulmonary vein *(arrow)* follows an abnormal pathway toward the mediastinum. Images caudal to this should show that the remnant of the left upper pulmonary vein coursing toward the left atrium is very fine and that the vertical vein does not flow toward the coronary sinus. *(Reprinted with the permission of Grenier P: Imagerie Thoracique de l'Adulte. Paris, Flammarion, 2006.)*

PATHOLOGY

- Persistence of connection between pulmonary and systemic venous return systems is noted toward the right side of the heart.
- Pulmonary arterial blood flow is redistributed toward PAPVR, resulting in dilatation of efferent vessels receiving anomalous vein.
- PAPVR results in left-to-right shunt; because the shunt only involves a portion of venous return from lung, it represents ≤25% of cardiac output.

INCIDENCE/PREVALENCE AND EPIDEMIOLOGY

- Isolated PAPVR in absence of congenital cardiac disease or other malformations is seen in 0.4%-0.7% of adults.
- Right-sided PAPVRs are twice as common as left-sided ones.

Suggested Readings

Chowdhury UK, Kothary SS, Airan B, et al: Right pulmonary artery to left atrium communication. *Ann Thorac Surg* 80:365-370, 2005.

Remy-Jardin M, Remy J, Mayo JR, Müller NL: *CT Angiography of the Chest*. Philadelphia, 2001, Lippincott Williams & Wilkins.

Zylak CJ, Eyler WR, Spizarny DL, Stone CH: Developmental lung anomalies in the adult: Radiologic-pathologic correlation. *Radio-Graphics* 22:S25-S43, 2002.

Unilateral Small Hilum

DEFINITION: Conditions that may have a unilateral small hilum include proximal interruption of pulmonary artery, scimitar syndrome, pulmonary vein stenosis or atresia, and Swyer-James-McLeod syndrome.

IMAGING

Radiography
Findings
- Proximal interruption of the pulmonary artery: a small lung is evident, with similar lucency to normal side, no air trapping, absent ipsilateral hilum, and prominent contralateral hilum.
- Hypogenetic right lung (scimitar) syndrome: right lung is small and commonly there is a vertically oriented curvilinear (scimitar) vein that is convex inferolaterally, increasing in diameter from superior to inferior.
- Pulmonary vein atresia or stenosis: there is a small lung with small hilum without evidence of bronchial obstruction or air trapping.
- Swyer-James-McLeod syndrome: unilateral hyperlucent lung with normal or reduced volume is evident on the inspiratory radiograph, and air trapping is present on the expiratory radiograph.

Utility
- Usually first imaging modality.
- Presence of air trapping on expiratory radiograph helpful in distinguishing Swyer-James-McLeod syndrome and partial bronchial obstruction from unilateral small lung and hilum due to congenital vascular abnormality.

CT
Findings
- Proximal interruption of the pulmonary artery: interrupted artery, thickening of bronchial walls, bronchial dilatation, late opacification of intrapulmonary vessels.
- Hypogenetic right lung (scimitar) syndrome: hypoplastic right lung, left-to-right shunt.
- Stenosis and atresia of pulmonary veins: on contrast-enhanced CT (CT angiography) juxta-atrial atresia/stenosis of pulmonary veins and small corresponding pulmonary arteries with late opacification via systemic-to-pulmonary artery shunting; retrograde opacification of ipsilateral pulmonary arteries; septal lines due to interstitial edema.
- Swyer-James-McLeod syndrome: unilateral hyperlucent lung with normal or decreased volume; decreased attenuation and vascularity; commonly bronchiectasis; air trapping on expiratory CT.

DIAGNOSTIC PEARLS

- Proximal interruption of the pulmonary artery: break in continuity of pulmonary arterial circulation, late opacification of intrapulmonary vessels, and hypoplastic lung.
- Scimitar syndrome: right lung malformation and anomalous right pulmonary vein resembling a scimitar.
- Stenosis and atresia of pulmonary veins: hypoplastic lung and ipsilateral interstitial pulmonary edema.
- Swyer-James-McLeod syndrome: unilateral hyperlucent lung with normal or decreased volume and air trapping on expiration.

Utility
- CT allows definitive diagnosis and recognition of associated findings.
- CT should be performed in all cases to establish confident diagnosis and for thorough and precise evaluation of anomaly, particularly because surgical repair may be contemplated, even in young adult patients.
- Multiplanar and 3D image reconstructions are required for optimal depiction of findings.

Nuclear Medicine
Findings
- Proximal interruption of the pulmonary artery: ventilation-perfusion scanning demonstrates complete absence of perfusion, associated with hypoventilation and normal "wash-out" delay.
- Stenosis and atresia of pulmonary veins: ventilation-perfusion scintigraphy may reveal "pseudo-pulmonary emboli" appearance with unmatched reduction in perfusion. Appearance of "pseudo-pneumonia" results if decrease in perfusion is matched by decrease in ventilation.

Utility
- Limited value in diagnosis

CLINICAL PRESENTATION

- Proximal interruption of pulmonary artery: pulmonary hypertension, recurrent infection, hemoptysis.

WHAT THE REFERRING PHYSICIAN NEEDS TO KNOW

- Presence of air trapping on expiratory radiography is helpful in distinguishing Swyer-James-McLeod syndrome and partial bronchial obstruction from unilateral small lung and hilum due to congenital vascular abnormality.
- In vast majority of cases diagnosis can be made on CT.

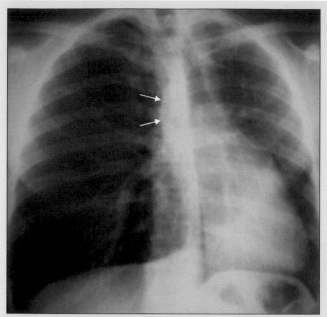

Figure 1. Proximal interruption of left pulmonary artery. Frontal chest radiograph demonstrates a reduction in volume of the left lung, accompanied by ipsilateral displacement of the trachea and heart and herniation of the right lung across the midline. The aortic arch (*arrows*) and the descending thoracic aorta are on the right side. The patient was a young adult being assessed for hemoptysis. *(Courtesy of Dr. Jacques Remy, Lille, France)*

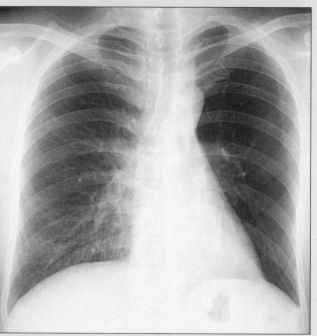

Figure 2. Swyer-James-McLeod syndrome. Chest radiograph shows hyperlucency and decreased vascularity of the left lung. The mediastinum is shifted to the left consistent with decreased left lung volume. The patient was a 40-year-old man.

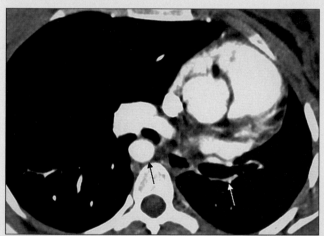

Figure 3. Proximal interruption of left pulmonary artery. CT angiography demonstrates the hypoplastic left lung. The left interlobar pulmonary artery is represented by a small vessel a few millimeters in diameter adjacent to the posterior aspect of the bronchus to the left upper lobe (*white arrow*). The descending thoracic aorta (*black arrow*) is situated on the right anterolateral aspect of the spine, posterior to the right bronchial tree. *(Courtesy of Dr. Jacques Remy, Lille, France)*

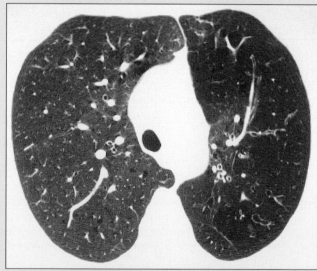

Figure 4. Swyer-James-McLeod syndrome. High-resolution CT shows decreased attenuation and vascularity of the left lung with associated bronchiectasis and mild volume loss leading to ipsilateral shift of the mediastinum and anterior junction line. The patient was a 61-year-old woman.

- Scimitar vein: recurrent respiratory tract infections, dyspnea on effort, chronic cough, chest pain, wheezing, recurrent hemoptysis; asymptomatic in 10%.
- Stenosis and atresia of pulmonary veins: clinical manifestations may be those of associated congenital cardiac anomaly, pulmonary arterial hypertension, and recurrent respiratory tract infections.
- Swyer-James-McLeod syndrome: patients asymptomatic or present with cough, recurrent chest infections, or hemoptysis.

DIFFERENTIAL DIAGNOSIS

- Fibrosing mediastinitis
- Proximal interruption of the pulmonary artery
- Partial anomalous pulmonary venous return: Scimitar syndrome (hypogenetic lung syndrome)
- Partial anomalous pulmonary venous return: Other forms
- Swyer-James-McLeod syndrome

PATHOLOGY

- Proximal interruption of pulmonary artery: because pulmonary blood flow influences lung development, interruption of pulmonary arterial supply in utero results in hypoplasia of lung. Dilatation of bronchi may presumably be result of decreased caliber of accompanying pulmonary arteries, which allows greater space for bronchi to expand.
- Scimitar vein: no known embryologic explanation takes into account all of malformations common to congenital hypogenetic lung syndrome.
- Stenosis and atresia of pulmonary veins: volume reduction of affected lung and interstitial pulmonary edema are commonly present.

- Swyer-James-McLeod syndrome: unilateral hyperlucent lung with normal or reduced volume, postinfectious bronchiolitis obliterans, and, commonly, bronchiectasis are noted.

INCIDENCE/PREVALENCE AND EPIDEMIOLOGY

- Proximal interruption of the pulmonary artery: is uncommon and usually diagnosed in childhood.
- Scimitar vein is the most common form of partial anomalous pulmonary venous return detected by radiography. It is usually sporadic but familial cases have been reported; age at detection depends on associated malformations and may vary from neonatal period to adulthood.
- Stenosis and atresia of pulmonary veins most often is discovered during infancy or childhood and rarely in adulthood. It is associated with congenital cardiac anomaly, pulmonary arterial hypertension, and recurrent bronchial and pulmonary infection.
- Swyer-James-McLeod syndrome is usually due to childhood infection, most commonly viral (particularly adenovirus) or *Mycoplasma* pneumonia.

Suggested Readings

Do KH, Goo JM, Im JG, et al: Systemic arterial supply to the lung in adults: Spiral CT findings. *RadioGraphics* 21:387-402, 2001.

Konen E, Raviv-Zilka L, Cohen RA, et al: Congenital pulmonary venolobar syndrome: Spectrum of helical CT findings with emphasis on computed reformatting. *RadioGraphics* 23:1175-1184, 2003.

Lucaya J, Gartner S, García-Peña P, et al: Spectrum of manifestations of Swyer-James-MacLeod syndrome. *J Comput Assist Tomogr* 22:592-597, 1998.

Ten Harkel ADJ, Blom NA, Ottenkamp J: Isolated unilateral absence of a pulmonary artery. *Chest* 122:1471-1477, 2002.

Zylak CJ, Eyler WR, Spizarny DL, Stone CH: Developmental lung anomalies in the adult: Radiologic-pathologic correlation. *RadioGraphics* 22:S25-S43, 2002.

Aberrant Pulmonary Veins

DEFINITION: An aberrant pulmonary vein is characterized by an abnormal course of a vein that drains into the left atrium.

IMAGING

Radiography
Findings
- Tubular opacities are more or less arciform or tortuous in configuration.
- Frequently these veins follow a "bucket handle" course, either in axial or sagittal planes.

Utility
- When two branches of the "bucket handle" approach each other, they can simulate a pulmonary arteriovenous malformation.

CT
Findings
- Abnormal course of the vein but normal drainage into the left atrium.
- Venous nature of abnormality recognized by absence of accompanying bronchus and by drainage into left atrium.

Utility
- Can confirm diagnosis
- Useful to describe other potentially associated anomalies
- May simulate a vascular malformation or pulmonary nodule

CLINICAL PRESENTATION

- Aberrant pulmonary veins are asymptomatic and are almost always discovered incidentally on chest radiograph or CT.

DIFFERENTIAL DIAGNOSIS

- Partial anomalous pulmonary venous return: Scimitar syndrome (hypogenetic lung syndrome)
- Partial anomalous pulmonary venous return: Other forms
- Pulmonary varices

DIAGNOSTIC PEARLS

- Abnormal venous pathway characterized by sinuous rather than smooth curvilinear course
- Abnormal course of vein that drains into left atrium
- Not associated with left-to-right shunt

PATHOLOGY

- Associated anomalies include hypoplastic, dilated or tortuous pulmonary artery; bronchopulmonary malformations (hypogenetic lung syndrome); abnormal systemic arteries; and partial anomalous pulmonary venous return in a different lung zone.

INCIDENCE/PREVALENCE AND EPIDEMIOLOGY

- This is an uncommon congenital malformation.
- Scimitar-mimicking syndromes may be associated with other anomalies classically encountered in hypogenetic lung syndrome.

Suggested Readings

Haramati LB, Moche IE, Rivera VT, et al: Computed tomography of partial anomalous pulmonary venous connection in adults. *J Comput Assist Tomogr* 27:743-749, 2003.

Marom EM, Herndon JE, Kim YH, McAdams HP: Variations in pulmonary venous drainage to the left atrium: Implications for radiofrequency ablation. *Radiology* 230:824-829, 2004.

Zylak CJ, Eyler WR, Spizarny DL, Stone CH: Developmental lung anomalies in the adult: Radiologic-pathologic correlation. *RadioGraphics* 22:S25-S43, 2002.

WHAT THE REFERRING PHYSICIAN NEEDS TO KNOW

- It is important to be aware of the existence of aberrant pulmonary veins to avoid diagnostic errors and anticipate surgical difficulties that their presence may cause.
- At time of right lower lobectomy, veins from the right middle lobe may be ligated inadvertently if tributaries of the right inferior pulmonary vein are not identified beforehand; resultant obstruction to venous return may cause pulmonary edema or venous infarction of this lobe.
- Aberrant pathways can simulate scimitar syndrome (from which term "pseudoscimitar syndrome" is derived).

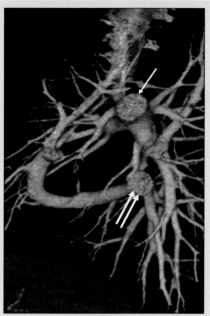

Figure 1. "Pseudoscimitar" syndrome. A volumetric reconstruction of the right lung shows a long vein with an abnormal trajectory descending from the lung apex toward the anteroinferior portion of the lung, then coursing almost horizontally before it terminates in the right inferior pulmonary vein (*double arrows*). The first portion of this aberrant pulmonary vein passes in front of the hilum, corresponding to the section of the right main pulmonary artery (*single arrow*). This is the classic appearance of a pseudoscimitar syndrome, in which the abnormal vein has a scimitar like trajectory but terminates within the left atrium. The patient was a young asymptomatic adult, with an abnormality discovered on a routine chest radiograph. *(Courtesy of Dr. Jacques Remy, Lille, France)*

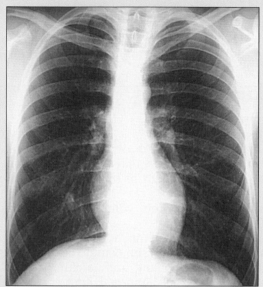

Figure 2. Aberrant pulmonary vein. Routine frontal radiograph in a young adult shows a large tubular opacity in the right lower lobe. *(Courtesy of Dr. Jacques Remy, Lille, France)*

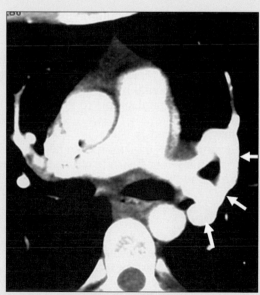

Figure 4. Aberrant pulmonary vein. CT image shows the aberrant intraparenchymal trajectory of a pulmonary vein in the left lung. The abnormal vein descends from the left upper lobe, crosses the left hilum from anterior to posterior (*arrows*), and then courses between the left interlobar pulmonary artery and the descending thoracic aorta, medial to the bronchus of the superior segment of the left lower lobe. At a more caudal level (not shown), this vein became confluent with the left inferior pulmonary vein and terminated in the left atrium. *(Courtesy of Dr. Jacques Remy, Lille, France)*

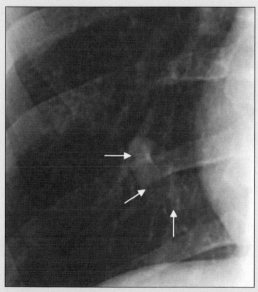

Figure 3. Aberrant pulmonary vein. Magnified view from a posteroanterior chest radiograph of right lower lung in a young adult shows a large tubular opacity in the right lower lobe (*arrows*). *(Courtesy of Dr. Jacques Remy, Lille, France)*

Proximal Interruption of the Pulmonary Artery

DEFINITION: Congenital malformation characterized by absence of mediastinal portion of the right or left pulmonary artery and intact intrapulmonary vessels.

IMAGING

Radiography
Findings
- Frontal chest radiograph demonstrates a reduction in volume of the affected lung, accompanied by ipsilateral displacement of the trachea and mediastinum.
- Ipsilateral hilum is absent; contralateral hilum is prominent.
- Signs of collateral systemic arterial system supplying abnormal lung include subpleural reticular opacities, smooth pleural thickening, and notching of ribs.
- Degree of lucency of abnormal lung is rarely different from that of contralateral lung; no air trapping occurs.

Utility
- Usually first imaging modality.
- Lack of increased lucency of involved lung and lack of air trapping shown on expiratory radiograph.
- Helpful in distinguishing proximal interruption of pulmonary artery from partial bronchial obstruction or Swyer-James-McLeod syndrome.

CT
Findings
- Unilateral atresia/absence of pulmonary artery.
- Small caliber of pulmonary vessels.
- Common associated findings: mosaic attenuation of lung parenchyma, thickened interlobular septa, bronchial wall thickening, cylindrical dilatation of proximal segmental or subsegmental bronchi.
- Collateral systemic arterial supply to the affected lung.

Utility
- Allows definitive diagnosis.
- Enables evaluation of morphologic functional effects of anomaly on heart, exclusion of cardiac malformation, and follow-up after surgical revascularization.

MRI
Findings
- Unilateral atresia/absence of pulmonary artery
- Small caliber of pulmonary vessels

DIAGNOSTIC PEARLS

- Atresia of mediastinal portion of right or left pulmonary artery.
- Intact but very small intrapulmonary vessels.
- Small lung

Utility
- Does not form part of routine workup because of limited spatial resolution.

CLINICAL PRESENTATION

- Pulmonary hypertension: dyspnea, hemoptysis, chest pain
- Recurrent pulmonary infections

DIFFERENTIAL DIAGNOSIS

- Pulmonary stenosis
- Swyer-James-Macleod syndrome
- Takayasu arteritis
- Fibrosing mediastinitis

PATHOLOGY

- There is a break in pulmonary arterial tree continuity beyond which pulmonary arteries are still present but appear small.
- Interruption of pulmonary arterial blood supply in utero results in hypoplasia of the lung.

INCIDENCE/PREVALENCE AND EPIDEMIOLOGY

- Uncommon congenital abnormality.
- Diagnosis usually made in childhood.
- Frequently associated with congenital heart defects, most common of which are ventricular septal defects and tetralogy of Fallot.
- Usually occurs as isolated malformation when first seen in adults.
- Occurs more frequently on the right side than on the left.
- Often associated with contralateral aortic arch.

WHAT THE REFERRING PHYSICIAN NEEDS TO KNOW

- Diagnosis can be made on CT or MRI.
- In children and young adults, revascularization of interrupted pulmonary artery can be attempted by reimplantation/bypass of affected segment.
- If caliber of artery is too narrow, temporary palliative anastomosis can be attempted to encourage further development of the vessel.
- When malformation is not detected until later adulthood, treatment is symptomatic.

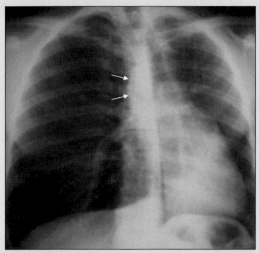

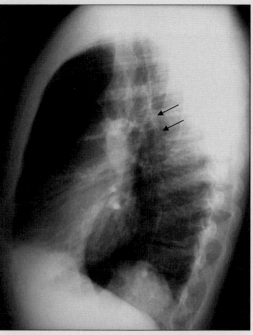

Figure 1. Proximal interruption of left pulmonary artery. Frontal chest radiograph demonstrates a reduction in volume of the left lung, accompanied by ipsilateral displacement of the trachea and heart and herniation of the right lung across the midline. The aortic arch (*arrows*) and the descending thoracic aorta are on the right side. The patient was a young adult being assessed for hemoptysis. *(Courtesy of Dr. Jacques Remy, Lille, France)*

Figure 2. Proximal interruption of left pulmonary artery. Lateral chest radiograph shows a very small left interlobar pulmonary artery (*arrows*) adjacent to the posterior aspect of the left main-stem bronchus. The patient was a young adult being assessed for hemoptysis. *(Courtesy of Dr. Jacques Remy, Lille, France)*

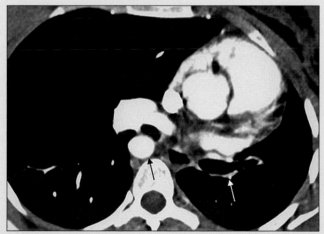

Figure 3. Proximal interruption of left pulmonary artery. CT angiography demonstrates the hypoplastic left lung. The left interlobar pulmonary artery is represented by a small vessel a few millimeters in diameter adjacent to the posterior aspect of the bronchus to the left upper lobe (*white arrow*). The descending thoracic aorta (*black arrow*) is situated on the right anterolateral aspect of the spine, posterior to the right bronchial tree. *(Courtesy of Dr. Jacques Remy, Lille, France)*

Suggested Readings

Castañer E, Gallardo X, Rimola J, et al: Congenital and acquired pulmonary artery anomalies in the adult? Radiologic overview. *RadioGraphics* 26:349-371, 2006.

Mahnken AH, Wildberger JE, Spüntrup E, Hübner D: Unilateral absence of the left pulmonary artery associated with coronary-to-bronchial artery anastomosis. *J Thorac Imaging* 15:187-190, 2000.

Ryu DS, Spirn PW, Trotman-Dickenson B, et al: HRCT findings of proximal interruption of the right pulmonary artery. *J Thorac Imaging* 19:171-175, 2004.

Sakai S, Murayama S, Soeda H, et al: Unilateral proximal interruption of the pulmonary artery in adults? CT findings in eight patients. *J Comput Assist Tomogr* 26:777-783, 2002.

Valvular Pulmonary Stenosis

DEFINITION: Stenosis of the pulmonary artery is due to a commissural fusion of the pulmonary cusps and results in a bicuspid pulmonary valve and valvular dysplasia.

IMAGING

Radiography
Findings
- Enlargement of main and left pulmonary arteries
- Can simulate mediastinal mass or enlarged left hilar lymph nodes
- Proximal dilatation of left main pulmonary artery limited to its upper lobe branches or extending to involve left interlobar pulmonary artery
- Cardiac silhouette not enlarged
- Variable convex bulging of middle arc of left-sided heart border
- Normal or small right hilum

Utility
- Usually first imaging modality used
- Of limited value in diagnosis

CT Angiography
Findings
- Pulmonary valve stenosis and dilatation of main pulmonary artery and left pulmonary artery
- If stenosis due to commissural fusion: pulmonary valves appear moderately thickened and dome shaped; can be identified even without electrocardiographic gating
- Leaflets much more thickened in valvular dysplasia
- Hypertrophic trabeculations and thickened myocardium predominate in right ventricular outflow tract; marked during systole (CT with electrocardiographic gating)
- Valvular dysplasia: valvular annulus and main pulmonary artery moderately hypoplastic

Utility
- Image reconstructions in systolic phase reformatted in short axis of main pulmonary artery provide good depiction of pulmonary valves.

MRI
Findings
- Pulmonary valve stenosis and dilatation of main pulmonary artery and left pulmonary artery

Utility
- Comparable to CT in demonstrating stenosis
- Lower spatial resolution than CT in demonstrating pulmonary valves

DIAGNOSTIC PEARLS
- Pulmonary valve stenosis
- Post-stenotic dilatation of the main and left pulmonary arteries
- Thickening of the pulmonary valves
- Right ventricular hypertrophy

CLINICAL PRESENTATION
- Asymptomatic or presents as progressive dyspnea
- Can cause systolic murmur in pulmonary outflow tract
- Echocardiographic signs of right ventricular hypertrophy

DIFFERENTIAL DIAGNOSIS
- Pulmonary arterial hypertension
- Pulmonary artery aneurysm
- Mediastinal lymphadenopathy

PATHOLOGY
- Stenosis is due to commissural fusion of pulmonary cusps causing thickened, dome-like pulmonary valve, bicuspid pulmonary valve, and valvular dysplasia.
- "Trilogy of Fallot": hypertrophy of right ventricle and right-to-left shunt across patent foramen ovale are due to pulmonary arterial stenosis.
- Stenosis of pulmonary valves: systole of right ventricle causes post-stenotic jet in main pulmonary artery.
- Elevated post-systolic pressure on right ventricle leads to muscular hypertrophy of right ventricle.

INCIDENCE/PREVALENCE AND EPIDEMIOLOGY
- Uncommon
- May not be diagnosed until adulthood

Suggested Reading
Steiner RM, Reddy GP, Flicker S: Congenital cardiovascular disease in the adult patient: Imaging update. *J Thorac Imaging* 17:1-17, 2002.

WHAT THE REFERRING PHYSICIAN NEEDS TO KNOW
- Stenosis of the pulmonary valve may be detected incidentally in an asymptomatic patient.
- Need for treatment depends on effects of pulmonary stenosis on cardiac function and pressure gradient across the stenosis.
- Surgical commissurotomy is increasingly being replaced by balloon angioplasty.

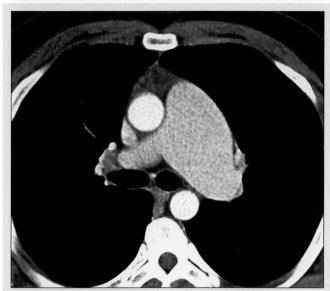

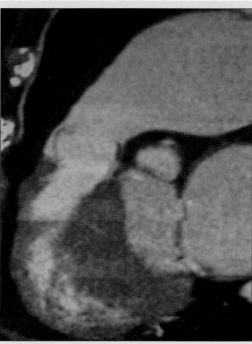

Figure 1. **Pulmonary valvular stenosis.** CT angiography demonstrates dilatation of the main pulmonary artery and of the proximal portion of the left main pulmonary artery. The right main pulmonary artery is of normal caliber. This image was acquired at a level just above the plane of the pulmonary valves. *(Courtesy of Dr. Jacques Remy, Lille, France)*

Figure 2. **Pulmonary valvular stenosis.** CT image acquired with electrocardiographic gating and reconstructed during the phase of right ventricular systole demonstrates the dome-like appearance of the pulmonary valve leaflets, which are moderately thickened, and the post-stenotic dilatation of the left main pulmonary artery. The inflow portion of the right ventricle demonstrates step-like artifacts, resulting from the lack of reproducibility of the same systolic volumes between each image slice. The outflow tract has no artifacts. *(Courtesy of Dr. Jacques Remy, Lille, France)*

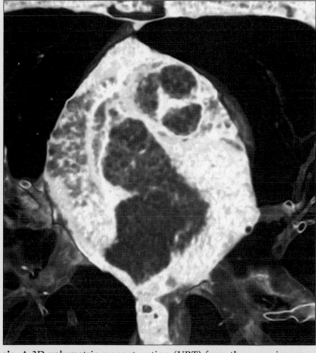

Figure 3. **Pulmonary valvular stenosis.** A 3D volumetric reconstruction (VRT) from the same image acquisition (see Fig. 1) at the level of the pulmonary valves demonstrates a tricuspid pulmonary valve with marked thickening of each pulmonary valve leaflet. *(Courtesy of Dr. Jacques Remy, Lille, France)*

Pulmonary Artery Sling

DEFINITION: Pulmonary artery sling refers to an anomalous origin of the left pulmonary artery from the right main pulmonary artery.

IMAGING

Radiography
Findings
- Opacity measuring approximately 2 cm in diameter in right tracheobronchial angle.
- Round opacity 10-15 mm in diameter indenting the posterior aspect of the trachea.
- Almost complete superimposition of the left main pulmonary artery on the right main pulmonary artery.

Utility
- Of limited value in diagnosis

CT
Findings
- Left pulmonary artery originates from posterior aspect of right main pulmonary artery and courses toward the left hilum between trachea and esophagus.
- When reaching the left hilum, it adopts a normal intrapulmonary course.
- Associated tracheobronchial malformations include tracheal bronchus to right upper lobe; distal tracheal hypoplasia; right main-stem bronchus stenosis; and complete cartilaginous rings.

Utility
- CT allows confident diagnosis.
- Reformatted images are useful to identify moderate tracheal stenosis.

MRI
Findings
- Left pulmonary artery originates from posterior aspect of right main pulmonary artery and courses toward the left hilum between trachea and esophagus.

Utility
- MRI allows confident diagnosis.

CLINICAL PRESENTATION

- Patient is asymptomatic unless there is an association with congenital tracheal or bronchial stenosis (dyspnea or recurring pulmonary tract infections).

DIAGNOSTIC PEARLS

- Left pulmonary artery arises from posterior surface of right pulmonary artery.
- Left pulmonary artery courses toward the left hilum between the trachea and the esophagus.

DIFFERENTIAL DIAGNOSIS

- Radiographic findings are nonspecific
- Contrast-enhanced CT or MRI is diagnostic

PATHOLOGY

- Left main pulmonary artery develops as a collateral vessel of right main pulmonary artery.
- Left main pulmonary artery originates from posterior aspect of right main pulmonary artery and courses above the right main-stem bronchus.
- It takes a pathway to the left between the trachea and esophagus before reaching the left hilum.

INCIDENCE/PREVALENCE AND EPIDEMIOLOGY

- Rare
- Great majority of cases detected in childhood
- Associated with other congenital malformations, most commonly of the tracheobronchial tree and of the heart

Suggested Readings

Chen SJ, Lee WJ, Lin MT, et al: Left pulmonary artery sling complex: Computed tomography and hypothesis of embryogenesis. *Ann Thorac Surg* 84:1645-1650, 2007.

Malmgren N, Laurin S, Lundstrom NR: Pulmonary artery sling: Diagnosis by magnetic resonance imaging. *Acta Radiol* 29:7-9, 1988.

Park SP, Im JG, Jung JW, Yeon KM: Anomalous left pulmonary artery with complete cartilaginous ring. *J Comput Assist Tomogr* 21:478-480, 1997.

Zylak CJ, Eyler WR, Spizarny DL, Stone CH: Developmental lung anomalies in the adult: Radiologic-pathologic correlation. *RadioGraphics* 22:S25-S43, 2002.

WHAT THE REFERRING PHYSICIAN NEEDS TO KNOW

- Diagnosis can be made on CT and MRI.
- Need for treatment depends on effects of pulmonary artery stenosis on cardiac function and pressure gradient across the stenosis.

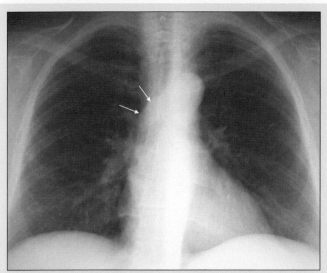

Figure 1. Aberrant retrotracheal left main pulmonary artery (pulmonary artery sling). Chest radiograph performed for evaluation of moderate dyspnea on effort shows an abnormal opacity in the right tracheobronchial angle (*arrows*). The opacity represents the course of a retrotracheal left main pulmonary artery within this angle (see Figs. 2 and 3). *(Courtesy of Dr. Jacques Remy, Lille, France)*

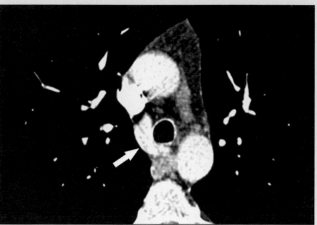

Figure 2. Aberrant retrotracheal left main pulmonary artery (pulmonary artery sling). CT image is at the level of the most superior portion of the left main pulmonary artery (*arrow*), which courses around the right lateral and posterior aspects of the morphologically normal trachea. *(Courtesy of Dr. Jacques Remy, Lille, France)*

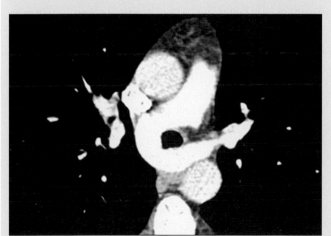

Figure 3. Aberrant retrotracheal left main pulmonary artery (pulmonary artery sling). CT image at a slightly more caudal level demonstrates the entire course of the left main pulmonary artery. It arises from the posterior aspect of the proximal portion of the right main pulmonary artery, passes around the right lateral and posterior aspects of the trachea, and then courses toward the left hilum. *(Courtesy of Dr. Jacques Remy, Lille, France)*

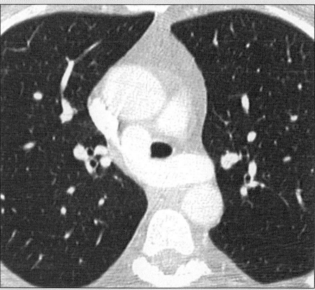

Figure 4. Aberrant retrotracheal left main pulmonary artery (pulmonary artery sling). CT image at the level of the aberrant pulmonary artery demonstrates the reduction in diameter of the trachea at the level of the ectopic pulmonary artery. These cases (Figs. 2 to 4) represent "ring-sling" syndromes. *(Courtesy of Dr. Jacques Remy, Lille, France)*

Pulmonary Infection

Part 8

COMMUNITY ACQUIRED AND NOSOCOMIAL PNEUMONIA

Community-Acquired Pneumonia

DEFINITION: Community-acquired pneumonia refers to pneumonia occurring in a patient who is not hospitalized or residing in a long-term care facility for >14 days before initial symptoms.

IMAGING

Radiography

Findings

- Lobar pneumonia: homogeneous airspace consolidation involving adjacent segments of lobe.
- Bronchopneumonia: patchy or confluent areas of consolidation involving one or more segments of single lobe or multiple lobes.
- Peribronchial thickening and ill-defined reticulonodular opacities with or without associated focal areas of consolidation in infectious bronchiolitis and early bronchopneumonia.
- Round pneumonia: focal spherical area of consolidation.

Utility

- According to American Thoracic Society (ATS) guidelines, posteroanterior (and lateral when possible) chest radiography should be obtained whenever pneumonia is suspected in adults.
- Initial examination is usually sufficiently specific to preclude need for additional imaging.
- Findings are informative with regard to extent of pneumonia, presence of cavitation, associated conditions, pleural effusion, and alternative diagnosis.

CT

Findings

- Lobar pneumonia: homogeneous airspace consolidation involving adjacent segments of a lobe.
- Bronchopneumonia (lobular pneumonia): centrilobular nodules and "tree-in-bud" pattern due to associated bronchiolitis; poorly defined focal nodular opacities measuring 5-10 mm in diameter (airspace nodules).

DIAGNOSTIC PEARLS

- Lobar pneumonia: nonsegmental, homogeneous consolidation involving predominantly or exclusively one lobe with visible air bronchograms.
- Bronchopneumonia: patchy areas of consolidation that may be lobular, subsegmental or segmental, although may coalesce to involve entire lobe.
- Interstitial pneumonia: extensive peribronchial thickening and ill-defined reticulonodular opacities; associated patchy subsegmental/plate-like atelectasis/focal areas of consolidation.
- Chest radiograph plays major role in confirming presence of pneumonia but is of limited value in making a specific diagnosis.

- Bronchopneumonia: lobular, subsegmental or segmental ground-glass opacities or areas of consolidation involving one or more segments of single lobe or multiple lobes.
- Centrilobular nodules and "tree-in-bud pattern" seen in infectious bronchiolitis due to viruses, *Mycoplasma,* bacteria, or fungi.

Utility

- Seldom indicated in community-acquired pneumonia.
- Helpful in detection, differential diagnosis, and management of patients with pulmonary or pleural complications.

CLINICAL PRESENTATION

- Acute respiratory symptoms (cough, sputum production, and/or dyspnea) accompanied by fever and auscultatory findings (abnormal breath sounds and crackles).

WHAT THE REFERRING PHYSICIAN NEEDS TO KNOW

- Chest radiography has pivotal role in confirming or excluding pneumonia but is of limited value in determining specific etiology of community-acquired pneumonia.
- In the absence of clinical information, the radiologist cannot reliably distinguish between pneumonia and other pulmonary processes.
- ATS guidelines recommendation: posteroanterior (and lateral when possible) chest radiography be performed in all adults with clinically suspected pneumonia.
- CT seldom warranted in diagnosis of community-acquired pneumonia; main role is in evaluation of patients with suspected complications such as empyema or necrotizing pneumonia.

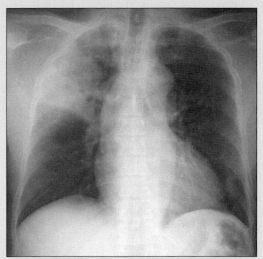

Figure 1. Lobar pneumonia. Chest radiograph in a 48-year-old man with clinical symptoms suggestive of pneumonia demonstrates lobar right upper lobe consolidation with air bronchograms and sharp demarcation by the minor fissure.

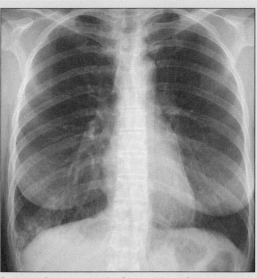

Figure 2. Bronchopneumonia due to *Mycoplasma pneumoniae.* Chest radiograph in a 34-year-old woman with cough and malaise shows multiple small patchy opacities in both lower lobes.

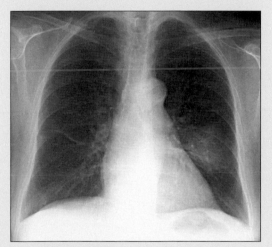

Figure 3. Round pneumonia. Chest radiograph in a 56-year-old woman with proven pneumococcal pneumonia shows an area of homogeneous round consolidation in the left lung.

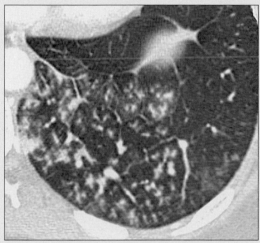

Figure 4. Bronchopneumonia due to *Mycoplasma pneumoniae.* View of the left lower lobe from a CT scan in a 34-year-old woman with cough and malaise shows small centrilobular nodules, ground-glass opacities, and airspace nodules.

DIFFERENTIAL DIAGNOSIS

- Aspiration pneumonia
- Organizing pneumonia
- Chronic eosinophilic pneumonia
- Bronchioloalveolar cell carcinoma
- Pulmonary lymphoma
- Acute pulmonary embolism

PATHOLOGY

- Lobar pneumonia: organism is inhaled or aspirated into peripheral airspaces, where bacteria injure alveolar wall, resulting in local inflammation and progressive consolidation.

- Bronchopneumonia: infectious organisms deposited on epithelium of bronchi produce acute bronchial inflammation with epithelial ulcerations and fibrino-purulent exudate formation; inflammatory reaction rapidly spreads through airways' walls and into contiguous pulmonary lobules.

INCIDENCE/PREVALENCE AND EPIDEMIOLOGY

- Pneumonia is leading cause of death due to infectious disease and sixth most common cause of death in United States.

- Estimated 4 million cases of community-acquired pneumonia occur annually in United States.
- Between 485,000 and 1 million patients each year are hospitalized in the United States for treatment of community-acquired pneumonia.
- Most common organisms in lobar pneumonia are *Streptococcus pneumoniae* and *Klebsiella pneumoniae*.
- Most common organisms in bronchopneumonia are *Staphylococcus aureus*, gram-negative organisms, and anaerobes.

Suggested Readings

Apisarnthanarak A, Mundy LM: Etiology of community-acquired pneumonia. *Clin Chest Med* 26:47-55, 2005.

Bartlett JG, Dowell SF, Mandell LA, et al: Practice guidelines for the management of community-acquired pneumonia in adults. Infectious Diseases Society of America. *Clin Infect Dis* 31:347-382, 2000.

Herold CJ, Sailer JG: Community-acquired and nosocomial pneumonia. *Eur Radiol* 14(Suppl 3):E2-E20, 2004.

Lutfiyya MN, Henley E, Chang LF, Reyburn SW: Diagnosis and treatment of community-acquired pneumonia. *Am Fam Physician* 73:442-450, 2006.

Sharma S, Maycher B, Eschun G: Radiological imaging in pneumonia: Recent innovations. *Curr Opin Pulm Med* 13:159-169, 2007.

Washington L, Palacio D: Imaging of bacterial pulmonary infection in the immunocompetent patient. *Semin Roentgenol* 42:122-145, 2007.

Nosocomial Pneumonia

DEFINITION: Nosocomial pneumonia is hospital-acquired pneumonia that occurs ≥ 48 hours after admission.

IMAGING

Radiography

Findings

- Bronchopneumonia: patchy areas of consolidation, which may be lobular, subsegmental, or segmental, although they may coalesce to involve entire lobe or cavitate.
- Lung abscess: single or multiple masses usually measuring 2-6 cm in diameter, often cavitated; internal margins of abscesses smooth (90%) or shaggy (10%); air-fluid levels possible.
- Necrotizing pneumonia: initially small lucencies within area of consolidated lung, with enlargement of lobe, outward bulging of fissure ("bulging fissure" sign), then lucencies coalescing into large cavity.

Utility

- Posteroanterior (and lateral when possible) chest radiography should be obtained whenever pneumonia is suspected according to American Thoracic Society guidelines.
- Radiography provides important information regarding extent of pneumonia, presence of complications.
- Although certain radiologic patterns are highly suggestive of pneumonia, chest radiography is of limited value in determining specific etiology.
- Manifestations are often delayed, which is particularly important in nosocomial infections (radiographs are often performed within hours of onset of symptoms).
- Radiographic abnormalities may be particularly delayed in immunocompromised patients.

CT

Findings

- Bronchopneumonia: centrilobular nodules and branching opacities ("tree-in-bud" pattern) due to bronchiolitis, progressing to airspace nodules, lobular, subsegmental, segmental, or confluent areas of consolidation.
- Lung abscesses: masses with low attenuation in central region or cavitation and rim enhancement after intravenous administration of a contrast agent.

Utility

- Can be helpful in detection, differential diagnosis, and management of patients with pulmonary or pleural complications.

DIAGNOSTIC PEARLS

- Vast majority of nosocomial pneumonias manifest as bronchopneumonia.
- Radiographic abnormalities are often delayed particularly in immunocompromised patients.
- Radiologic manifestations of nosocomial pneumonia are often indistinguishable from other pulmonary complications commonly seen in these patients.

- Findings suggestive of pneumonia evident up to 5 days earlier than chest radiographs.
- Recommended in cases of clinically suspected infection and normal or nonspecific radiographic findings, assessment of suspected complications, and suspicion of underlying lesion.

CLINICAL PRESENTATION

- Characteristic clinical findings of pneumonia consist of fever, cough, and purulent sputum.
- Signs and symptoms of pneumonia may be milder or even absent in the elderly.

DIFFERENTIAL DIAGNOSIS

- Acute respiratory distress syndrome (ARDS)
- Organizing pneumonia
- Acute pulmonary embolism and infarction
- Atelectasis
- Pulmonary hemorrhage

PATHOLOGY

- Nosocomial pneumonia most commonly manifests as bronchopneumonia.
- Bronchopneumonia occurs when infectious organisms are deposited on epithelium of bronchi and produce acute bronchial inflammation with epithelial ulcerations and fibrinopurulent exudate formation.

WHAT THE REFERRING PHYSICIAN NEEDS TO KNOW

- Main role of chest radiograph is in confirming presence of parenchymal disease in patients with clinically suspected pneumonia.
- Main role of CT is in evaluation of immunocompromised patients with suspected pulmonary infection but normal or nonspecific radiographic findings and suspected complications.
- Radiographic appearance of consolidation may be delayed particularly in patients with neutropenia, functional defects of granulocytes due to diabetes, alcoholism, or uremia.

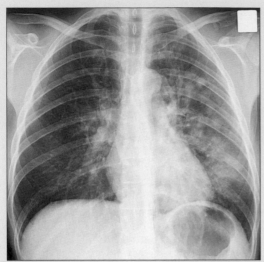

Figure 1. Bronchopneumonia. Posteroanterior chest radiograph shows patchy consolidation in the left upper and lower lobes. Note inhomogeneous increased opacity of the left side of the heart compared with the region of the right atrium consistent with consolidation in the retrocardiac region of the left lower lobe. The patient was a 36-year-old woman with bronchopneumonia.

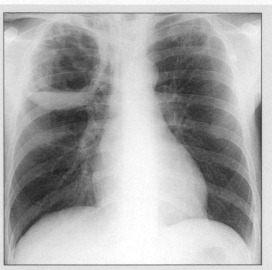

Figure 2. Lung abscess. Posteroanterior chest radiograph shows large cavity with air-fluid level in the right upper lobe. Also noted are small poorly defined areas of consolidation in the upper lobe. The patient was a 39-year-old man. Blood cultures grew *Salmonella*.

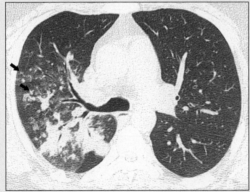

Figure 3. Bronchopneumonia. High-resolution CT image at the level of the upper zone shows centrilobular nodular and branching opacities ("tree-in-bud" pattern) (*arrows*), airspace nodules, focal areas of consolidation, and ground-glass opacities. The areas of consolidation have the size and shape consistent with involvement of one or more adjacent lobules (lobular pneumonia). The abnormalities involve the right upper, middle, and lower lobes and, to lesser extent, the left lower lobe. The patient was a 39-year-old man with acute myelogenous leukemia and bacterial bronchopneumonia.

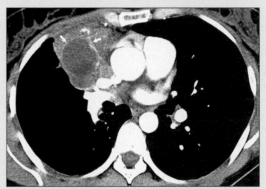

Figure 4. Lung abscess. Contrast-enhanced CT demonstrates large area of dense consolidation in the right upper lobe abutting the mediastinum. The consolidation contains a focal area of decreased attenuation with rim enhancement (*arrows*) characteristic of lung abscess. The patient was a 43-year-old woman with lung abscess secondary to *Haemophilus aphrophilus*.

INCIDENCE/PREVALENCE AND EPIDEMIOLOGY

- Pneumonia develops in 0.5% to 1.0% of hospitalized patients; mortality in such patients is higher, being estimated at approximately 30%.
- Pneumonia is particularly common after surgery and in patients undergoing mechanical ventilation.
- Causes include *S. aureus* (15% or more), *Pseudomonas aeruginosa* (20%), *Legionella* species (1%-40%), *K. pneumoniae* (15%), and *E. coli* (5% to 20%).

Suggested Readings

Depuydt P, Myny D, Blot S: Nosocomial pneumonia: Aetiology, diagnosis and treatment. *Curr Opin Pulm Med* 12:192-197, 2006.

Herold CJ, Sailer JG: Community-acquired and nosocomial pneumonia. *Eur Radiol* 14(Suppl 3):E2-E20, 2004.

Hubmayr RD, Burchardi H, Elliot M, et al: Statement of the 4th International Consensus Conference in Critical Care on ICU-Acquired Pneumonia. Chicago, May 2002, Illinois, Intensive Care Med 28:1521-1536, 2002.

Ostendorf U, Ewig S, Torres A: Nosocomial pneumonia. *Curr Opin Infect Dis* 19:327-338, 2006.

Porzecanski I, Bowton DL: Diagnosis and treatment of ventilator-associated pneumonia. *Chest* 130:597-604, 2006.

Pneumonia in the Immunocompromised Host

DEFINITION: Pneumonia that occurs in patient with impaired immune function has higher propensity for diffuse and bilateral disease.

IMAGING

Radiography

Findings

- Focal, multifocal, or confluent consolidation.
- Necrotizing pneumonia with cavity formation may occur particularly in infection by gram-negative organisms or *Staphylococcus aureus*.
- *Pneumocystis jiroveci* (formerly *Pneumocystis carinii*) pneumonia: bilateral perihilar or diffuse finely granular or ground-glass opacities that may progress to consolidation.
- CMV pneumonia: bilateral diffuse areas of parenchymal opacification; multiple pulmonary nodules typically <5 mm.

Utility

- Posteroanterior (and lateral when possible) chest radiography should be obtained whenever pneumonia is suspected according to American Thoracic Society guidelines.
- Radiography provides important information regarding extent of pneumonia and presence of complications.
- Although certain radiologic patterns are highly suggestive of pneumonia, chest radiography is of limited value in determining specific etiology.

CT

Findings

- Bacterial pneumonia: focal, multifocal, or confluent consolidation; associated findings often including ground-glass opacities, centrilobular nodules, tree-in-bud pattern, cavitation, and pleural effusion.
- *Pneumocystis* pneumonia: diffuse ground-glass opacities, sometimes in geographic distribution, with predilection for central, perihilar, upper lobe lung regions; "crazy-paving" pattern.
- *Aspergillus* bronchiolitis and bronchopneumonia: centrilobular nodules, tree-in-bud pattern, bronchopneumonia.
- Angioinvasive aspergillosis: typically manifests as multiple nodules with halo of ground-glass attenuation (CT halo sign).

DIAGNOSTIC PEARLS

- Bronchopneumonia: consolidation initially involves mainly peribronchiolar region but gradually extends to involve entire lobules, subsegments, and segments.
- Cavitation, lymphadenopathy, abscess formation, necrotizing pneumonia, pneumatocele, pleural effusion, empyema, and nodules occur.
- There is a higher propensity for multilobar and bilateral disease.
- Type and severity of immune defect will determine type of infection most likely to occur.

- CMV pneumonia: bilateral parenchymal consolidation, ground-glass opacities, nodules <10 mm that may have halo of ground-glass attenuation (CT halo sign).

Utility

- Useful if chest radiograph is normal or equivocal and pulmonary disease is suspected.
- May demonstrate parenchymal abnormalities in up to 50% of neutropenic patients with normal chest radiographs with suspected pneumonia.
- May show findings suggestive of pneumonia up to 5 days earlier than chest radiographs.

CLINICAL PRESENTATION

- Fever, cough, wheezing, and dyspnea are reported.
- Signs and symptoms may be greatly muted or absent in an immunocompromised host.
- HIV patients with bacterial pneumonia have acute onset of fever, pleuritic chest pain, productive cough, and purulent sputum.
- HIV patients with *Pneumocystis* pneumonia typically present after having symptoms for more than 1 week to 1 month.

WHAT THE REFERRING PHYSICIAN NEEDS TO KNOW

- In most situations, radiographic and CT findings are nonspecific and do not allow confident diagnosis of specific pathogen or disease process.
- Type and severity of immune defect will determine type of infection most likely to occur.
- Respiratory viral infections in the immunocompromised have a higher rate of nosocomial spread with a greater likelihood of spread to involve the lower respiratory tract and higher mortality.

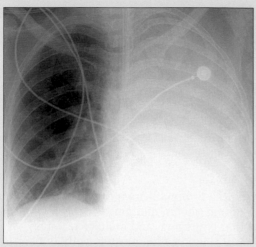

Figure 1. **Severe pneumococcal pneumonia in HIV patient:** chest radiograph demonstrates complete opacification of the left thorax *(Courtesy of Dr. Joel E. Fishman, University of Miami)*

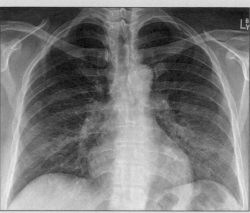

Figure 2. *Pneumocystis* **pneumonia.** Chest radiograph in a 42-year-old woman with newly diagnosed AIDS and *Pneumocystis* pneumonia shows symmetric, bilateral, hazy, increased opacity (ground-glass opacity).

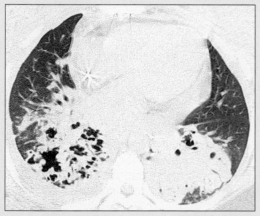

Figure 3. *P. aeruginosa and S. aureus* **pneumonia:** High-resolution CT image of a 22-year-old double-lung transplant recipient shows necrotizing pneumonia in both lower lobes. *(Courtesy of Dr. Ann Leung, Stanford University)*

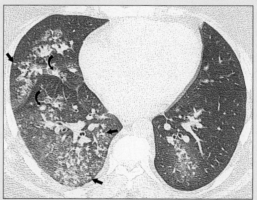

Figure 4. **Bronchopneumonia.** High-resolution CT image at the level of the lower lung zone shows centrilobular nodular and branching opacities ("tree-in-bud" pattern) *(straight arrows)*, airspace nodules *(curved arrows)*, focal areas of consolidation, and ground-glass opacities. The areas of consolidation have the size and shape consistent with involvement of one or more adjacent lobules (lobular pneumonia). The abnormalities involve the right upper, middle and lower lobes, and, to lesser extent, the left lower lobe. The patient was a 39-year-old man with acute myelogenous leukemia and bacterial bronchopneumonia.

DIFFERENTIAL DIAGNOSIS

- Drug-induced lung disease
- Pulmonary edema
- Pulmonary hemorrhage
- Lymphoma
- Pulmonary embolism and infarction

PATHOLOGY

- Microorganisms reach the lower respiratory tract via three routes: airways, vasculature, and direct spread from extrapulmonary sites.
- Bronchopneumonia occurs when infectious organisms are deposited on epithelium of bronchi, produce acute bronchial inflammation with epithelial ulcerations and fibrinopurulent exudate formation.
- Cavitation particularly with gram-negative organisms, *Staphylococcus aureus,* and invasive aspergillosis.
- *Pneumocystis* pneumonia: extensive ground-glass attenuation corresponds to presence of intra-alveolar exudate, consisting of surfactant, fibrin, cellular debris, and organisms.

INCIDENCE/PREVALENCE AND EPIDEMIOLOGY

- Bacteria are most common cause of infections.
- In neutropenic patient population, *Pseudomonas aeruginosa, Streptococcus pneumoniae,* and *Escherichia coli* are most common pathogens isolated during episodes of bacteremic pneumonia.

- In solid organ transplant population, nosocomial pneumonias caused by gram-negative organisms or *Staphylococcus aureus* occur almost exclusively as a perioperative complication.
- *Pneumocystis* pneumonia remains the most common opportunistic infection in patients infected with HIV and may also occur in patients receiving chemotherapy or long courses of corticosteroids.
- CMV is most common viral pathogen associated with life-threatening pulmonary infection in immunocompromised host.

Suggested Readings

Franquet T: Respiratory infection in the AIDS and immunocompromised patient. *Eur Radiol* 14(Suppl 3):E21-E33, 2004.

Haramati LB, Jenny-Avital ER: Approach to the diagnosis of pulmonary disease in patients infected with the human immunodeficiency virus. *J Thorac Imaging* 13:247-260, 1998.

Heussel CP, Kauczor HU, Ullmann AJ: Pneumonia in neutropenic patients. *Eur Radiol* 14:256-271, 2004.

Maki DD: Pulmonary infections in HIV/AIDS. *Semin Roentgenol* 35:124-139, 2002.

Oh YW, Effman EL, Godwin JD: Pulmonary infections in immunocompromised hosts: The importance of correlating the conventional radiologic appearance with the clinical setting. *Radiology* 217:647-656, 2000.

Lobar Pneumonia

DEFINITION: Lobar pneumonia is characterized histologically by filling of alveolar airspaces of one lobe by an exudate of edema fluid and neutrophils that crosses segmental boundaries.

IMAGING

Radiography
Findings
- Homogeneous airspace consolidation involving adjacent segments of lobe.
- Consolidation occurring initially in periphery of lung beneath visceral pleura and usually abutting an interlobar fissure with spreading centrally across segmental boundaries and possible eventual involvement of entire lobe.
- Bronchi usually patent, resulting in air bronchograms within areas of consolidation.

Utility
- Confirms presence of parenchymal disease in patients with clinically suspected pneumonia.
- Has high sensitivity and specificity in the detection and exclusion of community-acquired pneumonia.
- Of limited value in determining the specific etiology of pneumonia.
- Manifestations of pneumonia often delayed.
- Appearance of radiographic abnormalities particularly delayed in patients with neutropenia.

CT
Findings
- Homogeneous airspace consolidation involving adjacent segments of lobe
- Consolidation occurring initially in periphery of lung beneath visceral pleura and usually abutting an interlobar fissure with spreading centrally across segmental boundaries and possible eventual involvement of entire lobe
- Ground-glass opacities denoting incomplete filling of alveoli often seen adjacent to the airspace consolidation
- Air bronchograms

DIAGNOSTIC PEARLS
- Homogeneous airspace consolidation involving adjacent segments of a lobe.
- Consolidation occurring initially in periphery of lung beneath visceral pleura and usually abutting an interlobar fissure with spreading centrally across segmental boundaries and possible eventual involvement of entire lobe.

Utility
- Better depiction with high-resolution CT than with radiography of pattern and distribution of pneumonia.
- Has greater sensitivity than radiography in demonstrating the presence of pulmonary abnormalities.
- Seldom required in the evaluation of patients with suspected or proven bacterial pneumonia.
- Recommended in patients with clinical suspicion of infection with normal or nonspecific radiographic findings.
- Useful in assessment of suspected complications of pneumonia or suspicion of an underlying lesion such as pulmonary carcinoma.
- Indicated in patients with pneumonia and persistent or recurrent pulmonary opacities.

CLINICAL PRESENTATION
- Fever
- Cough
- Purulent sputum
- Pleuritic chest pain
- Hemoptysis
- In elderly: signs and symptoms of pneumonia often milder or even absent

---

WHAT THE REFERRING PHYSICIAN NEEDS TO KNOW

- Complications associated with bacterial pneumonia include abscess formation, necrotizing pneumonia, pneumatocele formation, pleural effusion, and empyema.
- Treatment of pneumonia depends on the organism causing infection, patient's immune status, and severity of symptoms.
- Vast majority of cases respond to oral antibiotics.
- Radiographic appearance of consolidation is delayed in neutropenic patients and patients with functional defects of granulocytes due to diabetes, alcoholism, and uremia.

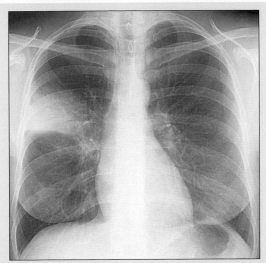

Figure 1. Lobar pneumonia. Posteroanterior chest radiograph shows focal area of consolidation in the right upper lobe abutting the minor fissure. Patent bronchi (air bronchograms) are seen within the area of consolidation. The patient was a 43-year-old woman with lobar pneumonia due to *Streptococcus pneumoniae.*

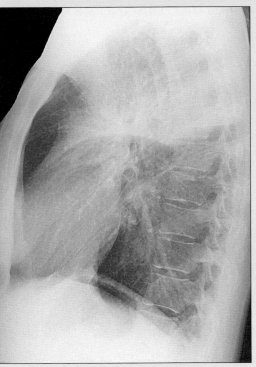

Figure 2. Lobar pneumonia. Lateral view demonstrates that the consolidation involves the anterior and posterior segments of the right upper lobe. Because the consolidation crosses the boundaries between two adjacent segments it is known as nonsegmental or lobar consolidation. The patient was a 43-year-old woman with lobar pneumonia due to *Streptococcus pneumoniae.*

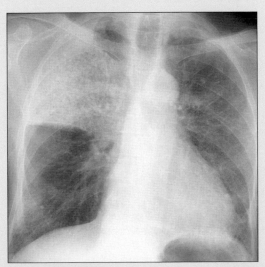

Figure 3. Lobar pneumonia. Posteroanterior chest radiograph show diffuse right upper lobe consolidation. The patient was a 79-year-old man with lobar pneumonia due to *Streptococcus pneumoniae.*

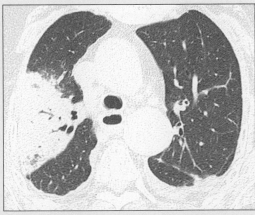

Figure 4. Lobar pneumonia. High-resolution CT image shows consolidation in the right upper lobe abutting the minor fissure and containing several air bronchograms. Incidental note is made of esophageal dilatation and a small left pleural effusion. The patient was an 80-year-old man with lobar pneumonia due to *Streptococcus pneumoniae.*

DIFFERENTIAL DIAGNOSIS

- Bronchopneumonia
- Obstructive pneumonitis
- Aspiration pneumonia

PATHOLOGY

- Lobar pneumonia is characterized histologically by filling of alveolar airspaces by exudate of edema fluid and neutrophils.
- Consolidation begins in periphery of lung adjacent to visceral pleura and spreads centripetally via interalveolar pores and small airways.
- Airspace filling typically extends across pulmonary segments (nonsegmental consolidation), sometimes to involve entire lobe.
- Most important pathogenetic feature is rapid production of edema fluid.
- Vast majority of cases are caused by bacteria: *Streptococcus pneumoniae, Klebsiella pneumoniae, Legionella pneumophila, Haemophilus influenzae,* and *Mycobacterium tuberculosis.*

INCIDENCE/PREVALENCE AND EPIDEMIOLOGY

- Pneumonia is a common cause of morbidity and mortality.
- In the United States there are an estimated 4 million cases of community-acquired pneumonia annually, resulting in approximately 600,000 hospitalizations.

- *Streptococcus pneumoniae* is the most common cause of community-acquired pneumonia requiring hospitalization.
- The vast majority of cases of lobar pneumonia are community acquired and due to *S. pneumoniae;* other causes include *K. pneumoniae, L. pneumophila, H. influenzae,* and *M. tuberculosis.*
- Nosocomial pneumonia including pneumonia due to *S. pneumoniae* or *K. pneumoniae* usually manifests in pattern of bronchopneumonia.

Suggested Readings

Herold CJ, Sailer JG: Community-acquired and nosocomial pneumonia. *Eur Radiol* 14(Suppl 3):E2-E20, 2004.

Marrie TJ: Pneumococcal pneumonia: Epidemiology and clinical features. *Semin Respir Infect* 14:227-236, 1999.

Ruiz M, Ewig S, Marcos MA, et al: Etiology of community-acquired pneumonia: Impact of age, comorbidity, and severity. *Am J Respir Crit Care Med* 160:397-405, 1999.

Waite S, Jeudy J, White CS: Acute lung infections in normal and immunocompromised hosts. *Radiol Clin North Am* 44:295-315, 2006:ix.

Washington L, Palacio D: Imaging of bacterial pulmonary infection in the immunocompetent patient. *Semin Roentgenol* 42:122-145, 2007.

Woodhead M: Community-acquired pneumonia in Europe: Causative pathogens and resistance patterns. *Eur Respir J* (Suppl 36):20s-27s, 2002.

Bronchopneumonia

DEFINITION: Bronchopneumonia differs pathogenetically from lobar pneumonia by production of a relatively small amount of fluid and rapid exudation of numerous polymorphonuclear leukocytes in relation to small membranous and respiratory bronchioles.

IMAGING

Radiography
Findings
- Patchy areas of consolidation involving one or more segments of single lobe or multiple lobes.
- Poorly defined focal nodular opacities measuring 5-10 mm in diameter (airspace nodules).
- Cavitation common, particularly in patients with extensive consolidation.
- Results in loss of volume of affected segments or lobes.
- Air bronchograms seldom evident.

Utility
- Confirms presence of parenchymal disease in patients with clinically suspected pneumonia.
- Has high sensitivity and specificity in detection and exclusion of community-acquired pneumonia.
- Of limited value in determining specific cause of pneumonia.

CT
Findings
- Centrilobular nodules and branching opacities ("tree-in-bud" pattern) are due to infectious bronchiolitis.
- Patchy airspace nodules (centrilobular lesions with poorly defined margins measuring 4-10 mm in diameter) are seen.
- Small foci of consolidation (airspace nodules) may progress to lobular, subsegmental, or segmental areas of consolidation.
- Areas of consolidation may be patchy or confluent and unilateral or bilateral but usually involve two or more lobes.
- Single or multiple cavitations may occur, pleural effusion and empyema, and hilar lymphadenopathy may occur.

Utility
- With high-resolution, allows better depiction of pattern and distribution of pneumonia than radiography.
- Has greater sensitivity than radiography in demonstrating presence of pulmonary abnormalities.
- Seldom required in evaluation of patients with suspected or proven bacterial pneumonia.

DIAGNOSTIC PEARLS

- Patchy areas of consolidation involving one or more segments of a single lobe or multiple lobes.
- Centrilobular nodules and tree-in-bud pattern on high-resolution CT.

- Recommended in patients with clinical suspicion of infection with normal or nonspecific radiographic findings.
- Useful in assessment of suspected complications of pneumonia or suspicion of an underlying lesion such as pulmonary carcinoma.
- Indicated in patients with pneumonia and persistent or recurrent pulmonary opacities.

CLINICAL PRESENTATION

- Fever
- Cough
- Purulent sputum
- Pleuritic chest pain
- Hemoptysis
- Signs and symptoms of pneumonia milder or even absent in the elderly

DIFFERENTIAL DIAGNOSIS

- Lobar pneumonia
- Organizing pneumonia
- Tuberculosis
- Septic embolism
- Pulmonary hemorrhage

PATHOLOGY

- Bacterial pneumonia is usually acquired by aspiration or inhalation of microorganisms.
- Production of a relatively small amount of fluid occurs.

WHAT THE REFERRING PHYSICIAN NEEDS TO KNOW

- Complications associated with bacterial pneumonia include abscess formation, necrotizing pneumonia, pneumatocele formation, pleural effusion, and empyema.
- Treatment of pneumonia depends on the organism causing the infection, the patient's immune status, and the severity of symptoms.
- Radiographic appearance of consolidation is delayed in neutropenic patients and in patients with functional defects of granulocytes due to diabetes, alcoholism, or uremia.

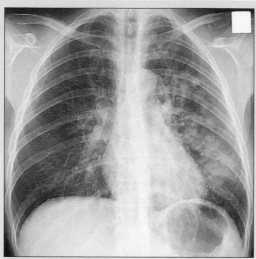

Figure 1. **Bronchopneumonia.** Posteroanterior chest radiograph shows patchy consolidation in the left upper and lower lobes. Note inhomogeneous increased opacity of the left side of the heart compared with the region of the right atrium consistent with consolidation in the retrocardiac region of the left lower lobe. The patient was a 36-year-old woman with bronchopneumonia.

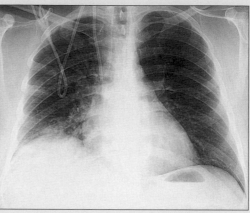

Figure 2. **Bronchopneumonia.** Chest radiograph shows poorly defined nodular opacities and small foci of consolidation in the right lung. A central venous line is in place. The patient was a 29-year-old man with acute myelogenous leukemia and *Streptococcus pneumoniae* pneumonia.

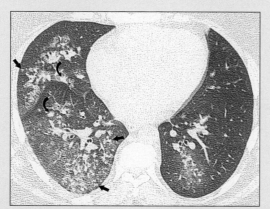

Figure 3. **Bronchopneumonia.** High-resolution CT image at the level of the lower lung zone shows centrilobular nodular and branching opacities ("tree-in-bud" pattern) (*straight arrows*), airspace nodules (*curved arrows*), focal areas of consolidation, and ground-glass opacities. The areas of consolidation have the size and shape consistent with involvement of one or more adjacent lobules (lobular pneumonia). The patient was a 39-year-old man with acute myelogenous leukemia and bacterial bronchopneumonia.

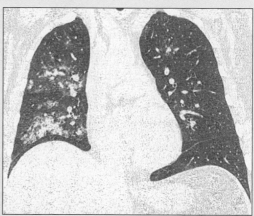

Figure 4. **Bronchopneumonia.** Coronal reformatted CT image demonstrates centrilobular nodular opacities and small foci of consolidation in the right upper and middle lobes and, to lesser extent, left upper lobe. The patient was a 29-year-old man with acute myelogenous leukemia and *Streptococcus pneumoniae* pneumonia.

- There is rapid exudation of numerous polymorphonuclear leukocytes, in relation to small membranous and respiratory bronchioles.
- Neutrophils appear to limit spread of organisms, resulting in a patchy appearance of the disease.
- Consolidation initially involves mainly peribronchiolar region but gradually extends to involve entire lobules, subsegments and segments.
- Several lobes may be involved.

INCIDENCE/PREVALENCE AND EPIDEMIOLOGY

- Pneumonia is a common cause of morbidity and mortality.
- In the United States there are an estimated 4 million cases of community-acquired pneumonia annually, resulting in approximately 600,000 hospitalizations.
- Overall mortality rate is approximately 14%.

- Pneumonia develops in 0.5% to 1.0% of hospitalized patients.
- Bronchopneumonia may be due to a variety of bacterial organisms, fungi, or viruses.
- Common causes include *Staphylococcus aureus*, *Escherichia coli*, *Pseudomonas aeruginosa*, *Haemophilus influenzae*, and anaerobes.

Suggested Readings

Apisarnthanarak A, Mundy LM: Etiology of community-acquired pneumonia. *Clin Chest Med* 26:47-55, 2005.

Herold CJ, Sailer JG: Community-acquired and nosocomial pneumonia. *Eur Radiol* 14(Suppl 3):E2-E20, 2004.

Lutfiyya MN, Henley E, Chang LF, Reyburn SW: Diagnosis and treatment of community-acquired pneumonia. *Am Fam Physician* 73:442-450, 2006.

Sharma S, Maycher B, Eschun G: Radiological imaging in pneumonia: Recent innovations. *Curr Opin Pulm Med* 13:159-169, 2007.

Washington L, Palacio D: Imaging of bacterial pulmonary infection in the immunocompetent patient. *Semin Roentgenol* 42:122-145, 2007.

Common Complications of Pneumonia

DEFINITION: Complications with bacterial pneumonia include abscess formation, necrotizing pneumonia, pneumatocele formation, pleural effusion, and empyema.

IMAGING

Radiography

Findings

- Lung abscesses: single or multiple masses usually measuring 2-6 cm in diameter that are often cavitated.
- Internal margins of abscesses appearing smooth (90%) or shaggy (10%).
- Necrotizing pneumonia: initially small lucencies within area of consolidated lung associated with lobar enlargement and outward bulging of fissure.
- Lucencies that rapidly coalesce into a large cavity containing fluid and sloughed lung.
- Pneumatoceles: single or multiple thin-walled, gas-filled spaces in areas of consolidation or ground-glass opacities.
- Pleural effusion.

Utility

- Often first imaging modality in patients with suspected complication of pneumonia.

CT

Findings

- Lung abscesses: single/multiple masses with low-attenuation central region or cavitation and rim enhancement after intravenous administration of a contrast agent.
- Smooth or shaggy-appearing abscess wall.
- Pneumatoceles: thin-walled, gas-filled spaces in areas of ground-glass opacity or consolidation in patients with acute pneumonia that resemble bullae, increase in size over days or weeks, and resolve over weeks to months.
- Pleural effusion.
- Pleural thickening and enhancement in empyema (may be absent in early stages).

Utility

- Helpful in assessment of suspected complications of pneumonia or suspicion of an underlying lesion such as pulmonary carcinoma
- Superior to the radiograph in demonstrating presence of abscess formation, pleural effusion, and empyema.

CLINICAL PRESENTATION

- Fever
- Cough
- Purulent sputum

DIAGNOSTIC PEARLS

- Lung abscess: single or multiple masses often cavitated with smooth or shaggy-appearing wall.
- Pneumatoceles: thin-walled, gas-filled spaces in areas of ground-glass opacity or consolidation.
- Intravenous contrast particularly helpful in demonstrating presence of abscess and empyema.

- Pleuritic chest pain
- Hemoptysis

PATHOLOGY

- Complications associated with bacterial pneumonia include abscess formation, necrotizing pneumonia, pneumatocele formation, pleural effusion, and empyema.
- Lung abscess is an inflammatory mass within lung parenchyma, the central part of which has undergone purulent liquefaction necrosis.
- A pneumatocele is a thin-walled, gas-filled space within the lung, usually occurring in association with acute pneumonia and almost invariably transient. It results from drainage of a necrotic lung parenchyma focus followed by check-valve airway obstruction subtending it, enabling air to enter the parenchymal space during inspiration but preventing its egress during expiration.
- Pneumatoceles appear in recovery phase of pneumonia, may result in pneumothorax, and usually resolve over weeks or months.

INCIDENCE/PREVALENCE AND EPIDEMIOLOGY

- Most common cause of lung abscess is aspiration.
- Most commonly affected areas are the posterior segment of an upper lobe or the superior segment of a lower lobe.
- Common causes of lung abscess are anaerobic bacteria (e.g., *Fusobacterium nucleatum* and *Bacteroides* species), *Staphylococcus aureus*, *Pseudomonas aeruginosa*, and *Klebsiella pneumoniae*.

WHAT THE REFERRING PHYSICIAN NEEDS TO KNOW

- Complications occur more commonly in immunosuppressed and debilitated patients.
- CT is superior to the radiograph in demonstrating pulmonary and pleural complications of pneumonia.

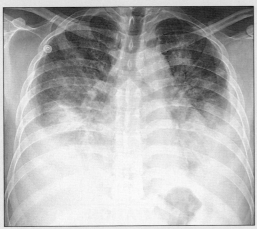

Figure 1. *Staphylococcus aureus* **pneumonia.** Chest radiograph shows extensive bilateral areas of consolidation and pleural effusions. The patient was a 38-year-old man with community-acquired staphylococcal pneumonia.

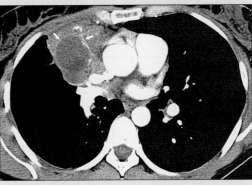

Figure 2. Lung abscess. Contrast-enhanced CT demonstrates large area of dense consolidation in the right upper lobe abutting the mediastinum. The consolidation contains a focal area of decreased attenuation with rim enhancement (*arrows*) characteristic of lung abscess. The patient was a 43-year-old woman with lung abscess secondary to *Haemophilus aphrophilus.*

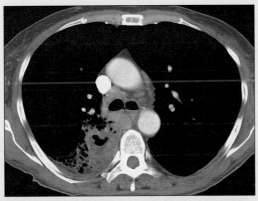

Figure 3. Lung abscess and empyema due to anaerobic infection. Contrast-enhanced CT image shows abscess in the right lower lobe. Also evident are enlarged paratracheal lymph nodes and a small right pleural effusion. Culture of pleural fluid confirmed presence of empyema by anaerobic organisms. The patient was a 57-year-old woman.

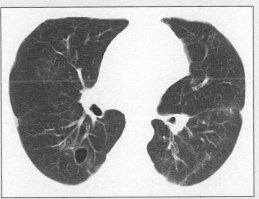

Figure 4. Pneumatocele after *S. pneumoniae* **pneumonia.** CT scan in a 47-year-old man with resolving *S. pneumoniae* bronchopneumonia shows thin-walled cystic lesion (pneumatocele) in right lower lobe, patchy bilateral ground-glass opacities, and a few poorly defined centrilobular nodules.

■ Pneumatoceles are most commonly associated with *S. aureus* pneumonia in infants and children and with *Pneumocystis jiroveci* pneumonia in adults.

Suggested Readings

Feuerstein I, Archer A, Pluda JM, et al: Thin-walled cavities, cysts, and pneumothorax in *Pneumocystis carinii* pneumonia: Further observations with histopathologic correlation. *Radiology* 174: 697-702, 1990.

Imamoglu M, Cay A, Kosucu P, et al: Pneumatoceles in postpneumonic empyema: An algorithmic approach. *J Pediatr Surg* 40: 1111-1117, 2005.

Klein JS, Schultz S, Heffner JE: Interventional radiology of the chest: Image-guided percutaneous drainage of pleural effusions, lung abscess, and pneumothorax. *AJR Am J Roentgenol* 164:581-588, 1995.

Mori T, Ebe T, Takahashi M, et al: Lung abscess: Analysis of 66 cases from 1979 to 1991. *Intern Med* 32:278-284, 1993.

Quigley MJ, Fraser RS: Pulmonary pneumatocele: Pathology and pathogenesis. *AJR Am J Roentgenol* 150:1275-1277, 1988.

Romano L, Pinto A, Merola S, et al: Intensive-care unit lung infections: The role of imaging with special emphasis on multi-detector row computed tomography. *Eur J Radiol* 65:333-339, 2008.

Rubin SA, Winer-Muram HT, Ellis JV: Diagnostic imaging of pneumonia and its complications in the critically ill patient. *Clin Chest Med* 16:45-59, 1995.

Sharma S, Maycher B, Eschun G: Radiological imaging in pneumonia: Recent innovations. *Curr Opin Pulm Med* 13:159-169, 2007.

Vilar J, Domingo ML, Soto C, Cogollos J: Radiology of bacterial pneumonia. *Eur J Radiol* 51:102-113, 2004.

Pneumonia (*Streptococcus pneumoniae*)

DEFINITION: Pneumonia caused by *Streptococcus pneumoniae* may occur after aspiration of organisms from a focus of colonization in the nasopharynx.

IMAGING

Radiography

Findings

- Homogeneous consolidation that crosses segmental boundaries (nonsegmental) but involves only one lobe (lobar pneumonia).
- Spherical focus of consolidation that simulates a mass (round pneumonia), seen more commonly in children.
- Consolidation that abuts against a visceral pleural space, either interlobar or over convexity of the lung.
- Other patterns: patchy unilateral or bilateral areas of consolidation (bronchopneumonia) and mixed air-space and reticulonodular opacities.
- Lobar expansion with bulging of interlobar fissure.
- Pleural effusion in approximately 10% of patients.

Utility

- First and usually only imaging modality used in the initial assessment and follow-up.

CT

Findings

- Homogeneous consolidation that crosses segmental boundaries (nonsegmental) but involves only one lobe (lobar pneumonia).
- Spherical focus of consolidation that simulates a mass (round pneumonia); occurs more commonly in children.
- Consolidation that abuts against a visceral pleural space, either interlobar or over convexity of the lung.
- Other patterns: patchy unilateral or bilateral areas of consolidation (bronchopneumonia) and mixed air-space and reticulonodular opacities.
- Lobar expansion with bulging of interlobar fissure.
- Ipsilateral hilar or mediastinal lymphadenopathy.
- Pleural effusion in approximately 10% of patients.

Utility

- Seldom adds any clinically relevant information in patients with characteristic radiographic and clinical findings and thus seldom warranted.
- Helpful in patients with suspected complications such as cavitation, empyema, and bronchopleural fistula seen on a radiograph.

DIAGNOSTIC PEARLS

- May result in lobar pneumonia or bronchopneumonia.
- May result in lobar expansion with bulging of interlobar fissure.
- Most commonly identified pathogen in community-acquired pneumonia.

CLINICAL PRESENTATION

- Abrupt in onset
- Fever
- Chills
- Cough
- Pleuritic chest pain
- In elderly: classic features possibly absent

DIFFERENTIAL DIAGNOSIS

- Lobar pneumonia caused by other organisms
- Bronchopneumonia caused by other organisms
- Organizing pneumonia
- Obstructive pneumonitis

PATHOLOGY

- *Streptococcus pneumoniae* (pneumococcus) is a gram-positive bacterium that is oval or lancet shaped and usually arranged in pairs.
- Pattern is most commonly of homogeneous airspace (lobar) pneumonia and less commonly of bronchopneumonia and round pneumonia (most commonly in children).
- Risk factors include extremes of age, chronic heart or lung disease, immunosuppression, alcoholism, institutionalization, and prior splenectomy.

INCIDENCE/PREVALENCE AND EPIDEMIOLOGY

- *S. pneumoniae* is most commonly identified pathogenic organism in patients admitted to a hospital for pneumonia, accounting for 40% of all isolated species.

WHAT THE REFERRING PHYSICIAN NEEDS TO KNOW

- Pneumonia may be confused with, or confounded by, other common medical problems (e.g., congestive heart failure, pulmonary thromboembolism, malignancy).
- Majority of patients respond rapidly to antibiotic therapy.
- In some cases the pneumonia may progress rapidly in spite of apparently adequate treatment.

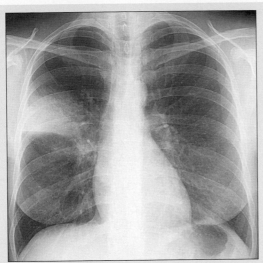

Figure 1. Lobar pneumonia. Posteroanterior chest radiograph shows focal area of consolidation in the right upper lobe abutting the minor fissure. Patent bronchi (air bronchograms) are seen within the area of consolidation. The patient was a 43-year-old woman with lobar pneumonia due to *S. pneumoniae.*

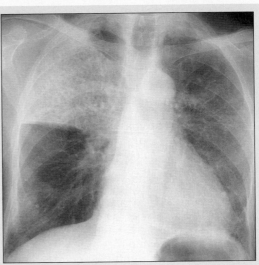

Figure 2. Lobar pneumonia. Posteroanterior chest radiograph show diffuse right upper lobe consolidation. The patient was a 79-year-old man with lobar pneumonia due to *S. pneumoniae.*

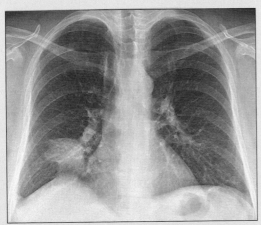

Figure 3. Round pneumonia due to *S. pneumoniae*. Chest radiograph shows mass-like area of consolidation in the right lower lobe (*arrow*). The patient was a 41-year-old man with *S. pneumoniae* pneumonia.

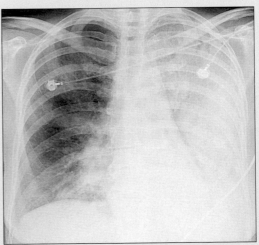

Figure 4. Bronchopneumonia caused by *S. pneumoniae* pneumonia. Chest radiograph demonstrates diffuse dense consolidation of the left lung and patchy areas of consolidation in the right lung. The patient was a previously healthy 49-year-old woman with sputum and blood cultures positive for *S. pneumoniae.*

■ It is the most commonly identified pathogen in community-acquired pneumonia, accounting for approximately 40% of identified organisms.

■ Complications, such as cavitation and pneumatocele formation, are uncommon.

Suggested Readings

Klugman KP, Feldman C: *Streptococcus pneumoniae* respiratory tract infections. *Curr Opin Infect Dis* 14:173-179, 2001.

Ortqvist A, Hedlund J, Kalin M: *Streptococcus pneumoniae*: Epidemiology, risk factors, and clinical features. *Semin Respir Crit Care Med* 26:563-574, 2005.

Porath A, Schlaeffer F, Pick N, et al: Pneumococcal community-acquired pneumonia in 148 hospitalized adult patients. *Eur J Clin Microbiol Infect Dis* 16:863-870, 1997.

Sharma S, Maycher B, Eschun G: Radiological imaging in pneumonia: Recent innovations. *Curr Opin Pulm Med* 13:159-169, 2007.

Stein DL, Haramati LB, Spindola-Franco H, et al: Intrathoracic lymphadenopathy in hospitalized patients with pneumococcal pneumonia. *Chest* 127:1271-1275, 2005.

Vilar J, Domingo ML, Soto C, Cogollos J: Radiology of bacterial pneumonia. *Eur J Radiol* 51:102-113, 2004.

Washington L, Palacio D: Imaging of bacterial pulmonary infection in the immunocompetent patient. *Semin Roentgenol* 42:122-145, 2007.

Pneumonia (*Staphylococcus aureus*)

DEFINITION: Pneumonia that is caused by infection with *Staphylococcus aureus*.

IMAGING

Radiography
Findings
- Characteristic pattern of presentation as bronchopneumonia (lobular pneumonia).
- Poorly defined focal nodular opacities measuring 5-10 mm in diameter (airspace nodules).
- Patchy or confluent areas of consolidation involving one or more segments of a single lobe or multiple lobes.
- Abscess formation: solitary and typically have an irregular shaggy inner wall.
- Pneumatocele formation, spontaneous pneumothorax, pleural effusions, empyemas.
- Septic embolism and multiple nodules or masses throughout lungs.

Utility
- First and foremost imaging modality in the initial assessment and follow-up.

CT
Findings
- Centrilobular nodules and branching opacities ("tree-in-bud" pattern) and lobular, subsegmental, or segmental areas of consolidation.
- Areas of consolidation may be patchy or confluent and unilateral or bilateral but usually involve two or more lobes.
- Abscess formation and pleural effusion.
- Septic embolism and multiple nodules usually measuring 1-3 cm in diameter that frequently cavitate.
- Pulmonary artery occlusion by septic emboli/thrombus resulting in hemorrhage and/or infarction and less well-defined/wedge-shaped foci of disease.
- Subpleural wedge-shaped areas of consolidation, often with central areas of necrosis or frank cavitation.
- Pleural effusion, empyema.

Utility
- Evaluation of patients with suspected cavitation or empyema.

CLINICAL PRESENTATION

- Abrupt onset
- Fever
- Pleuritic chest pain
- Cough and expectoration of purulent yellow or brown sputum, sometimes streaked with blood

DIAGNOSTIC PEARLS

- Patchy unilateral or bilateral consolidation
- Rapid progression
- Centrilobular nodules and "tree-in-bud" pattern on CT
- Abscess formation and empyema
- Pneumatocele formation particularly in children

DIFFERENTIAL DIAGNOSIS

- Bronchopneumonia caused by other organisms
- Organizing pneumonia
- Drug reaction

PATHOLOGY

- *Staphylococcus aureus* is a gram-positive coccus that appears on smear in pairs, short chains, tetrads, or clusters.
- It is distinguished from other staphylococcal species by its production of coagulase, a plasma-clotting enzyme.
- Bronchopneumonia is commonly associated with abscess formation.

INCIDENCE/PREVALENCE AND EPIDEMIOLOGY

- *S. aureus* is an uncommon cause of community-acquired pneumonia, accounting for only about 3% of all cases.
- It is a common pathogenic organism in nosocomial pneumonia, found in 15% or more of all cases.
- There has been an increase in the incidence of methicillin-resistant *S. aureus* (MRSA) infections in patients admitted to intensive care units.
- Bacteremic *S. aureus* pneumonia is found most commonly in patients in intensive care units and in intravenous drug users.

Suggested Readings

Al-Ujayli B, Nafziger DA, Saravolatz L: Pneumonia due to *Staphylococcus aureus* infection. *Clin Chest Med* 16:111-120, 1995.

George DL: Epidemiology of nosocomial pneumonia in intensive care unit patients. *Clin Chest Med* 16:29-44, 1995.

Kaye MG, Fox MJ, Bartlett JG, et al: The clinical spectrum of *Staphylococcus aureus* pulmonary infection. *Chest* 97:788-792, 1990.

Sharma S, Maycher B, Eschun G: Radiological imaging in pneumonia: Recent innovations. *Curr Opin Pulm Med* 13:159-169, 2007.

WHAT THE REFERRING PHYSICIAN NEEDS TO KNOW

- *S. aureus* is an important cause of nosocomial pneumonia, especially in the intensive care unit.
- Methicillin-resistant *S. aureus* (MRSA) infections are an important cause of nosocomial pneumonia.
- MRSA has also been recently described in community-acquired pneumonia.

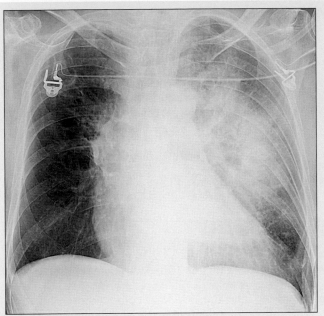

Figure 1. *S. aureus* **pneumonia.** Chest radiograph at hospital admission shows dense consolidation in the left lung and poorly defined opacities in the right upper lobe. The patient was a 51-year-old man with community-acquired staphylococcal pneumonia.

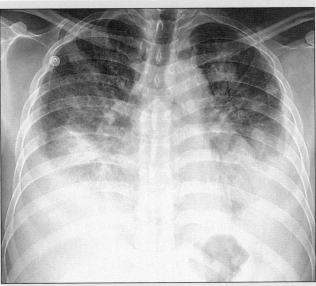

Figure 2. *S. aureus* **pneumonia.** Chest radiograph shows extensive bilateral areas of consolidation and pleural effusions. The patient was a 38-year-old man with community-acquired staphylococcal pneumonia.

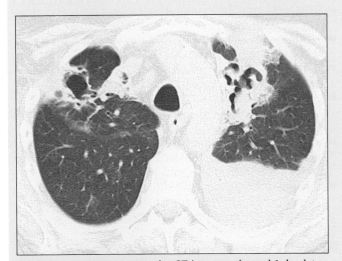

Figure 3. *S. aureus* **pneumonia.** CT image performed 1 day later than radiograph in Figure 1 shows foci of consolidation and abscesses in the upper lobes and dense consolidation in the left lower lobe. The patient was a 51-year-old man with community-acquired staphylococcal pneumonia.

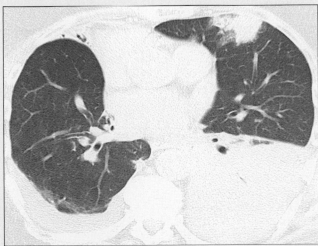

Figure 4. *S. aureus* **pneumonia.** CT image at a lower level shows consolidation in the lingula, dense consolidation in the left lower lobe, and small right pleural effusion. Also noted is right lung volume loss with consolidation in the right middle lobe. The patient was a 51-year-old man with community-acquired staphylococcal pneumonia.

Sista RR, Oda G, Barr J: Methicillin-resistant *Staphylococcus aureus* infections in ICU patients. *Anesthesiol Clin North Am* 22:405-435, 2004.

Spencer RC: Predominant pathogens found in the European Prevalence of Infection in Intensive Care Study. *Eur J Clin Microbiol Infect Dis* 15:281-285, 1996.

Washington L, Palacio D: Imaging of bacterial pulmonary infection in the immunocompetent patient. *Semin Roentgenol* 42:122-145, 2007.

Pneumonia (*Legionella*)

DEFINITION: Pneumonia caused by infection with *Legionella* species.

IMAGING

Radiography
Findings
- Lobar, focal, or multifocal areas of consolidation.
- Occasionally, focus is round (round pneumonia).
- Single or multiple nodules are seen in addition to consolidation involving part or all of one or more lobes.
- Immunocompromised individuals have high rate of cavitation and hilar lymphadenopathy.
- Pleural effusion may occur at the peak of the illness.

Utility
- First and foremost imaging modality in the assessment and follow-up of patients with pneumonia

CT
Findings
- Most commonly, multifocal and bilateral areas of consolidation and ground-glass opacities are evident; less commonly, the infection is unilateral or lobar.
- The infection may have peribronchial or peripheral predominance.
- Occasionally, the focus is round (round pneumonia).
- Ground-glass opacities may surround areas of consolidation ("CT halo" sign).
- Pleural effusion is present in the majority of patients, usually ipsilateral to the consolidation.
- Ipsilateral hilar and/or mediastinal lymphadenopathy is common.

Utility
- Helpful in patients with complicated pneumonia and in patients with normal or nonspecific radiographic findings

CLINICAL PRESENTATION

- Fever
- Cough, initially dry and later productive
- Malaise, myalgia
- Confusion, headaches
- Diarrhea
- Pleuritic chest pain (30%)

DIFFERENTIAL DIAGNOSIS

- Pneumonia caused by other organisms
- Organizing pneumonia

DIAGNOSTIC PEARLS

- Homogeneous lobar consolidation
- Progression to involve multiple lobes
- Tendency for rapid progression despite antibiotic therapy

- Aspiration pneumonia
- Pulmonary carcinoma

PATHOLOGY

- Findings of pneumonia
- *Legionella* organisms are weakly staining, gram-negative coccobacilli.
- Aspiration after upper airway colonization is an important source of infection in hospitals, long-term care facilities, and rehabilitation centers.

INCIDENCE/PREVALENCE AND EPIDEMIOLOGY

- Most common human pathogen is *Legionella pneumophila*.
- Accounts for 2% to 25% of patients with community-acquired pneumonias that require hospitalization.
- Reported incidence of nosocomial pneumonia from *Legionella* species varies from 1% to 5%.
- Legionnaires disease shows a propensity for older men, with the male-to-female ratio being on the order of 2 or 3:1.
- Most cases of nosocomial infection occur in patients with preexisting conditions such as malignancy, renal failure, and transplantation.
- Chronic obstructive pulmonary disease and malignancy often are present in patients who become infected in the community.

Suggested Readings

Coletta FS, Fein AM: Radiological manifestations of *Legionella/Legionella*-like organisms. *Semin Respir Infect* 13:109-115, 1998.
Kroboth FJ, Yu VL, Reddy SC, Yu AC: Clinicoradiographic correlation with the extent of legionnaire disease. *AJR Am J Roentgenol* 141:263-268, 1983.

WHAT THE REFERRING PHYSICIAN NEEDS TO KNOW

- Progression of pneumonia is rapid, with most of lobe becoming involved within 3 or 4 days, despite appropriate antibiotic therapy.
- Risk factors include elderly age, male gender, malignancy, and organ transplant.
- Complications include cavitation, hilar lymphadenopathy, and pleural effusion.

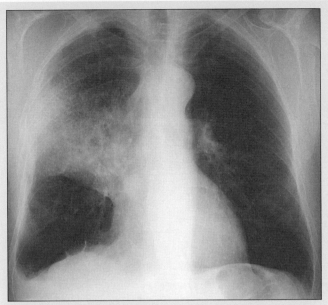

Figure 1. *Legionella* **pneumonia.** Chest radiograph shows lobar consolidation in the right upper lobe. The patient was a 77-year-old man with *Legionella pneumophila* pneumonia.

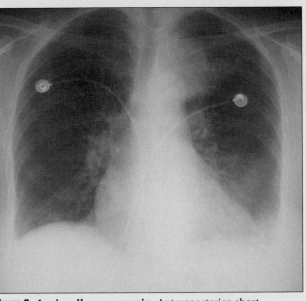

Figure 2. *Legionella* **pneumonia.** Anteroposterior chest radiograph shows a focus of dense consolidation in the left upper lobe and poorly defined, localized, patchy areas of consolidation in the lower lobes. The patient was a 66-year-old woman. Cultures from bronchoscopy specimens grew *Legionella micdadei*.

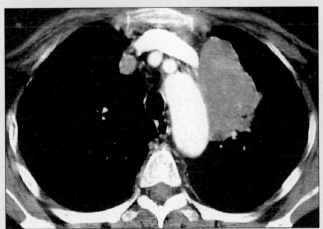

Figure 3. *Legionella* **pneumonia.** Contrast-enhanced CT scan demonstrates dense, mass-like consolidation in the left upper lobe immediately adjacent to the aortic arch. The patient was a 66-year-old woman. Cultures from bronchoscopy specimens grew *Legionella micdadei*.

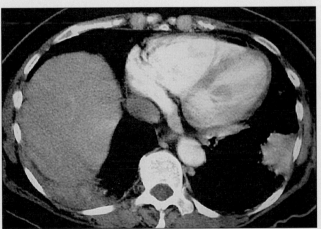

Figure 4. *Legionella* **pneumonia.** CT image at the level of the dome of the right hemidiaphragm demonstrates focal areas of consolidation in the lower lobes. The patient was a 66-year-old woman. Cultures from bronchoscopy specimens grew *Legionella micdadei*.

Lieberman D, Porath A, Schlaeffer F, et al: *Legionella* species community-acquired pneumonia: A review of 56 hospitalized adult patients. *Chest* 109:1243-1249, 1996.

Meenhorst PL, Mulder JD: The chest x-ray in *Legionella* Pneumonia (legionnaires' disease). *Eur J Radiol* 3:180-186, 1983.

Muder RR, Reddy SC, Yu VL, Kroboth FJ: Pneumonia caused by Pittsburgh pneumonia agent: Radiologic manifestations. *Radiology* 150:633-637, 1984.

Sakai F, Tokuda H, Goto H, et al: Computed tomographic features of *Legionella pneumophila* pneumonia in 38 cases. *J Comput Assist Tomogr* 31:125-131, 2007.

Stout JE, Yu VL: Legionellosis. *N Engl J Med* 337:682-687, 1997.

Stout JE, Yu VL: Hospital-acquired legionnaires' disease: New developments. *Curr Opin Infect Dis* 16:337-341, 2003.

Yagyu H, Nakamura H, Tsuchida F, et al: Chest CT findings and clinical features in mild *Legionella* pneumonia. *Intern Med* 42:477-482, 2003.

Pneumonia (Gram-Negative Organisms)

DEFINITION: Pneumonia caused by gram-negative bacilli.

IMAGING

Radiography

Findings

- *M. catarrhalis* pneumonia: patchy unilateral or bilateral consolidation involving mainly the lower lobes.
- Community-acquired *Klebsiella pneumoniae* pneumonia: homogeneous lobar consolidation with air bronchograms and tendency for abscess formation.
- Lobar consolidation with or without "bulging fissure" sign.
- Nosocomial *K. pneumoniae* pneumonia: bronchopneumonia and a greater tendency for abscess and cavity formation.
- *E. coli* and *P. aeruginosa* pneumonia: bronchopneumonia, consisting of multifocal bilateral areas of consolidation.
- Pleural effusion, abscess formation.
- *Legionella* pneumonia: areas of consolidation that enlarge to occupy all, or a large portion, of lobe or to involve contiguous lobes or become bilateral.

Utility

- First and often only imaging modality required in the initial assessment and follow-up.

CT

Findings

- *Klebsiella* pneumonia: enhancing homogeneous areas and poorly marginated low-density areas with multiple small cavities, suggesting necrotizing pneumonia.
- Nosocomial *P. aeruginosa* pneumonia: consolidation, nodular opacities including centrilobular nodules, and "tree-in-bud" pattern.
- Ground-glass opacities, necrosis, and unilateral pleural effusions.

Utility

- Superior to radiography in demonstrating presence of cavitation and other complications.

CLINICAL PRESENTATION

- *M. catarrhalis:* fever and productive cough.
- *K. pneumoniae* and *E. coli* pneumonia: onset usually acute, with fever, productive cough, dyspnea, and pleuritic chest pain.

DIAGNOSTIC PEARLS

- *Klebsiella*: lobar pneumonia or bronchopneumonia
- Gram-negative bacilli: multifocal bilateral consolidation
- *Legionella:* homogeneous lobar consolidation
- *Moraxella:* patchy unilateral or bilateral consolidation

- *P. aeruginosa* pneumonia: presentation typically acute but pleuritic chest pain uncommon.
- *Legionella* pneumonia: fever, cough (initially dry and later productive), malaise, myalgia, confusion, headaches, and diarrhea.

DIFFERENTIAL DIAGNOSIS

- Pneumonia due to other organisms
- Tuberculosis
- Aspiration
- Organizing pneumonia

PATHOLOGY

- *Moraxella catarrhalis* (previously known as *Neisseria catarrhalis*) is an intracellular gram-negative, kidney-shaped diplococcus that is an important cause of pneumonia in patients with chronic obstructive pulmonary disease, the elderly, and the immunocompromised; it is also responsible for outbreaks of nosocomial pneumonia, which occur predominantly in the winter.
- Gram-negative bacilli are important causes of nosocomial pneumonia and, under certain conditions, community-acquired pneumonia.
- *Legionella* organisms are weakly staining, gram-negative coccobacilli.

INCIDENCE/PREVALENCE AND EPIDEMIOLOGY

- *M. catarrhalis* is responsible for approximately 5% of nursing home–acquired pneumonias and 10% of pneumonias in the elderly.

WHAT THE REFERRING PHYSICIAN NEEDS TO KNOW

- Complications of *Klebsiella* and *Pseudomonas* pneumonia include abscess formation, parapneumonic effusion, and empyema.
- Complications of *Legionella* pneumonia include cavitation, hilar lymphadenopathy, and pleural effusion.
- The main role of the chest radiograph is to demonstrate the presence of parenchymal findings consistent with pneumonia and the presence of complications such as cavitation and pleural effusion.
- Radiography plays a limited role in the differential diagnosis of pneumonia.
- CT is superior to radiography in demonstrating the presence of complications such as abscess formation and empyema.

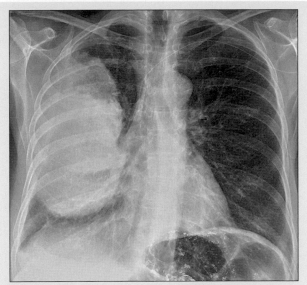

Figure 1. *Klebsiella* **pneumonia with "bulging fissure" sign.** Posteroanterior chest radiograph shows dense consolidation in the right upper and middle lobes. The patient was a 58-year-old woman with severe right upper and middle lobe pneumonia.

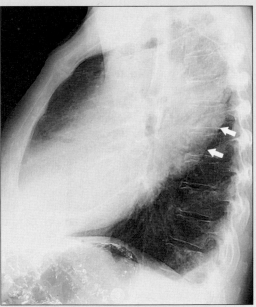

Figure 2. *Klebsiella* **pneumonia.** Lateral radiograph demonstrates posterior convexity of the major fissure (*arrows*) ("bulging fissure" sign) characteristic of lobar expansion. Also noted are small right pleural effusion and residual barium in the splenic flexure. The patient was a 58-year-old woman with severe right upper and middle lobe pneumonia.

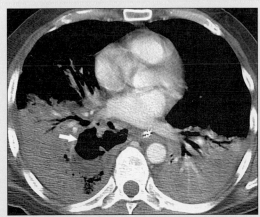

Figure 3. *Klebsiella* **pneumonia with abscess formation.** High-resolution CT shows extensive consolidation in the lower lobes and right lower lobe cavity (*arrow*). The patient was a 50-year-old man with bronchopneumonia due to *K. pneumoniae*.

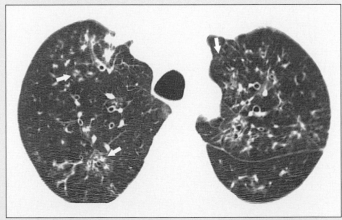

Figure 4. *Pseudomonas* **bronchiolitis and bronchopneumonia.** High-resolution CT at the level of the upper lobes shows bilateral centrilobular nodular and branching opacities ("tree-in-bud" pattern) (*arrows*) consistent with bronchiolitis. Also noted are bilateral ground-glass opacities and small areas of consolidation in the right upper lobe consistent with bronchopneumonia. The patient was a 68-year-old man with Hodgkin disease. Blood cultures grew *P. aeruginosa*.

- Overall, 90%-95% of patients with *M. catarrhalis* infection have underlying cardiopulmonary disease, and >70% are smokers or ex-smokers.
- *K. pneumoniae* accounts for 1%-5% of all cases of community-acquired pneumonia and approximately 15% of cases of nosocomial pneumonia.
- *K. pneumoniae* pneumonia occurs predominantly in men, many of whom are chronic alcoholics or have underlying chronic bronchopulmonary disease.
- *E. coli* accounts for approximately 4% of cases of community-acquired pneumonia and 5%-20% of cases of pneumonia acquired in a hospital or nursing home.
- *P. aeruginosa* pneumonia is the most common and most lethal form of nosocomial pulmonary infection; it is the cause of approximately 20% of nosocomial pneumonia in adult patients in intensive care units.

Suggested Readings

Dunn M, Wunderink RG: Ventilator-associated pneumonia caused by *Pseudomonas* infection. *Clin Chest Med* 16:95-109, 1995.

Gomez J, Banos V, Ruiz Gomez J, et al: Prospective study of epidemiology and prognostic factors in community-acquired pneumonia. *Eur J Clin Microbiol Infect Dis* 15:556-560, 1996.

Korvick JA, Hackett AK, Yu VL, Muder RR: *Klebsiella* pneumonia in the modern era: Clinicoradiographic correlations. *South Med J* 84:200-204, 1991.

Leeper KV Jr: Severe community-acquired pneumonia. *Semin Respir Infect* 11:96-108, 1996.

Maloney SA, Jarvis WR: Epidemic nosocomial pneumonia in the intensive care unit. *Clin Chest Med* 16:209-223, 1995.

Mundy LM, Auwaerter PG, Oldach D, et al: Community-acquired pneumonia: Impact of immune status. *Am J Respir Crit Care Med* 152:1309-1315, 1995.

Sakai F, Tokuda H, Goto H, et al: Computed tomographic features of *Legionella pneumophila* pneumonia in 38 cases. *J Comput Assist Tomogr* 31:125-131, 2007.

Schmidt AJ, Stark P: Radiographic findings in *Klebsiella* (Friedlander's) pneumonia: The bulging fissure sign. *Semin Respir Infect* 13:80-82, 1998.

Shah RM, Wechsler R, Salazar AM, Spirn PW: Spectrum of CT findings in nosocomial *Pseudomonas aeruginosa* pneumonia. *J Thorac Imaging* 17:53-57, 2002.

Sharma S, Maycher B, Eschun G: Radiological imaging in pneumonia: Recent innovations. *Curr Opin Pulm Med* 13:159-169, 2007.

Washington L, Palacio D: Imaging of bacterial pulmonary infection in the immunocompetent patient. *Semin Roentgenol* 42:122-145, 2007.

Winer-Muram HT, Jennings SG, Wunderink RG, et al: Ventilator-associated *Pseudomonas aeruginosa* pneumonia: Radiographic findings. *Radiology* 195:247-252, 1995.

Pneumonia (Anaerobes)

DEFINITION: Pneumonia caused by anaerobic bacteria.

IMAGING

Radiography
Findings
- Bronchopneumonia: ranging from localized segmental or round areas of consolidation to patchy bilateral consolidation to extensive confluent multilobar consolidation.
- Cavitation in 20%-60% of cases.
- Parenchymal abnormalities: consolidation with or without cavitation and lung abscess or necrotizing pneumonia.
- Lung abscess: circumscribed cavity with relatively little surrounding consolidation.
- Necrotizing pneumonia: areas of consolidation containing single or multiple cavities.
- Occasionally, hilar/mediastinal lymph node enlargement associated with an abscess.

Utility
- Usually first imaging modality used in the assessment of patients with suspected pneumonia.

CT
Findings
- Patchy or confluent unilateral or bilateral consolidation (bronchopneumonia).
- Involves mainly dependent lung regions of upper and lower lobe.
- Abscess formation and cavitation and pleural effusion and empyema.
- Occasionally, hilar/mediastinal lymph node enlargement associated with an abscess.
- Pleural effusion.
- Pleural effusion, thickening, and enhancement in empyema.

Utility
- Superior to radiography in demonstrating presence of cavitation and other complications

CLINICAL PRESENTATION
- History of impaired consciousness associated with general anesthesia, acute cerebrovascular accident, epileptic seizure, drug ingestion, or alcoholism.
- Fever: present in 70%-80% of patients; low grade.
- Cough: initially nonproductive until cavitation occurs.
- Foul-smelling sputum suggestive of diagnosis.
- Insidious protracted course over several weeks or even months; overall mean duration of 2-3 weeks.

DIAGNOSTIC PEARLS
- Patchy or confluent unilateral or bilateral consolidation.
- Involves mainly dependent lung regions of upper and lower lobes.
- Commonly associated with abscess formation and empyema.

DIFFERENTIAL DIAGNOSIS
- Pneumonia due to other organisms
- Obstructive pneumonitis
- Tuberculosis
- Pulmonary carcinoma

PATHOLOGY
- Polymicrobial infection may be causative.
- Distribution of pneumonia from aspiration of material contaminated by anaerobic organisms reflects gravitational flow.
- Posterior segments of upper lobes or superior segments of lower lobes are involved when aspiration occurs in a patient in a recumbent position.
- Basal segments of the lower lobes are involved when aspiration occurs in an erect patient.

INCIDENCE/PREVALENCE AND EPIDEMIOLOGY
- Anaerobic bacteria isolated in 20%-35% of all patients admitted to hospital with pneumonia.
- Second only to *S. pneumoniae* as a cause of community-acquired pneumonia requiring hospitalization.
- Important cause of nosocomial pneumonia.
- Common organisms: *Fusobacterium* species and *Bacteroides* species.

WHAT THE REFERRING PHYSICIAN NEEDS TO KNOW
- Important cause of nosocomial pneumonia.
- History of impaired consciousness of any cause.
- Commonly associated with abscess formation.

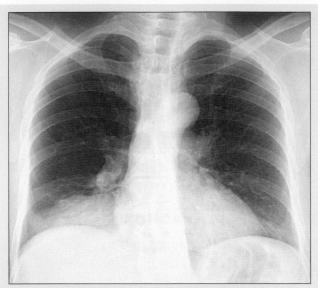

Figure 1. Pneumonia due to anaerobic infection.
Posteroanterior chest radiograph shows dense round consolidation in the posterior basal segment of the right lower lobe. Note small left pleural effusion. The patient was a 61-year-old man. Cultures grew *Prevotella loescheii,* an anaerobic bacterium.

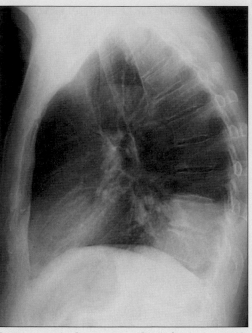

Figure 2. Pneumonia due to anaerobic infection. Lateral chest radiograph shows dense round consolidation in the posterior basal segment of the right lower lobe. Note small left pleural effusion. The patient was a 61-year-old man. Cultures grew *Prevotella loescheii,* an anaerobic bacterium.

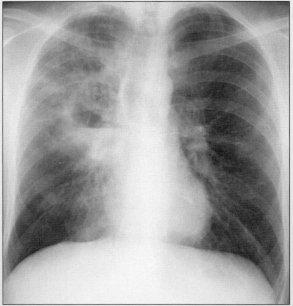

Figure 3. Lung abscess due to anaerobic infection.
Posteroanterior chest radiograph shows patchy areas of consolidation in the right upper and lower lobes and a cavity with a fluid level in the superior segment of the right lower lobe. The patient was a 24-year-old alcoholic male with pneumonia and lung abscess due to anaerobic bacteria.

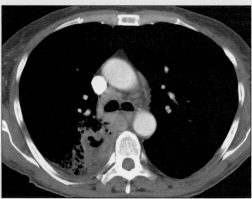

Figure 4. Lung abscess and empyema due to anaerobic infection. Contrast-enhanced CT image shows abscess in the right lower lobe. Also evident are enlarged paratracheal lymph nodes and a small right pleural effusion. Culture of pleural fluid confirmed presence of empyema by anaerobic organisms. The patient was a 57-year-old woman.

Suggested Readings

Bartlett JG: Anaerobic bacterial infections of the lung and pleural space. *Clin Infect Dis* 16(Suppl 4):S248-S255, 1993.

Dore P, Robert R, Grollier G, et al: Incidence of anaerobes in ventilator-associated pneumonia with use of a protected specimen brush. *Am J Respir Crit Care Med* 153:1292-1298, 1996.

Levison ME: Anaerobic pleuropulmonary infection. *Curr Opin Infect Dis* 14:187-191, 2001.

Mansharamani N, Balachandran D, Delaney D, et al: Lung abscess in adults: Clinical comparison of immunocompromised to non-immunocompromised patients. *Respir Med* 96:178-185, 2002.

Washington L, Palacio D: Imaging of bacterial pulmonary infection in the immunocompetent patient. *Semin Roentgenol* 42:122-145, 2007.

Pneumonia (*Nocardia*)

DEFINITION: Pneumonia caused by infection with *Nocardia* species, most commonly *N. asteroides.*

IMAGING

Radiography
Findings
- Homogeneous nonsegmental airspace consolidation that is usually peripheral, abuts the adjacent pleura, and is often extensive.
- Less commonly, consolidation may be patchy and inhomogeneous.
- Consolidation tends to involve multiple lobes and shows no predilection for lower lobes.
- Multifocal peripheral nodules or masses with irregular margins may also be seen.
- Cavitation may occur within areas of consolidation, nodular opacities, or masses.
- Pleural effusion is common, and empyema may occur.
- Extension to pericardium or mediastinum occurs occasionally.

CT
Findings
- Multifocal areas of consolidation, ground-glass opacities.
- Localized areas of low attenuation with rim enhancement suggestive of abscess formation.
- Cavitation.
- Pleural involvement common, including pleural effusion, empyema, and pleural thickening.
- Chest wall extension.
Utility
- Helpful in assessing extent of disease and as guide to obtain material for definitive diagnosis.

CLINICAL PRESENTATION

- Low-grade fever
- Productive cough
- Weight loss
- Exacerbations and remissions over periods of days to weeks
- Chronic clinical course, with duration of symptoms before diagnosis of ≥3 weeks

DIAGNOSTIC PEARLS

- Homogeneous peripheral multilobar (nonsegmental) consolidation.
- Localized area of low attenuation or cavitation within the consolidation due to abscess formation.

DIFFERENTIAL DIAGNOSIS

- Pneumonia due to other organisms
- Septic embolism
- Pulmonary metastases
- Pulmonary carcinoma

PATHOLOGY

- Filling of alveolar airspaces with exudate and neutrophils.
- Presence of *Nocardia* organisms, most commonly *N. asteroides.*
- *Nocardia* are aerobic gram-positive bacilli found in the soil and distributed throughout the world.

INCIDENCE/PREVALENCE AND EPIDEMIOLOGY

- This infection is uncommon.
- Nocardiosis is more common in males than in females (male-to-female ratio 2:1 to 3:1).
- Nocardial pneumonia is more common in immunocompromised patients, particularly those with lymphoma, with organ transplant, on corticosteroid therapy, or with AIDS.

Suggested Readings

Feigin DS: Nocardiosis of the lung: Chest radiographic findings in 21 cases. *Radiology* 159:9-14, 1986.
Yildiz O, Doganay M: Actinomycoses and *Nocardia* pulmonary infections. *Curr Opin Pulm Med* 12:228-234, 2006.
Yoon HK, Im JG, Ahn JM, Han MC: Pulmonary nocardiosis: CT findings. *J Comput Assist Tomogr* 19:52-55, 1995.

WHAT THE REFERRING PHYSICIAN NEEDS TO KNOW

- Risk factors: male gender, immune compromise.
- Complications: cavitation (35% of cases) and pleural effusion.

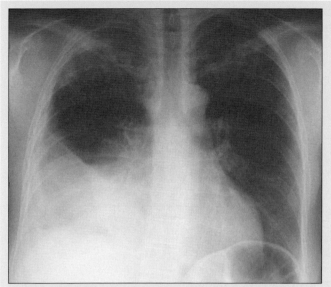

Figure 1. Pleuropulmonary nocardiosis. Posteroanterior chest radiograph shows areas of consolidation in the upper lobes and right middle lobe and a right pleural effusion. *Nocardia asteroides* was recovered from both bronchoalveolar lavage and pleural fluid. The patient was a previously healthy 36-year-old man who presented with severe pleuritic chest pain.

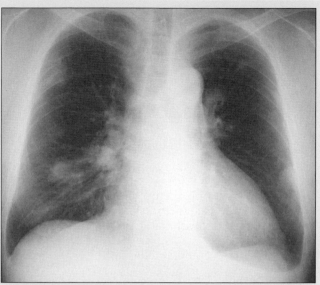

Figure 2. Nocardia pneumonia. Posteroanterior chest radiograph demonstrates bilateral nodular opacities and small left pleural effusion. *N. asteroides* was recovered on bronchoalveolar lavage. The patient was a 41-year-old man on immunosuppressive therapy after renal transplantation who presented with fever and cough.

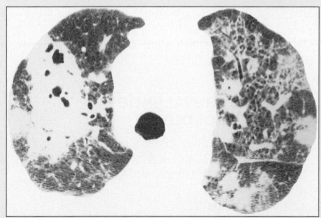

Figure 3. Nocardia pneumonia. CT images at the level of the aortic arch shows bilateral areas of consolidation, multiple cavities, extensive ground-glass opacities superimposed on centrilobular emphysema, and small bilateral pleural effusions. The patient was a 51-year-old man with *N. asteroides* pneumonia. *(Courtesy of Dr. Jim Barrie, University of Alberta Medical Centre, Edmonton, Canada)*

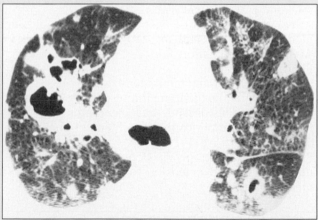

Figure 4. Nocardia pneumonia. CT images at the level of the main bronchi show bilateral areas of consolidation, multiple cavities, extensive ground-glass opacities superimposed on centrilobular emphysema, and small bilateral pleural effusions. The patient was a 51-year-old man with *N. asteroides* pneumonia. *(Courtesy of Dr. Jim Barrie, University of Alberta Medical Centre, Edmonton, Canada)*

Actinomycosis

DEFINITION: Actinomycosis is a chronic granulomatous infection characterized by suppuration, sulfur granules, abscess formation, and sinus tracts caused by *Actinomyces* species, most commonly *A. israelii.*

IMAGING

Radiography

Findings

- Unilateral, peripheral, and patchy consolidation is evident.
- Consolidation tends to involve mainly lower lobes.
- A mass that is sometimes cavitated may be present.
- Patients with chronic pleuropulmonary actinomycosis may develop extensive fibrosis.
- Pleural effusion occasionally is the only radiographic manifestation.
- Chest wall involvement, including soft tissue mass and rib abnormalities, may occur but is uncommon.

Utility

- Usually first imaging modality used in evaluation of patients.
- Of limited value in the diagnosis.

CT

Findings

- Focal/patchy areas of consolidation containing central areas of low attenuation/cavitation associated with thickening of adjacent pleura.
- After use of a contrast agent: ring-like rim enhancement around central areas of low attenuation.
- Airspace consolidation.
- Pleural effusion.
- Hilar or mediastinal lymphadenopathy.
- Chest wall involvement, including soft tissue mass and rib abnormalities possible but uncommon.
- Mediastinal and pericardial involvement uncommon.

Utility

- Superior to radiography in demonstrating presence of lung abscess and extension to pleura, chest wall, or mediastinum.

CLINICAL PRESENTATION

- Initial clinical manifestations are nonproductive cough and low-grade fever.
- Cough becomes productive or purulent and, in many cases, blood-streaked sputum occurs.
- Pleuritic chest pain commonly develops as infection spreads to pleura and chest wall.

DIAGNOSTIC PEARLS

- Unilateral, peripheral, and patchy consolidation
- Focal/patchy areas of consolidation containing central areas of low attenuation/cavitation
- Thickening of pleura adjacent to consolidation
- Majority of patients are alcoholic men

DIFFERENTIAL DIAGNOSIS

- Bronchopneumonia
- Fungal infection
- Organizing pneumonia
- Aspiration pneumonia
- Carcinoma

PATHOLOGY

- *Actinomyces* species are anaerobic filamentous bacteria (most common: *A. israelii*).
- *Actinomyces* is a normal inhabitant of the human oropharynx.
- This organism is frequently found in dental caries and at gingival margins of persons who have poor oral hygiene, and actinomycosis is believed to be acquired by the spread of organisms from these sites.

INCIDENCE/PREVALENCE AND EPIDEMIOLOGY

- Actinomycosis is uncommon.
- Most common pathogen is *Actinomyces israelii.*
- Majority of patients are alcoholic men.

Suggested Readings

Hsieh MJ, Liu HP, Chang JP, Chang CH: Thoracic actinomycosis. *Chest* 104:366-370, 1993.

Kim TS, Han J, Koh WJ, et al: Thoracic actinomycosis: CT features with histopathologic correlation. *AJR Am J Roentgenol* 186:225-231, 2006.

Kwong JS, Müller NL, Godwin JD, et al: Thoracic actinomycosis: CT findings in eight patients. *Radiology* 183:189-192, 1992.

Mabeza GF, Macfarlane J: Pulmonary actinomycosis. *Eur Respir J* 21:545-551, 2003.

WHAT THE REFERRING PHYSICIAN NEEDS TO KNOW

- Complications include extension to pleura with thickening, effusion, and empyema and extension to mediastinum, pericardium, and chest wall.
- Risk factors include poor oral hygiene and alcoholism.
- CT frequently demonstrates areas of low attenuation within consolidation due to abscess formation.

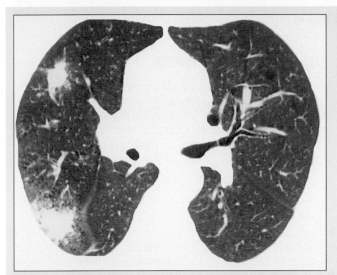

Figure 1. **Pleuropulmonary actinomycosis.** High-resolution CT image shows focal areas of consolidation in the right upper lobe and mild bilateral emphysema. The patient was a 59-year-old alcoholic man with surgically confirmed pleuropulmonary actinomycosis.

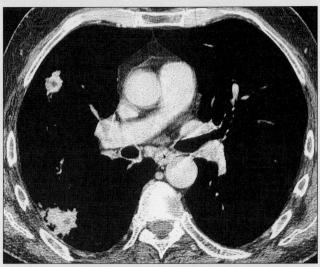

Figure 2. **Pleuropulmonary actinomycosis.** High-resolution CT image performed after intravenous administration of contrast material demonstrates localized areas of low attenuation within the consolidation consistent with abscess formation. The patient was a 59-year-old alcoholic man with surgically confirmed pleuropulmonary actinomycosis.

Septic Embolism

DEFINITION: Infected emboli to the lungs resulting in multiple abscesses.

IMAGING

Radiography

Findings
- Presence of nodules usually measuring 1-3 cm in diameter that are frequently cavitated.
- Nodules often most numerous in lower lobes.

Utility
- First and often only imaging modality used in the initial assessment and follow-up of patients.

CT

Findings
- Nodules usually measuring 1-3 cm in diameter are present and frequently cavitate.
- On cross-sectional CT images, nodules often appear to have vessel leading into them ("feeding vessel" sign).
- Pulmonary arteries course around nodule; vessels appearing to enter nodule usually are pulmonary veins draining the nodule.
- Subpleural wedge-shaped areas of consolidation are seen, often with central areas of necrosis or frank cavitation.
- After administration of an intravenous contrast agent, the periphery of the infarct enhances.

Utility
- CT is superior to radiography in demonstrating presence of nodules and cavitation.
- "Feeding vessel" sign is a misnomer and of limited value in the diagnosis of septic embolism.

CLINICAL PRESENTATION

- Fever
- Cough
- Purulent sputum
- Pleuritic chest pain
- Hemoptysis
- In elderly: signs and symptoms of pneumonia possibly milder or absent

PATHOLOGY

- Lung abscesses may result from systemic spread of infection (septic embolism).

DIAGNOSTIC PEARLS

- Presence of nodules usually measuring 1-3 cm in diameter that are frequently cavitated.
- Nodules often most numerous in the lower lobes.
- Subpleural wedge-shaped areas of consolidation, often with central areas of necrosis or frank cavitation on CT.

- Emboli can originate in variety of sites: cardiac valves (endocarditis), peripheral veins (thrombophlebitis), and infected venous catheters or pacemaker wires.
- Common feature in all these sites is endothelial damage associated with formation of friable thrombus containing organisms (usually bacteria).
- Pulmonary artery occlusion by septic emboli results in hemorrhage and/or infarction and pleural-based areas of consolidation.

INCIDENCE/PREVALENCE AND EPIDEMIOLOGY

- Septic embolism occurs most commonly in patients with infected venous catheters or pacemaker leads and in intravenous drug users.
- Common organisms include *Staphylococcus aureus*, *Streptococcus viridans*, gram-negative bacteria, and *Aspergillus*.

Suggested Readings

Dodd JD, Souza CA, Müller NL: High-resolution MDCT of pulmonary septic embolism: Evaluation of the feeding vessel sign. *AJR Am J Roentgenol* 187:623-629, 2006.

Huang RM, Naidich DP, Lubat E, et al:Septic pulmonary emboli: CT-radiographic correlation. *AJR Am J Roentgenol* 153:41-45, 1989.

Kuhlman JE, Fishman EK, Teigen C: Pulmonary septic emboli: Diagnosis with CT. *Radiology* 174:211-213, 1990.

Kwon WJ, Jeong YJ, Kim KI, et al:Computed tomographic features of pulmonary septic emboli: Comparison of causative microorganisms. *J Comput Assist Tomogr* 31:390-394, 2007.

WHAT THE REFERRING PHYSICIAN NEEDS TO KNOW

- Septic embolism should be suspected in patients with intravenous lines who develop fever and pulmonary nodules.
- CT is superior to radiography in demonstrating presence and extent of septic emboli.

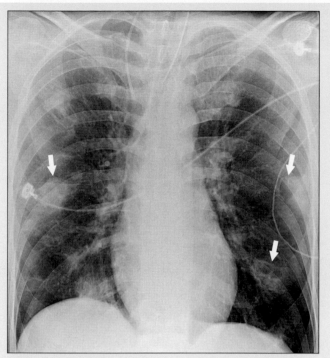

Figure 1. Septic embolism. Chest radiograph shows several bilateral nodules some of which are cavitated (*arrows*). Also noted are endotracheal tube, central venous line, and electrocardiographic leads.

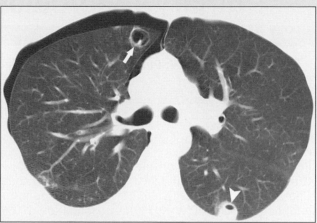

Figure 2. Septic embolism. CT image at the level of the right upper lobe bronchus shows a thin-walled cavity in the right upper lobe (*arrow*) and cavitated nodule in the left lower lobe (*arrowhead*). Also noted are a right pneumothorax and a few centrilobular nodules in the posterior segment of the right upper lobe. The patient was a 41-year-old male intravenous drug user with septic emboli caused by *Staphylococcus aureus*.

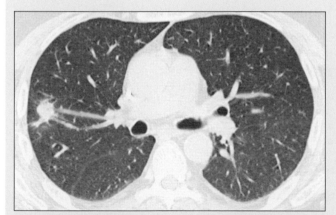

Figure 3. Septic embolism with apparent "feeding vessel" sign. Cross-sectional high-resolution CT image shows two vessels apparently coursing into a nodule ("feeding vessel" sign).

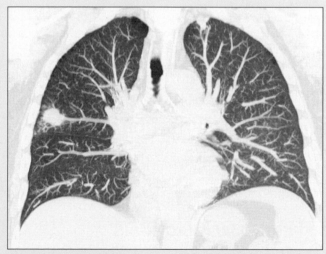

Figure 4. Septic embolism with apparent "feeding vessel" sign. Coronal maximum intensity projection image demonstrates that the only vessel in close contact with the nodule is a draining vein. Another nodule also drained by a vein is present in the left lung apex.

Primary Tuberculosis

DEFINITION: Pulmonary disease that develops after initial exposure to *Mycobacterium tuberculosis.*

IMAGING

Radiography
Findings
- Parenchymal focus of consolidation.
- Unilateral hilar or paratracheal enlarged lymph node.
- Characteristic findings in children: hilar or mediastinal lymphadenopathy (90%-95%), consolidation (70%), pleural effusion (5%-10%).
- Characteristic findings in adults: consolidation (90%), hilar or mediastinal lymphadenopathy (10%-30%), pleural effusion (30%-40%).

Utility
- Usually the only imaging modality required in initial evaluation and follow-up of patients.

CT
Findings
- Lobar or segmental consolidation.
- Consolidation that may be patchy, linear, nodular, or mass-like.
- Enlarged hilar or mediastinal lymph nodes with diffuse low attenuation or central low attenuation and rim enhancement.
- Pleural effusion.

Utility
- Used in clinically suspected patients with normal or equivocal radiograph.
- More sensitive in detection and characterization of subtle parenchymal disease and mediastinal lymphadenopathy.

CLINICAL PRESENTATION

- Usually asymptomatic
- Mild or progressive dry cough
- Systemic symptoms including fever, fatigue, weight loss, night sweats

DIFFERENTIAL DIAGNOSIS

- Non-Hodgkin lymphoma
- Hodgkin lymphoma

DIAGNOSTIC PEARLS

- Parenchymal consolidation
- Unilateral hilar or paratracheal lymphadenopathy
- Low attenuation lymph-nodes with rim enhancement

- Lobar pneumonia
- Bronchopneumonia

PATHOLOGY

- *Mycobacterium tuberculosis:* aerobic, nonmobile, non–spore-forming rod that is highly resistant to drying, acid, and alcohol.
- Inhalation of *M. tuberculosis,* causing infection and formation of pulmonary granulomas.
- Transmitted person to person via droplet nuclei containing the organism and spread mainly by coughing.
- Granulomas: may enlarge, undergo necrosis and/or heal.
- Cessation of bacterial proliferation at 2-10 weeks by cell-mediated immunity and delayed hypersensitivity.
- May progress into active disease without healing (progressive primary tuberculosis).

INCIDENCE/PREVALENCE AND EPIDEMIOLOGY

- >10 million new cases and >2 million deaths worldwide each year.
- Majority of cases occur in Southeast Asia and Africa.
- Risk is greatest with altered host cellular immunity (e.g., HIV infection).
- Active cases infect 10-15 people annually.

Suggested Readings

De Backer AI, Mortelé KJ, De Keulenaer BL, Parizel PM: Tuberculosis: Epidemiology, manifestations, and the value of medical imaging in diagnosis. *JBR-BTR* 89:243-250, 2006.
Lee KS, Song KS, Lim TH, et al: Adult-onset pulmonary tuberculosis: Findings on chest radiographs and CT scans. *AJR Am J Roentgenol* 160:753-758, 1993.

WHAT THE REFERRING PHYSICIAN NEEDS TO KNOW

- The strongest risk factor for tuberculosis is HIV infection.
- Primary tuberculosis occurs most commonly in children but increasingly is seen in adults.
- Patients may have active tuberculosis and a normal chest radiograph.
- Prevalence of normal radiographs in patients with tuberculosis is highest with miliary disease and severe immune compromise.

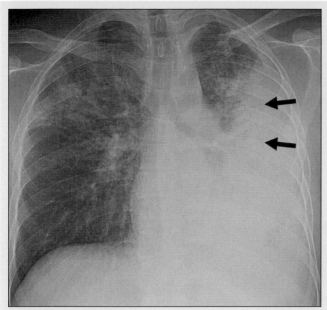

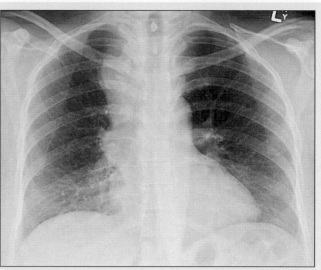

Figure 2. **Primary tuberculosis in a 46-year-old woman.** Chest radiograph showing a large homogeneous right mediastinal soft tissue opacity. CT showed extensive paratracheal lymphadenopathy.

Figure 1. **Primary tuberculosis with consolidation and lymph node enlargement in a 24-year-old man.** Chest radiograph showing parenchymal consolidation containing air bronchograms (*arrows*) in the left upper and lower lobes with relative sparing of the lung apex. The left apical soft tissue widening suggests an associated left pleural effusion. Also note the parenchymal opacity and small nodular lesions in right upper lung zone. (*Courtesy of Dr. Kyung Soo Lee, Seoul, Korea*)

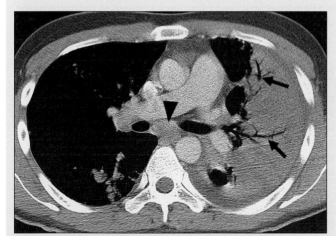

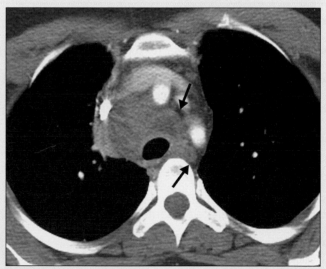

Figure 3. **Primary tuberculosis with consolidation and lymph node enlargement in a 24-year-old man.** A contrast medium–enhanced CT image at the level of the bronchus intermedius shows parenchymal consolidation containing air bronchograms (*arrows*) in the left lung. Also note the subcarinal lymph node enlargement (*arrowhead*), left pleural effusion, and some small nodular opacities in the contralateral right lung. (Courtesy of Dr. *Kyung Soo Lee, Seoul, Korea*)

Figure 4. **Primary tuberculosis in a 46-year-old woman.** Contrast medium–enhanced CT image demonstrating extensive paratracheal lymphadenopathy. Note the presence of enlarged lymph nodes with a low-attenuation center and rim enhancement (*arrows*), a characteristic feature of primary tuberculosis.

Leung AN: Pulmonary tuberculosis: The essentials. *Radiology* 210:307-322, 1999.

Leung AN, Müller NL, Pineda PR, FitzGerald JM: Primary tuberculosis in childhood: Radiographic manifestations. *Radiology* 182: 87-89, 1992.

Powell DA, Hunt WG: Tuberculosis in children: An update. *Adv Pediatr* 53:279-322, 2006.

Postprimary Tuberculosis

DEFINITION: Pulmonary disease that results from reactivation of a previous focus of tuberculosis or re-infection.

IMAGING

Radiography
Findings
- Focal or patchy heterogeneous consolidation or poorly defined nodules and linear opacities (fibronodular pattern).
- Single or multiple cavities with air-fluid levels.
- Mainly apical and posterior segments of upper lobes and superior segments of lower lobes.
- Distant nodules representing endobronchial spread.
- Tuberculoma: smoothly marginated or spiculated nodule.
- Multiple small nodular densities (1-3 mm) in miliary pattern.
- Pleural effusion.
- Hilar or mediastinal lymphadenopathy in 5%-10%. More common in immunocompromised patient.

Utility
- Used for initial evaluation and follow-up of patients.
- May be normal or show only mild or nonspecific findings.

CT
Findings
- Centrilobular nodules and branching linear and nodular opacities ("tree-in-bud" pattern).
- Patchy or lobular areas of consolidation with cavitation.
- Mainly apical and posterior segments of upper lobes and superior segments of lower lobes.
- Endobronchial spread shown by multilobar centrilobular and "tree-in-bud" opacities.
- Cavities usually thick walled; thin walls seen in patients undergoing treatment.
- Hilar or mediastinal lymphadenopathy in 5%-10%; nodes often of low attenuation and may show rim enhancement after intravenous administration of a contrast agent.
- Tuberculoma: peripherally enhancing, smoothly marginated or spiculated nodule; may have calcification and cavitation.
- Miliary: multiple randomly distributed nodules (1-3 mm diameter); may have associated septal lines.

Utility
- Used in clinically suspected patients with normal or equivocal radiograph.

- More sensitive in detection and characterization of subtle parenchymal disease and mediastinal lymphadenopathy.

Positron Emission Tomography
Findings
- Tuberculoma: increased FDG uptake in nodule.
Utility
- Of limited value in distinguishing active tuberculosis from neoplasm.

CLINICAL PRESENTATION
- May be asymptomatic
- Mild or progressive dry cough or productive cough
- Fever, fatigue, weight loss, night sweats

DIFFERENTIAL DIAGNOSIS
- Bronchopneumonia
- Lobar pneumonia
- Pulmonary lymphoma
- Infectious bronchiolitis
- Wegener granulomatosis
- *Mycobacterium avium-intracellulare* complex

PATHOLOGY
- *Mycobacterium tuberculosis:* aerobic, nonmobile, non–spore-forming rod that is highly resistant to drying, acid, and alcohol.
- Progressive extension and enlargement of foci of inflammation and necrosis.

WHAT THE REFERRING PHYSICIAN NEEDS TO KNOW
- The strongest risk factor for tuberculosis is HIV infection.
- Patients may have active tuberculosis and a normal chest radiograph.
- Normal radiographs occur most often with miliary disease and in severely immunocompromised patients.

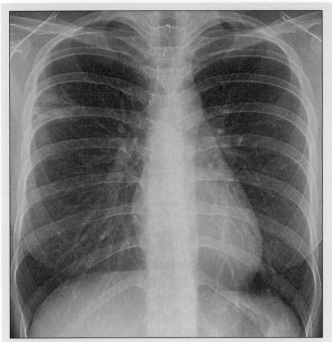

Figure 1. Postprimary tuberculosis. Chest radiograph shows a focal parenchymal opacity and small nodular clustering in the right upper lobe. *(Courtesy of Dr. Kyung Soo Lee, Seoul, Korea)*

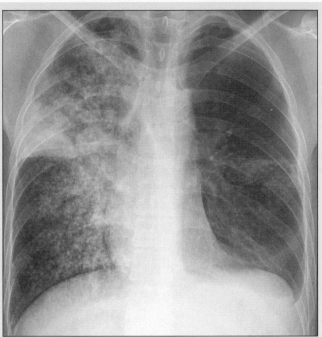

Figure 2. Postprimary tuberculosis. Chest radiograph shows extensive areas of small nodular clustering in both lungs. Also note the segmental consolidation in the right upper lobe and a left pleural effusion. *(Courtesy of Dr. Kyung Soo Lee, Seoul, Korea)*

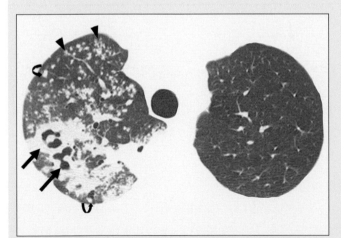

Figure 3. Cavitary postprimary tuberculosis in a 30-year-old man. CT scan at the level of the great vessels shows cavitating (*arrows*) and noncavitating consolidation, "tree-in-bud" opacities (*arrowheads*) and variably sized nodular lesions (*curved arrows*) in the right upper lobe. *(Courtesy of Dr. Kyung Soo Lee, Seoul, Korea)*

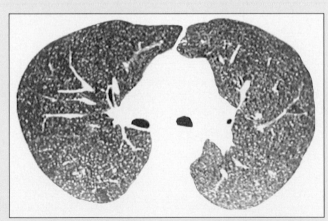

Figure 4. Miliary tuberculosis in a 27-year-old woman. A CT scan at the level of the main bronchi demonstrates the random distribution of numerous small nodules. *(Courtesy of Dr. Kyung Soo Lee, Seoul, Korea).*

- Erosion of cavity into bronchus with resultant endobronchial spread.
- Necrotizing granulomas.

INCIDENCE/PREVALENCE AND EPIDEMIOLOGY

- >10 million new tuberculosis cases, with >2 million deaths worldwide every year.
- Majority of cases occur in Southeast Asia and Africa.
- Risk of active tuberculosis is greatest with altered host cellular immunity (e.g., HIV infection).
- Reactivation of latent infection occurs in 5% of infected population.

Suggested Readings

Kim HY, Song KS, Goo JM, et al: Thoracic sequelae and complications of tuberculosis. *RadioGraphics* 21:839-858, 2001;discussion 859-860.

Krysl J, Korzeniewska-Koesela M, Müller NL, FitzGerald JM: Radiologic features of pulmonary tuberculosis: An assessment of 188 cases. *Can Assoc Radiol J* 45:101-107, 1994.

Kwong JS, Carignan S, Kang EY, et al: Miliary tuberculosis: Diagnostic accuracy of chest radiography. *Chest* 110:339-342, 1996.

Lee JY, Lee KS, Jung KJ, et al: Pulmonary tuberculosis: CT and pathologic correlation. *J Comput Assist Tomogr* 24:691-698, 2000.

Leung AN: Pulmonary tuberculosis: The essentials. *Radiology* 210:307-322, 1999.

Maartens G, Wilkinson RJ: Tuberculosis. *Lancet* 370:2030-2043, 2007.

Murayama S, Murakami J, Hashimoto S, et al: Noncalcified pulmonary tuberculomas: CT enhancement patterns with histological correlation. *J Thorac Imaging* 10:91-95, 1995.

Sequelae and Long-Term Complications of Tuberculosis

DEFINITION: Complications and sequelae that result from pulmonary tuberculosis.

IMAGING

Radiography

Findings

- Parenchymal nodules or consolidation.
- Fibrosis and calcifications, atelectasis, scarring, architectural distortion.
- Pleural effusion, thickening (fibrothorax), calcification.
- Acute respiratory distress syndrome: extensive bilateral ground-glass opacities or consolidation with miliary or endobronchial pattern.
- Cysts: airspaces with well-defined walls; may be in background of consolidation.
- Constrictive pericarditis: enlargement of cardiopericardial silhouette, extensive pericardial calcification, pleural effusions.
- Tuberculous spondylitis: paraspinal soft tissue densities.

Utility

- Used for initial evaluation and follow-up of patients.
- May be normal or show only mild or nonspecific findings.

CT

Findings

- Parenchymal consolidation with multiple cysts.
- Reticulonodular pattern (fibronodular tuberculosis).
- Architectural distortion, fibrosis, and scarring; mildly enlarged and calcified lymph nodes.
- Bronchiectasis: unilateral or bilaterally asymmetric, usually most severe in upper lobe.
- Tracheobronchial stenosis: thickening of bronchial wall and luminal narrowing.
- Rasmussen aneurysm: focal dilatation of pulmonary artery often associated with cavity.
- Constrictive pericarditis: pericardial effusion and thickening; extensive pericardial calcification; distortion of right ventricle; pleural effusions.
- Empyema necessitatis: fluid collections in pleura and chest wall.
- Tuberculous spondylitis: paraspinal soft tissue mass with bony destruction.

Utility

- Used in clinically suspected patients with normal or equivocal radiograph.

DIAGNOSTIC PEARLS

- Bronchiectasis and bronchial stenosis
- Progressive consolidation
- Chronic pleural effusion
- Cavitation and intracavitary mass
- Pulmonary artery aneurysm

- More sensitive in detection and characterization of subtle parenchymal disease and mediastinal lymphadenopathy.
- Superior to radiography in demonstrating pulmonary, pleural, cardiac, and chest wall complications.

Angiography

Findings

- Rasmussen aneurysm: focal dilatation of pulmonary artery

Utility

- Usually only performed before coil embolization

MRI

Findings

- Tuberculous spondylitis: paraspinal soft tissue mass may show intraspinal extension
- Superior to CT in demonstrating extent of tuberculous spondylitis and extension into spinal canal

CLINICAL PRESENTATION

- May be asymptomatic
- Mild or progressive dry cough or productive cough
- Fever, fatigue, weight loss, night sweats
- Hemoptysis due to bronchiectasis, aspergilloma, or Rasmussen aneurysm

DIFFERENTIAL DIAGNOSIS

- Bronchopneumonia
- Lobar pneumonia
- Lung cancer
- Wegener granulomatosis
- *Mycobacterium avium-intracellulare* complex

WHAT THE REFERRING PHYSICIAN NEEDS TO KNOW

- The strongest risk factor for tuberculosis is HIV infection.
- Patients may have active tuberculosis and normal chest radiograph.
- The most common sequelae of previous tuberculosis are areas of scarring, bronchiectasis, calcified parenchymal focus, and calcified ipsilateral lymph nodes.

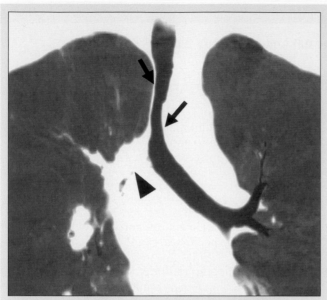

Figure 1. **Tracheobronchial tuberculosis in a 31-year-old woman.** Minimum intensity projection image shows luminal narrowing of the lower portion of the trachea (*arrows*) and an obliterated lumen of the right main bronchus (*arrowhead*). *(Courtesy of Dr. Kyung Soo Lee, Seoul, Korea)*

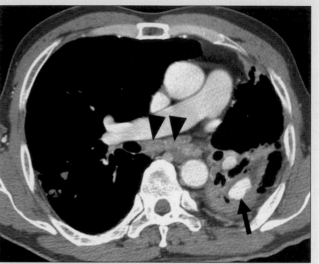

Figure 2. **Rasmussen aneurysm in a 60-year-old man with chronic destructive pulmonary tuberculosis.** A contrast-enhanced CT scan at the level of the bronchus intermedius shows a contrast-filling aneurysm (*arrow*) within parenchymal consolidation in a superior segment of the left lower lobe. Also note the enlarged subcarinal lymph nodes (*arrowheads*). *(Courtesy of Dr. Yeon Joo Jeong, Pusan National University Hospital, Pusan, Korea.)*

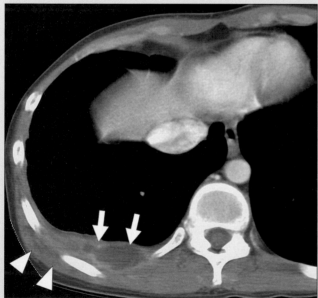

Figure 3. **Tuberculous empyema necessitatis in a 29-year-old woman.** CT scan image demonstrates a fluid collection in the extrapleural subcostal tissue (*arrows*) and in the right chest wall (*arrowheads*). *(Courtesy of Dr. Kyung Soo Lee, Seoul, Korea)*

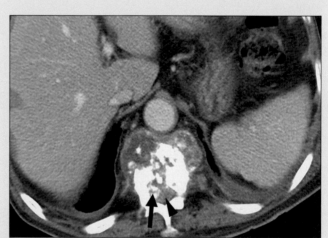

Figure 4. **Tuberculous spondylitis in a 79-year-old man.** A contrast-enhanced CT scan at the level of the caudate lobe of the liver shows a calcified, heterogeneous, and low-attenuation soft tissue opacity in the paraspinal region bilaterally, along with associated destruction of the vertebral body. Also note the intraspinal extension (*arrow*) of the soft tissue abnormality with associated cord (*arrowhead*) compression. *(Courtesy of Dr. Kyung Soo Lee, Seoul, Korea)*

PATHOLOGY

- *Mycobacterium tuberculosis* is an aerobic, nonmobile, non–spore-forming rod that is highly resistant to drying, acid, and alcohol.
- Active *M. tuberculosis* infection has lymphatic and hematogenous spread.
- Progressive extension of foci of inflammation and necrosis occurs.
- Healing may result in fibrosis, scar formation, calcification, and architectural distortion.
- Other complications include bronchiectasis, bronchial stenosis, aspergilloma, Rasmussen aneurysm, fibrothorax, empyema, empyema necessitatis, and constrictive pericarditis.

INCIDENCE/PREVALENCE AND EPIDEMIOLOGY

- >10 million new tuberculosis cases and >2 million deaths worldwide each year.
- Majority of tuberculosis occurs in Southeast Asia and Africa.

- Most common sequelae of previous tuberculosis are areas of scarring, bronchiectasis, calcified parenchymal focus, and calcified ipsilateral lymph nodes.
- Chronic cavitation and bronchiectasis due to previous tuberculosis are the most common underlying causes of aspergilloma.

Suggested Readings

Choi JA, Hong KT, Oh YW, et al: CT manifestations of late sequelae in patients with tuberculous pleuritis. *AJR Am J Roentgenol* 176:441-445, 2001.

Im JG, Itoh H, Shim YS, et al: Pulmonary tuberculosis: CT findings—early active disease and sequential change with antituberculous therapy. *Radiology* 186:653-660, 1993.

Kim HY, Song KS, Goo JM, et al: Thoracic sequelae and complications of tuberculosis. *RadioGraphics* 21:839-858, 2001; discussion 859-860.

Kim Y, Lee KS, Yoon JH, et al: Tuberculosis of the trachea and main bronchi: CT findings in 17 patients. *AJR Am J Roentgenol* 168:1051-1056, 1997.

Poey C, Verhaegen F, Giron J, et al: High resolution chest CT in tuberculosis: Evolutive patterns and signs of activity. *J Comput Assist Tomogr* 21:601-607, 1997.

PART 11 NONTUBERCULOUS (ATYPICAL) MYCOBACTERIAL INFECTION

Mycobacterium avium-intracellulare Complex

DEFINITION: Pulmonary disease that occurs secondary to infection with *Mycobacterium avium-intracellulare* complex.

IMAGING

Radiography

Findings
- Cavitary form: focal consolidation with thin-walled cavities; may be superimposed on chronic lung disease.
- Mild form (Lady Windermere syndrome): small nodules or foci of consolidation with bronchiectatic changes.
- Hot tub lung: patchy ground-glass opacities and small poorly defined nodules.

Utility
- Initial modality and used for follow-up
- Wide spectrum and severity of findings
- May be normal and usually nonspecific
- Radiographic progression of months or years
- Radiographic manifestations of cavitary form indistinguishable from those of tuberculosis

CT

Findings
- Cavitary form: cavitary lesions or cavitation in small nodules.
- Often underlying chronic lung disease.
- Bronchiectatic form: Mild multilobar cylindrical bronchiectasis with right middle lobe and lingular predominance.
- Small nodules in random, centrilobular or "tree-in-bud" pattern; or small foci of consolidation.
- Areas of decreased attenuation pattern reflecting obliterative small airways disease possible.
- Hot tub lung: ill-defined, low attenuation, centrilobular nodules, patchy ground-glass opacities, and air trapping.
- Uncommon features: fibrosis, pleural thickening or effusion, mediastinal lymphadenopathy.

Utility
- More sensitive than radiography.
- Findings nonspecific, but combination of findings highly suggestive in patients with Lady Windermere syndrome.
- High-resolution CT manifestations of cavitary form indistinguishable from those of tuberculosis.

DIAGNOSTIC PEARLS

- Bronchiectasis and nodules in the middle lobe and/or lingula.
- Slowly progressive bronchiectasis and tree-in-bud pattern.
- Focal consolidation and cavitation superimposed on top of chronic lung disease.
- Hot tub lung: ground-glass opacities with centrilobular nodules and air trapping.

- High-resolution CT findings of hot tub lung similar to those of hypersensitivity pneumonitis.

CLINICAL PRESENTATION

- May be asymptomatic
- Symptoms of pulmonary infection
- Unexplained exacerbation of symptoms in patient with chronic disease
- Hot tub lung: subacute dry cough and dyspnea in hot tub user

DIFFERENTIAL DIAGNOSIS

- Postprimary tuberculosis
- Bronchopneumonia
- Hypersensitivity pneumonitis

PATHOLOGY

- Spectrum of pulmonary infection secondary to *Mycobacterium avium-intracellulare* complex.
- Cavitary form: upper lobe cavitary lesions, granulomatous inflammation with caseation necrosis.
- Bronchiectatic form: granulomatous inflammation, bronchiectasis.
- Hot tub lung: infection by aerosolized droplets with resultant granulomatous hypersensitivity reaction.

WHAT THE REFERRING PHYSICIAN NEEDS TO KNOW

- Decision to treat infection is complex and influenced by patient-based factors.
- Sensitivity to drug treatment is highly variable.
- CT is particularly helpful in demonstrating slowly progressive parenchymal disease and bronchiectasis in patients with bronchiectatic form of infection.

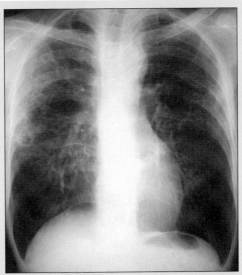

Figure 1. *M. avium-intracellulare* **complex.** Chest radiograph demonstrates widespread consolidation and a cavitating lesion in the right mid lung zone in a patient with *M. avium-intracellulare* complicating severe chronic obstructive pulmonary disease. *(Courtesy of Dr. David M. Hansell, London, UK)*

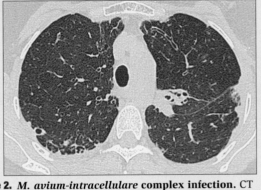

Figure 2. *M. avium-intracellulare* **complex infection.** CT through the lung apices shows mild cylindrical bronchiectasis, a few bilateral centrilobular nodules, a small cavitating lesion in the periphery of the right apex, and small foci of consolidation. Note the loss of volume in the left upper lobe. *(Courtesy of Dr. David M. Hansell, London, UK)*

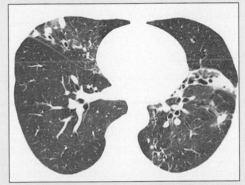

Figure 3. *M. avium-intracellulare* **complex infection with a "Lady Windermere" distribution.** CT image at the level of right inferior pulmonary vein shows bilateral bronchiectasis. Ground-glass opacities and mild consolidation are present in the right middle lobe, lingula, and left lower lobe. Also evident are small nodular opacities and a few "tree-in-bud" opacities. The patient was a 67-year-old woman.

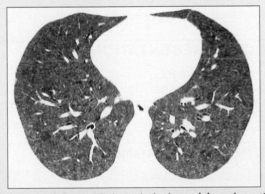

Figure 4. **Hot tub lung.** CT through the lower lobes of a patient with biopsy-proven hot tub lung shows diffuse ground-glass opacity and indistinct small nodules measuring 1-2 mm in diameter and resembling subacute hypersensitivity pneumonitis.

INCIDENCE/PREVALENCE AND EPIDEMIOLOGY

- Incidence of nontuberculous mycobacterial infection: 0.5-10 per 100,000 population.
- Cavitary form: tendency to affect males with smoking-related chronic lung disease.
- Bronchiectatic form: affects females > age 50 years with no preexisting disease or patients with underlying bronchiectasis.
- Hot tub lung: affects otherwise fit and relatively healthy hot tub users.

Suggested Readings

Diagnosis and treatment of disease caused by nontuberculous mycobacteria. This official statement of the American Thoracic Society was approved by the Board of Directors, March 1997. Medical Section of the American Lung Association. *Am J Respir Crit Care Med* 156:21-25, 1997.

Hartman TE, Jensen E, Tazelaar HD, et al: CT findings of granulomatous pneumonitis secondary to *Mycobacterium avium-intracellulare* inhalation: "Hot tub lung." *AJR Am J Roentgenol* 188:1050-1053, 2007.

Hartman TE, Swensen SJ, Williams DE: *Mycobacterium avium-intracellulare* complex: Evaluation with CT. *Radiology* 187:23-26, 1993.

Hollings NP, Wells AU, Wilson R, Hansell DM: Comparative appearances of non-tuberculous mycobacteria species: A CT study. *Eur Radiol* 12:2211-2217, 2002.

Jeong YJ, Lee KS, Koh WJ, et al: Nontuberculous mycobacterial pulmonary infection in immunocompetent patients: Comparison of thin-section CT and histopathologic findings. *Radiology* 231:880-886, 2004.

Waller EA, Roy A, Brumble L, et al: The expanding spectrum of *Mycobacterium avium* complex–associated pulmonary disease. *Chest* 130:1234-1241, 2006.

Unusual Nontuberculous Mycobacteria

DEFINITION: Pulmonary disease that occurs secondary to infection with various nontuberculous *Mycobacterium* species.

IMAGING

Radiography
Findings
- Consolidation
- Cavities with or without air-fluid levels
- Small nodules

Utility
- Initial modality and used for follow-up
- Wide spectrum and severity of findings: can be normal
- Findings resemble those of reactivation tuberculosis

CT
Findings
- Consolidation with cavities
- Bronchiectasis
- Centrilobular nodules and "tree-in-bud" pattern
- May have background of chronic lung disease

Utility
- CT is more sensitive than radiography.
- Findings resemble those of tuberculosis.

CLINICAL PRESENTATION

- May be asymptomatic
- Symptoms of pulmonary infection
- Rapid decline in patients with existing disease (e.g., cystic fibrosis)

DIFFERENTIAL DIAGNOSIS

- Postprimary tuberculosis
- *Mycobacterium avium-intracellulare* complex

PATHOLOGY

- Pulmonary infection secondary to various ubiquitous environmental opportunistic nontuberculous *Mycobacterium* species.
- Severity of disease largely determined by immune status or supervening infection.

DIAGNOSTIC PEARLS

- Consolidation with cavitation
- Small nodules with variable pattern
- Background of chronic parenchymal disease

INCIDENCE/PREVALENCE AND EPIDEMIOLOGY

- Incidence of nontuberculous mycobacterial infection is 0.5-10 per 100,000 population.
- Prevalence differs globally (e.g., *M. malmoense* is common in Europe; *M. kansasii* occurs in southern United States).
- *M. kansasii* is second most common pathogen in nontuberculous mycobacterial infection.
- *M. kansasii* infection is seen in HIV-positive individuals and middle-aged men.

Suggested Readings

Diagnosis and treatment of disease caused by nontuberculous mycobacteria. This official statement of the American Thoracic Society was approved by the Board of Directors, March 1997. Medical Section of the American Lung Association. *Am J Respir Crit Care Med* 156:21-25, 1997.

Ellis SM, Hansell DM: Imaging of non-tuberculous (atypical) mycobacterial pulmonary infection. *Clin Radiol* 57:661-669, 2002.

Erasmus JJ, McAdams HP, Farrell MA, Patz EF: Pulmonary nontuberculous mycobacterial infection: Radiologic manifestations. *RadioGraphics* 19:1487-1503, 1999.

Hollings NP, Wells AU, Wilson R, Hansell DM: Comparative appearances of non-tuberculous mycobacteria species: A CT study. *Eur Radiol* 12:2211-2217, 2002.

WHAT THE REFERRING PHYSICIAN NEEDS TO KNOW

- Decision to treat infection is complex and influenced by patient-based factors.
- Sensitivity to drug treatment is highly variable.

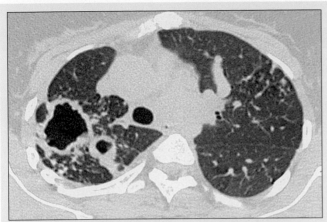

Figure 1. *M. kansasii* **infection.** CT image through the upper lobes of a patient with background centrilobular emphysema and *M. kansasii* infection demonstrates thick-walled cavities at the right lung apex and bilateral centrilobular nodular opacities. The appearance is similar to that of reactivation tuberculosis. *(Courtesy of Dr. David M. Hansell, London, UK)*

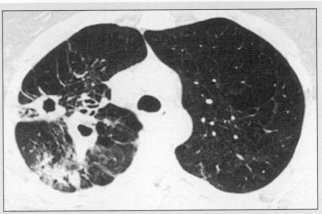

Figure 2. *M. xenopi* **infection.** CT image through the lung apices shows cavitating lesions on a background of severe centrilobular emphysema. *(Courtesy of Dr. David M. Hansell, London, UK)*

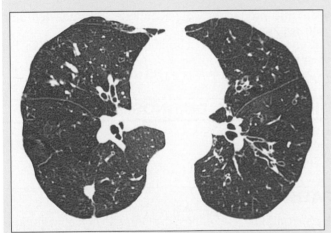

Figure 3. **Cystic fibrosis and** *M. chelonae* **infection.** CT image at the level of inferior pulmonary veins of a patient with *M. chelonae* infection shows extensive bronchiectasis and right lower lobe nodule. *(Courtesy of Dr. David M. Hansell, London, UK)*

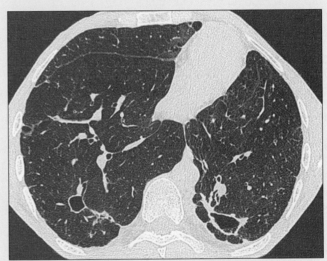

Figure 4. *M. szulgai* **infection in an HIV-infected patient.** CT image shows multiple cavitating lesions in a HIV-infected patient. *(Courtesy of Dr. David M. Hansell, London, UK)*

Aspergillosis

DEFINITION: Aspergillosis is a lung infection caused by *Aspergillus* fungi.

IMAGING

Radiography
Findings
- Aspergilloma: upper lobe rounded or oval, mobile mass within cavity with surrounding crescent of air (air crescent sign).
- Allergic bronchopulmonary aspergillosis: bronchiectasis seen as "finger-in-glove" or tube-like opacities corresponding to mucus plugs in dilated central bronchi.
- Segmental or lobar consolidation in chronic necrotizing aspergillosis.
- Poorly defined bilateral nodular opacities evident in airway-invasive aspergillosis.
- Angioinvasive aspergillosis: multiple, ill-defined nodular opacities; air crescent sign.

Utility
- Helpful in detecting disease and monitoring of treatment.

CT
Findings
- Upper lobe mass within a cavity in aspergilloma.
- Bronchiectasis with mucus plugs resulting in branching opacities that may have increased attenuation.
- Segmental or lobar consolidation in chronic necrotizing aspergillosis.
- "Tree-in-bud" appearance in airway-invasive aspergillosis.
- Angioinvasive aspergillosis: nodules without and with halo of ground-glass attenuation (CT halo sign).

Utility
- Detects aspergilloma too small to be seen on radiography.
- More sensitive and specific than radiography in the diagnosis of invasive aspergillosis.

CLINICAL PRESENTATION

- Hemoptysis (aspergilloma, chronic necrotizing aspergillosis)
- Wheezing, expectoration of mucus plugs (allergic bronchopulmonary aspergillosis)

DIAGNOSTIC PEARLS

- Aspergilloma: upper lobe, rounded or oval, mobile mass within cavity with surrounding crescent of air (air crescent sign).
- Allergic bronchopulmonary aspergillosis: central and predominantly upper lobe bronchiectasis seen as "finger-in-glove" or tube-like opacities corresponding to mucus plugs in dilated central bronchi.
- Airway-invasive aspergillosis: tree-in-bud pattern and patchy consolidation.
- Angioinvasive aspergillosis: nodules with halo of ground-glass attenuation (CT halo sign).

- Chronic productive cough, fatigue, dyspnea (chronic necrotizing aspergillosis)
- Bronchiolitis and bronchopneumonia (airway-invasive aspergillosis)
- Fever (angioinvasive aspergillosis)

DIFFERENTIAL DIAGNOSIS

- Bronchopneumonia
- Bronchiectasis
- Septic embolism

PATHOLOGY

- Aspergilloma is composed of fungal mycelia, inflammatory cells, fibrin, mucus, and tissue debris and develops in preexisting lung cavity.
- Airway colonization causes persistent inflammation and fibrosis leading to bronchiectasis, mucoid impaction, and parenchymal scarring in allergic bronchopulmonary aspergillosis.
- Airway-invasive aspergillosis is characterized by presence of fungi deep to airway basement membrane.
- Angioinvasive aspergillosis is caused by hyphal invasion of blood vessels resulting in infarction and necrosis.

WHAT THE REFERRING PHYSICIAN NEEDS TO KNOW

- Allergic bronchopulmonary aspergillosis occurs mainly in patients with asthma or cystic fibrosis and results from hypersensitivity reaction to *Aspergillus* antigens.
- Nodules with a halo of ground-glass attenuation on CT in severely neutropenic patients are highly suggestive of angioinvasive aspergillosis.
- CT is superior to chest radiography in the diagnosis of *Aspergillus*-related airway or parenchymal disease.

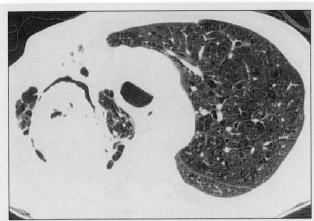

Figure 1. Aspergilloma. A 59-year-old woman with previous right mastectomy and right upper lobectomy presented with cough and weight loss. High-resolution CT scan shows a large mycetoma within the cavity. *Aspergillus fumigatus* was recovered at bronchoscopy.

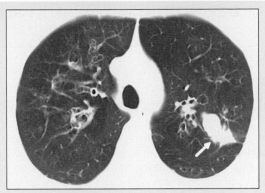

Figure 2. Allergic bronchopulmonary aspergillosis. A 31-year-old man presented with a history of asthma, recurrent pneumonias, and expectoration of brownish mucus plugs. CT image shows bilateral central bronchiectasis and a left upper lobe mucus plug (*arrow*). (*Courtesy of Dr. Thomas E. Hartman, Mayo Clinic, Rochester, MN*)

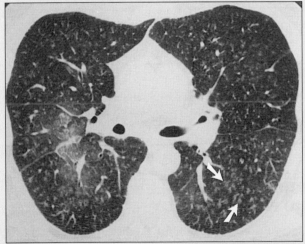

Figure 3. *Aspergillus* **bronchiolitis and bronchopneumonia.** High-resolution CT scan shows localized area of ground-glass attenuation in the right lung and bilateral, poorly defined small nodular opacities, and branching opacities ("tree-in-bud") (*arrows*). Open-lung biopsy showed *Aspergillus* bronchiolitis and bronchopneumonia. The patient was a 52-year old man who had undergone bone marrow transplantation. (*From Müller NL, Fraser RS, Colman NC, Paré PD: Radiologic Diagnosis of Diseases of the Chest. Philadelphia, WB Saunders, 2001.*)

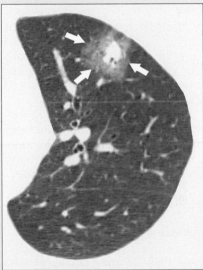

Figure 4. CT halo sign in invasive pulmonary aspergillosis. Magnified view of the left lung from a high-resolution CT shows nodule with surrounding ground-glass attenuation (CT halo sign) (*arrows*). The patient was a 33-year-old man with acute leukemia, severe neutropenia, and angioinvasive pulmonary aspergillosis.

INCIDENCE/PREVALENCE AND EPIDEMIOLOGY

- *Aspergillus* is most common cause of fungus ball.
- Allergic bronchopulmonary aspergillosis occurs in 7%-14% of corticosteroid-dependent asthmatics and 6% of patients with cystic fibrosis.
- Semi-invasive or chronic necrotizing aspergillosis primarily occurs in patients with underlying chronic lung disease, with chronic debilitating illness, or on prolonged corticosteroid therapy.
- Airway-invasive aspergillosis occurs most commonly in neutropenic patients.
- Angioinvasive aspergillosis primarily affects severely immunocompromised patients with neutropenia.

Suggested Readings

Chong S, Lee KS, Yi CA, et al: Pulmonary fungal infection: Imaging findings in immunocompetent and immunocompromised patients. *Eur J Radiol* 59:371-383, 2006.

Franquet T, Muller NL, Gimenez A, et al: Spectrum of pulmonary aspergillosis: Histologic, clinical, and radiologic findings. *Radio-Graphics* 21:825-837, 2001.

Waite S, Jeudy J, White CS: Acute lung infections in normal and immunocompromised hosts. *Radiol Clin North Am* 44:295-315, 2006.

Wheat LJ, Goldman M, Sarosi G: State-of-the-art review of pulmonary fungal infections. *Semin Respir Infect* 17:158-181, 2002.

Blastomycosis

DEFINITION: Blastomycosis is infection caused *Blastomyces dermatitidis.*

IMAGING

Radiography
Findings
- Varied and nonspecific findings: consolidation, masses, nodules, cavitation, and interstitial changes.
- Most common appearance: patchy or confluent segmental or subsegmental airspace consolidation, which often has ill-defined margins; air bronchograms.

Utility
- Findings often resemble those of community-acquired pneumonia but granulomatous infection should be suspected if findings progress or are slow to resolve.
- Masses may be confused with bronchogenic carcinoma.
- Chest radiography helps detect disease.

CT
Findings
- Pulmonary masses that frequently contain air bronchograms.
- Nodules < 2 cm in diameter, perihilar location of parenchymal disease, satellite lesions, and consolidation.
- Lymphadenopathy.

Utility
- Chest CT is more sensitive than radiography and better depicts findings and possible complications.
- Complementary use of chest radiography and CT is helpful in monitoring treatment response.

Positron Emission Tomography
Findings
- Increased uptake in FDG-PET
Utility
- False-positive PET/CT may occur, as with any infection.

CLINICAL PRESENTATION

- Mild flu-like symptoms.
- Acute pneumonia with fever, productive cough, pleuritic chest pain, arthralgias, and myalgias.

DIAGNOSTIC PEARLS

- Pulmonary masses containing air bronchograms.
- Patchy or confluent airspace consolidation with ill-defined margins, air bronchograms, and usually segmental or subsegmental.
- Endemic regions: southeastern and south central United States, Central Canada, South America.

- Verrucous skin lesion with raised, irregular border drainage or ulcerative lesion with sharp, heaped-up border and exudate at its base.

DIFFERENTIAL DIAGNOSIS

- Community-acquired pneumonia
- Tuberculosis
- Pulmonary carcinoma
- Pulmonary metastases

PATHOLOGY

- Immunocompetent patients most often develop bronchopneumonia with regional lymph node involvement.
- Extension into pleura or chest wall may occur in immunocompromised patients.

INCIDENCE/PREVALENCE AND EPIDEMIOLOGY

- Infection is most common in North America, particularly occurring in the southeastern and south central states and parts of the Midwest in the United States and in central Canada.
- Endemic regions also found in Africa, Central America, and South America.
- Fungus proliferates in warm, moist soil of wooded areas rich in organic debris.
- Patients with underlying lung disease or immunocompromised patients are at risk for more serious forms of infection.

WHAT THE REFERRING PHYSICIAN NEEDS TO KNOW

- Endemic fungal pneumonias may mimic community-acquired bronchopneumonia, whereas masses may be confused with bronchogenic carcinoma.
- Fungal infection should be suspected in a patient with bronchopneumonia that does not respond to typical antibiotic therapy.
- History of travel to or residence in an endemic region is important in diagnosis.
- Endemic areas are mainly the southeastern and south central states and parts of the Midwest in the United States and in central Canada.

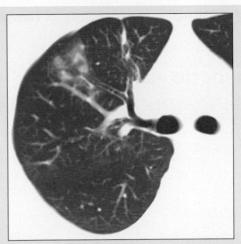

Figure 1. A 41-year-old man presented with myalgias, fever, and fatigue. CT images reveal ill-defined nodular opacities and small areas of consolidation (see Fig. 2), with air bronchograms in the right upper lobe. Bronchial washings grew out *Blastomyces dermatitidis. (Courtesy of Drs. Rebecca M. Lindell and Thomas E. Hartman, Mayo Clinic, Rochester, MN)*

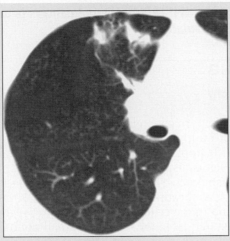

Figure 2. A 41-year-old male with myalgias, fever and fatigue. CT images reveal ill-defined nodular opacities (see Fig. 1) and small areas of consolidation, with air bronchograms in the right upper lobe. Bronchial washings grew out *Blastomyces dermatitidis. (Courtesy of Drs. Rebecca M. Lindell and Thomas E. Hartman, Mayo Clinic, Rochester, MN)*

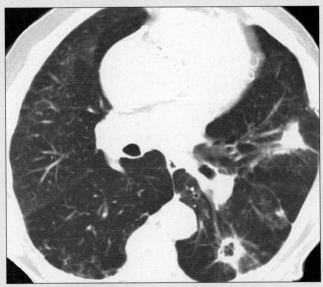

Figure 3. An 80-year-old diabetic man presents with worsening chronic cough with blood-streaked sputum. CT image shows a 25-mm cavitated irregular nodule and a 9-mm nodule in the left lower lobe. Also noted is an irregular 2.5-mm nodule in the lingula. Serology was positive for *Blastomyces. (Courtesy of Drs. Rebecca M. Lindell and Thomas E. Hartman, Mayo Clinic, Rochester, MN)*

Suggested Readings

Chong S, Lee KS, Yi CA, et al: Pulmonary fungal infection: Imaging findings in immunocompetent and immunocompromised patients. *Eur J Radiol* 59:371-383, 2006.

Fang W, Washington L, Kumar N: Imaging manifestations of blastomycosis: A pulmonary infection with potential dissemination. *RadioGraphics* 27:641-655, 2007.

Waite S, Jeudy J, White CS: Acute lung infections in normal and immunocompromised hosts. *Radiol Clin North Am* 44:295-315, 2006.

Wheat LJ, Goldman M, Sarosi G: State-of-the-art review of pulmonary fungal infections. *Semin Respir Infect* 17:158-168, 2002.

Histoplasmosis

DEFINITION: Histoplasmosis is fungal infection caused by inhalation of microconidia of *Histoplasma capsulatum.*

IMAGING

Radiography
Findings
- Patchy airspace consolidation.
- Single or multiple small nodules.
- Chronic histoplasmosis: unilateral or bilateral upper lobe opacities usually extending to pleura.
- Histoplasmoma: slowly enlarging nodule, with or without calcifications, measuring up to 30 mm, usually found in lower lobe peripherally.
- Disseminated infection: multiple small nodules.
- Widened mediastinum on chest radiograph seen in mediastinal granuloma, fibrosing mediastinitis.
Utility
- Chest radiograph normal in most patients

CT
Findings
- Unilateral or bilateral upper lobe consolidation and ground-glass opacities.
- Histoplasmoma commonly demonstrates diffuse, central, or laminated patterns of calcification.
- Satellite nodules and centrilobular nodules (sometimes with "tree-in-bud" pattern).
- Fibrosing mediastinitis: hilar or mediastinal mass, diffuse mediastinal soft tissue infiltration, calcification, bronchial narrowing, obstruction or narrowing of superior vena cava and pulmonary artery.
- Miliary nodules with poorly or sharply defined margins.
Utility
- Volumetric chest CT with thin-section images more sensitive in detecting disseminated histoplasmosis.
- CT superior to radiography in demonstrating calcification of histoplasmoma.
- CT performed almost routinely in the assessment of patients suspected of having fibrosing mediastinitis.

Positron Emission Tomography
Findings
- Increased metabolism of pulmonary nodule is seen in acute disease and occasionally in chronic disease.
- Histoplasmomas may also have increased glucose metabolism and result in false-positive PET scans.

DIAGNOSTIC PEARLS
- Endemic areas: central and eastern North America
- Histoplasmoma: slowly enlarging nodule, with or without calcifications, measuring up to 30 mm, usually found peripherally in lower lobe
- Fibrosing mediastinitis: hilar or mediastinal mass-like area of calcification with associated narrowing of bronchus, pulmonary artery, or superior vena cava

- Fibrosing mediastinitis or mediastinal granuloma may have false-positive results on PET imaging.
Utility
- Both malignancy and infection may result in a positive scan.

CLINICAL PRESENTATION
- Acute histoplasmosis: flu-like illness with fever, dry cough, and fatigue.
- Chronic histoplasmosis: productive cough, fever, dyspnea, fatigue, weight loss, hemoptysis.
- Disseminated histoplasmosis: respiratory distress, hepatic and renal failure, shock, and coagulopathy.
- Histoplasmomas typically asymptomatic.
- Broncholithiasis: nonproductive cough, hemoptysis; less commonly, fever, chills, pain from postobstructive pneumonitis; expectoration of broncholith.

DIFFERENTIAL DIAGNOSIS
- Postprimary tuberculosis
- Pulmonary metastases
- Community-acquired pneumonia
- Pulmonary carcinoma

PATHOLOGY
- Diagnosis requires identification of yeast-like forms in tissue.
- Chronic infection is characterized most commonly by necrotizing granuloma with tendency to calcify.

WHAT THE REFERRING PHYSICIAN NEEDS TO KNOW
- Central, laminar, or diffuse calcification within nodule and calcification within lymph node helps identify nodule as calcified granuloma.
- History of travel to or residence in an endemic region is important in diagnosis.
- Bronchopneumonia that dose not respond to typical antibiotic therapy in endemic regions is suggestive of the diagnosis.
- Fungal infections may mimic bronchogenic carcinoma or metastases.

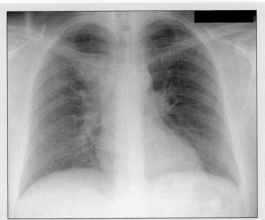

Figure 1. Acute histoplasmosis. A 39-year-old man presented with a 2-week history of cough and fever. Chest radiograph shows consolidation in the right upper lobe medially. Bronchoscopic biopsy revealed histoplasmosis. *(Courtesy of Drs. Rebecca M. Lindell and Thomas E. Hartman, Mayo Clinic, Rochester, MN)*

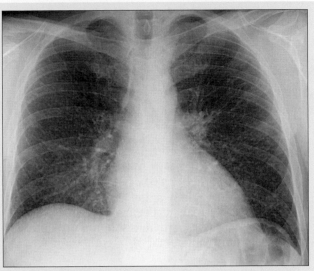

Figure 2. Disseminated histoplasmosis in a 41-year-old man with AIDS. Chest radiograph shows diffuse bilateral miliary pulmonary nodules. *(Courtesy of Drs. Rebecca M. Lindell and Thomas E. Hartman, Mayo Clinic, Rochester, MN)*

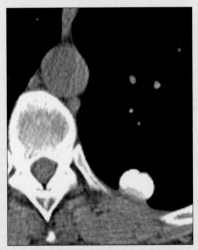

Figure 3. Calcified granuloma secondary to histoplasmosis in a 43-year-old asymptomatic woman living in an area endemic for histoplasmosis. CT image shows densely calcified nodule in the left lower lobe. The patient also had calcified left hilar nodes (not shown) *(Courtesy of Drs. Rebecca M. Lindell and Thomas E. Hartman, Mayo Clinic, Rochester, MN)*

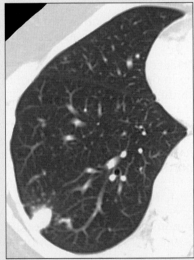

Figure 4. Histoplasmoma. A 51-year-old woman presented with an incidental nodule on routine chest radiograph. A 5-mm CT scan shows a peripheral right lower lobe nodule with tiny surrounding satellite nodules *(Courtesy of Drs. Rebecca M. Lindell and Thomas E. Hartman, Mayo Clinic, Rochester, MN)*

- Disseminated form results from progression of primary infection or from reactivation of prior infection in disseminated histoplasmosis.
- As sequela to histoplasmosis, chronic fibrotic process may develop in mediastinum (fibrosing mediastinitis).

INCIDENCE/PREVALENCE AND EPIDEMIOLOGY

- Endemic regions include central and eastern North America, especially in Ohio, Mississippi, and St. Lawrence River Valleys.
- Over half of adults living in endemic areas are infected with *H. capsulatum*.
- Chronic pulmonary histoplasmosis occurs almost exclusively in middle-aged men with emphysema.

- Immune-competent patients most often develop bronchopneumonia with regional lymph node involvement.
- Patients with underlying lung disease or immunocompromised patients are at risk for more serious forms of infection.
- Disseminated histoplasmosis is considered an opportunistic infection affecting immunocompromised individuals.
- Mediastinal granuloma is more common than fibrosing mediastinitis.

Suggested Readings

Chong S, Lee KS, Yi CA, et al: Pulmonary fungal infection: Imaging findings in immunocompetent and immunocompromised patients. *Eur J Radiol* 59:371-383, 2006.

Waite S, Jeudy J, White CS: Acute lung infections in normal and immunocompromised hosts. *Radiol Clin North Am* 44:295-315, 2006.

Wheat LJ, Goldman M, Sarosi G: State-of-the-art review of pulmonary fungal infections. *Semin Respir Infect* 17:158-181, 2002.

Coccidioidomycosis

DEFINITION: Coccidioidomycosis is a pulmonary disease caused by the dimorphic fungus *Coccidioides immitis*.

IMAGING

Radiography

Findings

- Primary infection: single or multiple foci of airspace consolidation, nodules with cavitation and air-fluid level
- Hilar or mediastinal lymphadenopathy, in association with lung parenchymal findings
- Pleural effusion, usually small
- Chronic infection: thin-walled cavitation, single or, less commonly, multiple peripheral pulmonary nodules
- Pleural effusion, empyema, or pneumothorax

Utility

- First and often only imaging modality used in the evaluation of these patients.

CT

Findings

- Acute/primary coccidioidomycosis: consolidations or nodules, which may be associated with satellite nodules.
- Chronic/persistent coccidioidomycosis: solitary nodule of 10-20 mm in diameter in periphery of upper lobes.
- Nodule with thin-wall cavity.
- Hilar or mediastinal lymphadenopathy in association with parenchymal findings.
- Some nodules with surrounding ground-glass attenuation (CT halo sign) due to granulomatous inflammation or hemorrhage.
- Focal areas of ground-glass opacity and focal consolidation (chronic type).

Utility

- Chest CT is more sensitive than radiography in depicting findings and complications of chronic coccidioidomycosis.
- Chest CT is helpful if diagnosis is uncertain or if patient does not improve as expected or develops complications.

CLINICAL PRESENTATION

- Acute infection is usually asymptomatic or mild.
- Symptoms typically develop 1-4 weeks after exposure: cough, fever, chest pain, fatigue, anorexia, headache.

DIAGNOSTIC PEARLS

- Single or multiple foci of consolidation or nodules (acute)
- Nodule with low attenuation center
- Thin-walled ("grapeskin") cavitary nodule
- Endemic regions: southwestern United States and northern Mexico

---

- Infection is usually self-limited, resolving over 3-6 weeks.
- Chronic infection is usually asymptomatic or mild but may develop into severe pneumonia (fever, productive cough, night sweats, hemoptysis).

DIFFERENTIAL DIAGNOSIS

- Lung cancer
- Bronchopneumonia
- Tuberculosis
- Pulmonary metastases

PATHOLOGY

- Infection is caused by inhalation of fungal arthrospores or arthroconidia.
- *C. immitis* in tissues has characteristic appearance of round to oval spherule containing endospores.
- Histologic reaction is usually initially an acute suppurative pneumonitis followed by granulomatous inflammation and necrotizing granulomas.

INCIDENCE/PREVALENCE AND EPIDEMIOLOGY

- Causative organism is the dimorphic fungus *Coccidioides immitis*, which is found in soil and endemic in southwestern United States, northern Mexico, and in regions of Central and South America.
- Incidence of pulmonary coccidioidomycosis is highest in late summer and early fall, when soil is driest.
- Approximately 5% of cases of primary coccidioidomycosis become chronic.

WHAT THE REFERRING PHYSICIAN NEEDS TO KNOW

- History of travel to or residence in an endemic region is important in diagnosis.
- Fungal infection should be suspected in a patient with bronchopneumonia that does not respond to typical antibiotic therapy.
- Fungal infections may mimic bronchogenic carcinoma or metastases.

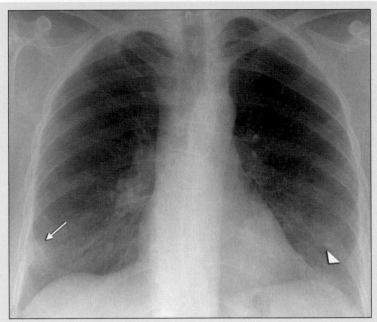

Figure 1. Disseminated coccidioidomycosis. A 50-year-old woman developed a rash, fatigue, productive cough, fever, and headache while vacationing in Arizona. Posteroanterior radiograph shows a 3-cm nodule (*arrow*) in the right lower lobe with associated right hilar lymphadenopathy and a small nodule (*arrowhead*) in the left lower lung. (*Courtesy of Drs Rebecca M. Lindell and Thomas E. Hartman, Mayo Clinic, Rochester, MN*)

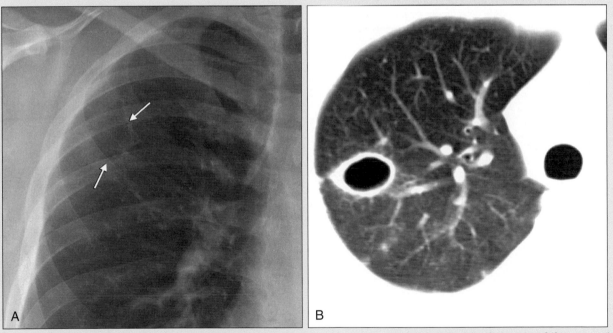

Figure 2. Chronic coccidioidomycosis. A 33-year-old man with chronic productive cough developed acute chest pain while on vacation in Arizona. Chest radiograph (**A**) showed a 3.3-cm subtle thin-walled cavity (*arrows*) in the right upper lobe that was confirmed on CT scan (**B**). Cultures from sputum and bronchial washings grew *Coccidioides immitis*. (*Courtesy of Drs Rebecca M. Lindell and Thomas E. Hartman, Mayo Clinic, Rochester, MN*)

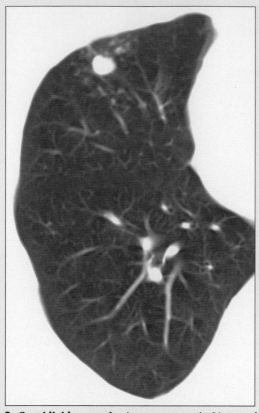

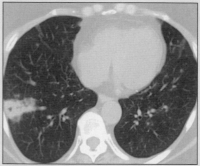

Figure 4. **Disseminated coccidioidomycosis.** A 50-year-old woman developed a rash, fatigue, productive cough, fever, and headache while vacationing in Arizona. CT image demonstrates a cavitated nodule with surrounding infiltrate versus focal consolidation in the right lower lobe. There are associated air bronchograms. Several small nodules are scattered in both lungs. CSF serology was positive for coccidioidomycosis (see also Fig. 1). (*Courtesy of Drs. Rebecca M. Lindell and Thomas E. Hartman, Mayo Clinic, Rochester, MN*)

Figure 3. **Coccidioidomycosis.** An asymptomatic 64-year-old man from Arizona had a nodule detected on a routine chest radiograph. A chest radiograph (not shown) 1 year earlier was negative. Chest CT image demonstrates a 13-mm nodule surrounded by tiny satellite nodules in the right middle lobe. Surgical resection revealed caseating granulomas and coccidioidomycosis. (*Courtesy of Drs. Rebecca M. Lindell and Thomas E. Hartman, Mayo Clinic, Rochester, MN*)

Suggested Readings

Chong S, Lee KS, Yi CA, et al: Pulmonary fungal infection: Imaging findings in immunocompetent and immunocompromised patients. *Eur J Radiol* 59:371-383, 2006.

Waite S, Jeudy J, White CS: Acute lung infections in normal and immunocompromised hosts. *Radiol Clin North Am* 44:295-315, 2006.

Wheat LJ, Goldman M, Sarosi G: State-of-the-art review of pulmonary fungal infections. *Semin Respir Infect* 17:158-181, 2002.

Opportunistic Fungal Infections

DEFINITION: Opportunistic fungal infections include aspergillosis, candidiasis, cryptococcosis and zygomycosis.

IMAGING

Radiography
Findings
- Angioinvasive aspergillosis: round, subsegmental or segmental consolidation; multiple, ill-defined nodular opacities; cavitation common.
- Airway-invasive aspergillosis (*Aspergillus* bronchiolitis and bronchopneumonia): poorly defined nodular opacities, patchy areas of consolidation.
- Candidiasis: nodules and/or consolidation.
- Zygomycosis: unilateral or bilateral airspace consolidation that may progress rapidly; solitary or multiple nodules that may cavitate.
- Cryptococcosis: single or multiple nodules/masses with varied margins that may cavitate; may have consolidation, lymphadenopathy, or pleural effusions.

Utility
- Initial radiologic modality
- Of limited value in the differential diagnosis

CT
Findings
- Angioinvasive aspergillosis: multiple nodules usually 0.5-3.0 cm in diameter and frequently surrounded by rim of ground-glass attenuation (CT halo sign) and cavitated; may have air crescent sign.
- Airway-invasive aspergillosis (*Aspergillus* bronchiolitis and bronchopneumonia): centrilobular nodules, "tree-in-bud" pattern, patchy areas of consolidation.
- Pulmonary candidiasis: nodules, ground-glass opacities, foci of consolidation; nodules may have CT halo sign.
- Zygomycosis: consolidation, nodules or masses; may have CT halo sign.
- Cryptococcosis: single or multiple nodules/masses with varied margins that may cavitate; consolidation, lymphadenopathy, or pleural effusions possible.

Utility
- Superior to chest radiography in showing pattern and distribution of disease and presence of nodules and cavitation.

DIAGNOSTIC PEARLS
- Nodules with halo of ground-glass attenuation in neutropenic patient are highly suggestive of angioinvasive aspergillosis.
- Angioinvasive aspergillosis results in multiple lung nodules whereas airway-invasive aspergillosis results in bronchiolitis and bronchopneumonia.
- Pulmonary candidiasis is uncommon and usually only seen in patients with systemic candidemia.

CLINICAL PRESENTATION
- Fever
- Cough
- Hemoptysis
- Dyspnea

DIFFERENTIAL DIAGNOSIS
- Bacterial or viral pneumonia
- Tuberculosis
- Septic embolism
- Pulmonary hemorrhage
- Lymphoma

PATHOLOGY
- Immunocompromised patients are at risk for serious forms of infection such as dissemination, chronic infection, and extension into pleura or chest wall.
- Airway-invasive aspergillosis is characterized by presence of fungi deep to airway basement membrane.
- Angioinvasive aspergillosis is caused by hyphal invasion of blood vessels resulting in infarction and hemorrhage.
- Respiratory infection results from overgrowth of endogenous *Candida,* but nosocomial transmission may occur.
- Cryptococcal infection occurs via inhalation of *Cryptococcus neoformans.*

WHAT THE REFERRING PHYSICIAN NEEDS TO KNOW
- Knowledge of underlying lung disease, corticosteroid use, and immune status is important for diagnosis.
- The radiographic findings are nonspecific.
- CT is superior to radiography in demonstrating the presence of parenchymal abnormalities and suggesting the possibility of opportunistic fungal infection.
- CT halo sign (rim of ground-glass opacity surrounding nodule or mass) in neutropenic patient is highly suggestive of invasive aspergillosis; less common causes include candidiasis and mucormycosis.
- The radiologic findings of airway-invasive aspergillosis (*Aspergillus* bronchiolitis and bronchopneumonia) mimic those of other infectious causes.

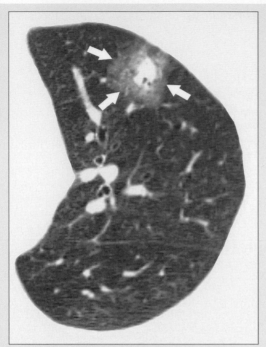

Figure 1. Invasive pulmonary aspergillosis. Magnified view of the left lung from a high-resolution CT shows a nodule with surrounding ground-glass attenuation (CT halo sign, *arrows*). The patient was a 33-year-old man with acute leukemia, severe neutropenia, and angioinvasive pulmonary aspergillosis.

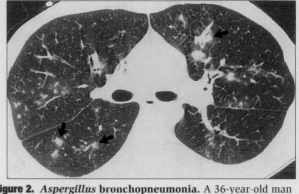

Figure 2. *Aspergillus* **bronchopneumonia.** A 36-year-old man presented with fever and cough after allogeneic bone marrow transplantation. High-resolution CT image shows focal areas of consolidation in a predominantly peribronchial distribution (*arrows*), and several small centrilobular nodules. Transbronchial biopsy showed *Aspergillus fumigatus* and pneumonia. (*From Müller NL, Fraser RS, Colman NC, Paré PD: Radiologic Diagnosis of Diseases of the Chest. Philadelphia, WB Saunders, 2001.*)

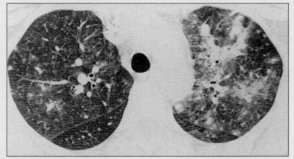

Figure 3. *Candida* **pneumonia.** High-resolution CT scan shows nodules of various sizes, focal areas of consolidation, and ground-glass attenuation. The patient was a 27-year-old woman who developed *Candida* pneumonia after bone marrow transplantation. (*From Müller NL, Fraser RS, Colman NC, Paré PD: Radiologic Diagnosis of Diseases of the Chest. Philadelphia, WB Saunders, 2001.*)

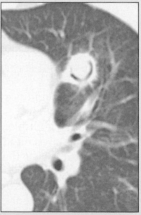

Figure 4. Zygomycosis. A 58-year-old neutropenic man undergoing chemotherapy for acute myelogenous leukemia presented with fever and cough with pain. CT image shows cavitated left upper lobe nodule. Cultures grew *Zygomycetes*. (*Courtesy of Dr. Thomas E. Hartman, Mayo Clinic, Rochester, MN*)

INCIDENCE/PREVALENCE AND EPIDEMIOLOGY

- Airway-invasive aspergillosis occurs most commonly in neutropenic and AIDS patients.
- Angioinvasive aspergillosis primarily affects severely immunocompromised patients with neutropenia.
- Pulmonary candidiasis is rare opportunistic infection caused by *Candida albicans* and less commonly by *C. tropicalis* or *C. krusei*.
- Cryptococcosis is caused by *Cryptococcus neoformans*, which is a thin-walled, non-mycelial, budding encapsulated yeast.
- Zygomycosis (mucormycosis, phycomycosis) is an uncommon and often fatal opportunistic fungal infection.

Suggested Readings

Chong S, Lee KS, Yi CA, et al: Pulmonary fungal infection: Imaging findings in immunocompetent and immunocompromised patients. *Eur J Radiol* 59:371-383, 2006.

Franquet T, Müller NL, Giménez A, et al: Spectrum of pulmonary aspergillosis: Histologic, clinical, and radiologic findings. *Radio-Graphics* 21:825-837, 2001.

Franquet T, Müller NL, Lee KS, et al: Pulmonary candidiasis after hematopoietic stem cell transplantation: Thin-section CT findings. *Radiology* 236:332-337, 2005.

Greene RE, Schlamm HT, Oestmann JW, et al: Imaging findings in acute invasive pulmonary aspergillosis: Clinical significance of the halo sign. *Clin Infect Dis* 44:373-379, 2007.

Pneumonia *(Mycoplasma)*

DEFINITION: Pneumonia that is caused by *Mycoplasma pneumoniae.*

IMAGING

Radiography
Findings
- Patchy unilateral or bilateral areas of consolidation, small nodular opacities, and unilateral or bilateral reticular or reticulonodular opacities.
- Involves lower lobes, mainly.
- Pleural effusions possible but usually small and unilateral.

Utility
- First and usually only imaging modality in diagnosis and follow-up of patients with community-acquired pneumonia.

CT
Findings
- Centrilobular nodular and branching linear opacities ("tree-in-bud" pattern) in patchy distribution.
- Bronchial wall thickening, ground-glass opacities, consolidation in lobular or segmental distribution.
- Ground-glass opacities commonly in a lobular distribution.
- Patchy unilateral or asymmetric bilateral distribution, but may be diffuse.
- May be associated with areas of decreased attenuation and vascularity, air trapping, and, in severe cases, hyperinflation.

Utility
- Helpful in symptomatic patients with normal or non-specific radiographic findings.

CLINICAL PRESENTATION

- Onset is insidious with fever, sore throat, cough, headache, and malaise.
- Cough is initially nonproductive but may become associated with mucoid or purulent sputum.
- Extensive pneumonia may result in shortness of breath.

DIAGNOSTIC PEARLS

- *Mycoplasma pneumoniae* is the most common cause of community-acquired pneumonia in 5- to 20-year-olds.
- May occur in epidemics in enclosed populations such as college students and military garrisons.
- Patchy unilateral or bilateral areas of consolidation and small nodular opacities.
- Associated findings may include myringitis, meningoencephalitis, and hemolytic anemia.

- Associated findings may include myringitis, meningoencephalitis, thrombocytopenic purpura, hemolytic anemia, pericarditis, myocarditis and a rash associated with high fever, stomatitis, and ophthalmia (Stevens-Johnson syndrome).

DIFFERENTIAL DIAGNOSIS

- Pneumonia caused by other organisms
- Organizing pneumonia
- Aspiration pneumonia
- Tuberculosis

PATHOLOGY

- *Mycoplasma* is a bacterium that lacks a cell wall and grows in an extracellular location; it is the smallest free-living organism that can be cultured on artificial media.
- Predominant pulmonary abnormality is bronchiolitis.
- Pneumonia is characterized by inflammatory infiltrate in bronchiolar wall and neutrophil-rich luminal exudates.
- Transmission of organism is usually from person to person by droplet inhalation secondary to coughing.
- Less common histologic manifestations include diffuse alveolar damage, organizing pneumonia, obliterative bronchiolitis, and bronchiectasis.

WHAT THE REFERRING PHYSICIAN NEEDS TO KNOW

- Most common radiographic manifestations of *Mycoplasma* pneumonia consist of patchy areas of consolidation and reticular or reticulonodular opacities.
- Chest radiograph and CT are of limited value in distinguishing *Mycoplasma* pneumonia from other causes of pneumonia.
- Majority of patients with *Mycoplasma* pneumonia recover completely; however, a small percentage, particularly children, develop bronchiectasis and obliterative bronchiolitis.
- It has been estimated that 20%-30% of cases of bronchiolitis obliterans in children are secondary to *Mycoplasma* pneumonia.
- Diagnosis is usually made based on clinical findings, normal white blood cell count, abnormal chest radiograph, and antibody assays.

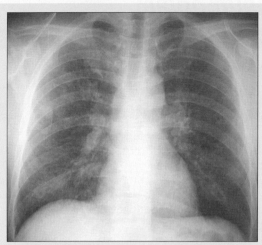

Figure 1. Posteroanterior chest radiograph shows poorly defined reticulonodular pattern and ground-glass opacities in the right lung and poorly defined small nodular opacities in the left lung. The patient was a 37-year-old man with *Mycoplasma* pneumonia.

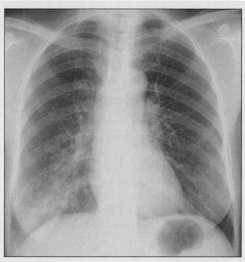

Figure 2. Posteroanterior chest radiograph shows poorly defined nodular opacities and foci of consolidation in the right lower lobe. The patient was a 48-year-old man with *Mycoplasma* pneumonia. (*Courtesy of Dr. Atsushi Nambu, Department of Radiology, University of Yamanashi, Yamanashi, Japan.*)

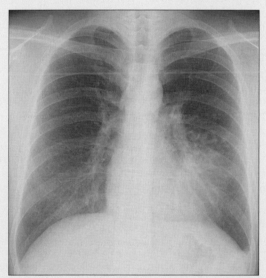

Figure 3. Posteroanterior chest radiograph shows consolidation in the lingula and small left pleural effusion. The patient was a 25-year-old man with *Mycoplasma* pneumonia. (*Courtesy of Dr. Atsushi Nambu, Department of Radiology, University of Yamanashi, Yamanashi, Japan.*)

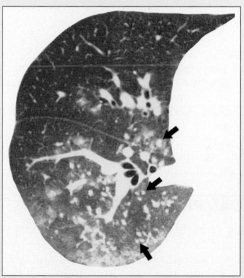

Figure 4. View of the right lung from a high-resolution CT demonstrates centrilobular nodules (*arrows*) in the right middle and lower lobes and patchy ground-glass opacities. The patient was a 44-year-old man with *Mycoplasma* pneumonia. (*Courtesy of Dr. Atsushi Nambu, Department of Radiology, University of Yamanashi, Yamanashi, Japan.*)

INCIDENCE/PREVALENCE AND EPIDEMIOLOGY

- It is the most common cause of community-acquired pneumonia in 5- to 20-year-olds and accounts for 10%-15% of pneumonias in adults.
- Epidemics have been described in enclosed populations such as college students, prisoners, and military garrisons.
- Simultaneous cases may also occur within single households.
- Infections occur throughout the year, with a peak during the autumn and early winter in temperate regions.

Suggested Readings

Blasi F, Tarsia P, Aliberti S, et al: *Chlamydia pneumoniae* and *Mycoplasma pneumoniae*. *Semin Respir Crit Care Med* 26:617-624, 2005.

Cunha BA: The atypical pneumonias: Clinical diagnosis and importance. *Clin Microbiol Infect* 12(Suppl 3):12-24, 2006.

Lee I, Kim TS, Yoon HK: *Mycoplasma pneumoniae* pneumonia: CT features in 16 patients. *Eur Radiol* 16:719-725, 2006.

Reittner P, Müller NL, Heyneman L, et al: *Mycoplasma pneumoniae* pneumonia: Radiographic and high-resolution CT features in 28 patients. *AJR Am J Roentgenol* 174:37-41, 2000.

Waites KB, Talkington DF: *Mycoplasma pneumoniae* and its role as a human pathogen. *Clin Microbiol Rev* 17:697-728, 2004.

Pneumonia (*Chlamydia pneumoniae*)

DEFINITION: Pulmonary disease that is caused by infection with *Chlamydia pneumoniae*.

IMAGING

Radiography
Findings
- Reticulonodular opacities and focal, segmental, or sublobar areas of consolidation are seen.
- Radiographic abnormalities tend to progress from predominantly reticulonodular opacities to mixed reticulonodular and airspace opacities during course of infection.
- Areas of consolidation may be patchy and unilateral or bilateral, consistent with bronchopneumonia or, less commonly, sublobar or lobar.

Utility
- Usually the only imaging modality performed in these patients.
- Manifestations tend to be mild but are otherwise nonspecific.

CT
Findings
- Ground-glass opacities and consolidation are seen.
- Patchy, poorly defined areas of opacities are more consistent with bronchopneumonia.
- Centrilobular nodules and bronchial wall thickening may occur.

Utility
- Findings indistinguishable from those of pneumonia due to other organisms.

CLINICAL PRESENTATION

- Patients present with sore throat, nonproductive cough, and fever.
- Majority of patients have hoarseness due to laryngitis.
- Clinical course may vary from mild, self-limiting illness to severe pneumonia in the elderly or in patients with comorbidities.

DIFFERENTIAL DIAGNOSIS

- Pneumonia caused by other organisms
- Organizing pneumonia
- Aspiration pneumonia
- Tuberculosis

DIAGNOSTIC PEARLS

- Usually mild.
- Most common in children and in adults with chronic airway disease.
- Radiographic abnormalities tend to progress from predominantly reticulonodular opacities to mixed reticulonodular and airspace opacities during course of infection.

PATHOLOGY

- *Chlamydia pneumoniae* is the causative organism.
- Chlamydiae are obligate intracellular bacteria that can only grow in host cells and not in artificial culture media.
- Pathologic features are poorly documented because infection is usually mild.

INCIDENCE/PREVALENCE AND EPIDEMIOLOGY

- *C. pneumoniae* is common cause of community-acquired pneumonia, accounting for 12%-20% of cases.
- Pneumonia occurs most commonly in children and in adults with underlying chronic airway disease such as chronic obstructive pulmonary disease or cystic fibrosis.
- Outbreaks of pneumonia due to *C. pneumoniae* have been described in nursing homes.

Suggested Readings

Blasi F, Tarsia P, Aliberti S, et al: *Chlamydia pneumoniae* and *Mycoplasma pneumoniae*. *Semin Respir Crit Care Med* 26:617-624, 2005.

Cunha BA: The atypical pneumonias: Clinical diagnosis and importance. *Clin Microbiol Infect* 12(Suppl 3):12-24, 2006.

Marrie TJ, Poulin-Costello M, Beecroft MD, Herman-Gnjidic Z: Etiology of community-acquired pneumonia treated in an ambulatory setting. *Respir Med* 99:60-65, 2005.

McConnell CT Jr, Plouffe JF, File TM, et al: Radiographic appearance of *Chlamydia pneumoniae* (TWAR strain) respiratory infections. CBPIS Study Group. Community-based Pneumonia Incidence Study. *Radiology* 192:819-824, 1994.

Okada F, Ando Y, Wakisaka M, et al: *Chlamydia pneumoniae* pneumonia and *Mycoplasma pneumoniae* pneumonia: Comparison of clinical findings and CT findings. *J Comput Assist Tomogr* 29:626-632, 2005.

WHAT THE REFERRING PHYSICIAN NEEDS TO KNOW

- In majority of cases diagnosis is made based on clinical findings, abnormal findings on a chest radiograph, and positive serologic microimmunofluorescent assay.
- Treatment is with antibiotics, most commonly tetracycline or erythromycin or their derivatives.

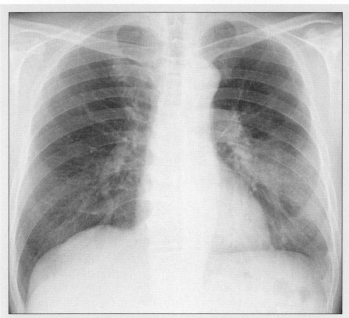

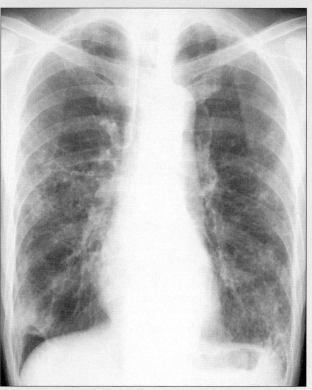

Figure 1. *Chlamydia* **pneumonia.** Posteroanterior chest radiograph shows poorly defined consolidation and ground-glass opacities in the left lower lobe. The patient was a 62-year-old man. (*Courtesy of Dr. Atsushi Nambu, Department of Radiology, University of Yamanashi, Yamanashi, Japan.*)

Figure 2. *Chlamydia* **pneumonia.** Posteroanterior chest radiograph shows bilateral poorly defined ground-glass opacities and small nodular opacities. Also noted are increased lung volumes due to chronic obstructive pulmonary disease. The patient was a 79-year-old man. (*Courtesy of Dr. Atsushi Nambu, Department of Radiology, University of Yamanashi, Yamanashi, Japan.*)

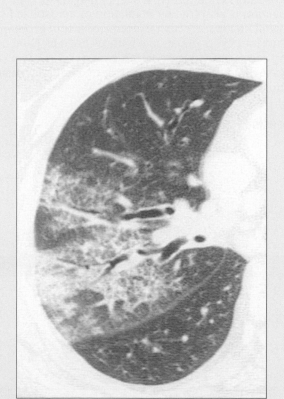

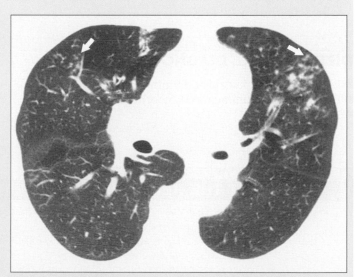

Figure 3. *Chlamydia* **pneumonia.** View of the right lung from a high-resolution CT shows ground-glass opacities and mild consolidation in the right middle lobe. The patient was an 84-year-old woman. (*Courtesy of Dr. Atsushi Nambu, Department of Radiology, University of Yamanashi, Yamanashi, Japan.*)

Figure 4. *Chlamydia* **pneumonia.** High-resolution CT shows bilateral centrilobular nodules (*arrows*) and patchy ground-glass opacities. The patient was a 66-year-old woman. (*Courtesy of Dr. Atsushi Nambu, Department of Radiology, University of Yamanashi, Yamanashi, Japan.*)

Psittacosis

DEFINITION: Pulmonary disease caused by infection with *Chlamydia psittaci*.

IMAGING

Radiography
Findings
- Patchy reticular pattern radiating from hila or involving lung bases, homogeneous ground-glass opacities, and patchy areas of consolidation (bronchopneumonia) or lobar consolidation (lobar pneumonia) are seen.
- Interval between first abnormal radiograph and complete resolution averages about 6 weeks, with range of 1-20 weeks.

Utility
- Manifestations are variable.

CT
Findings
- Ground-glass opacities and patchy areas of consolidation (bronchopneumonia) or lobar consolidation (lobar pneumonia)
- Centrilobular nodules and "tree-in-bud" pattern

Utility
- Nonspecific findings

CLINICAL PRESENTATION

- Incubation period is 1 to 2 weeks.
- Signs and symptoms include fever, sore throat, myalgia, headache, dry cough, dyspnea, and pleuritic chest pain.
- Hepatosplenomegaly and superficial lymph node enlargement may be present.

DIFFERENTIAL DIAGNOSIS

- Lobar pneumonia caused by other microorganisms
- Bronchopneumonia caused by other microorganisms
- Tuberculosis

DIAGNOSTIC PEARLS

- Patchy reticular pattern radiating from hila or involving lung bases, homogeneous ground-glass opacities, and segmental or lobar areas of consolidation
- History of recent exposure to birds, most commonly parrots, parakeets, and poultry.

PATHOLOGY

- Histologic features consist of bronchiolitis and pneumonia, which may be lobular or lobar.
- Severe cases demonstrate diffuse alveolar damage.
- *Chlamydia psittaci* is an obligate intracellular bacterium that can only grow in host cells and not in artificial culture media.

INCIDENCE/PREVALENCE AND EPIDEMIOLOGY

- Psittacosis is usually acquired by exposure to infected birds, most commonly parrots, parakeets, and poultry.
- Infection is acquired by inhalation of aerosolized chlamydial elementary bodies excreted in bird feces.
- Majority (85%) of patients with psittacosis have a history of recent exposure to birds.
- Disease can occur sporadically or in epidemics, usually among poultry workers.

Suggested Readings

Blasi F, Tarsia P, Aliberti S, et al: *Chlamydia pneumoniae* and *Mycoplasma pneumoniae. Semin Respir Crit Care Med* 26:617-624, 2005.

Cunha BA: The atypical pneumonias: Clinical diagnosis and importance. *Clin Microbiol Infect* 12(Suppl 3):12-24, 2006.

WHAT THE REFERRING PHYSICIAN NEEDS TO KNOW

- In patients with severe pneumonia, clinical and radiologic findings may resemble those of pneumococcal pneumonia.
- Diagnosis should be suspected clinically in patients who become ill after contact with a sick psittacine bird (parrot or parakeet).
- Diagnosis is based on elevated tube agglutination tests for *C. psittaci* in nonimmune or previously unexposed patients.
- Treatment is with antibiotics, most commonly tetracycline or erythromycin or their derivatives.

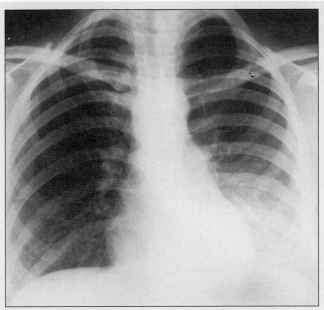

Figure 1. Posteroanterior radiograph reveals homogenous consolidation of the basal segments of the left lower lobe associated with slight loss of volume; an air bronchiogram is not visualized, and there is no evidence of left hilar lymph node enlargement. This 34-year-old woman had recently acquired a parakeet; *Chlamydia psittaci* was recovered from the sputum. (From Fraser RS, Müller NL, Colman N, Paré PD [eds]: *Fraser and Paré's Diagnosis of Diseases of the Chest.* 4th ed. Philadelphia, Pa: WB Saunders, pp 1017-1019, 1999.)

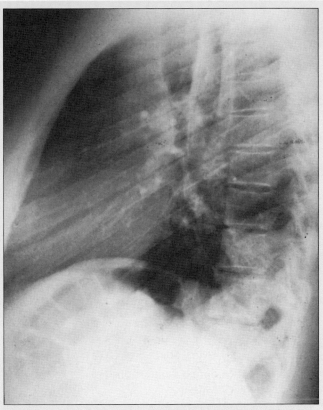

Figure 2. Lateral radiograph reveals homogenous consolidation of the basal segments of the left lower lobe associated with slight loss of volume; an air bronchiogram is not visualized, and there is no evidence of left hilar lymph node enlargement. This 34-year-old woman had recently acquired a parakeet; *Chlamydia psittaci* was recovered from the sputum. (From Fraser RS, Müller NL, Colman N, Paré PD [eds]: *Fraser and Paré's Diagnosis of Diseases of the Chest.* 4th ed. Philadelphia, Pa: WB Saunders, pp 1017-1019, 1999.)

Pneumonia (Influenza Virus)

DEFINITION: Pneumonia that is caused by influenza virus.

IMAGING

Radiography
Findings
- Poorly defined, patchy areas of consolidation, which become rapidly confluent
- Nodular areas of consolidation
- Reticulonodular opacities
- Usually involves mainly the lower lobes
Utility
- Chest radiograph is usually the only imaging modality used to assess patients with suspected or proven influenza viral pneumonia.
- The radiologic findings are similar to those of pneumonia due to other organisms.

CT
Findings
- Patchy or confluent consolidation
- Ground-glass opacities
- Centrilobular nodules and tree-in-bud pattern nodules
- "Crazy-paving" pattern
Utility
- May be helpful in assessing complications, particularly related to superimposed infection such as abscess formation or empyema.

CLINICAL PRESENTATION

- Rapid onset of dry cough, myalgia, chills, headache, conjunctivitis, and fever
- Infection often mild but can be overwhelming and rapidly fatal
- Most severe cases characterized by predisposing condition (e.g., cardiac disease, pregnancy, cystic fibrosis, or immunodeficiency)
- Infants and the elderly at particular risk for serious disease

DIFFERENTIAL DIAGNOSIS

- Pneumonia (*Mycoplasma*)
- Pneumonia (Cytomegalovirus)
- Pneumonia (*Staphylococcus aureus*)

DIAGNOSTIC PEARLS

- Reticulonodular pattern
- Focal areas of consolidation that become rapidly confluent
- Risk factors for primary influenza viral pneumonia include old age and cardiopulmonary disease.
- Influenza outbreaks tend to occur during the winter in temperate climates and during the rainy season in the tropics and subtropics.

- Pneumonia (*Streptococcus pneumoniae*)
- Organizing pneumonia

PATHOLOGY

- Death can result from severe influenza pneumonia or from superinfection by bacteria.
- Histology of fatal influenza pneumonia is diffuse alveolar damage.
- Parenchyma shows variably severe interstitial mononuclear inflammatory infiltrate; consolidation of airspaces by edema, hemorrhage, and fibrin; and hyaline membranes.
- Less severe cases of pneumonia may result in findings of mild acute lung injury and organizing pneumonia.

INCIDENCE/PREVALENCE AND EPIDEMIOLOGY

- Pneumonia is uncommon but serious complications of influenza are usually caused by influenza virus type A and occasionally by influenza virus type B organisms.
- Influenza can occur in pandemics, in epidemics, or sporadically in individual or small clusters of patients.
- Type A influenza viruses cause almost all severe epidemics and all pandemics and are generally transmitted from person to person by droplet infection.

WHAT THE REFERRING PHYSICIAN NEEDS TO KNOW

- Differential diagnosis includes other viral and bacterial respiratory pathogens.
- Diagnosis of influenza virus infection can be confirmed by direct immunofluorescence, enzyme-linked immunosorbent assay, viral culture, and polymerase chain reaction.
- Viral culture and polymerase chain reaction have the highest sensitivity and specificity in diagnosis.
- Bacterial superinfection is common.

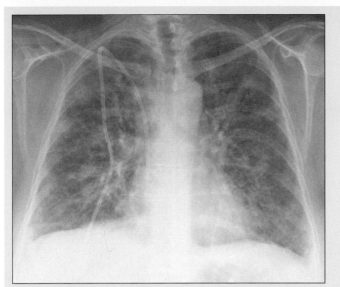

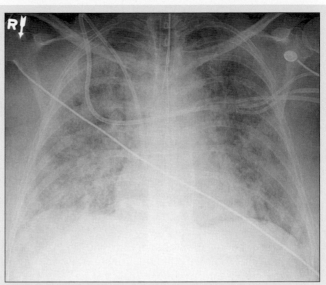

Figure 1. Influenza virus pneumonia. Chest radiograph shows patchy bilateral areas of consolidation, poorly defined nodular opacities, ground-glass opacities, and small bilateral pleural effusions. Also noted is a central venous line. The patient was a 45-year-old man who developed influenza virus pneumonia after hematopoietic stem cell transplantation.

Figure 2. Influenza virus pneumonia. Chest radiograph made 1 day after radiograph in Figure 1 shows marked progression of the abnormalities with development of extensive bilateral areas of consolidation. The patient was a 45-year-old man who developed influenza pneumonia after hematopoietic stem cell transplantation.

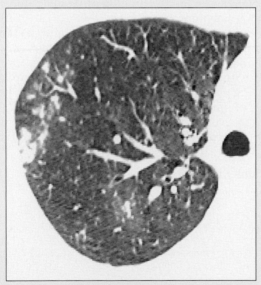

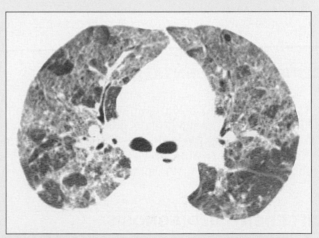

Figure 4. Influenza virus pneumonia. High-resolution CT scan shows extensive bilateral ground-glass opacities with superimposed fine linear opacities ("crazy-paving" pattern) and small bilateral pleural effusions. The patient was a 45-year-old man who developed influenza virus pneumonia after hematopoietic stem cell transplantation (see also Figures 1 and 2).

Figure 3. Influenza virus pneumonia. View of the right upper lobe from a high-resolution CT scan shows centrilobular nodular opacities and small foci of consolidation in the right upper lobe. The patient was a 33-year-old man who developed influenza virus pneumonia after hematopoietic stem cell transplantation.

- Influenza affects approximately 20% of children and 5% of adults each year worldwide.
- Influenza outbreaks tend to occur on an annual basis, typically during winter in temperate climates.
- In tropical and subtropical areas, they occur either during the rainy season or throughout the year.

Suggested Readings

Kim EA, Lee KS, Primack SL, et al: Viral pneumonias in adults: Radiologic and pathologic findings. *RadioGraphics* 22:S137-S149, 2002.

Nicholson KG, Wood JM, Zambon M: Influenza. *Lancet* 362: 1733-1745, 2003.

Shorman M, Moorman JP: Clinical manifestations and diagnosis of influenza. *South Med J* 96:737-739, 2003.

Pneumonia (Cytomegalovirus)

DEFINITION: Pulmonary parenchymal disease that is causd by cytomegalovirus (CMV) and typically occurs in immunocompromised hosts.

IMAGING

Radiography
Findings
- Bilateral ground-glass opacities, patchy consolidation, poorly defined nodules, or reticulonodular pattern.

Utility
- Usually the initial modality employed but has limited sensitivity and specificity.

CT
Findings
- Bilateral parenchymal abnormalities consisting of variable combinations of patchy consolidation, ground-glass opacities, and nodules < 10 mm.
- Nodules of random, subpleural or centrilobular distribution sometimes associated with halo of ground-glass attenuation (CT halo sign).
- Bronchial wall thickening.

Utility
- In immunocompromised patients, pneumonia can be identified on high-resolution CT approximately 5 days before abnormalities become visible on chest radiography.
- CT is useful when infection is suspected despite a negative or equivocal radiograph.

CLINICAL PRESENTATION

- Fever is the most common presenting sign in an immunocompromised host with pulmonary infection. Other findings include cough and dyspnea.
- In both solid organ and hematopoietic stem cell transplant populations, infection typically arises between 30 and 100 days after transplantation.

DIFFERENTIAL DIAGNOSIS

- *Pneumocystis* pneumonia
- Aspergillosis
- Bacterial pneumonia

DIAGNOSTIC PEARLS

- Bilateral patchy ground-glass opacities and consolidation
- Centrilobular nodules
- On microscopy, typical cytoplasmic and nuclear inclusions in inflamed tissues
- Occurs most commonly between 30 and 100 days following solid organ or hematopoietic stem cell transplantation

PATHOLOGY

- Typical nuclear and cytoplasmic inclusions are found in cells within inflamed tissue.
- Bronchiolitis and bronchopneumonia.

INCIDENCE/PREVALENCE AND EPIDEMIOLOGY

- Cytomegalovirus is the most common viral pathogen associated with life-threatening pulmonary infection in an immunocompromised host.
- Occurs most commonly between 30 and 100 days following solid organ or hematopoietic stem cell transplantation.
- CMV is the most common viral pulmonary pathogen in AIDS patients and affects patients with advanced levels of immunosuppression (CD4 < 100/mm³).
- Highly active antiretroviral therapy (HAART) has substantially reduced all manifestations of CMV in AIDS patients.

Suggested Readings

Boiselle PM, Aviram G, Fishman JE: Update on lung disease in AIDS. *Semin Roentgenol* 37:54-71, 2001.
Franquet T, Lee KS, Müller NL: Thin-section CT findings in 32 immunocompromised patients with cytomegalovirus pneumonia who do not have AIDS. *AJR Am J Roentgenol* 181:1059-1063, 2003.
Kim EA, Lee KS, Primack SL, et al: Viral pneumonias in adults: Radiologic and pathologic findings. *RadioGraphics* 22:S137-S149, 2002.

WHAT THE REFERRING PHYSICIAN NEEDS TO KNOW

- Diagnosis should be suspected particularly in patients with fever 30 to 100 days after stem cell transplantation.
- Radiologic findings are nonspecific, most commonly consisting of variable combinations of ground-glass opacities, patchy consolidation, and small nodules.
- Typical microscopic finding of nuclear and cytoplasmic inclusions is required to confirm true infection as opposed to colonization.
- Diagnostic yield of bronchoscopic procedures is higher when parenchymal disease involves central one third of lung parenchyma.

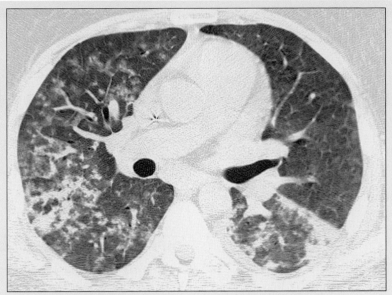

Figure 1. Cytomegalovirus pneumonia. High-resolution CT image of a 41-year-old hematopoietic stem cell transplant recipient shows centrilobular nodules associated with patchy ground-glass opacities and focal areas of consolidation.

Kotloff RM, Ahya VN, Crawford SW: Pulmonary complications of solid organ and hematopoietic stem cell transplantation. *Am J Respir Crit Care* 170:22-48, 2004.

Oh YW, Effman EL, Godwin JD: Pulmonary infections in immuno-compromised hosts: The importance of correlating the conventional radiologic appearance with the clinical setting. *Radiology* 217:647-656, 2000.

Pneumonia (SARS)

DEFINITION: Severe acute respiratory syndrome (SARS) is a pneumonia resulting from infection with SARS coronavirus.

IMAGING

Radiography
Findings
- Focal or multifocal patchy or confluent areas of consolidation are seen.
- At presentation 20%-40% of patients with SARS have normal radiographs.

Utility
- Radiography is essential imaging modality in diagnosis of SARS.

CT
Findings
- Most common findings consist of focal, multifocal, or diffuse ground-glass opacities or areas of consolidation.
- Interlobular septal or intralobular interstitial thickening is often seen superimposed on ground-glass opacities ("crazy-paving" pattern).

Utility
- High-resolution CT is helpful in evaluation of patients with normal radiographs by demonstrating parenchymal abnormalities in virtually all cases.
- Findings common in other pneumonias (e.g., branching nodular and linear opacities; hilar, mediastinal lymphadenopathy; pleural effusion) are uncommon in SARS.

CLINICAL PRESENTATION

- Mean incubation period is 6 days (range: 2-10).
- There is a history of close contact within 10 days with another person with SARS.
- Presenting symptoms include fever, chills, dry cough, myalgia, and headache, with progression to acute respiratory distress syndrome (ARDS).
- Laboratory findings include lymphopenia, evidence of disseminated intravascular coagulation, and elevated blood lactate dehydrogenase and creatine kinase levels.

DIAGNOSTIC PEARLS

- Focal unilateral or multifocal unilateral or bilateral areas of consolidation.
- Consolidation tends to involve predominantly peripheral lung regions and middle and lower lung zones.
- Criteria for diagnosis: respiratory illness, radiographic evidence of pneumonia, close contact within 10 days with another person with SARS.

DIFFERENTIAL DIAGNOSIS

- Community-acquired pneumonia
- Bronchopneumonia
- *Pneumocystis* pneumonia
- Pneumonia (*Staphylococcus aureus*)
- Pneumonia (*Streptococcus pneumoniae*)
- Pneumonia (influenza virus)

PATHOLOGY

- Predominant pattern of lung injury in autopsy specimens was diffuse alveolar damage.
- Cases of 10 or fewer days' duration demonstrated acute-phase diffuse alveolar damage.
- Cases of more than 10 days' duration exhibited organizing-phase diffuse alveolar damage, superimposed with bacterial bronchopneumonia.

INCIDENCE/PREVALENCE AND EPIDEMIOLOGY

- Disease is transmitted by droplets or direct inoculation from contact with infected surfaces.
- SARS first emerged in southern China in 2002.
- Once it reached Hong Kong, disease spread rapidly to other parts of the world by international air travel.
- Within approximately 8 months, SARS affected 8422 patients and resulted in 916 deaths (case-fatality rate of 11%).

WHAT THE REFERRING PHYSICIAN NEEDS TO KNOW

- During the epidemic, presence of consolidation or ground-glass opacities in patients with history of exposure was considered highly suggestive of diagnosis.
- Radiologic findings are nonspecific, resembling those of other viral, bacterial, and fungal pneumonias.
- Diagnosis of SARS is based on clinical, epidemiologic, and laboratory criteria, which include respiratory illness, radiographic evidence of pneumonia, and close contact within 10 days with another infected person.
- Laboratory confirmation of diagnosis can be made by detection of antibody to SARS-CoV or detection of SARS-CoV or isolation of SARS-CoV.

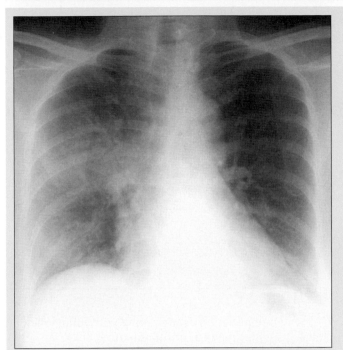

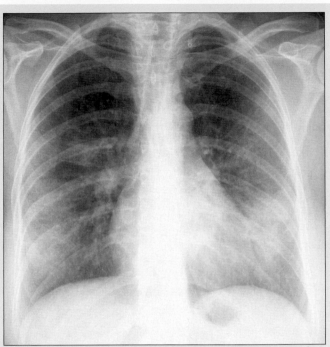

Figure 1. **Severe acute respiratory syndrome (SARS).** Chest radiograph shows area of consolidation in the right perihilar region and ground-glass opacities in the right middle and lower lung zones. The patient was a 64-year-old woman. (*From Müller NL, et al. Severe acute respiratory syndrome: Radiographic and CT findings. AJR Am J Roentgenol 181:3-8, 2003, with permission.*)

Figure 2. **Severe acute respiratory syndrome (SARS).** Chest radiograph shows patchy bilateral areas of consolidation. The patient was a 44-year-old woman. (*From Müller NL, et al: Severe acute respiratory syndrome: Radiographic and CT findings. AJR Am J Roentgenol 181:3-8, 2003, with permission*).

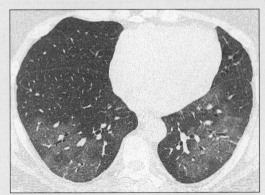

Figure 3. **Severe acute respiratory syndrome (SARS).** High-resolution CT image shows patchy bilateral ground-glass opacities in the lower lobes. The patient was a 48-year-old woman.

- Most of the infections occurred in hospitals, laboratories involved in diagnosis or research on the organism, and nursing homes.
- Only a few sporadic cases of SARS have been reported since 2003.
- The natural reservoir of the organism is believed to be wild animals such as raccoons, ferrets, and civets.

Suggested Readings

Chan-Yeung M, Xu RH: SARS: Epidemiology. *Respirology* 8(Suppl): S9-S14, 2003.

Müller NL, Ooi GC, Khong PL, Nicolaou S: Severe acute respiratory syndrome: Radiographic and CT findings. *AJR Am J Roentgenol* 181:3-8, 2003.

Müller NL, Ooi GC, Khong PL, et al: High-resolution CT findings of severe acute respiratory syndrome at presentation and after admission. *AJR Am J Roentgenol* 182:39-44, 2004.

Poon LL, Guan Y, Nicholls JM, et al: The etiology, origins, and diagnosis of severe acute respiratory syndrome. *Lancet* 4:663-671, 2004.

Wong KT, Antonio GE, Hui DS, et al: Severe acute respiratory syndrome: Radiographic appearances and pattern of progression in 138 patients. *Radiology* 228:401-406, 2003.

Viral Bronchiolitis

DEFINITION: Viral bronchiolitis is infection of the bronchioles by viruses, most commonly by respiratory syncytial viruses (RSV), influenza viruses, parainfluenza viruses, and adenoviruses.

IMAGING

Radiography

Findings
- Hyperinflation mainly in infants.
- Poorly defined nodular opacities in adults.
- Progression to bronchopneumonia resulting in unilateral or bilateral areas of consolidation in children and adults.

Utility
- Almost always the only imaging modality required in assessment and follow-up.

CT

Findings
- Centrilobular nodules.
- Branching nodular opacities ("tree-in-bud" pattern).
- Areas of decreased attenuation and vascularity particularly in children.
- Unilateral or bilateral areas of consolidation due to viral bronchopneumonia.

Utility
- May show parenchymal abnormalities in patients with normal or nonspecific radiographic findings.
- Seldom indicated.
- Useful mainly in immunocompromised patients with clinical findings suggestive of bronchiolitis or pneumonia but normal or nonspecific radiographic findings.

CLINICAL PRESENTATION

- Cough
- Fever
- Dyspnea

DIFFERENTIAL DIAGNOSIS

- Pneumonia (*Mycoplasma*)
- Bronchiolitis due to inhalation of gases and fumes
- Aspiration bronchiolitis
- Infectious bronchiolitis due to other causes

DIAGNOSTIC PEARLS

- Hyperinflation typical in infants.
- Centrilobular nodules, "tree-in-bud" pattern typical on high-resolution CT in adults.
- May progress to bronchopneumonia.
- Symptomatic viral bronchiolitis in adults occurs mainly in immunocompromised patients, in the elderly, and in patients with underlying cardiopulmonary disease.

PATHOLOGY

- Airway inflammation occurs along with filling of small airways with mucus and inflammatory cells.
- Other findings may include ulceration and necrosis of the airway epithelium (necrotizing bronchitis and bronchiolitis).
- Possible residual sequela, particularly of adenovirus bronchiolitis/bronchopneumonia in children, is Swyer-James-McLeod syndrome (bronchiectasis, bronchiolitis obliterans, unilateral hyperlucent lung).

INCIDENCE/PREVALENCE AND EPIDEMIOLOGY

- Viruses are the most common cause of respiratory infection and may result in rhinitis, pharyngitis, laryngotracheitis, bronchitis, and bronchiolitis.
- Older patients and patients with underlying cardiopulmonary disease are at higher risk for bronchitis, bronchiolitis, and pneumonia.
- Parainfluenza viruses account for high proportion of cases of pneumonia, acute bronchiolitis, and tracheobronchitis (croup) in young children.
- Respiratory syncytial virus is the most common cause of bronchiolitis in the first few years of life.

WHAT THE REFERRING PHYSICIAN NEEDS TO KNOW

- Radiographic findings in adults are similar to those of infectious bronchiolitis and bronchopneumonia caused by other organisms.
- Infection can be diagnosed using rapid antigen detection tests, viral culture, polymerase chain reaction, and acute and convalescent antibody titers.
- Long-term sequelae of adenovirus bronchiolitis in children include bronchiectasis, bronchiolitis obliterans, and unilateral hyperlucent lung (Swyer-James-McLeod) syndrome.

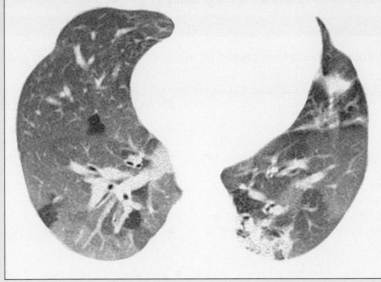

Figure 1. **Adenovirus pneumonia.** High-resolution CT scan shows focal areas of consolidation in the lingula and left lower lobe, ground-glass opacities, and small foci of decreased attenuation and vascularity. The patient was a young child with adenoviral bronchopneumonia. (*Courtesy of Dr. Kyung Soo Lee, Samsung Medical Center, Seoul, Korea.*)

Suggested Readings

Kanne JP, Godwin JD, Franquet T, et al: Viral pneumonia after hematopoietic stem cell transplantation: High-resolution CT findings. *J Thorac Imaging* 22:292-299, 2007.

Kim EA, Lee KS, Primack SL, et al: Viral pneumonias in adults: Radiologic and pathologic findings. *RadioGraphics* 22:S137-S149, 2002.

Shorman M, Moorman JP: Clinical manifestations and diagnosis of influenza. *South Med J* 96:737-739, 2003.

Echinococcosis (Hydatid Disease)

DEFINITION: Pulmonary disease caused by infection with *Echinococcus granulosus.*

IMAGING

Radiography

Findings

- Sharply circumscribed, spherical or oval nodules or masses are seen.
- "Water lily sign" is seen when membrane floats in residual intracystic fluid after rupture into airway.
- "Meniscus or air crescent sign" is seen when cyst communicates with bronchus producing thin peripheral radiolucency.
- Transdiaphragmatic extension of liver cysts may result in elevation of hemidiaphragm, pleural effusion, and lower lobe atelectasis or consolidation.

Utility

- First imaging modality performed in suspected cases.
- May show evidence of involvement of adjacent structures.

CT

Findings

- Round or oval smoothly marginated fluid-filled cysts with thin, enhancing walls.
- Intracystic fluid with attenuation values close to 0 Hounsfield units.
- Detached or collapsed endocyst membranes ("water lily" sign), collapsed daughter cyst membranes, and intact daughter cysts.
- Rupture resulting in adjacent consolidation and poor definition of cyst margins.
- Transdiaphragmatic extension of liver cyst resulting in elevation of hemidiaphragm, pleural effusion, pleural cysts, and pulmonary invasion.

Utility

- Used to differentiate fluid-filled hydatid cysts from solid tumors.

DIAGNOSTIC PEARLS

- Smoothly marginated oval or round single or multiple cysts; "daughter" cysts.
- "Water lily" sign of ruptured cyst.
- Coexistence of liver cyst with similar appearance.
- Pastoral form mainly in Mediterranean region, Middle East, South America, Australia, and New Zealand.
- Sylvatic form mainly in Alaska and Canada.

- May show coexistence of liver and lung cysts.
- Identifies pathognomonic features in ruptured or complicated hydatid cysts.

MRI

Findings

- Cyst of low signal intensity on T1-weighted images.
- Homogeneous cyst of high signal intensity on T2-weighted images.

Utility

- Identifies same features as CT
- Used in young patients because of lack of radiation exposure

CLINICAL PRESENTATION

- Most patients are asymptomatic but have mild eosinophilia.
- Cyst rupture, either spontaneously or as result of secondary infection, may result in abrupt onset of cough, expectoration, and fever; occasionally acute hypersensitivity reaction occurs, with urticaria, pruritus, and, in some cases, hypotension.

WHAT THE REFERRING PHYSICIAN NEEDS TO KNOW

- Chest radiograph is usually the first imaging modality performed but CT or MRI is required to identify cystic nature of lesions.
- In patients with suspected hydatid cysts and young patients with nodules or masses, MRI is modality of choice.
- Main differential diagnosis is with other conditions that may result in fluid-filled lung lesions, particularly bronchogenic cysts and fluid-filled bullae.
- Distinguishing features include presence of blood eosinophilia, which usually is mild and present in 25%-50% of cases.
- Laboratory aids in diagnosis include indirect hemagglutination, latex agglutination, complement fixation, and enzyme-linked immunosorbent assay.
- Laboratory diagnostics are more sensitive for liver cysts, but specificity is limited by cross reaction with other parasites.

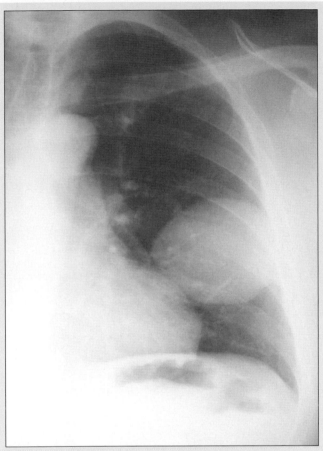

Figure 1. **Hydatid cyst.** View of the left lung from a chest radiograph shows a smoothly marginated 6-cm-diameter mass. The patient was a 51-year-old asymptomatic man who hunted for several years in northern Canada.

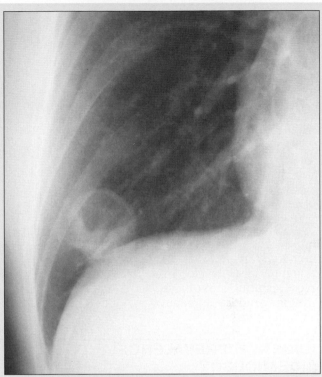

Figure 2. **Hydatid cyst with water lily sign.** View of the right lung from a posteroanterior chest radiograph shows thin-walled cystic lesion with air-fluid level. Note poorly defined opacity immediately above the fluid level. The patient was a 36-year-old man who was a hunter in northern Canada.

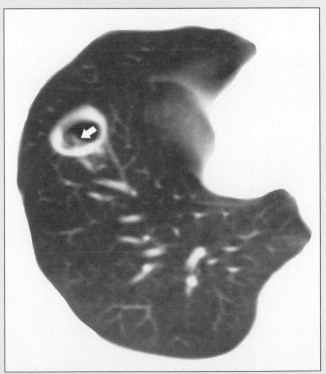

Figure 4. **Hydatid cyst.** View of the right lung from a CT shows thin-walled cyst containing soft tissue floating on the fluid ("water-lily" sign). The patient was a 36-year-old man who was a hunter in northern Canada (see also Fig. 2).

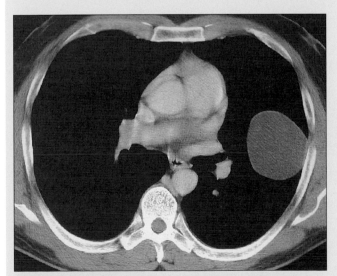

Figure 3. **Hydatid cyst.** Contrast-enhanced CT image demonstrates a cystic lesion containing fluid with attenuation values similar to water (0 HU). The patient was a 51-year-old asymptomatic man who hunted for several years in northern Canada (see also Fig. 1).

DIFFERENTIAL DIAGNOSIS

- Bronchogenic cyst
- Fluid-filled bulla
- Lung mass on the radiograph

PATHOLOGY

- Humans acquire disease by direct contact with definite hosts (most commonly dogs) or by ingestion of eggs in water, food, and soil.
- Eggs hatch in duodenum into larvae that pass via portal system to liver, where most are trapped.
- Most of those that escape are, in turn, trapped in pulmonary alveolar capillaries.
- Cyst has laminated outer membrane (exocyst) and thin inner layer of cells (endocyst) that produces intracystic fluid and larval protoscoleces.
- Daughter cysts develop from exocyst or free protoscoleces, resulting in multicystic structure.
- Cyst may rupture spontaneously or as result of secondary infection.

INCIDENCE/PREVALENCE AND EPIDEMIOLOGY

- Pastoral form is more common and seen mainly in Mediterranean region, Eastern Europe, South America, Middle East, Australia, and New Zealand.

- Intermediate hosts in pastoral form are usually sheep, cows, or pigs; definite hosts are dogs.
- Sylvatic form is more common in Alaska and northern Canada.
- Intermediate hosts in sylvatic form are moose, deer, and caribou; definite hosts are dogs, wolves, and coyotes.
- In pastoral variety, 65%-70% of cysts occur in liver and 15%-30% occur in lungs.
- Lung cysts are more common than liver cysts in sylvatic variety.

Suggested Readings

Fraser RS, Colman N, Müller NL, Paré PD: Infectious disease of the lungs. In Fraser RS, Colman N, Müller NL, Paré PD (eds): *Synopsis of Diseases of the Chest*, Philadelphia, 2005, Elsevier Saunders, pp 222-336.

Jerray M, Benzarti M, Garrouche A, et al: Hydatid disease of the lungs: Study of 386 cases. *Am Rev Respir Dis* 146:185-189, 1992.

Martinez S, Restrepo CS, Carrillo JA, et al: Thoracic manifestations of tropical parasitic infections: A pictorial review. *RadioGraphics* 25:135-155, 2005.

Saksouk FA, Fahl MH, Rizk GK: Computed tomography of pulmonary hydatid disease. *J Comput Assist Tomogr* 10:226-232, 1986.

von Sinner WN: New diagnostic signs in hydatid disease: Radiography, ultrasound, CT and MRI correlated to pathology. *Eur J Radiol* 12:150-159, 1991.

Paragonimiasis

DEFINITION: Pulmonary disease can result from infection by flukes of the genus *Paragonimus.*

IMAGING

Radiography

Findings
- Nodule or focal areas of consolidation.
- Thin-walled cystic lesions seen in areas of consolidation or isolated thin-walled ring shadows.
- Worms in cysts seen as crescent-shaped or oval opacity along internal periphery.
- Irregular tracks or burrows up to 5 mm in diameter connecting adjacent cysts in some cases.

Utility
- Usually first and often only imaging modality used.

CT

Findings
- Most common finding: subpleural or subfissural nodules frequently containing necrotic low-attenuation area or cavitation.
- Adjacent focal fibrotic pleural thickening (important diagnostic clue).
- May also have ground-glass opacities, bronchiectasis adjacent to nodule, and focal areas of consolidation.
- Subpleural streaky opacity 2-7 mm thick and 5-60 mm long connecting pleura and nodule, adjacent cysts, or cysts and bronchus.
- Pleural effusion or hydropneumothorax in 30%-60%.
- Hilar or mediastinal lymphadenopathy in 10%.

Utility
- Recommended in selected cases for further characterization of pattern and extent of abnormalities.

Positron Emission Tomography

Findings
- Positive uptake on FDG-PET

Utility
- Same findings as in lung cancer. Not useful in differential diagnosis.

DIAGNOSTIC PEARLS

- Single or multiple nodules or cystic lesions.
- Areas of consolidation with possible "burrow tracks."
- Subpleural location on CT.
- Endemic regions are East and Southeast Asia, South America, and Africa.

CLINICAL PRESENTATION

- Chronic intermittent hemoptysis or blood-tinged sputum and cough.
- May have episodic chest pain due to pleurisy and fever.
- Hemoptysis: sporadic occurrence for months or years in absence of other signs or illness.

DIFFERENTIAL DIAGNOSIS

- Postprimary tuberculosis
- Pulmonary carcinoma

PATHOLOGY

- Single or multiple 1- to 4-cm cystic spaces contain reddish brown mucinous fluid and usually a single adult parasite.
- Adult parasite induces cyst formation, nodules, and bronchiectasis.
- Erosion into draining airway may result in expectoration of cyst contents or pneumonia.

WHAT THE REFERRING PHYSICIAN NEEDS TO KNOW

- Chest radiography is usually the first and often only imaging modality used in assessment of these patients.
- CT, however, is recommended in selected cases for further characterization of pattern and extent of abnormalities.
- Paragonimiasis frequently results in clinical symptoms and radiologic findings that resemble those of pulmonary tuberculosis.
- Diagnosis is by finding of eggs in sputum samples, bronchial washings, or lung biopsy specimens or by serologic tests (e.g., enzyme-linked immunosorbent assay).

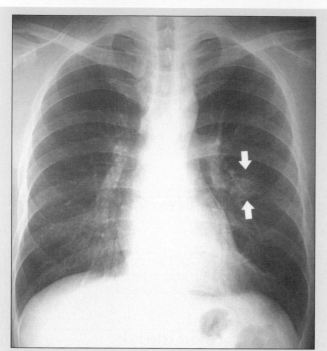

Figure 1. Paragonimiasis: single opacity. Posteroanterior chest radiograph shows a poorly defined nodular opacity in the lingula (*arrows*). The diagnosis of paragonimiasis was confirmed by open-lung biopsy in this 39-year-old South Korean man seen for left chest pain (see also Fig. 4). (*Courtesy of Dr. Kyung Soo Lee, Samsung Medical Center, Seoul, Korea.*)

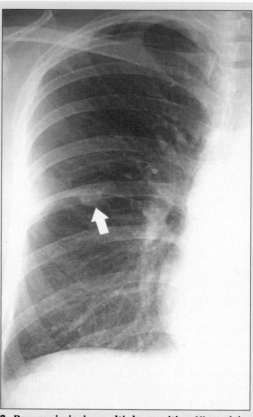

Figure 2. Paragonimiasis: multiple opacities. View of the right lung from a chest radiograph shows poorly defined opacities in the right mid-lung zone (*arrow*). The diagnosis was confirmed by enzyme-linked immunosorbent assay and transthoracic needle aspiration, which demonstrated characteristic ova. The patient was a 38-year-old South Korean man evaluated for vague chest pain and cough (see also Fig. 3). (*Courtesy of Dr. Kyung Soo Lee, Samsung Medical Center, Seoul, Korea.*)

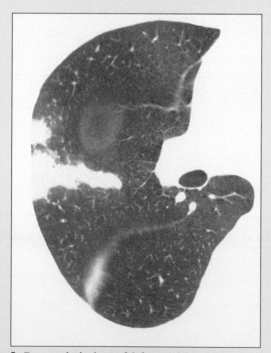

Figure 3. Paragonimiasis: multiple opacities. CT image demonstrates subpleural nodular opacities and focal area of consolidation. The diagnosis was confirmed by enzyme-linked immunosorbent assay and transthoracic needle aspiration, which demonstrated characteristic ova. The patient was a 38-year-old South Korean man evaluated for vague chest pain and cough (see also Fig. 2). (*Courtesy of Dr. Kyung Soo Lee, Samsung Medical Center, Seoul, Korea.*)

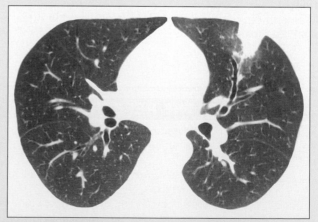

Figure 4. Paragonimiasis: single opacity. CT image demonstrates a subsegmental pleural-based area of consolidation surrounded by a halo of ground-glass attenuation. The appearance is consistent with a pulmonary infarct. The diagnosis of paragonimiasis was confirmed by open-lung biopsy in this 39-year-old South Korean man seen for left chest pain (see also Fig. 1). (*Courtesy of Dr. Kyung Soo Lee, Samsung Medical Center, Seoul, Korea.*)

INCIDENCE/PREVALENCE AND EPIDEMIOLOGY

- Most common etiologic agent is *Paragonimus westermani.*
- Paragonimiasis affects approximately 20 million people.
- Endemic areas are East Asia, Southeast Asia, Latin America, and Africa.

Suggested Readings

Im JG, Chang KH, Reeder MM: Current diagnostic imaging of pulmonary and cerebral paragonimiasis, with pathological correlation. *Semin Roentgenol* 32:301-324, 1997.

Kim TS, Han J, Shim SS, et al: Pleuropulmonary paragonimiasis: CT findings in 31 patients. *AJR Am J Roentgenol* 185:616-621, 2005.

Martinez S, Restrepo CS, Carrillo JA, et al: Thoracic manifestations of tropical parasitic infections: A pictorial review. *RadioGraphics* 25:135-155, 2005.

Schistosomiasis

DEFINITION: Pulmonary disease that results from infection by trematodes of the genus *Schistosoma*.

IMAGING

Radiography
Findings
- Small, poorly defined nodular lesions or reticulonodular pattern or bilateral ground-glass opacities.
- Enlarged central pulmonary arteries, if infection is chronic.

Utility
- First and often only imaging modality used in the evaluation of these patients.

CT
Findings
- Areas of consolidation or nodules surrounded by ground-glass opacities (CT halo sign).
- "Reverse halo sign" when patchy consolidation surrounds ground-glass opacities.
- Enlarged central pulmonary arteries, if infection is chronic.

CLINICAL PRESENTATION

- Acute syndrome (Katayama fever) presents as fever, cough, diarrhea, and hives.
- Leukocytosis and eosinophilia are almost invariable.
- Chronic cases are characterized by progressive shortness of breath, chest pain, fatigue, palpitations, and cough secondary to pulmonary hypertension.
- Extrathoracic manifestations, which are invariably present, include hepatic or urinary symptoms.
- Infection with *S. mansoni* or *S. japonicum* results in symptoms and signs of cirrhosis and hepatosplenomegaly.
- *S. haematobium* infestation is associated with dysuria and hematuria.

DIAGNOSTIC PEARLS

- Patchy, migratory areas of consolidation related to migration of schistosomules through pulmonary circulation (Katayama fever).
- Extrathoracic disease (hepatomegaly, cirrhosis, hematuria).
- Evidence of pulmonary arterial hypertension (enlarged pulmonary artery, rapid tapering, cardiomegaly).
- Endemic regions are mainly South America for *S. mansoni*; China, Phillipines, and Japan for *S. japonicum*; and Middle East for *S. hematobium*.

DIFFERENTIAL DIAGNOSIS

- Simple pulmonary eosinophilia (Loeffler syndrome)
- Pneumonia

PATHOLOGY

- Humans acquire infestation by drinking, swimming, working, or washing in fresh water containing infective cercariae that penetrate the skin.
- Worms pass via venous circulation to pulmonary capillaries and through these to the systemic circulation.
- Worms migrate to superior mesenteric (*S. japonicum*), inferior mesenteric (*S. mansoni*), or vesical (*S. haematobium*) veins.
- Tissue damage results from release of eggs into host tissues with subsequent immunologic reaction, inflammation, and fibrosis.
- Eggs may reach lungs directly through inferior vena cava or, once liver has become cirrhotic as result of *Schistosoma*-related fibrosis, via anastomotic channels.
- Once they reach the lungs, most embolized eggs become impacted in pulmonary arterioles.

WHAT THE REFERRING PHYSICIAN NEEDS TO KNOW

- Parasites are a common cause of lung disease particularly in the tropics and in immigrants from endemic regions.
- Schistosomiasis may result in eosinophilic lung disease and pulmonary arterial hypertension.
- Patients may have acute symptoms related to migration of large number of schistosomules through the pulmonary circulation and present with fever, cough, diarrhea, and hives (Katayama fever).
- The most important pulmonary manifestation of schistosomiasis is pulmonary arterial hypertension.
- Diagnosis of pulmonary arterial hypertension is suggested by clinical findings or chest radiograph and confirmed by echocardiography.
- Radiologic manifestations of pleuropulmonary disease related to parasites are relatively nonspecific.
- Diagnosis of schistosomiasis is usually confirmed by demonstration of ova in specimens (stool, urine) or at rectal biopsy.

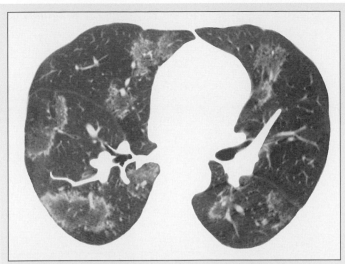

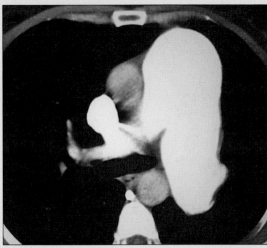

Figure 1. Schistosomiasis: parenchymal abnormalities. High-resolution CT image shows patchy bilateral ground-glass opacities. Ring-like areas of consolidation outline some of the ground-glass opacities (reverse halo sign). The diagnosis of schistosomiasis was confirmed by open-lung biopsy that showed granulomatous inflammation surrounding *Schistosoma* eggs. (*Courtesy of Dr. Gustavo Meirelles, São Paulo, Brazil.*)

Figure 2. Pulmonary arterial hypertension secondary to schistosomiasis. Contrast-enhanced CT image in a patient with long-standing schistosomiasis shows markedly enlarged central pulmonary arteries. (*Courtesy of Dr. Claudia Figueiredo, São Paulo, Brazil.*)

INCIDENCE/PREVALENCE AND EPIDEMIOLOGY

- Schistosomiasis affects 150-200 million people and causes 500,000 deaths annually.
- Endemic area for *S. mansoni* includes Caribbean islands and South America (particularly Brazil).
- Endemic area for *S. japonicum* includes China, Japan, and the Philippines.
- Endemic area for *S. hematobium* includes Middle East and central and southern Africa.
- Increased emigration from these regions has resulted in increased prevalence of the disease in nonendemic areas.

Suggested Readings

Fraser RS, Colman N, Müller NL, Paré PD: Infectious disease of the lungs. In Fraser RS, Colman N, Müller NL, Paré PD (eds): *Synopsis of Diseases of the Chest*, Philadelphia, 2005, Elsevier Saunders, pp 222-336.

Martinez S, Restrepo CS, Carrillo JA, et al: Thoracic manifestations of tropical parasitic infections: A pictorial review. *RadioGraphics* 25:135-155, 2005.

Morris W, Knauer CM: Cardiopulmonary manifestations of schistosomiasis. *Semin Respir Infect* 12:159-170, 1997.

Schwartz E, Rozenman J, Perelman M: Pulmonary manifestations of early schistosome infection among nonimmune travelers. *Am J Med* 109:718-722, 2000.

The Immunocompromised Patient

Part 17

ACQUIRED IMMUNODEFICIENCY SYNDROME (AIDS)

Bacterial Infection

DEFINITION: HIV-positive patients have increased prevalence of bacterial tracheobronchitis, bronchiolitis, and pneumonia.

IMAGING

Radiography

Findings

- Focal consolidation, in either segmental or lobar distribution, occurs, with higher propensity for multilobar and bilateral disease than in immunocompetent patients.
- Solitary or multiple lung nodules are seen.
- *Staphylococcus aureus* is frequently associated with septic emboli among intravenous drug abusers and usually presents as multiple cavitary nodules.
- Extensive bronchiolitis may create apparent interstitial pattern of reticulonodular opacities that represent impacted bronchioles.
- Infection with *Nocardia* includes nodules and areas of consolidation, which may be mass-like; cavitation, lymphadenopathy, and pleural effusions may be present.
- *Rhodococcus equi* pneumonia usually presents as one or more foci of cavitary consolidation, often with upper lobe predominance; empyema and lymphadenopathy are additional features.

Utility

- Chest radiography is the mainstay of diagnosis and follow-up of bacterial pneumonia.

CT

Findings

- Infectious bronchiolitis: centrilobular opacities arranged in "tree-in-bud" pattern, manifested by small Y- and V-shaped opacities.
- Bacterial pneumonia: patchy or confluent consolidation, lobular, segmental, or, less commonly, lobar distribution.
- Mildly enlarged mediastinal and hilar lymph nodes (usually < 2 cm).
- *Nocardia* infection: nodules and areas of consolidation, which may be patchy or mass-like.
- *Rhodococcus equi* pneumonia: usually presents as one or more foci of cavitary consolidation, often with an upper lobe predominance.
- Bacillary angiomatosis is manifested by endobronchial lesions, nodules, pleural effusions, densely enhancing lymphadenopathy, and chest wall masses.

DIAGNOSTIC PEARLS

- Focal consolidation, either segmental or lobar with high propensity for multilobar and bilateral disease.
- Infectious bronchiolitis: centrilobular opacities arranged in "tree-in-bud" pattern, manifested by small Y- and V-shaped opacities in lung periphery.
- Focal or multifocal and commonly asymmetric distribution of consolidation in bacterial pneumonia is distinct from the diffuse bilateral symmetric distribution of predominantly ground-glass opacities in *Pneumocystis* pneumonia.

Utility

- Useful when chest radiographic findings are atypical and culture/serology has failed to identify organism.
- Identifies presence of mild or subtle disease suggesting bacterial or other cause.
- Identifies lymphadenopathy, cavitation, pleural fluid or empyema, and other differential features that may be occult on a chest radiograph.

CLINICAL PRESENTATION

- Signs and symptoms of bacterial pneumonia by usual agents are the same as in non–HIV-infected patients.
- Onset is relatively rapid with productive cough, chills, fever, pleuritic chest pain, and dyspnea (< 1 week before patient seeks medical attention).
- *Rhodococcus equi* infection manifests as indolent course of cough, fever, and dyspnea.
- Bacillary angiomatosis presents as angiomatous skin lesions that mimic Kaposi sarcoma, fever, night sweats, cough, and occasional hemoptysis.
- Laboratory evaluation of HIV-infected patients with bacterial pneumonia usually shows leukocytosis but leukopenia can occur.
- Serum lactate dehydrogenase levels are typically normal or only mildly elevated.

WHAT THE REFERRING PHYSICIAN NEEDS TO KNOW

- Bacterial pneumonia is often associated with an acute onset of fever, pleuritic chest pain, productive cough, and purulent sputum.
- Bacterial pneumonia can usually be well assessed on the chest radiograph.
- CT is used when diagnosis cannot be arrived at with clinical and radiography findings.

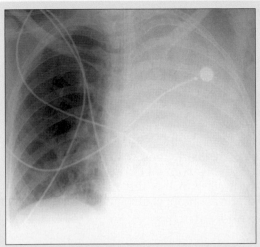

Figure 1. Pneumococcal pneumonia. Chest radiograph demonstrates complete opacification of the left thorax. (*Courtesy of Dr. Joel E. Fishman, University of Miami*)

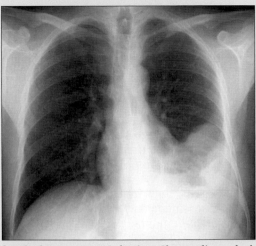

Figure 2. *Rhodococcus equi* infection. Chest radiograph shows a lingular consolidation with left pleural effusion. (*Courtesy of Dr. Joel E. Fishman, University of Miami*)

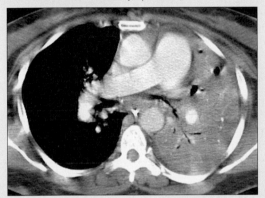

Figure 3. Pneumococcal pneumonia. Contrast-enhanced CT demonstrates diffuse hypodense consolidation without pleural effusion. (*Courtesy of Dr. Joel E. Fishman, University of Miami*)

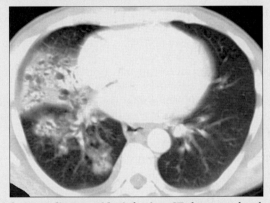

Figure 4. *Nocardia asteroides* infection. CT shows patchy alveolar opacities with air bronchograms in the right middle and lower lobes. (*Courtesy of Dr. Joel E. Fishman, University of Miami*)

DIFFERENTIAL DIAGNOSIS

- *Pneumocystis* pneumonia
- Tuberculosis
- Lymphoma

PATHOLOGY

- Infectious bronchitis, bronchiolitis, and pneumonia.
- Most common etiologic agents: *Streptococcus pneumoniae, Hemophilus influenzae,* and *S. aureus.*
- Patients with advanced immunosuppression are vulnerable to unusual infections, including those caused by *Nocardia asteroides, R. equi, Bartonella henselae,* and *B. quintana.*
- Bacillary angiomatosis (*Bartonella henselae* and *B. quintana*) is characterized by neovascular proliferation involving multiple sites in the body.

INCIDENCE/PREVALENCE AND EPIDEMIOLOGY

- Bacterial respiratory infections are currently the most common respiratory diseases in HIV-infected individuals in developed countries.

- HIV infection is associated with a 10- to 25-fold increased incidence of bacterial pneumonia compared with the general community.
- *Streptococcus pneumoniae* is the most common bacterial cause of community-acquired pneumonia among HIV-infected adults (20% of all bacterial pneumonias).
- HIV-infected intravenous drug users and those who smoke illicit drugs (cocaine, crack, marijuana) have an increased risk of bacterial pneumonia.

Suggested Readings

Boiselle PM, Aviram G, Fishman JE: Update on lung disease in AIDS. *Semin Roentgenol* 37:54-71, 2002.

Castaner E, et al: Radiologic approach to the diagnosis of infectious pulmonary diseases in patients infected with the human immunodeficiency virus. *Eur J Radiol* 51:114-129, 2004.

Haramati LB, Jenny-Avital ER: Approach to the diagnosis of pulmonary disease in patients infected with the human immunodeficiency virus. *J Thorac Imaging* 13:247-260, 1998.

Maki DD: Pulmonary infections in HIV/AIDS. *Semin Roentgenol* 35:124-139, 2000.

Waite S, Jeudy J, White CS: Acute lung infections in normal and immunocompromised hosts. *Radiol Clin North Am* 44:295-315, 2006:ix.

Pneumocystis Pneumonia

DEFINITION: Pneumonia caused by *Pneumocystis jiroveci* is the most common opportunistic infection in patients with AIDS.

IMAGING

Radiography
Findings
- Bilateral symmetric granular appearance or ground-glass opacities that progress to consolidation.
- Perihilar or upper lobe predominance.
- Upper lobe cystic lesions.

Utility
- First and usually only imaging modality required in the initial assessment and follow-up of patients with *Pneumocystis* pneumonia.
- Is normal in approximately 5% of patients.

CT
Findings
- Bilateral symmetric ground-glass opacities.
- Lobular sparing can lead to geographic appearance.
- Superimposed linear opacities result in "crazy paving" pattern.
- Less common manifestations: upper lobe distribution of parenchymal opacities and cystic lesions.
- Presence of cysts (pneumatoceles) that may lead to spontaneous pneumothorax or resolve with therapy.

Utility
- CT is more sensitive than chest radiography for detecting *Pneumocystis* pneumonia.
- CT is helpful in evaluating symptomatic patients with normal or equivocal radiographic findings.
- Presence of extensive bilateral ground-glass opacities in patients with AIDS is highly suggestive of *Pneumocystis* pneumonia.
- When "tree-in-bud" appearance is present on high-resolution CT, *Pneumocystis* pneumonia infection is unlikely.

CLINICAL PRESENTATION

- Onset is insidious with fever, dry cough, and dyspnea.
- Tachypnea, tachycardia, and cyanosis are evident, but lung auscultation reveals few abnormalities.
- Patients with AIDS who develop *Pneumocystis* pneumonia almost always have <200 CD4 cells/mm^3 and often <100 cells/mm^3.
- On average, symptoms are present for about a month before patients seek medical attention.

DIAGNOSTIC PEARLS

- Bilateral perihilar or diffuse finely granular or ground-glass pattern on the radiograph.
- Bilateral symmetric ground-glass opacities that may be patchy or diffuse and may have a geographic distribution.
- Cystic lesions seen on CT in approximately 30% of cases; involve mainly the upper lobes.
- Most prevalent opportunistic infection in patients with AIDS.

- Reduced arterial oxygen pressure, increased alveolar-arterial oxygen gradient, and respiratory alkalosis are evident.

DIFFERENTIAL DIAGNOSIS

- Bacterial infection
- Cytomegalovirus pneumonia
- Drug reaction
- Hypersensitivity pneumonitis

PATHOLOGY

- Intra-alveolar exudate, consisting of surfactant, fibrin, cellular debris, and *Pneumocystis* organisms.

INCIDENCE/PREVALENCE AND EPIDEMIOLOGY

- Most prevalent opportunistic infection in HIV-infected patients.
- One of the leading causes of morbidity and mortality among persons with AIDS.
- Single most common opportunistic pulmonary HIV infection in the United States.
- Responsible for approximately 25% of pneumonia cases in HIV infection.

WHAT THE REFERRING PHYSICIAN NEEDS TO KNOW

- Chest radiograph often shows characteristic findings.
- High-resolution CT may show findings suggestive of *Pneumocystis* pneumonia in patients with a normal chest radiograph.
- Proper specimens are usually obtained from induced sputum or fiberoptic bronchoscopy with bronchoalveolar lavage.

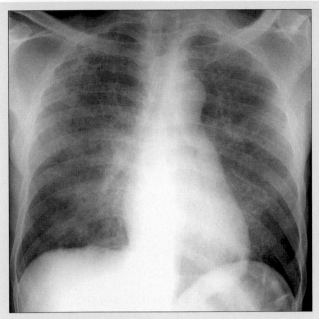

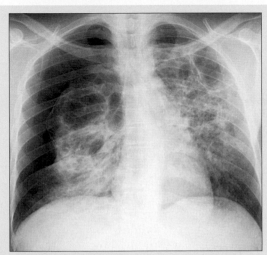

Figure 1. *Pneumocystis* **pneumonia.** Chest radiograph demonstrates bilateral hazy increased opacity. (*Courtesy of Dr. Joel E. Fishman, University of Miami*)

Figure 2. *Pneumocystis* **pneumonia.** Chest radiograph demonstrates bilateral interstitial and airspace opacities, multiple cysts, and a right pneumothorax. (*Courtesy of Dr. Joel E. Fishman, University of Miami*)

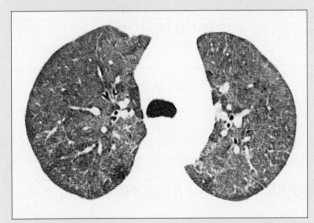

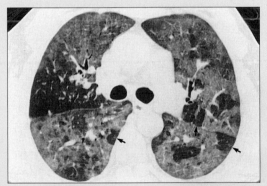

Figure 3. *Pneumocystis* **pneumonia.** High-resolution CT at the level of the upper lobes shows extensive bilateral ground-glass opacities.

Figure 4. *Pneumocystis* **pneumonia.** High-resolution CT in a 46-year-old man who had AIDS shows bilateral areas of ground-glass attenuation. There is sharp demarcation between normal and abnormal lung parenchyma, with the areas of spared lung parenchyma having a size and configuration that corresponds to that of secondary pulmonary lobules (*arrows*). (*From Müller NL, Fraser RS, Colman NC, Paré PD: Radiologic Diagnosis of Diseases of the Chest. Philadelphia, WB Saunders, 2001.*)

Suggested Readings

Boiselle PM, Aviram G, Fishman GE: Update on lung disease in AIDS. *Semin Roentgenol* 37:54-71, 2002.

Castaner E, et al: Radiologic approach to the diagnosis of infectious pulmonary diseases in patients infected with the human immuno-deficiency virus. *Eur J Radiol* 51:114-129, 2004.

Haramati LB, Jenny-Avital ER: Approach to the diagnosis of pulmonary disease in patients infected with the human immunodeficiency virus. *J Thorac Imaging* 13:247-260, 1998.

Maki DD: Pulmonary infections in HIV/AIDS. *Semin Roentgenol* 35:124-139, 2000.

McGuinness G: Changing trends in the pulmonary manifestations of AIDS. *Radiol Clin North Am* 35:1029-1082, 1997.

Tuberculosis

DEFINITION: A person with AIDS has increased risk of developing active infection with *Mycobacterium tuberculosis*.

IMAGING

Radiography

Findings

- Early in HIV infection: parenchymal opacities, occasionally cavitary, often located within apical, posterior, and superior segments of the lungs.
- With decreased CD4 counts (< 200 cells/mm³): mid and lower lobe consolidation, pleural effusion, and lymph node enlargement.
- In progressive primary infection: diffuse lung disease, multiple pulmonary nodules, mediastinal lymphadenopathy, miliary spread, and lower likelihood of cavitary disease.
- With advanced levels of immune suppression: chest radiographs normal in up to 20% of HIV-positive patients with TB.
- With immune reconstitution syndrome: increased size of hilar and mediastinal lymph nodes.

Utility

- Imaging begins with chest radiograph in suspected cases of TB.
- Chest radiographic screening of asymptomatic, purified protein derivative (PPD)-negative AIDS patients for possible TB is not generally performed.
- Negative chest radiograph may predict poorer outcome in AIDS patients with TB.

CT

Findings

- Early in HIV infection: parenchymal opacities, occasionally cavitary, often located within apical, posterior, and superior segments of the lungs.
- In patients with decreased CD4 counts (< 200 cells/mm³): mid and lower lobe consolidation, pleural effusion, and lymph node enlargement.
- Enlarged lymph nodes that are often hypodense, with rim enhancement after intravenous administration of a contrast agent.
- Endobronchial spread, resulting in "tree-in-bud" pattern.
- Immune reconstitution syndrome: new enlarged lymph nodes or increase in size of hilar and mediastinal lymph nodes.

DIAGNOSTIC PEARLS

- Early in HIV infection: parenchymal opacities, occasionally cavitary, often located within apical, posterior, and superior segments of the lungs. Findings resemble postprimary tuberculosis.
- Patients with decreased CD4 counts (<200 cells/mm³): mid and lower lobe consolidation, pleural effusion, and lymph node enlargement. Findings resemble primary tuberculosis.
- Immune reconstitution syndrome in patients with tuberculosis is characterized by a marked increase in the hilar and mediastinal lymphadenopathy.

Utility

- CT is used in equivocal cases or when a symptomatic patient has a normal chest radiograph.
- Suspected lymphadenopathy on chest radiography is also indication for CT.
- Miliary disease is better characterized by CT than by radiography.

CLINICAL PRESENTATION

- Classic symptoms include cough, hemoptysis, night sweats, and weight loss.
- Symptoms are often present for more than 7 days before patients seek medical attention.
- Median CD4 count in HIV patients co-infected with TB is approximately 350 cells/mm³.
- In early HIV disease, TB skin tests are positive and the infection is confined to the lungs.

DIFFERENTIAL DIAGNOSIS

- Bacterial infection
- Lymphoma

PATHOLOGY

- Early in HIV infection: parenchymal opacities, occasionally cavitary, often located within apical, posterior, and superior segments of the lungs.

WHAT THE REFERRING PHYSICIAN NEEDS TO KNOW

- Because TB is both contagious and highly curable (except for multidrug-resistant strains), prompt diagnosis and treatment are essential.
- Diagnosis of TB can be difficult and time consuming, requiring multiple sputum samples and polymerase chain reaction testing to identify *M. tuberculosis*.
- Diagnosis in HIV-infected persons may be more difficult than in immunocompetent patients.

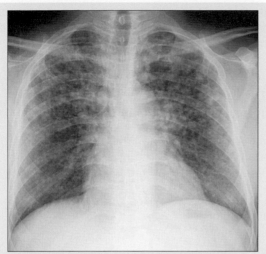

Figure 1. Tuberculosis. Chest radiograph demonstrates bilateral airspace nodular opacities with an upper lobe predominance (CD4 = 278 cells/mm^3). (*Courtesy of Dr. Joel E. Fishman, University of Miami*)

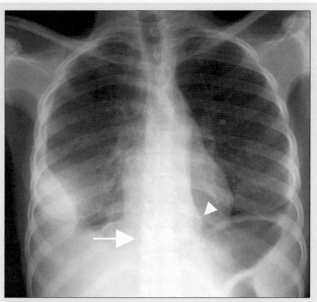

Figure 2. Tuberculosis. Chest radiograph shows bilateral pleural effusions and tuberculous infection of the T10 vertebral body (Pott's disease) (*arrow*) with paraspinal widening (*arrowhead*). (*Courtesy of Dr. Joel E. Fishman, University of Miami*)

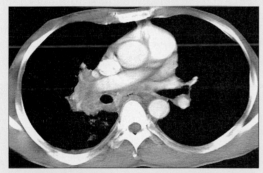

Figure 3. Tuberculosis. CT image shows hypodense right hilar lymphadenopathy (CD4 = 3 cells/mm^3). (*Courtesy of Dr. Joel E. Fishman, University of Miami*)

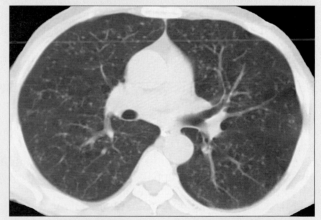

Figure 4. Tuberculosis. CT shows miliary nodules bilaterally. (*Courtesy of Dr. Joel E. Fishman, University of Miami*)

- Patients with decreased CD4 counts (< 200 cells/mm^3): mid and lower lobe consolidation, pleural effusion, and lymph node enlargement.
- With more severe immunosuppression: anergy, with only 20%-40% of patients able to produce a positive skin test for TB.

INCIDENCE/PREVALENCE AND EPIDEMIOLOGY

- One third of nearly 40 million people living with HIV/AIDS worldwide are co-infected with TB.
- Highest number of deaths and mortality per capita occur in Africa, where HIV has led to rapid growth of a TB epidemic.
- HIV-infected individuals have a 50- to 200-fold increased risk of TB compared with general population.
- TB can be associated with accelerated progression and higher mortality in HIV-infected persons.

- HIV infection increases the risk of developing active TB and TB recurrence among patients not receiving HAART.
- TB can occur at any stage of HIV infection.
- HIV-infected individuals at particularly high risk for TB are intravenous drug abusers and patients from areas where TB is endemic.

Suggested Readings

Boiselle PM, Aviram G, Fishman JE: Update on lung disease in AIDS. *Semin Roentgenol* 37:54-71, 2002.

Castaner E, et al: Radiologic approach to the diagnosis of infectious pulmonary diseases in patients infected with the human immunodeficiency virus. *Eur J Radiol* 51:114-129, 2004.

Haramati LB, Jenny-Avital ER, Alterman DD: Thoracic manifestations of immune restoration syndromes in AIDS. *J Thorac Imaging* 22:213-220, 2007.

Lazarous DG, O'Donnell AE: Pulmonary infections in the HIV-infected patient in the era of highly active antiretroviral therapy: An update. *Curr Infect Dis Rep* 9:228-232, 2007.

Maki DD: Pulmonary infections in HIV/AIDS. *Semin Roentgenol* 35:124-139, 2000.

Immune Reconstitution Syndrome

DEFINITION: It is transient clinical worsening due to recovery of the immune system and subsequent inflammation in response to latent or subclinical infection or malignancy that some patients with AIDS develop when they begin highly active antiretroviral therapy (HAART).

IMAGING

Radiography
Findings
- Tuberculosis and *Mycobacterium avium-intracellulare* complex–related immune reconstitution syndrome: new or increased mediastinal lymphadenopathy.
- New or increased lung parenchymal abnormalities: consolidation, nodules, or micronodules.
- Pleural effusions less common than nodal or parenchymal disease.
- Kaposi sarcoma: increase in the extent of the parenchymal nodular opacities.

Utility
- Findings generally appear 1-5 weeks after beginning HAART and resolve within months.

CT
Findings
- Tuberculosis and *M. avium-intracellulare* complex–related immune reconstitution syndrome: new or increased intrathoracic, axillary, and cervical lymphadenopathy.
- Nodes frequently with low attenuation centers and rim enhancement.
- New or increased pulmonary parenchymal disease, including consolidation, nodules, or micronodules.
- Pleural effusion.
- *Cryptococcus:* lymphadenopathy, frequently with low attenuation centers and rim enhancement.
- Kaposi sarcoma: increase in the extent of the parenchymal findings and lymphadenopathy.

Utility
- Follows chest radiography in cases of equivocal lymphadenopathy.

CLINICAL PRESENTATION

- Paradoxical deterioration in clinical status after initiation of HAART despite improved immune function due to exaggerated inflammatory response.

DIAGNOSTIC PEARLS

- Tuberculosis-related immune reconstitution syndrome: lymph node enlargement, often with central low attenuation centers, located in abdominal, axillary, and mediastinal locations.
- Lung parenchymal abnormalities: consolidation, nodules, or micronodules.
- Axillary, cervical, and/or intrathoracic lymphadenopathy.

- Onset usually within 6 weeks of HAART initiation.
- Factors associated with development of immune reconstitution syndrome: low initial CD4 count (usually < 50), close temporal relation between an opportunistic infection and HAART initiation, and marked decrease in HIV virus load.
- Symptoms subtle (fever, cough, and minor lymph node enlargement) or dramatic (respiratory failure or neurologic deterioration).
- Nonthoracic manifestations of immune reconstitution syndrome: cryptococcal meningitis, varicella zoster infection, and genital warts.

DIFFERENTIAL DIAGNOSIS

- Tuberculosis
- Kaposi sarcoma
- Lymphoma
- Drug reaction

PATHOLOGY

- Exaggerated inflammatory response
- Inciting pathogens: *Mycobacterium tuberculosis* (30% of cases), *M. avium-intracellulare* complex, *Cryptococcus, Pneumocystis,* cytomegalovirus, human herpesvirus 8 (Kaposi and Castleman disease)
- Hilar and mediastinal lymphadenopathy often with central necrosis.

WHAT THE REFERRING PHYSICIAN NEEDS TO KNOW

- Differential diagnosis: progressive disease due to nonadherence to treatment, single/multidrug-resistant mycobacterial infection, adverse drug reaction, concurrent opportunistic infection/malignancy.
- Proposed diagnostic criteria: atypical presentation of opportunistic infections in patients responding to antiretroviral therapy, falling plasma HIV RNA levels, increased blood CD4 count.
- Treatment with antimicrobial and/or anti-inflammatory therapy, with symptomatic use of corticosteroids if necessary.
- Resolution of the process within weeks or months without specific antibiotic therapy.
- Findings appearing 1-5 weeks after beginning HAART that resolve within months.

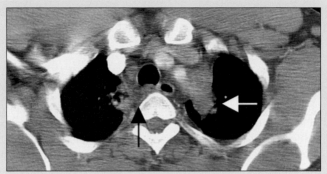

Figure 1. **Immune reconstitution syndrome in patient with tuberculosis.** CT demonstrates multiple hypodense superior mediastinal lymph nodes (*arrows*). (*Courtesy of Dr. Joel E. Fishman, University of Miami*)

INCIDENCE/PREVALENCE AND EPIDEMIOLOGY

- Mycobacteria (tuberculosis and nontuberculous) are most commonly implicated infectious organisms in immune reconstitution inflammatory syndrome (IRIS), accounting for almost 40% of cases reported.
- IRIS is associated with restoration of cutaneous delayed-type hypersensitivity reaction to tuberculin.
- Baseline CD4 count < 50 cells/mm^3 represents risk factor for IRIS.
- Infections by *Cryptococcus,* herpesviruses, hepatitis B and C viruses, and JC virus are also associated with infectious IRIS.

Suggested Readings

French MA, Price P, Stone SF: Immune restoration disease after antiretroviral therapy. *AIDS* 18:1615-1627, 2004.

Godoy MC, Rouse H, Brown JA, et al: Imaging features of pulmonary Kaposi sarcoma–associated immune reconstitution syndrome. *AJR Am J Roentgenol* 189:956-965, 2007.

Haramati LB, Jenny-Avital ER, Alterman DD: Thoracic manifestations of immune restoration syndromes in AIDS. *J Thorac Imaging* 22:213-220, 2007.

Hirsch HH, Kaufmann G, Sendi P, Battegay M: Immune reconstitution in HIV-infected patients. *Clin Infect Dis* 38:1159-1166, 2004.

Lazarous DG, O'Donnell AE: Pulmonary infections in the HIV-infected patient in the era of highly active antiretroviral therapy: An update. *Curr Infect Dis Rep* 9:228-232, 2007.

Martinez S, McAdams HP, Batchu CS: The many faces of pulmonary nontuberculous mycobacterial infection. *AJR Am J Roentgenol* 189:177-186, 2007.

Neoplasms

DEFINITION: Kaposi sarcoma is a low-grade mesenchymal tumor involving blood and lymphatic vessels, and non-Hodgkin lymphoma is the second most common malignancy in patients with AIDS.

IMAGING

Radiography
Findings
- Kaposi sarcoma: peribronchovascular interstitial thickening, poorly defined nodular opacities, septal lines, hilar and mediastinal lymphadenopathy, unilateral or bilateral pleural effusions.
- Lymphoma: multiple pulmonary nodules or masses, areas of consolidation, hilar and mediastinal lymphadenopathy, unilateral or bilateral pleural effusions.
- Bronchogenic carcinoma: central or peripheral mass, ipsilateral hilar and variable mediastinal lymphadenopathy, postobstructive consolidation/atelectasis.

Utility
- Most commonly obtained modality in AIDS patients with thoracic disease.

CT
Findings
- Kaposi sarcoma: bilateral and symmetric irregular ("flame shaped") nodules in peribronchovascular distribution; septal lines; lymphadenopathy (approximately 40% of cases); unilateral or bilateral pleural effusions; ground-glass opacities due to hemorrhage that may surround nodules ("CT halo sign")
- Lymphoma: nodules or masses ≤5 cm in diameter, smooth margins, sometimes with halo of ground-glass attenuation; mediastinal lymphadenopathy (~50% of cases); unilateral or bilateral pleural effusions
- Bronchogenic carcinoma: central or peripheral mass; lymphadenopathy (~30% of cases); postobstructive consolidation/atelectasis

Utility
- Superior to chest radiography in depiction of parenchymal findings and mediastinal lymphadenopathy.

MRI
Findings
- Lymphomatous involvement of heart in AIDS patients

DIAGNOSTIC PEARLS
- Kaposi sarcoma: peribronchovascular "flame-shaped" nodules, septal lines.
- Lymphoma: nodules or masses ≤5 cm in diameter, smooth margins.
- Bronchogenic carcinoma: presents as central or peripheral mass; spiculated margins.

Utility
- Lack of ionizing radiation
- Better tissue characterization using gadolinium as a contrast material

CLINICAL PRESENTATION
- Most common presenting symptoms of pulmonary Kaposi sarcoma are dyspnea and cough; hemoptysis and chest pain are less common.
- Non-Hodgkin lymphoma: most common symptoms are cough, dyspnea, and pleuritic chest pain.
- HIV-infected patients have similar clinical presentations of lung cancer as do non–HIV-infected patients.

PATHOLOGY
- Kaposi sarcoma: low-grade mesenchymal tumor involving blood and lymphatic vessels; affects skin and causes disseminated disease in variety of organs; both human herpesvirus type 8 and HIV may be involved in its development; lymphatic distribution with propensity to involve mainly the peribronchovascular interstitium.
- Diffuse non-Hodgkin B-cell type: aggressive, high-grade tumors that include poorly differentiated large and anaplastic lymphomas; most commonly extranodal involvement: lungs, central nervous system, gastrointestinal tract, liver, spleen, kidneys, and bone marrow.
- Pulmonary carcinoma: tendency for more aggressive behavior than in non-AIDS patients; adenocarcinoma most common cell type.

WHAT THE REFERRING PHYSICIAN NEEDS TO KNOW
- CD4 count is most widely used indicator of degree of immunosuppression in HIV-infected individuals and related directly to complications that occur.
- AIDS-related NHL usually affects patients with CD4+ levels <100 cells/mm^3.
- Kaposi sarcoma is most common in patients with advanced immunosuppression whose CD4 cell count is usually below 100 cells/mm^3.
- Bronchogenic carcinoma: CD4 cell count often shows moderate but not severe immunodeficiency.
- Most patients with lung cancer are symptomatic, and 75%-90% of patients present with advanced (stage III-IV) disease.

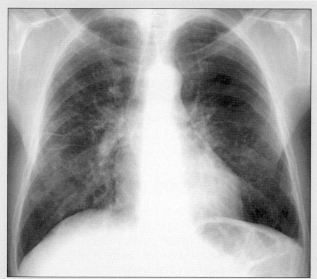

Figure 1. Kaposi sarcoma. Chest radiograph shows interstitial and peribronchovascular opacities bilaterally. (*Courtesy of Dr. Joel E. Fishman, University of Miami*)

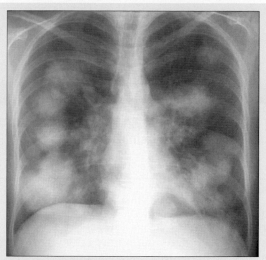

Figure 2. Pulmonary lymphoma. Chest radiograph shows multiple ill-defined pulmonary masses. (*From Boiselle PM, Aviram G, Fishman JE: Update on lung disease in AIDS. Semin Roentgenol 37:54-71, 2002.*)

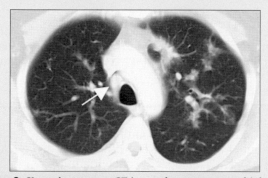

Figure 3. Kaposi sarcoma. CT image demonstrates multiple ill-defined pulmonary nodules and an enlarged paratracheal lymph node (*arrow*). (*Courtesy of Dr. Joel E. Fishman, University of Miami*)

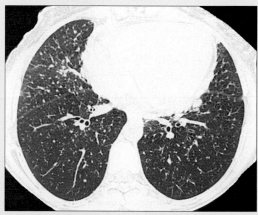

Figure 4. Lymphoma. High-resolution CT image reveals diffuse tiny pulmonary nodules. (*Courtesy of Dr. Joel E. Fishman, University of Miami*)

INCIDENCE/PREVALENCE AND EPIDEMIOLOGY

- Combination antiretroviral therapy and other factors have lead to significant decrease in incidence of Kaposi sarcoma in HIV-positive patients.
- Most often Kaposi sarcoma occurs in male homosexuals.
- Thoracic disease is found at autopsy in 45%-50% of patients with cutaneous AIDS-related Kaposi sarcoma and clinically detected in approximately 33%.
- Non-Hodgkin lymphoma is one of three AIDS-defining malignancies and the second most common, occurring in 2%-10% of HIV-infected individuals; it is twice as common in whites and males than in African-Americans and women.
- The prevalence of lung cancer seems to be higher in HIV-infected subjects than in the general population.
- Lung cancer manifests at an earlier age in the HIV population (mean age: 45 years).

Suggested Readings

Cadranel J, Garfield D, Lavolé A, et al: Lung cancer in HIV infected patients: Facts, questions and challenges. *Thorax* 61:1000-1008, 2006.

Kanmogne GD: Noninfectious pulmonary complications of HIV/AIDS. *Curr Opin Pulm Med* 11:208-212, 2005.

Marchiori E, Müller NL, Soares Souza A Jr, et al: Pulmonary disease in patients with AIDS: High-resolution CT and pathologic findings. *AJR Am J Roentgenol* 184:757-764, 2005.

Restrepo CS, Diethelm L, Lemos JA, et al: Cardiovascular complications of human immunodeficiency virus infection. *RadioGraphics* 26:213-231, 2006.

Restrepo CS, Martínez S, Lemos JA, et al: Imaging manifestations of Kaposi sarcoma. *RadioGraphics* 26:1169-1185, 2006.

Infection in the Immunocompromised Patient

DEFINITION: Pulmonary bacterial, fungal, and viral infections occur with increased prevalence in inmmunocompromised patients.

IMAGING

Radiography
Findings

- Bacterial, viral pneumonia: may range from normal to extensive bilateral areas of consolidation
- *Pneumocystis jiroveci* pneumonia: typically consists of bilateral perihilar or diffuse symmetric interstitial or ground-glass opacities; normal findings possible
- Invasive aspergillosis: single or multiple pulmonary nodules or masses or peripheral areas of consolidation with or without associated cavitation
- Pulmonary candidiasis: unilateral or bilateral lobar or segmental airspace disease
- Cytomegalovirus (CMV) pneumonia: bilateral parenchymal opacification associated with multiple pulmonary nodules typically < 5 mm

Utility

- Usually initial modality employed but has limited sensitivity and specificity

CT
Findings

- Bacterial and fungal pneumonia: patchy unilateral or bilateral areas of consolidation; may have associated parenchymal necrosis or pleural effusion.
- *Pneumocystis* pneumonia: diffuse ground-glass opacities, sometimes in geographic distribution; thin-walled cysts, intralobular and interlobular septal thickening ("crazy-paving" pattern).

DIAGNOSTIC PEARLS

- Invasive aspergillosis is the most common opportunistic fungal infection of the lung.
- In immunocompromised patients with severe neutropenia the presence of nodules with a CT halo sign is most suggestive of angioinvasive aspergillosis.
- The radiologic manifestations of viral, bacterial, and fungal pneumonia are similar and include centrilobular nodules, "tree-in-bud" pattern, and focal, multifocal, or confluent areas of consolidation.

- Aspergillosis: nodule or mass surrounded by rim of ground-glass attenuation (CT halo sign); air crescent sign; centrilobular nodules, peribronchial consolidation.
- Mucormycosis: solitary or multiple pulmonary nodules, areas of consolidation with or without cavitation, CT halo sign.
- Pulmonary candidiasis: multiple nodules (3-30 mm) distributed randomly or centrilobularly, involve lower lung zones; CT halo sign; consolidation.
- CMV pneumonia: consolidation, ground-glass opacities, nodules < 10 mm with random, subpleural or centrilobular distribution; CT halo sign.
- Respiratory syncytial viral pneumonia: areas of parenchymal opacification with associated findings of airway inflammation (centrilobular nodules, "tree-in-bud" pattern, bronchial wall thickening).

WHAT THE REFERRING PHYSICIAN NEEDS TO KNOW

- In an immunocompromised patient with fever the presence of multiple nodules or a "tree-in-bud" pattern is most suggestive of infection.
- In an immunocompromised patient consolidation is a nonspecific finding that may be seen in pneumonia, drug reaction, hemorrhage, edema, and infarction.
- Diagnostic yield of bronchoscopic procedures is higher when parenchymal disease involves central third of lung parenchyma.
- More peripheral parenchymal abnormalities typically require diagnosis by percutaneous or video-assisted thoracoscopic biopsy.
- Nature, severity, and duration of immune defect will determine specific types of infection most likely to occur.
- Owing to impaired inflammatory response, clinical symptoms may be minimal or absent.

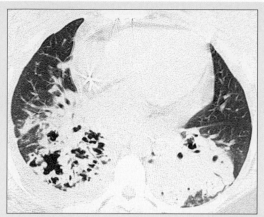

Figure 1. *Pseudomonas aeruginosa* and *Staphylococcus aureus* pneumonia. High-resolution CT image of a 22-year-old double-lung transplant recipient shows necrotizing pneumonia in both lower lobes. (*Courtesy of Dr. Ann Leung, Stanford University*)

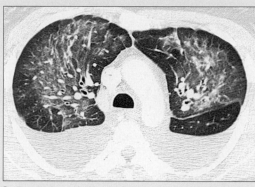

Figure 2. *Pneumocystis jiroveci* **pneumonia.** High-resolution CT image of a 48-year-old with acute leukemia shows bilateral ground-glass opacities. Also noted are bilateral pleural effusions. (*Courtesy of Dr. Ann Leung, Stanford University*)

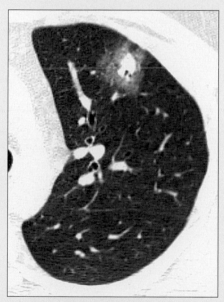

Figure 3. CT halo sign in invasive pulmonary aspergillosis. Magnified view of the left lung from a high-resolution CT shows nodule with surrounding ground-glass attenuation (CT halo sign). The patient was a 33-year-old man with acute leukemia, severe neutropenia, and angioinvasive pulmonary aspergillosis.

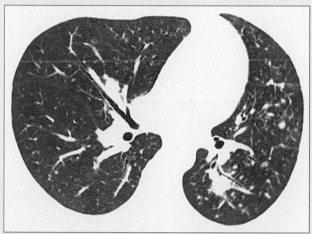

Figure 4. Respiratory syncytial virus pneumonia. High-resolution CT image of a 50-year-old woman with acute leukemia shows bilateral centrilobular nodules and peribronchial consolidation. (*Courtesy of Dr. Ann Leung, Stanford University*)

Utility

- High-resolution CT may demonstrate parenchymal abnormalities in up to 50% of neutropenic patients with normal chest radiographs.
- CT better characterizes disease, narrows the differential diagnosis, and guides selection of optimal type and sampling site of invasive diagnostic technique.

CLINICAL PRESENTATION

- In first month after transplantation, solid organ transplant recipients are most susceptible to bacterial infections and invasive aspergillosis.
- From months 1 to 6, opportunistic fungal infections and viruses, including CMV, become most frequent pathogens in solid organ transplant recipients.

- Fever is most common presenting sign in immunocompromised host with pulmonary infection.
- Owing to the impaired inflammatory response in this patient population, other signs and symptoms may be greatly muted or absent.
- Respiratory viruses typically cause coryza and cough; involvement of lower respiratory tract results in wheezing and dyspnea.
- Viral infections in an immunocompromised patient have a higher rate of nosocomial spread, with likelihood of spread to lower respiratory tract and higher mortality.
- Pulmonary invasive aspergillosis and mucormycosis are rapidly progressive.

PATHOLOGY

- CT halo sign (aspergillosis, candidiasis) pathologically corresponds to central fungal nodule surrounded by hemorrhage and coagulative necrosis.
- Angioinvasive aspergillosis results in infected hemorrhagic infacts while airway-invasive aspergillosis results in bronchiolitis and bronchopneumonia.
- Bacterial, viral, and fungal pneumonia usually manifest as bronchopneumonia.
- Parenchymal necrosis and cavitation may occur particularly in bacterial pneumonias due to gram-negative organisms or *Staphylococcus aureus*.

INCIDENCE/PREVALENCE AND EPIDEMIOLOGY

- Infections account for approximately 75% of cases of pulmonary complications in the immunocompromised host.
- Bacteria are most common cause of infections in the immunocompromised host with chemotherapy-induced neutropenia.
- Pneumocystis jiroveci pneumonia remains the most common opportunistic infection in patients infected with HIV.
- Patients receiving chemotherapy or long courses of corticosteroids are predisposed to P. jiroveci pneumonia.
- Invasive aspergillosis is the most common opportunistic fungal infection of the lung.
- Patient groups susceptible to pulmonary candidiasis include those with hematologic malignancies, those receiving chemotherapy, and transplant recipients.
- Cytomegalovirus is most common viral pathogen associated with life-threatening pulmonary infection in an immunocompromised host.

Suggested Readings

Fishman JA, Rubin RH: Infection in organ transplant recipients. *N Engl J Med* 338:1741-1751, 1998.
Kotloff RM, Ahya VN, Crawford SW: Pulmonary complications of solid organ and hematopoietic stem cell transplantation. *Am J Respir Crit Care* 170:22-48, 2004.
Oh YW, Effman EL, Godwin JD: Pulmonary infections in immunocompromised hosts: The importance of correlating the conventional radiologic appearance with the clinical setting. *Radiology* 217:647-656, 2000.

Noninfectious Complications in the Immunocompromised Patient

DEFINITION: Noninfectious complications in immunocompromised patients include drug toxicity, radiation pneumonitis, neoplastic disease, diffuse alveolar hemorrhage, lymphoproliferative disorder, rejection, pulmonary edema, and pulmonary embolism.

IMAGING

Radiography

Findings

- Drug toxicity: nonspecific patterns including bilateral consolidation, ground-glass opacities, poorly defined nodular opacities, and reticulation.
- Radiation pneumonitis: normal to parenchymal opacification (either ground-glass attenuation or consolidation).
- Diffuse alveolar hemorrhage: patchy or confluent bilateral ground-glass opacities or consolidation.
- Transfusion-related acute lung injury: bilateral parenchymal opacities typical of noncardiogenic pulmonary edema.
- Pulmonary edema: prominence of pulmonary vessels, peribronchial cuffing, septal (Kerley) lines, perihilar haze or consolidation, pleural effusion.
- Progression or recurrence of neoplastic disease: reticulonodular and reticular pattern, septal (Kerley) lines, nodular opacities.
- Acute lung rejection: normal findings or reticular or airspace opacities predominating in middle and lower lung zones.

Utility

- Usually first imaging modality used to assess presence of pulmonary disease.
- Radiographic findings often nonspecific.
- Chest radiographs normal in up to 10% of patients with proven pulmonary disease.

CT

Findings

- Drug-induced lung disease: various patterns including bilateral consolidation, ground-glass opacities, poorly defined nodular opacities, and reticulation.
- Radiation pneumonitis: parenchymal opacification, nodules, and focal consolidative opacities may be found within treatment port; ipsilateral pleural effusion.

DIAGNOSTIC PEARLS

- Radiation-induced lung injury: parenchymal opacification, and focal consolidative opacities within treatment port.
- Progression or recurrence of neoplastic disease: nodules, perilymphatic infiltration, parenchymal opacification.
- Drug-induced lung injury: various patterns depending of histology of injury, most commonly bilateral ground-glass opacities and/or consolidation.
- Diffuse alveolar hemorrhage: bilateral ground-glass opacities on CT.
- Pulmonary edema: ground-glass opacities, thickening of peribronchovascular interstitium, septal lines.
- Radiologic manifestations of the various noninfectious complications in immunocompromised patients are often nonspecific and may mimic infection.

- Diffuse alveolar hemorrhage: nonspecific, varied, from focal ground-glass opacities to diffuse bilateral consolidation.
- Lung transplant rejection: septal lines, interlobar fissure thickening, effusion, parenchymal opacification in acute cases; areas of decreased attenuation and vascularity, air trapping, bronchiectasis when chronic.
- Pulmonary edema: ground-glass opacities, thickening of peribronchovascular interstitium, interlobular septa.
- Acute pulmonary embolism: multiple filling defects within opacified pulmonary arterial system.
- Progression or recurrence of neoplastic disease: reticulonodular and reticular pattern, septal (Kerley) lines, nodular opacities, lymphadenopathy.

WHAT THE REFERRING PHYSICIAN NEEDS TO KNOW

- Noninfectious complications seen in immunocompromised patients include drug-induced lung disease, pulmonary edema, pulmonary embolism, radiation pneumonitis, progression or recurrence of neoplastic disease, lung transplant rejection, chronic graft-versus-host disease, and transfusion-related acute lung injury.
- Clinical and radiologic manifestations of various noninfectious complications in immunocompromised patients are often nonspecific and may mimic infection.
- CT is more sensitive than radiography in detection of subtle abnormalities and often helpful to better characterize disease and guide the type and site of invasive diagnostic procedure.

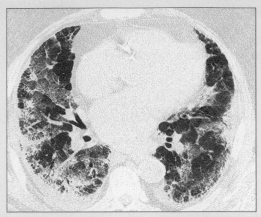

Figure 1. Bleomycin-induced diffuse alveolar damage. High-resolution CT image of a 75-year-old man with lymphoma shows peripheral areas of consolidation and patchy areas of ground-glass attenuation associated with an intralobular reticular pattern. (*Courtesy of Dr. Ann Leung, Stanford University*)

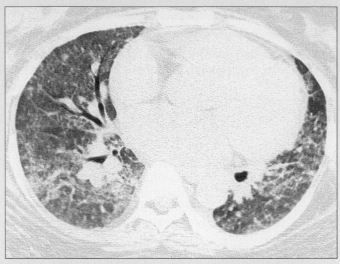

Figure 2. Diffuse alveolar hemorrhage. CT scan of a 38-year-old woman with systemic lupus erythematosus and cardiomegaly shows diffuse ground-glass opacities and a fine reticular pattern. (*Courtesy of Dr. Ann Leung, Stanford University*)

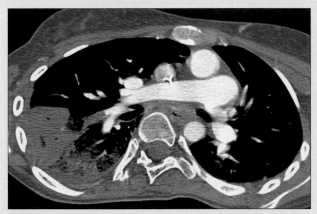

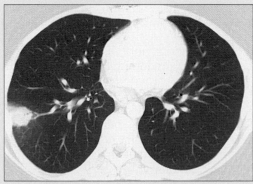

Figure 3. Pulmonary embolism. High-resolution CT scan in a 19-year-old heart transplant recipient shows an occlusive thrombus in the anterobasal segmental artery of the right lower lobe with associated distal consolidation due to pulmonary infarction and hemorrhage. (*Courtesy of Dr. Ann Leung, Stanford University*)

Figure 4. Post-transplant lymphoproliferative disorder. CT scan of a 27-year-old heart-lung transplant recipient shows a nodular area of consolidation in the periphery of the right lower lobe. (*Courtesy of Dr. Ann Leung, Stanford University*)

■ Post-transplant lymphoproliferative disorder: lung nodules sometimes with halo of ground-glass attenuation (CT halo sign), lymphadenopathy in 30%-40% of cases.

Utility

■ Superior to radiography in demonstrating presence, pattern, and distribution of pulmonary complications in immunocompromised patients.
■ High-resolution CT recommended in patients with clinically suspected pulmonary disease and normal or nonspecific radiographic findings.

CLINICAL PRESENTATION

■ Patients generally present with nonspecific symptoms of cough, dyspnea, and fever.
■ Radiation pneumonitis occurs 4-12 weeks after completion of radiotherapy.
■ Radiation fibrosis develops approximately 6 months after treatment; fibrosis is stable at 2 years.
■ Sirolimus toxicity occurs within 6 months of sirolimus initiation.

- Transfusion-related acute lung injury mirrors that of acute respiratory distress syndrome, with acute dyspnea and hypoxia.

DIFFERENTIAL DIAGNOSIS

- Infection in the immunocompromised patient

PATHOLOGY

- Drugs can produce virtually all histologic patterns of interstitial pneumonia, alveolar changes (including pulmonary edema, alveolar hemorrhage, diffuse alveolar damage), and pulmonary vasculitis.
- Lymphoproliferative disorder arises as sequela of immunosuppression leading to B-cell proliferation induced by Epstein-Barr virus.
- Pulmonary edema in immunocompromised host may be due to drug-induced cardiac dysfunction and fluid overload.
- Chronic lung transplant rejection and graft-versus-host disease result in bronchiolitis obliterans.

INCIDENCE/PREVALENCE AND EPIDEMIOLOGY

- Post-transplant lymphoproliferative disorder occurs in 1%-2% of all organ transplant recipients; risk is highest in first transplant year.
- Acute rejection: 60%-75% of lung recipients experience one or more episodes by first year.

- Pulmonary embolism: risk factors are immobilization, recent surgery, malignancy, preexisting cardiac, respiratory diseases, and history of venous thromboembolism.
- Diffuse alveolar hemorrhage: predisposed populations are those with leukemia, connective tissue disorders, vasculitis, and those who have received hematopoietic stem cell transplants.
- Incidence of drug toxicity varies by drug.

Suggested Readings

Choi YW, Munden RF, Erasmus JJ, et al: Effects of radiation therapy on the lung: Radiology appearances and differential diagnosis. *RadioGraphics* 24:985-998, 2004.

Collard HR, Schwarz MI: Diffuse alveolar hemorrhage. *Clin Chest Med* 25:583-592, 2004.

Hiorns MP, Screaton NJ, Müller NL: Acute lung disease in the immunocompromised host. *Radiol Clin North Am* 39:1137-1151, 2001.

Limper AH: Chemotherapy-induced lung disease. *Clin Chest Med* 25:53-64, 2004.

Peckham D, Elliott MW: Pulmonary infiltrates in the immunocompromised: Diagnosis and management. *Thorax* 57(Suppl 2):II3-II7, 2002.

Silva CI, Müller NL: Drug-induced lung diseases: Most common reaction patterns and corresponding high-resolution CT manifestations. *Semin Ultrasound CT MR* 27:111-116, 2006.

Triulzi DJ: Transfusion-related acute lung injury: An update. *Hematology Am Soc Hematol Educ Program* 497-501, 2006.

Whelan TPM, Hertz MI: Allograft rejection after lung transplantation. *Clin Chest Med* 26:599-612, 2005.

Pulmonary Complications of Hematopoietic Stem Cell Transplantation

DEFINITION: Lung complications of hematopoietic stem cell transplantation include opportunistic lung infections, diffuse alveolar hemorrhage, drug reactions, pulmonary edema, and bronchiolitis obliterans.

IMAGING

Radiography
Findings
- Bacterial pneumonia: variable, ranging from normal to bilateral diffuse areas of consolidation.
- Invasive aspergillosis: single or multiple pulmonary nodules, masses, or peripheral areas of consolidation with or without associated cavitation.
- Cytomegalovirus (CMV) pneumonia: bilateral areas of parenchymal opacification associated with multiple pulmonary nodules typically < 5 mm.
- Diffuse alveolar hemorrhage: interstitial to alveolar opacities in unilateral or bilateral distribution.
- Drug reaction: bilateral ground-glass opacities or consolidation.

Utility
- Initial modality employed but has limited sensitivity, specificity.
- Normal in up to 10% of patients with proven pulmonary disease.

CT
Findings
- Bacterial, fungal, or viral pneumonia: patchy or confluent areas of consolidation, ground-glass opacities, centrilobular nodules, "tree-in-bud" pattern.
- Airway-invasive aspergillosis (*Aspergillus* bronchiolitis and bronchopneumonia): centrilobular nodules, patchy consolidation.
- Angioinvasive aspergillosis: nodules frequently with a halo of ground-glass attenuation, air crescent sign (late manifestation), pleural-based wedge-shaped areas of consolidation.
- CMV pneumonia: bilateral parenchymal abnormalities including patchy consolidation and ground-glass opacities and nodules < 10 mm.
- Diffuse alveolar hemorrhage: nonspecific findings, varying from focal ground-glass opacities to diffuse areas of consolidation.
- Bronchiolitis obliterans: areas of decreased attenuation and vascularity, with bronchiectasis on inspiratory images and air trapping on expiratory high-resolution CT.

DIAGNOSTIC PEARLS
- Bacterial, fungal, or viral pneumonia: focal or patchy consolidation, ground-glass opacities, centrilobar nodules, "tree-in-bud" pattern.
- Angioinvasive aspergillosis: nodules with a rim of ground-glass attenuation (CT halo sign).
- CMV pneumonia: bilateral parenchymal abnormalities of consolidation and ground-glass opacities and nodules <10 mm.
- Bronchiolitis obliterans: areas of decreased attenuation and vascularity, with bronchiectasis on inspiratory images and air trapping on expiratory high-resolution CT.
- Drug reaction: bilateral ground-glass opacities with or without superimposed reticulation and/or consolidation.

- Drug reaction: bilateral ground-glass opacities with or without superimposed reticulation, consolidation.

Utility
- High-resolution CT more sensitive in detection of subtle abnormalities.
- Performed to better characterize disease, narrow differential diagnosis, and guide selection of optimal type and sampling site of invasive diagnostic technique.
- Expiratory high-resolution CT helpful in diagnosis of bronchiolitis obliterans (obliterative bronchiolitis).

CLINICAL PRESENTATION
- Fever most common presenting sign in an immunocompromised host with pulmonary infection.
- Diffuse alveolar hemorrhage: dyspnea, cough, low-grade fever; hemoptysis possible.
- Bronchiolitis obliterans: subtle increases in exertional dyspnea, progressive airflow obstruction.
- Drug reaction: acute, subacute, or chronic presentation with dry cough and progressive dyspnea.

WHAT THE REFERRING PHYSICIAN NEEDS TO KNOW
- Chest radiographs may be normal in up to 10% of patients with proven pulmonary disease.
- CT is more sensitive in detection of subtle abnormalities and is often helpful to better characterize disease and to guide type and site of invasive diagnostic procedure.
- Clinical and radiologic manifestations of pulmonary infection are often nonspecific.
- Infections account for approximately 75% of pulmonary complications in the immunocompromised host.

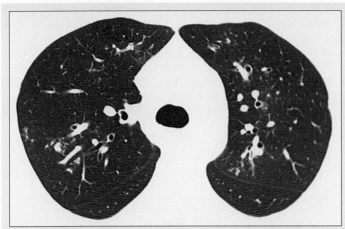

Figure 1. Airway-invasive aspergillosis. High-resolution CT image of a 29-year-old hematopoietic stem cell transplant recipient with graft-versus-host disease shows centrilobular nodules and bronchial wall thickening in the upper lobes. (*Courtesy of Dr. Ann Leung, Stanford University*)

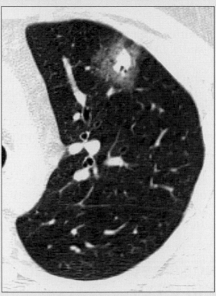

Figure 2. CT halo sign in invasive pulmonary aspergillosis. Magnified view of the left lung from a high-resolution CT scan shows a nodule with surrounding ground-glass attenuation (CT halo sign). The patient was a 33-year-old man with acute leukemia, severe neutropenia, and angioinvasive pulmonary aspergillosis.

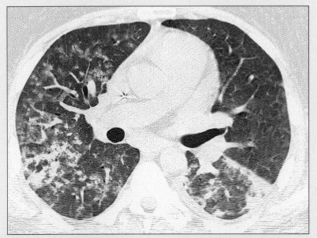

Figure 3. Cytomegalovirus pneumonia. High-resolution CT image of a 41-year-old hematopoietic stem cell transplant recipient shows centrilobular nodules associated with patchy ground-glass and focal consolidation. (*Courtesy of Dr. Ann Leung, Stanford University*)

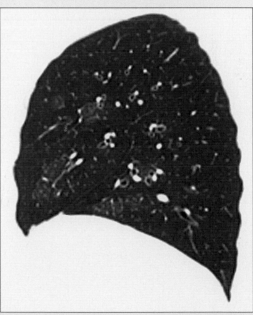

Figure 4. Bronchiolitis obliterans. Sagittal reformatted CT image of the right lung in a 57-year-old hematopoietic stem cell transplant recipient shows bronchial wall thickening, bronchiectasis, and a mosaic perfusion/attenuation pattern with areas of decreased attenuation and vascularity. (*Courtesy of Dr. Ann Leung, Stanford University*)

PATHOLOGY

- Recipients suffer from severe immune impairment that directly results from myeloablative preparatory regimens.
- Pre-engraftment period (days 0-30): neutropenia is dominant defect in host defense, predisposing patient to bacterial or fungal infections.
- Postengraftment period (days 31-100): infections occur secondary to cellular or humoral immunity defects, predisposing patient to viral infections.
- Late transplantation period (day 101 +): pulmonary infection is uncommon in patients who do not have graft-versus-host disease (chronic rejection).
- Diffuse alveolar hemorrhage occurs within first 2 weeks after hematopoietic stem cell transplantation.

INCIDENCE/PREVALENCE AND EPIDEMIOLOGY

- Pulmonary complications are common cause of morbidity and mortality in the immunocompromised host, with infections accounting for approximately 75% of these complications.

- Bacterial pneumonia is most prevalent during pre-engraftment period of profound neutropenia.
- Risk of diffuse alveolar hemorrhage is higher in autologous compared with allogeneic transplant recipients.
- Chronic airflow obstruction develops in 6%-26% and is most common late noninfectious pulmonary complication of allogeneic hematopoietic stem cell transplantation.

Suggested Readings

Collard HR, Schwarz MI: Diffuse alveolar hemorrhage. *Clin Chest Med* 25:583-592, 2004.

Kotloff RM, Ahya VN, Crawford SW: Pulmonary complications of solid organ and hematopoietic stem cell transplantation. *Am J Respir Crit Care* 170:22-48, 2004.

Oh YW, Effman EL, Godwin JD: Pulmonary infections in immunocompromised hosts: The importance of correlating the conventional radiologic appearance with the clinical setting. *Radiology* 217:647-656, 2000.

Pulmonary Complications of Lung and Heart-Lung Transplantation

DEFINITION: Lung complications of lung and heart-lung transplantation include opportunistic infection, drug-induced injury, rejection, and lymphoproliferative disorder.

IMAGING

Radiography

Findings

- Bacterial, fungal, and viral pneumonia: variable radiologic findings ranging from apparently normal radiograph to extensive bilateral areas of consolidation.
- Invasive aspergillosis: single or multiple pulmonary nodules or masses or peripheral areas of consolidation with or without associated cavitation.
- Cytomegalovirus (CMV) pneumonia: bilateral areas of parenchymal opacification associated with multiple pulmonary nodules typically <5 mm.
- Sirolimus-induced lung injury: patchy bilateral ground-glass, alveolar opacities sometimes associated with findings of fibrosis.
- Post-transplant lymphoproliferative disorder: single or multiple nodules, areas of parenchymal opacification, interlobular septal thickening, effusions.
- Acute rejection: normal in 50% of cases; reticular or airspace opacities.

Utility

- Initial modality employed but has limited sensitivity and specificity.
- Normal in up to 10% of patients with proven pulmonary disease.

CT

Findings

- Bacterial, fungal, and viral pneumonia: focal or confluent unilateral or bilateral areas of consolidation, ground-glass opacities, bronchial wall thickening, centrilobular nodules, "tree-in-bud" pattern, pleural effusion.
- Invasive aspergillosis: CT halo sign (early); air crescent sign (recovery phase).
- CMV pneumonia: bilateral parenchymal abnormalities: consolidation, ground-glass opacities, and nodules <10 mm.
- Sirolimus-induced lung injury: patchy bilateral ground-glass, alveolar opacities sometimes associated with findings of fibrosis.
- Post-transplant lymphoproliferative disorder: single or multiple nodules, areas of parenchymal opacification, interlobular septal thickening, lymphadenopathy, pleural effusions.
- Acute rejection: septal thickening, fissure thickening, pleural effusion, areas of parenchymal opacification.
- Chronic rejection: areas of decreased attenuation and vascularity and bronchiectasis on inspiratory high-resolution CT images and air trapping on expiratory CT.

Utility

- High-resolution CT more sensitive than radiography in detection of subtle abnormalities.
- Performed to better characterize disease, narrow differential diagnosis, and guide selection of optimal type and sampling site of invasive diagnostic technique.

CLINICAL PRESENTATION

- Fever is most common presenting sign in an immunocompromised host with pulmonary infection.
- Sirolimus-induced lung injury has nonspecific symptoms, including fever, fatigue, dyspnea, and cough.
- Acute lung rejection symptoms vary depending on grade of rejection.

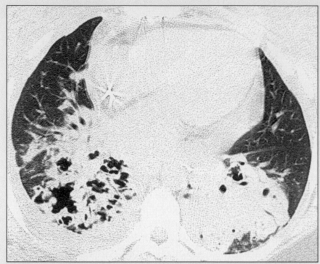

Figure 1. *Pseudomonas aeruginosa* and *S. aureus* pneumonia. High-resolution CT image of a 22-year-old double-lung transplant recipient shows necrotizing pneumonia in both lower lobes. (*Courtesy of Dr. Ann Leung, Stanford University*)

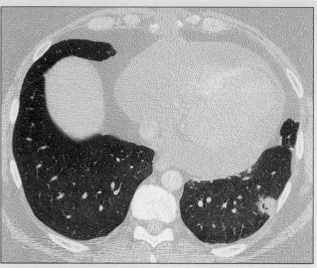

Figure 2. **Angioinvasive aspergillosis.** High-resolution CT image of a 48-year-old heart transplant recipient shows left lower lobe nodule with a peripheral linear cavitation (air crescent sign). (*Courtesy of Dr. Ann Leung, Stanford University*)

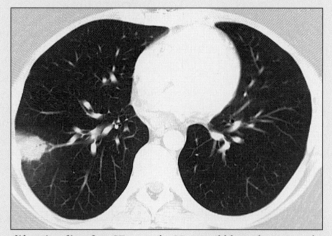

Figure 3. **Post-transplant lymphoproliferative disorder.** CT scan of a 27-year-old heart-lung transplant recipient shows a nodular area of consolidation in the periphery of the right lower lobe. (*Courtesy of Dr. Ann Leung, Stanford University*)

- Mild rejection is asymptomatic.
- Higher grades of rejection are associated with non-specific symptoms such as fever, cough, fatigue, and dyspnea.

DIFFERENTIAL DIAGNOSIS

- Pneumonia
- Drug reaction
- Pulmonary edema
- Acute lung rejection
- Lymphoma

PATHOLOGY

- In first month after transplantation, solid organ transplant recipients are most susceptible to bacterial infections.
- From months 1 to 6, opportunistic fungal infections and viruses, including CMV, become most frequent pathogens.
- After 6 months, risk of infection is similar to that of general population.
- Sirolimus is potent, relatively new immunosuppressive agent that is used to prevent rejection in solid organ transplants.

- Post-transplant lymphoproliferative disorders are direct sequelae of immunosuppression and related to B-cell proliferation induced by infection with Epstein-Barr virus.
- Chronic rejection in the form of bronchiolitis obliterans remains the major limitation to long-term survival in the lung transplant population.

INCIDENCE/PREVALENCE AND EPIDEMIOLOGY

- Pulmonary complications are common cause of morbidity and mortality in the immunocompromised host.
- Infections account for approximately 75% of pulmonary complications in the immunocompromised host.
- Aspergillosis occurs in approximately 5% of the solid organ transplant population within the first 6 months after operation.

- Sirolimus-induced lung injury is uncommon.
- Post-transplant lymphoproliferative disorders affect 1%-2% of all organ transplant recipients.
- Acute rejection is a common complication; 60%-75% of lung recipients experience one or more episodes by first year after transplantation.
- Chronic rejection accounts for 30% of all deaths after third postoperative year of lung transplantation.

Suggested Readings

Fishman JA, Rubin RH: Infection in organ transplant recipients. *N Engl J Med* 338:1741-1751, 1998.

Kotloff RM, Ahya VN, Crawford SW: Pulmonary complications of solid organ and hematopoietic stem cell transplantation. *Am J Respir Crit Care* 170:22-48, 2004.

Oh YW, Effman EL, Godwin JD: Pulmonary infections in immunocompromised hosts: The importance of correlating the conventional radiologic appearance with the clinical setting. *Radiology* 217:647-656, 2000.

Pulmonary Neoplasms

Lung Cancer: Adenocarcinoma

DEFINITION: Pulmonary adenocarcinomas are frequently histologically heterogeneous and consist of a mixture of histologic subtypes including acinar, papillary, bronchioloalveolar, and solid with formation of mucus.

IMAGING

Radiography
Findings
- Adenocarcinomas usually present as solitary spiculated nodules measuring <4 cm in diameter.
- Bronchoalveolar carcinoma is a subtype of adenocarcinoma that may present as a small focal area of ground-glass opacity or consolidation, as a solid nodule, or as multicentric or diffuse disease.

Utility
- Helpful in demonstrating presence of tumor

CT
Findings
- Adenocarcinomas may be solid or have mixed solid and ground-glass components and usually have spiculated margins. Pleural tags are commonly present.
- Small focal ("bubble") lucencies are often present, and cavitation may occur.
- Bronchioalveolar carcinoma may present as a small focal area of ground-glass opacity or consolidation, as a solid nodule, or as multicentric or diffuse disease; it commonly contains bubble lucencies.
- Focal soft tissue nodule with surrounding halo of ground-glass opacity (CT halo sign) may be seen in invasive adenocarcinoma; the greater the relative percentage of soft tissue, the greater the likelihood of invasive adenocarcinoma.

Utility
- Superior to radiography in the assessment of tumor extent

Positron Emission Tomography
Findings
- Increased uptake on FDG-PET
- Increased uptake of intrathoracic, chest wall, and extrathoracic metastases

Utility
- Superior to CT in the staging of pulmonary carcinoma
- PET/CT currently best imaging for assessment of presence of intrathoracic and extrathoracic metastases

DIAGNOSTIC PEARLS

- Adenocarcinomas may be solid or have mixed solid and ground-glass components.
- Small focal ("bubble") lucencies are often present.
- Adenocarcinomas most commonly have spiculated margins.
- False-negative PET may occur in bronchioloalveolar carcinomas and in adenocarcinomas with less than 1 cm diameter solid component on CT.

- False-negative PET occurs mainly in bronchioloalveolar carcinomas and adenocarcinomas with less than 1 cm diameter solid component on CT.

CLINICAL PRESENTATION
- Often asymptomatic
- Clinical symptoms: cough, dyspnea, hemoptysis, weight loss, and paraneoplastic syndromes

DIFFERENTIAL DIAGNOSIS
- Squamous cell carcinoma
- Large cell carcinoma
- Metastasis
- Hamartoma
- Carcinoid tumor
- Lymphoma
- Granuloma

PATHOLOGY
- There are four major subtypes of adenocarcinoma: acinar (gland forming), papillary, bronchioloalveolar, and solid with formation of mucus.
- Pulmonary adenocarcinomas are frequently histologically heterogeneous and consist of a mixture of the histologic subtypes.

WHAT THE REFERRING PHYSICIAN NEEDS TO KNOW
- Adenocarcinomas presenting in lung can be primary or metastatic.
- Metastatic adenocarcinomas can mimic the histologic appearance of primary lung adenocarcinomas.
- The radiologic findings are of limited value in distinguishing the various subtypes of pulmonary carcinoma.

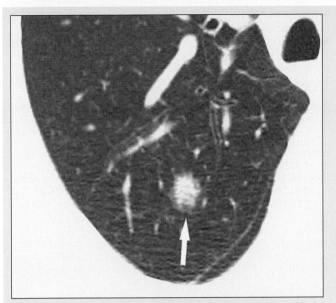

Figure 1. Adenocarcinoma with mixed attenuation. Magnified view of the right lung from a high-resolution CT shows nodule with predominantly solid component and with halo of ground-glass attenuation (CT halo sign) (*arrow*) in a patient with invasive pulmonary adenocarcinoma.

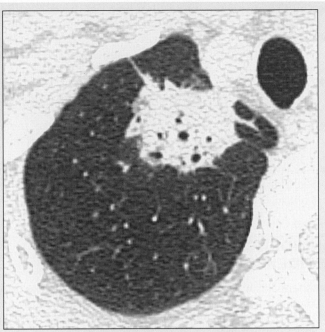

Figure 2. Bubble-like lucencies in adenocarcinoma. Magnified view of right upper lobe from a high-resolution CT scan shows nodule containing small round areas of low attenuation (bubble lucencies). The patient was a 79-year-old woman with adenocarcinoma.

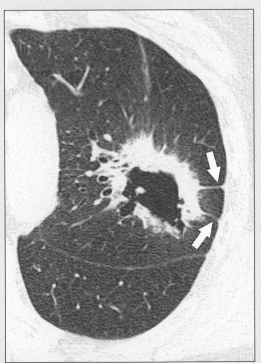

Figure 3. Pleural tags. A magnified view of the left lung shows a cavitating mass with spiculated margins. Linear opacities can be seen extending from the mass to the visceral pleura (pleural tag) (*arrows*). Note the slight tenting of the visceral pleura at the site of the pleural tag. The patient was a 67-year-old woman with pulmonary adenocarcinoma.

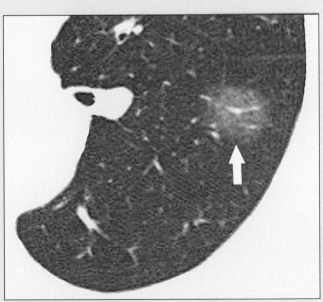

Figure 4. Bronchioloalveolar carcinoma. Magnified view of the left lung from a high-resolution CT shows solitary nodule composed only of ground-glass opacity (*arrow*). This was proven to be bronchioloalveolar carcinoma.

- Solid adenocarcinomas with mucin require at least five mucin-positive cells in at least two high-power fields.
- Nonmucinous bronchioalveolar carcinoma is composed of cuboidal cells proliferating along the alveolar septa.
- Mucinous bronchioalveolar carcinoma consists of tall columnar cells with abundant apical cytoplasmic mucin and small, basally oriented nuclei.
- Airspaces surrounding mucinous bronchioalveolar carcinoma are often filled with mucin, sometimes creating a colloid-like appearance.
- Bronchioalveolar carcinoma grows in a lepidic fashion along alveolar septa without vascular, stromal, or pleural invasion.

INCIDENCE/PREVALENCE AND EPIDEMIOLOGY

- Adenocarcinoma accounts for approximately one third of all lung cancers.
- It is the most common histologic type of lung cancer in most countries.

- The mixed subtype is the most common histologic lung presentation.
- Bronchioalveolar carcinoma is uncommon, accounting for less than 4% of all lung malignancies.

Suggested Readings

Beadsmoore CJ, Screaton NJ: Classification, staging and prognosis of lung cancer. *Eur J Radiol* 45:8-17, 2003.

Collins LG, Haines C, Perkel R, Enck RE: Lung cancer: Diagnosis and management. *Am Fam Physician* 75:56-63, 2007.

Hollings N, Shaw P: Diagnostic imaging of lung cancer. *Eur Respir J* 19:722-742, 2002.

Shiau MC, Bonavita J, Naidich DP: Adenocarcinoma of the lung: Current concepts in radiologic diagnosis and management. *Curr Opin Pulm Med* 13:261-266, 2007.

Lung Cancer: Bronchioloalveolar Cell Carcinoma and Atypical Adenomatous Hyperplasia

DEFINITION: Bronchioloalveolar cell carcinoma is a subtype of adenocarcinoma; atypical adenomatous hyperplasia is a preinvasive lesion of lung adenocarcinoma.

IMAGING

Radiography
Findings
- Atypical adenomatous hyperplasia: seldom visible on the radiograph
- Bronchioloalveolar carcinoma: solitary nodule; focal, multifocal, or confluent consolidation

CT
Findings
- Atypical adenomatous hyperlasia: typically pure focal ground-glass opacities that remain unchanged for several months and measure <5 mm in diameter.
- Bronchioloalveolar cell carcinoma: may present as small focal area of ground-glass opacity or consolidation, as solid nodule, or as multicentric or diffuse disease.
- Multicentric bronchioloalveolar carcinoma may result in areas of consolidation that typically have lower attenuation than chest wall muscle and contain visible pulmonary vessels (CT angiogram sign).

CLINICAL PRESENTATION

- Usually asymptomatic
- Occasionally may result in dyspnea and cough

DIFFERENTIAL DIAGNOSIS

- Lung cancer: Squamous cell carcinoma
- Lung cancer: Adenocarcinoma
- Infection

PATHOLOGY

- Atypical adenomatous hyperplasia is characterized by bronchioloalveolar proliferation usually millimeters in size; lesions are often multiple and may be associated with multicentric adenocarcinomas.
- Atypical adenomatous hyperplasia grows along alveoli and respiratory bronchioles, typically showing gaps between adjacent cells.

DIAGNOSTIC PEARLS

- Focal lesions of ground-glass opacity that remain unchanged for several months and measure <5 mm in diameter usually represent atypical adenomatous hyperplasia; lesions >5 mm are more likely to represent bronchioloalveolar carcinoma.
- Bronchioloalveolar carcinoma may present as ground-glass nodule, mixed ground-glass and solid nodule, solid nodule, or as patchy or confluent ground-glass opacities and consolidation.

- Bronchioloalveolar cell carcinoma has two types: nonmucinous type is composed of cuboidal cells proliferating along alveolar septa, whereas mucinous type consists of tall columnar cells with abundant apical cytoplasmic mucin and small basally oriented nuclei.
- Airspaces surrounding mucinous bronchioloalveolar cell carcinomas are often filled with mucin, sometimes creating a colloid-like appearance.
- Bronchioloalveolar cell carcinoma grows in lepidic fashion along alveolar septa without vascular, stromal, or pleural invasion.

INCIDENCE/PREVALENCE AND EPIDEMIOLOGY

- Atypical adenomatous hyperplasia is a preinvasive lesion of lung adenocarcinoma.
- Atypical adenomatous hyperplasia is reported to occur in 5.7%-21.4% of lung cancer specimens.
- Bronchioloalveolar cell carcinoma is uncommon, accounting for less than 4% of all lung malignancies.

WHAT THE REFERRING PHYSICIAN NEEDS TO KNOW
- Atypical adenomatous hyperplasia must be distinguished from the nonmucinous subtype of bronchioloalveolar cell carcinoma by cell uniformity, cellular crowding, and nuclear atypia.
- No adverse prognosis is shown for lung cancer patients with atypical adenomatous hyperplasia compared with those without atypical adenomatous hyperplasia.

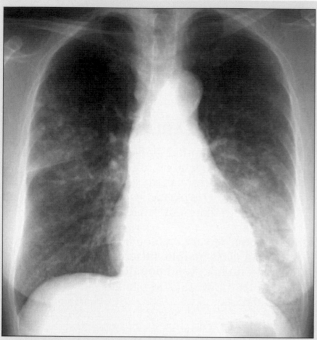

Figure 1. Bronchioloalveolar cell carcinoma. Posteroanterior chest radiograph shows patchy areas of consolidation in the right lung, confluent consolidation in the left lower lobe, and bilateral poorly defined nodules. The patient was a 63-year-old woman with bronchioloalveolar cell carcinoma.

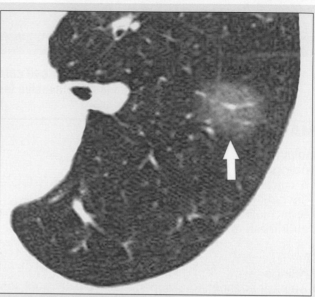

Figure 2. Ground-glass nodule. Magnified view of the left lung from a high-resolution CT shows solitary nodule appearing as a ground-glass opacity (*arrow*). This was proven to be a bronchioloalveolar carcinoma.

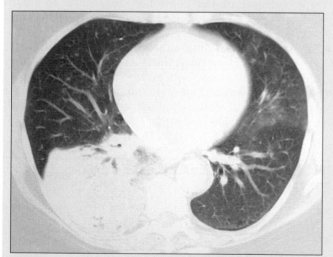

Figure 3. Bronchioloalveolar carcinoma and CT angiogram sign. CT image demonstrates consolidation in the right lower lobe, a few poorly defined nodular opacities bilaterally, and ground-glass opacities in the lingula.

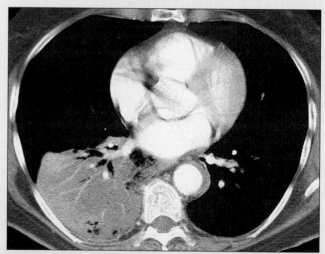

Figure 4. Bronchioloalveolar carcinoma and CT angiogram sign. Contrast-enhanced CT image demonstrates that some of the areas of consolidation have lower attenuation than the chest wall muscles and that opacified vessels are well seen within the consolidation (CT angiogram sign).

Suggested Readings

Gandara DR, Aberle D, Lau D, et al: Radiographic imaging of bronchioloalveolar carcinoma: Screening, patterns of presentation and response assessment. *J Thorac Oncol* 1(9 Suppl):S20-S26, 2006.

Raz DJ, Kim JY, Jablons DM: Diagnosis and treatment of bronchioloalveolar carcinoma. *Curr Opin Pulm Med* 13:290-296, 2007.

Yousem SA, Beasley MB: Bronchioloalveolar carcinoma: A review of current concepts and evolving issues. *Arch Pathol Lab Med* 131:1027-1032, 2007.

Lung Cancer: Large Cell Carcinoma

DEFINITION: Large cell carcinomas appear as sheets and nests of large polygonal cells with vesicular nuclei and prominent nucleoli.

IMAGING

Radiography
Findings
- Large mass usually in the periphery of lung
- May have smooth or spiculated margins
- May be associated with unilateral hilar or mediastinal lymphadenopathy

Utility
- Helpful in demonstrating presence of tumor

CT
Findings
- Large mass usually in the periphery of the lung
- Heterogeneous enhancement after intravenous administration of a contrast agent
- Unilateral hilar or mediastinal lymphadenopathy
- Atelectasis and obstructive pneumonitis in central tumors
- Invasion of the chest wall or vertebrae

Utility
- Superior to radiography in the assessment of tumor extent

MRI
Findings
- Large mass usually in the periphery of the lung
- Heterogeneous enhancement after intravenous administration of a contrast agent
- Unilateral hilar or mediastinal lymphadenopathy
- Atelectasis and obstructive pneumonitis in central tumors

Utility
- Comparable to CT in the assessment of tumor extent within the chest.
- Superior to CT in the assessment of vascular invasion.

Positron Emission Tomography
Findings
- Increased uptake on FDG-PET
- Increased uptake in intrathoracic, chest wall, and extrathoracic metastases

Utility
- FDG-PET and integrated PET/CT are superior to CT in the staging of pulmonary carcinoma.
- PET/CT is currently best imaging modality for assessment of presence of intrathoracic and extrathoracic metastases.

DIAGNOSTIC PEARLS
- Tumors tend to be large and necrotic and occur in periphery of lung
- Frequently associated with lymph node and distal metastases
- Account for 5%-10% of lung carcinomas

CLINICAL PRESENTATION
- May be asymptomatic
- Cough, hemoptysis, weight loss

DIFFERENTIAL DIAGNOSIS
- Lung cancer: Squamous cell carcinoma

PATHOLOGY
- Tumors usually occur in periphery of lung, but they can also be central tumors.
- Tumors are large and necrotic and appear as sheets and nests of large polygonal cells with vesicular nuclei and prominent nucleoli.
- Large cell neuroendocrine carcinoma has organoid, palisading, trabecular, or rosette-like growth patterns.

INCIDENCE/PREVALENCE AND EPIDEMIOLOGY
- Large cell carcinoma accounts for 5%-10% of all lung carcinomas.
- Large cell neuroendocrine carcinoma is the most common variant of large cell carcinoma, accounting for approximately 3% of surgically resected lung cancers.
- Survival for both small cell lung carcinoma and large cell neuroendocrine carcinoma is very poor with no significant difference demonstrated.

Suggested Readings

Beadsmoore CJ, Screaton NJ: Classification, staging and prognosis of lung cancer. *Eur J Radiol* 45:8-17, 2003.
Collins LG, Haines C, Perkel R, Enck RE: Lung cancer: Diagnosis and management. *Am Fam Physician* 75:56-63, 2007.
Hollings N, Shaw P: Diagnostic imaging of lung cancer. *Eur Respir J* 19:722-742, 2002.

WHAT THE REFERRING PHYSICIAN NEEDS TO KNOW
- Large cell carcinoma accounts for 5%-10% of all lung carcinomas.
- By definition, no specific squamous or glandular tissue should be seen.
- The tumors typically present as large peripheral masses and are associated with early metastases.

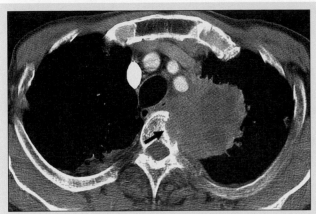

Figure 1. **Large cell lung cancer in a 72-year-old man.**
Enhanced transverse CT scan obtained at level of thoracic inlet
shows large heterogeneous left upper lobe mass (stage 4 tumor)
invading into vertebral body (*arrow*). (*Courtesy of Dr. Kyung Soo
Lee, Seoul, Korea*)

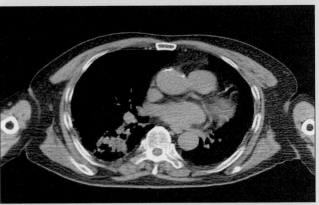

Figure 2. **Large cell carcinoma.** Rib metastasis detected at
integrated PET/CT but not at CT in a 72-year-old man. CT scan
shows mass in the superior segment of the right lower lobe.
(*Courtesy of Dr. Kyung Soo Lee, Seoul, Korea*)

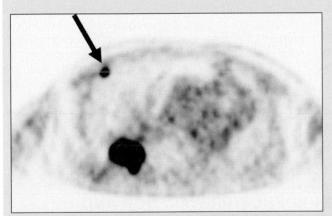

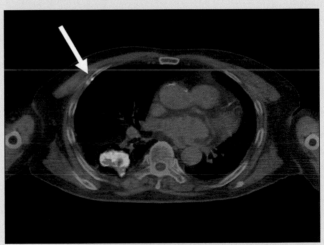

Figure 3. **Large cell carcinoma.** Rib metastasis detected at
integrated PET/CT but not at CT (see Fig. 2) in a 72-year-old
man. PET image shows increased FDG uptake (*arrow*) in rib and
lung mass. (*Courtesy of Dr. Kyung Soo Lee, Seoul, Korea*)

Figure 4. **Large cell carcinoma.** Rib metastasis detected at
integrated PET/CT but not at CT (see Fig. 2) in a 72-year-old
man. Integrated PET/CT image shows increased FDG uptake
(*arrow*) in rib and lung mass. (*Courtesy of Dr. Kyung Soo Lee,
Seoul, Korea*)

Lung Cancer: Small Cell Carcinoma

DEFINITION: Small cell lung cancer is characterized by tumor cells that have a small size, a round to fusiform shape, scant cytoplasm, finely granular nuclear chromatin, and absent or inconspicuous nucleoli.

IMAGING

Radiography
Findings
- Unilateral hilar and mediastinal lymphadenopathy

Utility
- Helpful in demonstrating presence of tumor

CT
Findings
- Extensive hilar and mediastinal lymphadenopathy
- Noncontiguous parenchymal mass in up to 40% of cases
- Extensive mediastinal invasion, which may result in obstruction of the superior vena cava (SVC syndrome)
- Extrathoracic metastases common at presentation

Utility
- Superior to radiography in the assessment of tumor extent

MRI
Findings
- Extensive hilar and mediastinal lymphadenopathy
- High signal intensity of tumor on T2-weighted images

Utility
- Comparable to CT in the assessment of tumor extent within the chest
- Superior to CT in the assessment of vascular invasion

Positron Emission Tomography
Findings
- Increased uptake on FDG-PET
- Increased uptake in intrathoracic, chest wall, and extrathoracic metastases

Utility
- FDG-PET and integrated PET/CT superior to CT in staging of pulmonary carcinoma
- PET/CT currently best imaging modality for assessment of presence of intrathoracic and extrathoracic metastases

CLINICAL PRESENTATION

- Patients typically present with disseminated disease.
- Most common symptoms are cough and dyspnea.
- Other common findings are weight loss, weakness, and chest pain.

DIAGNOSTIC PEARLS

- Perihilar mass
- Infiltration into bronchial submucosa and peribronchial tissue
- Extensive lymph node metastases
- Most common cause of superior vena cava syndrome

DIFFERENTIAL DIAGNOSIS

- Adenocarcinoma
- Large cell carcinoma
- Squamous cell carcinoma
- Lymphoma

PATHOLOGY

- Tumor is usually peribronchial and infiltrates bronchial submucosa and peribronchial tissue, causing circumferential compression and bronchial obstruction.
- Extensive lymph node metastases are common.
- Characterized by small tumor cells, round to fusiform shape, scant cytoplasm, finely granular nuclear chromatin, and absent or inconspicuous nucleoli.
- Necrosis is usually extensive, and mitotic rates are high.
- Growth pattern consists of diffuse sheets, but rosettes, peripheral palisading, organoid nesting, and ribbons are also common.

INCIDENCE/PREVALENCE AND EPIDEMIOLOGY

- Accounts for approximately 20% of lung cancers

Suggested Readings
Beadsmoore CJ, Screaton NJ: Classification, staging and prognosis of lung cancer. *Eur J Radiol* 45:8-17, 2003.
Collins LG, Haines C, Perkel R, Enck RE: Lung cancer: Diagnosis and management. *Am Fam Physician* 75:56-63, 2007.
Hollings N, Shaw P: Diagnostic imaging of lung cancer. *Eur Respir J* 19:722-742, 2002.
Jackman DM, Johnson BE: Small cell lung cancer. *Lancet* 366: 1385-1396, 2005.

WHAT THE REFERRING PHYSICIAN NEEDS TO KNOW

- Classic presentation of small cell lung carcinoma is as a hilar mass associated with extensive mediastinal lymphadenopathy.
- The tumor is usually peribronchial and infiltrates bronchial submucosa and peribronchial tissue, causing circumferential compression and bronchial obstruction.
- In most cases, diagnosis is established on transbronchial biopsy and/or cytology.
- Most patients present with disseminated disease.

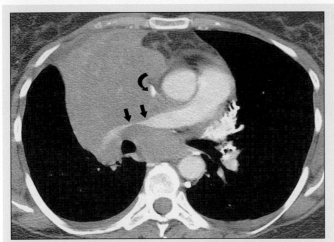

Figure 1. Small cell carcinoma with SVC syndrome. Contrast-enhanced CT shows a large mass in the right hilum and mediastinum with marked encasement of the right descending pulmonary artery (*straight arrows*) and near-complete occlusion of the superior vena cava (*curved arrow*). Note the presence of mediastinal venous collaterals as a result of the SVC obstruction. (*Courtesy of Dr. Jeffrey S. Klein, University of Vermont*)

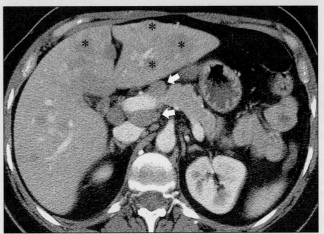

Figure 2. Small cell carcinoma with abdominal metastases. CT image at the level of the upper abdomen shows multiple liver lesions (*asterisks*) and enlarged porta hepatis lymph nodes (*arrows*). Liver biopsy revealed small cell carcinoma. (*Courtesy of Dr. Jeffrey S. Klein, University of Vermont*)

Lung Cancer: Squamous Cell Carcinoma

DEFINITION: Pulmonary squamous cell carcinoma consists of sheets of tumor cells that show intercellular bridging, squamous pearl formation, and individual cell keratinization.

IMAGING

Radiography
Findings
- Atelectasis of segment, lobe, or lung
- When associated with hilar mass may result in focal convexity (S sign of Golden)
- Peripheral nodule or mass; frequently cavitated

Utility
- Helpful in demonstrating presence of tumor

CT
Findings
- Endobronchial lesion with partial or complete distal obstruction
- Pulmonary, lobar, or segmental atelectasis
- Peripheral nodule or mass; frequently cavitated
- Hilar and mediastinal lymphadenopathy

Utility
- Superior to radiography in the assessment of tumor extent
- Superior to radiograph in showing endobronchial tumor in patients with atelectasis or obstructive pneumonitis

MRI
Findings
- Endobronchial lesion with partial or complete distal obstruction; tumor has high signal intensity on T2-weighted images
- Pulmonary, lobar, or segmental atelectasis
- Hilar and mediastinal lymphadenopathy

Utility
- Comparable to CT in the assessment of tumor extent within the chest
- Superior to CT in the assessment of vascular invasion

Positron Emission Tomography
Findings
- Increased uptake on FDG-PET
- Increased uptake of intrathoracic, chest wall, and extrathoracic metastases

Utility
- FDG-PET and integrated PET/CT are superior to CT in the staging of pulmonary carcinoma.
- PET/CT is currently best imaging modality for assessment of presence of intrathoracic and extrathoracic metastases.

DIAGNOSTIC PEARLS
- Endobronchial tumor with pulmonary, lobar, or segmental atelectasis
- Peripheral mass with cavitation
- Hilar and mediastinal lymphadenopathy

CLINICAL PRESENTATION
- Cough, dyspnea, hemoptysis, weight loss
- May be associated with paraneoplastic syndrome

DIFFERENTIAL DIAGNOSIS
- Adenocarcinoma
- Large cell carcinoma
- Endobronchial carcinoid tumor
- Metastasis
- Tuberculosis

PATHOLOGY
- Four major subtypes: papillary, clear cell, small cell, and basaloid
- Tumor consists of sheets of tumor cells that show intercellular bridging and individual cell keratinization
- Endobronchial tumors most commonly present in segmental bronchi; involvement of lobar and main-stem bronchus occurs by extension

INCIDENCE/PREVALENCE AND EPIDEMIOLOGY
- Squamous cell carcinoma accounts for 20%-30% of all lung cancers in the United States.

Suggested Readings

Beadsmoore CJ, Screaton NJ: Classification, staging and prognosis of lung cancer. *Eur J Radiol* 45:8-17, 2003.
Collins LG, Haines C, Perkel R, Enck RE: Lung cancer: Diagnosis and management. *Am Fam Physician* 75:56-63, 2007.
Hollings N, Shaw P: Diagnostic imaging of lung cancer. *Eur Respir J* 19:722-742, 2002.
Yang P, Allen MS, Aubry MC, et al: Clinical features of 5,628 primary lung cancer patients: Experience at Mayo Clinic from 1997 to 2003. *Chest* 128:452-462, 2005.

WHAT THE REFERRING PHYSICIAN NEEDS TO KNOW
- Squamous cell carcinoma should be suspected in patients with chronic segmental or lobar atelectasis or nonresolving segmental or lobar pneumonia.
- Squamous cell carcinoma also commonly occurs in the lung periphery, including the superior sulcus (Pancoast tumor).

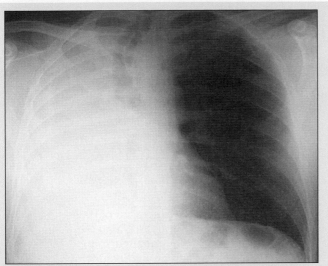

Figure 1. Squamous cell carcinoma with obstructive atelectasis of right lung. Chest radiograph shows opacification and decreased volume of the right hemithorax. The trachea and mediastinum are shifted to the right, and the left lung shows compensatory overinflation. The lack of air bronchograms within the opacified atelectatic right lung is consistent with obstructive atelectasis. The patient was a 44-year-old man with squamous cell carcinoma.

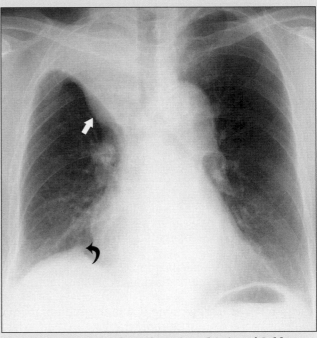

Figure 2. Right upper lobe atelectasis and S sign of Golden. Chest radiograph demonstrates right upper lobe atelectasis. Note focal downward bulge (*straight arrow*) in the medial portion of displaced minor fissure and a concave appearance of the lateral aspect of the minor fissure, resulting in a reverse-S configuration known as the S sign of Golden. Also note mild elevation and tenting (*curved arrow*) of the right hemidiaphragm.

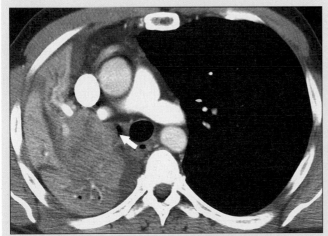

Figure 3. Squamous cell carcinoma with obstructive atelectasis of right lung. Contrast-enhanced CT demonstrates complete obstruction of the right main bronchus by tumor (*arrow*) and distal atelectasis and obstructive pneumonitis. The patient was a 44-year-old man (see Fig.1).

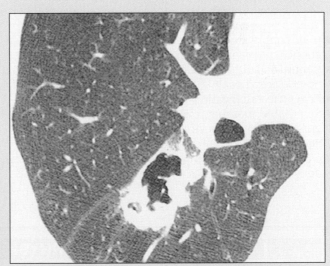

Figure 4. Squamous cell carcinoma. View of the right lung from a high-resolution CT shows right lower lobe mass with cavitation. The wall of the cavity is thick and has a nodular appearance. The patient was a 73-year-old man.

Part 20

LUNG CANCER: RADIOLOGIC MANIFESTATIONS AND DIAGNOSIS

Lung Cancer: Solitary Lung Nodule

DEFINITION: A solitary nodule, defined as a rounded opacity measuring up to 3 cm in diameter, is a common manifestation of lung cancer.

IMAGING

Radiography

Findings
- Rounded opacity measuring up to 3 cm in diameter
- Smooth margins seen more commonly in benign nodules; spiculated margins seen more commonly in malignant lesions.
- Central or diffuse calcification in a smoothly margined nodule is virtually diagnostic of a granuloma

Utility
- It can be used to determine if solitary pulmonary nodule was present on prior radiographs.
- Confirmation of stable nodule over 2 years or longer is strong evidence of benignity.
- Any growth in solitary pulmonary nodule or a nodule not evident on prior radiographs often requires CT for further evaluation.

CT

Findings
- Rounded opacity measuring up to 3 cm in diameter
- May have ground-glass opacity, mixed ground-glass and soft tissue, or soft tissue density
- May contain foci of calcification, cavitation, air bronchograms, or bubble lucencies
- Central and diffuse calcification in a smoothly marginated nodule are virtually diagnostic of a granuloma
- Eccentric calcification is consistent with carcinoma
- Spiculated margins favor carcinoma and smooth margins favor benign lesion

Utility
- CT features that are important to analyze include size, density, margins, 3D shape, and growth rate

DIAGNOSTIC PEARLS

- Most small (<10 mm) solitary pulmonary nodules detected on CT are benign.
- Most smooth solitary pulmonary nodules reflect benign conditions, whereas lobulated or irregular margins are suggestive of malignancy.
- Findings that favor carcinoma include: mixed solid and ground-glass nodules, bubble lucencies, large size, spiculated margins, and smoking history.
- Presence of central or diffuse calcifications in a smoothly marginated nodule is virtually diagnostic of a granuloma.

- Solitary pulmonary nodules 4-10 mm in diameter are often followed by short-interval follow-up CT scans to assess for growth
- CT is superior to radiographs to assess for presence of calcification
- Presence of foci of fat density within a smoothly marginated nodule is diagnostic of hamartoma

Ultrasonography

Findings
- Detects mass contiguous to chest wall

Utility
- Ultrasound-guided needle biopsy can provide material for histologic diagnosis in patients with peripherally situated nodules contacting chest wall

Positron Emission Tomography

Findings
- FDG uptake in mass or nonuptake.

WHAT THE REFERRING PHYSICIAN NEEDS TO KNOW

- Radiographic features of importance in evaluation of solitary pulmonary nodules include change in size over time, margins, and presence of calcification.
- CT is the main imaging procedure for evaluation of solitary pulmonary nodules or suspected lung cancer.
- CT features that are important to analyze include size, density, margins, 3D shape, and growth rate.
- Four conditions account for 95% of cases of solitary pulmonary nodules: granulomas, lung cancer, hamartomas, and intrapulmonary lymph nodes.
- Most smooth solitary pulmonary nodules reflect benign conditions, whereas lobulated or irregular margins are suggestive of malignancy.
- Imaging algorithm for evaluation of solitary pulmonary nodules incorporates clinical probability assessment with lesion characteristics seen on imaging studies.

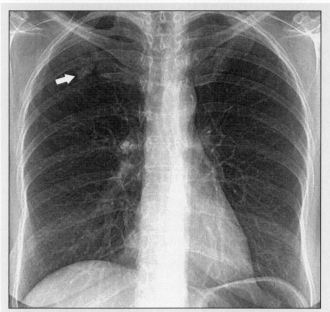

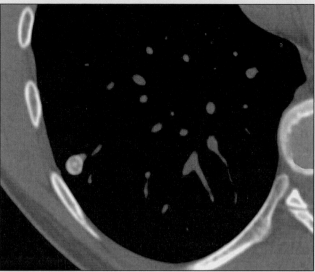

Figure 1. Solitary pulmonary nodule as carcinoma on chest radiograph. Chest radiograph shows a solitary right upper lobe nodule (*arrow*). CT-guided aspiration and subsequent resection showed adenocarcinoma. (*Courtesy of Dr. Jeffrey S. Klein, University of Vermont*)

Figure 2. Target calcification in granuloma. Targeted thin-section reconstruction through right lower lobe nodule shows concentric or target calcification most typical of a granuloma. (*Courtesy of Dr. Jeffrey S. Klein, University of Vermont*)

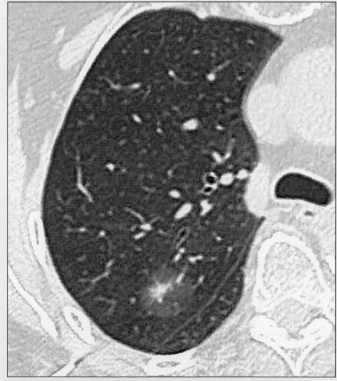

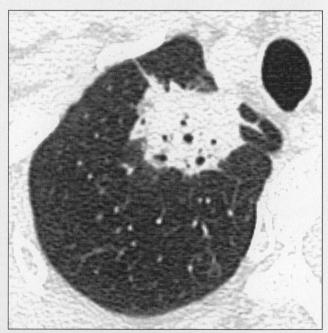

Figure 3. Mixed solid/ground-glass attenuation nodule reflecting adenocarcinoma. A mixed-attenuation lesion with central solid component and peripheral ground-glass attenuation is evident in the posterior segment of the right upper lobe. Biopsy revealed well-differentiated adenocarcinoma. (*Courtesy of Dr. Jeffrey S. K lein, University of Vermont*)

Figure 4. Bubble-like lucencies in adenocarcinoma. Magnified view of right upper lobe from a high-resolution CT image shows nodule containing small round areas of low attenuation ("bubble lucencies"). The patient was a 79-year-old woman with adenocarcinoma. (*Courtesy of Dr. Jeffrey S. Klein, University of Vermont*)

Utility

- With lesions >10 mm, positive PET has sensitivity of approximately 97% and specificity of 78% in detection of malignancy.
- Absolute standardized uptake value of malignant solitary pulmonary nodules is of prognostic value because higher values correlate with poor patient outcome.
- False-negative PET imaging may occur with bronchioloalveolar carcinoma and small well-differentiated adenocarcinomas.

CLINICAL PRESENTATION

- Most patients are asymptomatic.

DIFFERENTIAL DIAGNOSIS

- Pulmonary carcinoma
- Hamartoma
- Granuloma
- Carcinoid tumor
- Inflammatory pseudotumor

PATHOLOGY

- Four conditions account for 95% of cases of SPNs: granulomas, lung cancer, hamartomas, and intrapulmonary lymph nodes.

INCIDENCE/PREVALENCE AND EPIDEMIOLOGY

- Vast majority of asymptomatic solitary pulmonary nodules are benign lesions.
- Approximately 50% of SPNs that are resected prove to be malignant.

Suggested Readings

Gould MK, Maclean CC: Accuracy of positron emission tomography for diagnosis of pulmonary nodules and mass lesions: A meta-analysis. *JAMA* 285:914-924, 2001.

Henschke CI, Yankelevitz DF, Mirtcheva R, et al: CT screening for lung cancer: Frequency and significance of part-solid and nonsolid nodules. *AJR Am J Roentgenol* 178:1053-1057, 2002.

MacMahon H, Austin JHM, Gamsu G, et al: Guidelines for management of small pulmonary nodules detected on CT scans: A statement from the Fleischner Society. *Radiology* 237:395-400, 2005.

Revel M-P, Lefort C, Bissery A, et al: Pulmonary nodules: Preliminary experience with three-dimensional evaluation. *Radiology* 231:459-466, 2004.

Winer-Muram HT: The solitary pulmonary nodule. *Radiology* 239:34-49, 2006.

Yankelevitz DF, Reeves AP, Kostis WJ, et al: Small pulmonary nodules: Volumetrically determined growth rates based on CT evaluation. *Radiology* 217:251-256, 2000.

Lung Cancer: Superior Sulcus (Pancoast) Tumor

DEFINITION: Lung cancer that arises in the apical region of the lung has been termed *Pancoast* or *superior sulcus tumor.*

IMAGING

Radiography
Findings
- Asymmetric apical opacity, particularly if inferior margin is convex
- Associated rib or vertebral involvement

Utility
- Often first imaging modality used in the evaluation

CT
Findings
- Only specific findings of chest wall invasion is mass extending through intercostal space or associated with bone destruction.
- Local invasion of subclavian artery or brachial plexus is well depicted on coronal and sagittal reformatted multidetector CT images.

Utility
- Relationship of peripheral lung cancers to pleural surface and chest wall is usually well depicted on CT.
- Because normal pleura is not visible on CT, pleural invasion is only inferred when chest wall invasion is evident.

MRI
Findings
- Lung mass in apex
- Local invasion

Utility
- Superior to CT in the evaluation of superior sulcus tumors and extension into the chest wall
- Can assess for local invasion of subclavian artery and brachial plexus

CLINICAL PRESENTATION

- Horner syndrome (triad of miosis, partial ptosis, and hemifacial anhidrosis) from sympathetic chain involvement
- Shoulder pain and brachial plexopathy

DIAGNOSTIC PEARLS

- Asymmetric apical opacity, particularly if inferior margin is convex
- Mass at apical region of lung
- Specific finding of chest wall invasion: mass extending through intercostal space or associated with bone destruction

DIFFERENTIAL DIAGNOSIS

- Chest wall tumors

PATHOLOGY

- Squamous cell carcinoma and adenocarcinoma are most common cell types to present as Pancoast tumor.

INCIDENCE/PREVALENCE AND EPIDEMIOLOGY

- Account for less than 5% of pulmonary carcinomas

Suggested Readings

Rusch VW: Management of Pancoast tumours. *Lancet Oncol* 7: 997-1005, 2006.

Webb WR, Gatsonis C, Zerhouni EA, et al: CT and MR imaging in staging non-small cell bronchogenic carcinoma: Report of the Radiologic Diagnostic Oncology Group. *Radiology* 178:705-713, 1991.

WHAT THE REFERRING PHYSICIAN NEEDS TO KNOW

- Disease is suggested by asymmetric apical opacity, particularly if inferior margin is convex.
- Specific finding of chest wall invasion is mass extending through intercostal space or associated bone destruction.
- Chest wall invasive mass is radiographically difficult to distinguish from primary wall lesions, and biopsy is necessary for diagnosis.

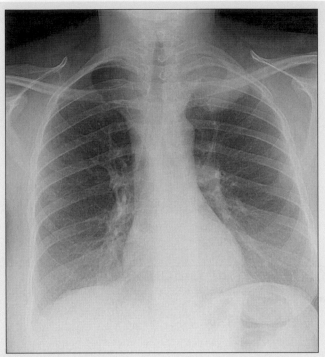

Figure 1. **Pancoast tumor.** Frontal chest radiograph shows a left apical mass. (*Courtesy of Dr. Jeffrey S. Klein, University of Vermont*)

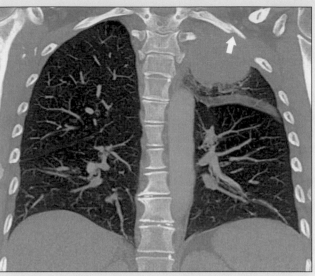

Figure 2. **Pancoast tumor.** Coronal MIP reconstruction from a multidetector CT demonstrates soft tissue mass in the left lung apex with erosion of the undersurface of the left first rib (*arrow*). Biopsy revealed non–small cell carcinoma. (*Courtesy of Dr. Jeffrey S. Klein, University of Vermont*)

Part 21

CARCINOID TUMORS, PULMONARY TUMORLETS, AND NEUROENDOCRINE HYPERPLASIA

Typical Carcinoid Tumors

DEFINITION: Bronchial carcinoid tumors are neuroendocrine neoplasms with immunohistologic features similar to the neuroendocrine (Kulchitsky) cells normally present in the tracheobronchial epithelium.

IMAGING

Radiography

Findings

- Most arise centrally in main, lobar, or segmental bronchi and occur as round or oval opacities with sharp margins.
- They frequently obstruct the airway, resulting in distal atelectasis and obstructive pneumonitis.
- Segmental atelectasis and pneumonitis may show periodic exacerbations and remissions.
- Peripheral carcinoid tumors present as solitary nodules that are homogeneous in density, sharply defined, round or oval, and slightly lobulated.
- Most typical carcinoid tumors measure 1 to 3 cm in diameter.

Utility

- Calcification or ossification is visible on radiographs in less than 5% of cases.

CT

Findings

- Endobronchial lesion is noted with or without distal obstructive pneumonitis or atelectasis or peripheral nodule.
- Partial bronchial obstruction may result in decreased attenuation and vascularity and air trapping on expiratory CT.
- Spherical or ovoid nodule or mass has a well-defined, slightly lobulated border.
- Calcification or ossification is more common in central than in peripheral tumors.
- Carcinoids have rich vascular stroma and often show marked, homogeneous enhancement on CT after intravenous administration of contrast material.
- Enlargement of hilar or mediastinal lymph nodes can occur (5%).

Utility

- CT is routinely done in assessment of patients with suspected or proven carcinoid tumor.

DIAGNOSTIC PEARLS

- Endobronchial tumor, smoothly marginated
- 1-3 cm diameter lung nodule homogenous in density, sharply defined, round or oval, and slightly lobulated
- Most common primary pulmonary neoplasm in children and adolescents

- Relationship of carcinoid with bronchus is best assessed on multidetector CT using thin sections ($\leq$1 mm collimation).
- Optimal assessment of tumor size and distinction from distal atelectasis requires use of intravenous contrast material.
- Findings usually can be well seen on standard cross-sectional images.
- Coronal and sagittal reformatted images may be helpful in some cases.

MRI

Findings

- Signal intensity similar to that of muscle on T1-weighted spin-echo images.
- Moderately high signal on T2-weighted spin-echo images and short T1 inversion recovery images.
- Marked signal enhancement during systemic phase of circulation on ultrafast contrast-enhanced MRI.

Utility

- Preferred modality in young patients and patients allergic to iodinated contrast agents.
- Useful in assessing presence and extent of local invasion.

Nuclear Medicine

Findings

- Positive uptake on scintigraphy with radiolabeled somatostatin analogue (^{123}I-octreotide).

WHAT THE REFERRING PHYSICIAN NEEDS TO KNOW

- Carcinoid tumors usually have typical appearance of a cherry-red intraluminal polypoid tumor at bronchoscopy.
- Diagnosis of carcinoid tumor often can be confirmed by bronchoscopic biopsy.
- Diagnosis of peripheral lesions can be established by transthoracic needle aspiration or biopsy.

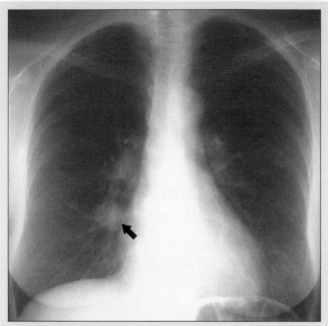

Figure 1. Peripheral typical carcinoid. Posteroanterior chest radiograph shows a 2.5-cm-diameter, smoothly marginated nodule in the right middle lobe (*arrow*). The patient was a 59-year-old woman with a typical carcinoid tumor.

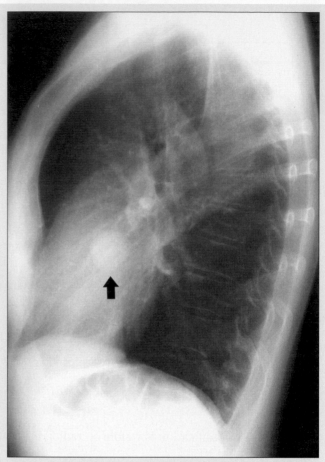

Figure 2. Peripheral typical carcinoid. Lateral chest radiograph shows a 2.5-cm-diameter, smoothly marginated nodule in the right middle lobe (*arrows*). The patient was a 59-year-old woman with a typical carcinoid tumor. Same patient as in Figure 1.

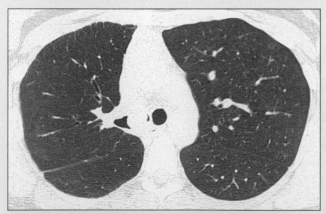

Figure 3. Endobronchial carcinoid tumor in a patient who presented with a history of asthma. Inspiratory high-resolution CT scan shows an endoluminal tumor in the right main bronchus. Note decreased size of right lung and diffuse decrease in attenuation and vascularity compared with the left lung. The patient was a 31-year-old woman with a typical carcinoid tumor. She presented with recurrent episodes of shortness of breath and tightness in the chest and had a clinical diagnosis of asthma.

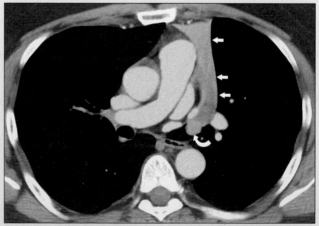

Figure 4. Endobronchial carcinoid tumor with obstructive atelectasis of the left upper lobe. Contrast-enhanced CT scan shows enhancing endobronchial tumor (*curved arrow*) and distal atelectasis (*straight arrows*).

Utility
- Allows identification of primary and metastatic tumors and is a useful tool for staging and follow-up.
- Superior to FDG-PET in assessment of these tumors.
- Helpful in assessing lymph node involvement and distal metastases.

Positron Emission Tomography
Findings
- Does not show increased metabolic activity
Utility
- Cannot distinguish typical carcinoid tumors from benign lesions

CLINICAL PRESENTATION

- Central carcinoid tumors present as cough and hemoptysis.
- Some patients have symptoms simulating asthma.
- Peripheral tumors are usually asymptomatic.
- Paraneoplastic syndromes are uncommon and include Cushing syndrome, acromegaly, and, rarely, carcinoid syndrome.

DIFFERENTIAL DIAGNOSIS

- Pulmonary carcinoma
- Granuloma
- Hamartoma

PATHOLOGY

- Carcinoid tumors are highly vascular and appear to compress rather than infiltrate adjacent normal tissue.
- Cytoplasm of individual tumor cells is usually moderate in amount.
- Nuclei show mild pleomorphism and small nucleoli; mitotic figures are scarce or absent; there is no necrosis.

- Neoplastic cells of carcinoid tumors have membrane receptors with high affinity for the neuroregulatory peptide somatostatin.
- Carcinoid tumors are positive for neuroendocrine markers such as chromogranin and synaptophysin.

INCIDENCE/PREVALENCE AND EPIDEMIOLOGY

- Bronchial carcinoid tumors are uncommon, accounting for only 1%-2% of all pulmonary neoplasms.
- Typical carcinoids account for 80%-90% of carcinoid tumors; 10%-20% are atypical carcinoids.
- Carcinoid tumor is the most common primary pulmonary neoplasm in children and adolescents.
- It is slightly more common in women.
- Mean age at presentation is 49 years.
- It is not associated with cigarette smoking.

Suggested Readings
Chong S, Lee KS, Chung MJ, et al: Neuroendocrine tumors of the lung: Clinical, pathologic, and imaging findings. *RadioGraphics* 26:41-57, 2006; discussion 57-58.

Ducrocq X, Thomas P, Massard G, et al: Operative risk and prognostic factors of typical bronchial carcinoid tumors. *Ann Thorac Surg* 65:1410-1414, 1998.

Jeung MY, Gasser B, Gangi A, et al: Bronchial carcinoid tumors of the thorax: Spectrum of radiologic findings. *RadioGraphics* 22:351-365, 2002.

Magid D, Siegelman SS, Eggleston JC, et al: Pulmonary carcinoid tumors: CT assessment. *J Comput Assist Tomogr* 13:244-247, 1989.

Nessi R, Basso Ricci P, Basso Ricci S, et al: Bronchial carcinoid tumors: Radiologic observations in 49 cases. *J Thorac Imaging* 6:47-53, 1991.

Rosado de Christenson ML, Abbott GF, Kirejczyk WM, et al: Thoracic carcinoids: Radiologic-pathologic correlation. *RadioGraphics* 19:707 736, 1999.

Valli M, Fabris GA, Dewar A, et al: Atypical carcinoid tumour of the lung: A study of 33 cases with prognostic features. *Histopathology* 24:363-369, 1994.

Diffuse Idiopathic Pulmonary Neuroendocrine Cell Hyperplasia

DEFINITION: Diffuse idiopathic pulmonary neuroendocrine cell hyperplasia is an extensive proliferation of neuroendocrine cells as clusters of cells or as linear arrays along the basement membrane.

IMAGING

Radiography
Findings
- Normal
- Increased lung volumes
- Decreased peripheral vascular markings

Utility
- Limited value in diagnosis

CT
Findings
- Obliterative bronchiolitis
- Areas of decreased attenuation and vascularity on inspiratory CT scans (mosaic perfusion pattern)
- Air trapping on expiratory CT
- Small nodules consistent with carcinoid tumorlets are seen in most of these patients

Utility
- Expiratory high-resolution CT is imaging modality of choice to demonstrate air trapping

CLINICAL PRESENTATION

- Signs and symptoms of progressive airway obstruction

PATHOLOGY

- Extensive proliferation of neuroendocrine cells as clusters of cells or as linear arrays along basement membrane.
- Obliterative bronchiolitis with submucosal fibrosis of affected airways in regions with and regions away from neuroendocrine hyperplasia.
- Obliterative bronchiolitis due to combination of intraluminal obstruction by hyperplastic neuroendocrine cells and peribronchiolar fibrosis.

DIAGNOSTIC PEARLS

- Areas of decreased attenuation and vascularity are evident on inspiratory CT scans (mosaic attenuation and perfusion pattern)
- Expiratory CT shows air trapping
- Multiple small nodules
- Diagnosis should be suspected in patients with findings of bronchiolitis obliterans and multiple noncalcified pulmonary nodules

- Progressive airway obstruction secondary to peptide secretory products or released by proliferating neuroendocrine cells.

INCIDENCE/PREVALENCE AND EPIDEMIOLOGY

- Rare condition
- Seen in association with concomitant pulmonary disease, the most common being carcinoid tumor
- Occurs most frequently in women 45 to 65 years old

Suggested Readings

Aguayo SM, Miller YE, Waldron J Jr, et al: Brief report: Idiopathic diffuse hyperplasia of pulmonary neuroendocrine cells and airways disease. *N Engl J Med* 327(18):1285-1288, 1992.

Brown MJ, English J, Müller NL: Bronchiolitis obliterans due to neuroendocrine hyperplasia: High-resolution CT–pathologic correlation. *AJR Am J Roentgenol* 168:1561-1562, 1997.

Davies SJ, Gosney JR, Hansell DM, et al: Diffuse idiopathic pulmonary neuroendocrine cell hyperplasia: An under-recognised spectrum of disease. *Thorax* 62(3):248-252, 2007.

Lee JS, Brown KK, Cool C, et al: Diffuse pulmonary neuroendocrine cell hyperplasia: Radiologic and clinical features. *J Comput Assist Tomogr* 26:180-184, 2002.

WHAT THE REFERRING PHYSICIAN NEEDS TO KNOW

- Diffuse pulmonary neuroendocrine hyperplasia and multiple pulmonary carcinoid tumorlets may be associated with obliterative bronchiolitis and progressive airway obstruction.
- Symptomatic obliterative bronchiolitis is more common in women.

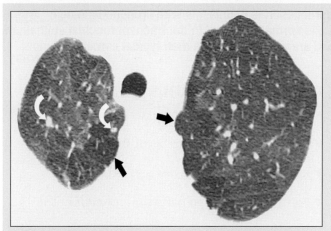

Figure 1. **Diffuse idiopathic pulmonary neuroendocrine cell hyperplasia,** carcinoid tumorlets and tumors, and obliterative bronchiolitis. Expiratory high-resolution CT scan at the lung apices shows areas of air trapping (*straight arrows*) and bilateral 2- to 8-mm, well-defined soft tissue nodules (*curved arrows*).

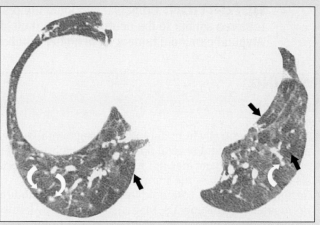

Figure 2. **Diffuse idiopathic pulmonary neuroendocrine cell hyperplasia,** carcinoid tumorlets and tumors, and obliterative bronchiolitis. Expiratory high-resolution CT scan at the lung bases shows areas of air trapping (*straight arrows*) and bilateral 2- to 8-mm, well-defined soft tissue nodules (*curved arrows*).

Atypical Carcinoid Tumors

DEFINITION: Bronchial carcinoid tumors are neuroendocrine neoplasms with immunohistologic features similar to the neuroendocrine (Kulchitsky) cells normally present in the tracheobronchial epithelium. Atypical carcinoid tumors have higher mitotic rate and are more aggressive than typical carcinoid tumors.

IMAGING

Radiography
Findings
- Most arise centrally in main, lobar, or segmental bronchi and occur as round or oval opacities with sharp margins
- Frequently obstruct airway, resulting in distal atelectasis and obstructive pneumonitis
- Peripheral atypical carcinoid tumors: solitary nodules or masses homogeneous in density, sharply defined, round or oval, and lobulated or spiculated margins
- Larger than typical tumors, sometimes attaining huge size
- Hilar and mediastinal lymph node enlargement

CT
Findings
- Endobronchial lesion with or without distal obstructive pneumonitis or atelectasis or peripheral nodule
- Spherical or ovoid nodule or mass with well-defined, lobulated, or spiculated margins
- Calcification or ossification, more common in central than in peripheral tumors
- Less uniform contrast enhancement than typical carcinoids
- Enlargement of hilar or mediastinal lymph nodes (50%)

Utility
- CT is routinely done in assessment of patients with suspected or proven carcinoid tumor.
- Relationship of carcinoid with bronchus is best assessed on multidetector CT using thin sections (≤1 mm collimation).
- Optimal assessment of tumor size and distinction from distal atelectasis requires the use of intravenous contrast material.
- Findings usually can be well seen on standard cross-sectional images.
- Coronal and sagittal reformatted images may be helpful in some cases.

MRI
Findings
- Signal intensity similar to that of muscle on T1-weighted spin-echo images
- Moderately high signal on T2-weighted spin-echo images and short T1 inversion recovery images
- Marked signal enhancement during systemic phase of circulation on ultrafast contrast-enhanced MRI

DIAGNOSTIC PEARLS
- Atypical carcinoid tumors tend to be larger than typical carcinoid tumors.
- Lymph node metastases occur in 50% of atypical carcinoids.
- Increased FDG uptake has been shown with atypical carcinoid.
- Positive uptake of somatostatin receptor noted.

Utility
- Preferred modality in young patients and patients allergic to contrast agents
- Useful in assessing presence and extent of local invasion, particularly when histologic examination of biopsy specimen has revealed atypical features

Nuclear Medicine
Findings
- Positive uptake on scintigraphy with radiolabeled somatostatin analogue (^{123}I-octreotide)

Utility
- Allows identification of primary and metastatic tumors and is a useful tool for staging and follow-up
- Superior to FDG-PET in assessment of these tumors
- Helpful in assessing lymph node involvement and distal metastases

PET
Findings
- Increased FDG uptake has been shown in some aggressive carcinoid tumors.

Utility
- FDG-PET may be falsely negative in carcinoid tumors.

CLINICAL PRESENTATION
- Central carcinoid tumors present as cough and hemoptysis.
- Some patients have symptoms simulating asthma.
- Peripheral tumors are usually asymptomatic.
- Paraneoplastic syndromes include Cushing syndrome, acromegaly, and, rarely, carcinoid syndrome.

WHAT THE REFERRING PHYSICIAN NEEDS TO KNOW
- Diagnosis is usually evident with hematoxylin-eosin staining and confirmed by immunohistochemical study using antibodies directed to components of neurosecretory granule.
- Diagnosis of carcinoid tumor often can be confirmed by bronchoscopic biopsy.
- Diagnosis of peripheral lesions can be established by transthoracic needle aspiration or biopsy.
- Atypical carcinoid tumors have worse prognosis than typical carcinoids; 50% have lymph node metastases at the time of initial evaluation, and 5-year survival rate is approximately 70%.

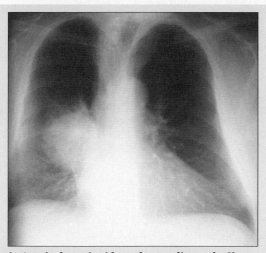

Figure 1. Atypical carcinoid on chest radiograph. Chest radiograph demonstrates a 6-cm-diameter mass in the right lower lobe. The patient was a 64-year-old man with atypical carcinoid tumor. At surgery the patient had right hilar lymph node metastases.

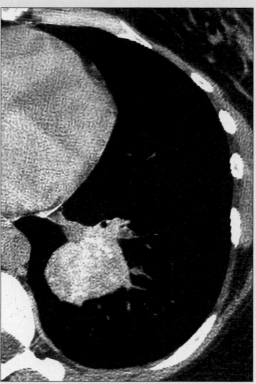

Figure 2. Calcified atypical carcinoid tumor. View of the left lung from a high-resolution CT scan demonstrates a 4-cm-diameter mass in the left lower lobe. Several small areas of calcification can be seen within the tumor. The patient was a 41 year old woman with atypical carcinoid tumor.

DIFFERENTIAL DIAGNOSIS

- Adenocarcinoma
- Small cell carcinoma
- Squamous cell carcinoma
- Hamartoma
- Granuloma

PATHOLOGY

- Architectural pattern is similar to that of typical carcinoid tumor but shows histologic and cytologic features suggesting an aggressive nature.
- Necrosis or mitotic rate of 2-10 per 10 high-power microscopic fields noted.
- Immunohistochemical study is usually positive for neuroendocrine markers, such as chromogranin and synaptophysin.
- Neoplastic cells of carcinoid tumors have membrane receptors with high affinity for neuroregulatory peptide somatostatin.

INCIDENCE/PREVALENCE AND EPIDEMIOLOGY

- Bronchial carcinoid tumors are uncommon, accounting for only 1%-2% of all pulmonary neoplasms.

- Atypical carcinoid tumors account for 10%-20% of carcinoid tumors, and low-grade typical carcinoids account for 80%-90% of cases.
- Atypical carcinoids are more common in males; mean age at presentation is 59 years.
- Approximately 90% are associated with a history of cigarette smoking.

Suggested Readings

Chong S, Lee KS, Chung MJ, et al: Neuroendocrine tumors of the lung: Clinical, pathologic, and imaging findings. *RadioGraphics* 26:41-57, 2006; discussion 57–58.

Hage R, de la Rivière AB, Seldenrijk CA, van den Bosch JM: Update in pulmonary carcinoid tumors: A review article. *Ann Surg Oncol* 10(6):697-704, 2003.

Jeung MY, Gasser B, Gangi A, et al: Bronchial carcinoid tumors of the thorax: Spectrum of radiologic findings. *RadioGraphics* 22:351-365, 2002.

Marty-Ane CH, Costes V, Pujol JL, et al: Carcinoid tumors of the lung: Do atypical features require aggressive management? *Ann Thorac Surg* 59:78-83, 1995.

Rosado de Christenson ML, Abbott GF, Kirejczyk WM, et al: Thoracic carcinoids: Radiologic-pathologic correlation. *RadioGraphics* 19:707-736, 1999.

Valli M, Fabris GA, Dewar A, et al: Atypical carcinoid tumour of the lung: A study of 33 cases with prognostic features. *Histopathology* 24:363-369, 1994.

Part 22

NEOPLASMS OF TRACHEOBRONCHIAL GLANDS

Adenoid Cystic Carcinoma of the Trachea and Bronchi

DEFINITION: This low-grade malignancy arises from the tracheobronchial glands and is characterized by uniform cells organized in cribriform pattern.

IMAGING

Radiography
Findings
- Normal findings can be seen.
- Lobulated, polypoid mass encroaches on airway lumen.
- Circumferential involvement resembles tracheal stenosis.
- Obstructive pneumonitis or atelectasis may be present.

Utility
- Initial imaging modality performed in suspected tracheal or bronchial abnormalities.
- Limitations of radiography in evaluation of trachea and main bronchi.

CT
Findings
- Lobulated, polypoid endoluminal mass has associated focal thickening of airway wall.
- Extensive thickening of tracheal or bronchial wall is seen less commonly.
- Obstructive pneumonitis or atelectasis may be present.

Utility
- CT is superior to radiography in identifying tumors and particularly helpful in assessing presence of extraluminal extent and mediastinal invasion.
- CT is performed almost routinely in the evaluation of these patients.
- Optimal evaluation is obtained with multidetector spiral CT performed using thin collimation (≤1 mm), multiplanar reformatted images.

MRI
Findings
- Lobulated, polypoid endoluminal mass with associated focal thickening of airway wall.

DIAGNOSTIC PEARLS
- Radiography: lobulated, polypoid mass that encroaches on airway lumen.
- CT: lobulated, polypoid endoluminal mass with associated focal thickening of airway wall.
- May result in extensive tracheal thickening and tracheal or bronchial stenosis.
- It is the second most common primary tumor of the trachea (after squamous cell carcinoma).

Utility
- Optimal evaluation of adenoid cystic carcinoma of trachea by MRI requires multiplanar imaging.

Positron Emission Tomography
Findings
- Increased uptake on FDG-PET.
- Degree of uptake influenced by grade of differentiation of tumor.

Utility
- PET/CT helpful in assessment of tumor extent.

CLINICAL PRESENTATION
- Cough
- Dyspnea
- Wheeze
- Stridor
- Hemoptysis
- Recurrent pneumonia

WHAT THE REFERRING PHYSICIAN NEEDS TO KNOW
- Symptoms of dyspnea and wheeze frequently lead to initial misdiagnosis of asthma.
- Differential diagnosis of polypoid intratracheal or intrabronchial lesions includes squamous cell carcinoma, carcinoid tumor, metastases, and papilloma.
- These various tumors cannot be reliably distinguished radiologically.
- Endoscopy typically reveals smooth-surfaced, sometimes lobulated tumor partly or completely occluding airway lumen.
- Definitive diagnosis usually requires bronchoscopy and biopsy.

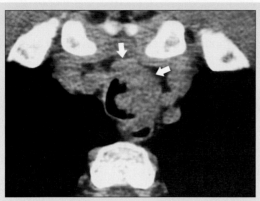

Figure 1. Adenoid cystic carcinoma of the trachea. Magnified view of CT image demonstrates a lobulated, polypoid endotracheal tumor with extensive involvement of the tracheal wall and extension into the adjacent mediastinum (*arrows*). The patient was a 36-year-old man.

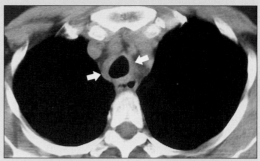

Figure 2. Adenoid cystic carcinoma of the trachea. CT image at the level of the great vessels shows diffuse thickening of the tracheal wall (*arrows*). The patient was a 54-year-old woman with adenoid cystic carcinoma.

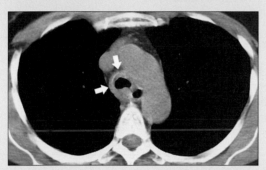

Figure 3. Adenoid cystic carcinoma of the trachea. CT image at the level of the aortic arch shows diffuse thickening of the tracheal wall (*arrows*). The patient was a 54-year-old woman with adenoid cystic carcinoma.

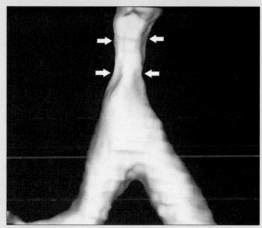

Figure 4. Adenoid cystic carcinoma of the trachea. Volumetric coronal reformatted image demonstrates the extent of the tracheal narrowing. The patient was a 54-year-old woman with adenoid cystic carcinoma.

DIFFERENTIAL DIAGNOSIS

- Mucoepidermoid carcinoma of the trachea and bronchi
- Squamous cell carcinoma
- Papilloma
- Carcinoid tumor

PATHOLOGY

- Low-grade malignancy consists of nests of uniform cells organized in cribriform pattern.
- Lesion usually grows into airway lumen, forming smooth-surfaced, polypoid mass.
- Submucosal extension, sometimes a considerable distance from tumor, may be seen.
- Mitotic activity and necrosis are uncommon.

INCIDENCE/PREVALENCE AND EPIDEMIOLOGY

- Uncommon neoplasm of tracheobronchial mucous glands (< 0.3% of all tracheobronchial tumors).

- Most common tracheobronchial gland neoplasm, accounting for 75% to 80% of cases.
- Second most common primary malignant tumor of trachea.
- Mean age at diagnosis: 45 to 50 years.
- Not associated with cigarette smoking.

Suggested Readings

Jeong SY, Lee KS, Han J, et al: Integrated PET/CT of salivary gland type carcinoma of the lung in 12 patients. *AJR Am J Roentgenol* 189:1407-1413, 2007.

Kwak SH, Lee KS, Chung MJ, et al: Adenoid cystic carcinoma of the airways: Helical CT and histopathologic correlation. *AJR Am J Roentgenol* 183:277-281, 2004.

Kwong JS, Müller NL, Miller RR: Diseases of the trachea and mainstem bronchi: Correlation of CT with pathologic findings. *RadioGraphics* 12:645-657, 1992.

McCarthy MJ, Rosado-de-Christenson ML: Tumors of the trachea. *J Thorac Imaging* 10:180-198, 1995.

Mucoepidermoid Carcinoma of the Trachea and Bronchi

DEFINITION: This tracheobronchial gland neoplasm is composed of cells that show both glandular (typically mucus production) and "epidermoid" features.

IMAGING

Radiography
Findings
- Solitary nodule or mass measuring 1.0 to 4.0 cm in diameter
- Lobar or segmental consolidation
- Atelectasis
- Central mass with associated obstructive pneumonitis or atelectasis

Utility
- Cannot reliably distinguish from other intratracheal or intrabronchial lesions

CT
Findings
- Homogeneous, smoothly oval or lobulated, slightly enhancing soft tissue nodule/mass measuring 1.0 to 4.0 cm in diameter
- Punctate calcification within tumor in approximately 50% of cases
- Close association with bronchus
- Associated findings: distal bronchial dilatation with mucoid impaction, postobstructive pneumonia, atelectasis, and air trapping
- If tumor involves trachea: polypoid intraluminal nodule
- Uncommon: hilar or mediastinal lymphadenopathy

Utility
- Superior to radiography in assessment of intraluminal tumor and extent of involvement of bronchial or tracheal wall and mediastinum
- Multidetector spiral CT with thin sections (≤1 mm) recommended
- Intravenous contrast possibly helpful in assessing extraluminal extent of tumor
- Cannot reliably distinguish from other intratracheal or intrabronchial tumors

Positron Emission Tomography
Findings
- Intraluminal mass with increased FDG uptake

Utility
- Helpful in assessing tumor extent, particularly when combined with CT (PET/CT)

DIAGNOSTIC PEARLS
- Uncommon tumor
- Radiologic findings are nonspecific
- May be endobronchial or present as a lung nodule adjacent to a bronchus

CLINICAL PRESENTATION
- Cough
- Hemoptysis
- Recurrent pneumonia
- Dyspnea

DIFFERENTIAL DIAGNOSIS
- Adenoid cystic carcinoma
- Squamous cell carcinoma
- Solitary lung nodule
- Papilloma
- Carcinoid tumor

PATHOLOGY
- Cells show both glandular and "epidermoid" features.
- Cells grow within the airway lumen and produce a polypoid mass with an intact or occasionally ulcerated surface epithelium.
- Peripheral extension within the bronchial lumen occurs sometimes.
- Low-grade: minimal nuclear pleomorphism and few mitotic figures; confined to bronchial wall.
- High-grade: nuclear pleomorphism, average 4 to 10 mitoses per high-power field, cellular necrosis, extends into peribronchial interstitium or adjacent lung parenchyma.

INCIDENCE/PREVALENCE AND EPIDEMIOLOGY
- Neoplasms of the tracheobronchial mucous glands are uncommon, accounting for less than 0.3% of all tracheobronchial tumors.

WHAT THE REFERRING PHYSICIAN NEEDS TO KNOW
- Polypoid intratracheal or intrabronchial lesions cannot be reliably distinguished radiologically.
- Definitive diagnosis of mucoepidermoid carcinoma usually requires biopsy or surgical resection.
- Optimal assessment of tumor extent requires volumetric multidetector CT with thin sections (preferably ≤1 mm) and multiplanar reformatted imaging.
- Differential diagnosis: squamous cell carcinoma, adenoid cystic carcinoma, metastases, and benign lesions such as papilloma.

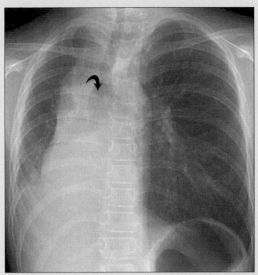

Figure 1. **Mucoepidermoid carcinoma originating in right main bronchus.** Chest radiograph shows poorly defined soft tissue mass in right main bronchus (*arrow*) and marked volume loss of the right lung with ipsilateral shift of the mediastinum and elevation of the right hemidiaphragm. (*Courtesy of Dr. Joungho Han, Department of Pathology, Samsung Medical Center, Sungkyunkwan University School of Medicine, Seoul, Korea.*)

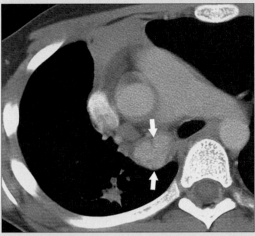

Figure 2. **Mucoepidermoid carcinoma originating in right main bronchus.** CT image photographed at soft tissue windows demonstrates large endobronchial tumor (*arrows*). Same patient as in Figure 1. (*Courtesy of Dr. Joungho Han, Department of Pathology, Samsung Medical Center, Sungkyunkwan University School of Medicine, Seoul, Korea.*)

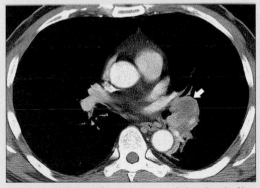

Figure 3. **Mucoepidermoid carcinoma originating in lingular bronchus.** CT image shows large tumor (*arrow*) originating from the lingular bronchus and extending into adjacent hilum and parenchyma. Also evident is associated volume loss of the left lung. The patient was a 48-year-old man with mucoepidermoid carcinoma. (*Courtesy of Dr. Kyung Soo Lee, Samsung Medical Center, Seoul, Korea.*)

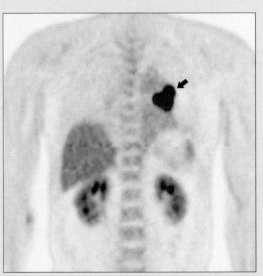

Figure 4. **Mucoepidermoid carcinoma originating in lingular bronchus.** PET image demonstrates marked FDG uptake (*arrow*). The patient was a 48-year-old man with mucoepidermoid carcinoma. Same patient as in Figure 3. (*Courtesy of Dr. Kyung Soo Lee, Samsung Medical Center, Seoul, Korea.*)

- They are the second most common form of tracheo-bronchial gland neoplasm.
- They make up less than 0.2% of pulmonary carcinomas.
- Patients vary in age from 3 months to 78 years, but nearly half are younger than 30 years.
- Five-year survival after surgery: 80% in low-grade types, 30% in high-grade types.
- Lesions are usually located in segmental bronchi and less commonly arise within the lobar or main bronchi or trachea.
- Punctate calcification within the tumors is evident on CT in 50% of cases.

Suggested Readings

Kim TS, Lee KS, Han J, et al: Mucoepidermoid carcinoma of the tracheobronchial tree: Radiographic and CT findings in 12 patients. *Radiology* 212:643-648, 1999.

Kwong JS, Müller NL, Miller RR: Diseases of the trachea and mainstem bronchi: Correlation of CT with pathologic findings. *Radio-Graphics* 12:645-657, 1992.

McCarthy MJ, Rosado-de-Christenson ML: Tumors of the trachea. *J Thorac Imaging* 10:180-198, 1995.

Tsuchiya H, Nagashima K, Ohashi S, Takase Y: Childhood bronchial mucoepidermoid tumors. *J Pediatr Surg* 32:106-109, 1997.

Vadasz P, Egervary M: Mucoepidermoid bronchial tumors: A review of 34 operated cases. *Eur J Cardiothorac Surg* 17:566-569, 2000.

Yousem SA, Hochholzer L: Mucoepidermoid tumors of the lung. *Cancer* 60:1346-1352, 1987.

Hamartoma

DEFINITION: A hamartoma is a benign neoplasm probably derived from bronchial wall mesenchymal cells characterized by the presence of cartilage, loose fibroblastic tissue, and, commonly, adipose tissue.

IMAGING

Radiography

Findings

- A smoothly marginated, well-circumscribed solitary nodule is seen without lobar predilection.
- Most nodules are smaller than 4.0 cm in diameter.
- Radiographic pattern of calcification may resemble popcorn.
- Endobronchial hamartomas manifest by effects of airway obstruction with distal atelectasis and obstructive pneumonitis.

Utility

- Calcification is visible on a chest radiograph in less than 10% of cases.
- Serial radiographs show slow growth.

CT

Findings

- Sharply defined, smoothly marginated nodule.
- Focal areas of fat density in 50% to 60% of cases.
- Multiple coarse foci of calcification or popcorn calcification.
- Nodules with soft tissue attenuation and single or multiple foci of calcification.
- Occasionally present as collection of multiple tiny nodules.
- Endotracheal and endobronchial hamartomas composed entirely of fat or mixture of fat and soft tissue or calcification.

Utility

- Allows confident diagnosis in 50%-60% of cases based on presence of foci of fat density within well-defined smoothly marginated nodule.

DIAGNOSTIC PEARLS

- Well-circumscribed, smoothly marginated solitary nodule
- Popcorn calcification is characteristic but uncommon
- Confident diagnosis can be made on CT in 50%-60% of patients by showing focal areas of fat density in smoothly marginated nodule

MRI

Findings

- Intermediate signal intensity is evident on T1-weighted images (higher than that of skeletal muscle, lower than fat).
- High signal intensity is noted on T2-weighted images.
- Tumor frequently contains septa that have high signal intensity on T1-weighted images and low intensity on T2-weighted images.
- Marked enhancement of septa separates tumors into less well-enhanced lobules (on gadolinium-enhanced T1-weighted images).
- Regions with less enhancement correspond to core cartilaginous tissue.
- Areas of marked contrast enhancement correspond to cleft-like branching mesenchymal connective tissue that dipped into cartilaginous core.

Utility

- Limited role in assessment

Positron Emission Tomography

Findings

- No significant uptake of FDG

WHAT THE REFERRING PHYSICIAN NEEDS TO KNOW

- Differential diagnosis must include all other pulmonary nodules, particularly carcinoma.
- Most pulmonary hamartomas occur in patients older than age 40 years.
- Most hamartomas manifest as a solitary nodule.
- Confident diagnosis can be made on CT in 50%-60% of patients by showing focal areas of fat density in smoothly marginated nodule.
- Presence of multiple coarse foci of calcification (popcorn calcification) is highly suggestive of diagnosis, but appearance is uncommon.
- Definitive diagnosis can be made by transthoracic core needle biopsy of peripheral hamartomas and bronchoscopic biopsy of endobronchial hamartomas.
- Adequate surgical excision results in cure in most patients.

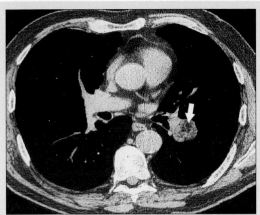

Figure 1. Pulmonary hamartoma: characteristic CT findings.
High-resolution CT scan shows smoothly marginated nodule containing focal areas of fat (*arrow*). This CT appearance is diagnostic of pulmonary hamartoma.

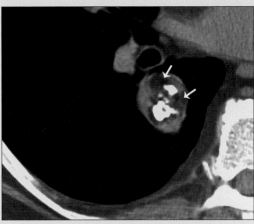

Figure 2. Pulmonary hamartoma. Magnified view of the right lower lobe from a CT scan shows smoothly marginated nodule containing several coarse foci of calcification (popcorn calcification) and foci of fat attenuation (*arrows*).

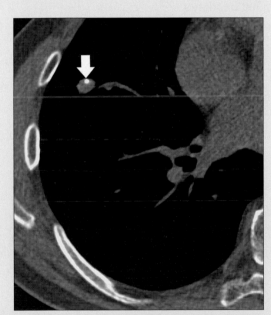

Figure 3. Pulmonary hamartoma with focus of calcification.
Magnified view of the right lung from a high-resolution CT scan shows smoothly marginated nodule with single eccentric focus of calcification (*arrow*).

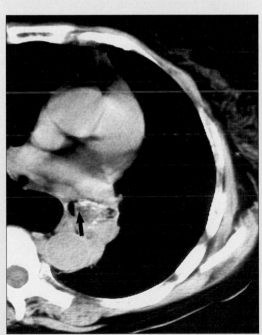

Figure 4. Endobronchial hamartoma. Magnified view of the left lung from a CT scan shows an endobronchial tumor with focal areas of fat attenuation (*arrow*) and calcification. Note associated left lower lobe atelectasis and ipsilateral shift of the mediastinum. The patient was a 62-year-old woman.

Utility

- Helpful in confirming benign nature of tumor particularly in patients in whom the CT findings are nonspecific.

CLINICAL PRESENTATION

- The patient is usually asymptomatic.
- Endobronchial hamartomas may result in bronchial obstruction and present as cough, hemoptysis, and recurrent pneumonia.

DIFFERENTIAL DIAGNOSIS

- Pulmonary carcinoma
- Pulmonary carcinoid tumor
- Granuloma

PATHOLOGY

- Benign neoplasms that are probably derived from bronchial wall mesenchymal cells.
- Multiple hamartomas may be part of Carney's syndrome (pulmonary chondroma, gastric epithelioid leiomyosarcoma, functioning extra-adrenal paraganglioma).
- Solitary, well-circumscribed, slightly lobulated tumors are located within parenchyma, usually in a peripheral location.
- Cut section: lobules of white, cartilaginous-appearing tissue.

- Histologically: lobules with central area of more or less well-developed cartilage surrounded by loose fibroblastic tissue.
- Adipose tissue, smooth muscle, and seromucinous bronchial glands also possible.
- Endobronchial hamartoma: fleshy, polypoid tumors attached to bronchial wall by narrow stalk; central portion: core of adipose tissue surrounded by compressed myxoid tissue.

INCIDENCE/PREVALENCE AND EPIDEMIOLOGY

- This is the most common benign pulmonary neoplasm (approximately 8% of primary lung tumors).
- Most cases occur in patients older than age 40 years with peak incidence in the seventh decade.
- Endobronchial hamartomas are less common than parenchymal lesions (5% of pulmonary hamartomas).

Suggested Readings

Erasmus JJ, Connolly JE, McAdams HP, et al: Solitary pulmonary nodules. I. Morphologic evaluation for differentiation of benign and malignant lesions. *RadioGraphics* 20:43-58, 2000.
Gaerte SC, Meyer CA, Winer-Muram HT, et al: Fat-containing lesions of the chest. *RadioGraphics* 22(Spec No):S61-S78, 2002.
Siegelman SS, Khouri NF, Scott W Jr, et al: Pulmonary hamartoma: CT findings. *Radiology* 160(2):313-317, 1986.

Inflammatory Pseudotumor

DEFINITION: Inflammatory pseudotumor is a fibroinflammatory lesion that is believed to result from an exaggerated response to tissue injury.

IMAGING

Radiography
Findings
- Solitary, peripheral, sharply circumscribed, lobulated nodule or mass is seen.
- Smooth or spiculated margins occur and size of mass ranges from 1 to >6 cm in diameter.
- Calcification is present occasionally, particularly in children.
- Cavitation is present rarely.
- Endobronchial tumors can cause obstructive pneumonitis and atelectasis.
- Hilar or mediastinal lymph node enlargement and pleural effusion occur occasionally.
- Lesion is usually detected as an incidental finding on a chest radiograph.
- Smoothly marginated nodule in child or adolescent is most suggestive of the diagnosis.
- Lesions in adults often have spiculated margins and mimic pulmonary carcinoma.

CT
Findings
- Smooth or spiculated margins
- Homogeneous or heterogeneous attenuation
- No enhancement or variable enhancement after intravenous administration of contrast medium
- Nodules usually closely associated with bronchus

Utility
- CT superior to radiography in demonstrating presence of calcification.

MRI
Findings
- Intermediate signal intensity on T1-weighted images
- High signal intensity on T2-weighted images
- Enhance after intravenous administration of gadolinium

DIAGNOSTIC PEARLS
- Most common primary lung mass in children and adolescents
- Most commonly smooth margins in children (plasma cell granuloma)
- Smoothly marginated nodule in child or adolescent is suggestive of diagnosis
- Most commonly spiculated margins in adults
- Radiologic findings in adults are nonspecific

Utility
- Limited value in the diagnosis

Positron Emission Tomography
Findings
- High-intensity uptake on FDG-PET, indicating high degree of metabolic activity
- High uptake on PET performed with rubidium-82, indicating the presence of increased perfusion.

Utility
- PET not helpful in distinguishing inflammatory pseudotumor from malignancy.

CLINICAL PRESENTATION
- Most patients are asymptomatic.
- Most common signs are cough, fever, dyspnea, and hemoptysis.

DIFFERENTIAL DIAGNOSIS
- Pulmonary carinoma
- Tuberculosis
- Histoplasmosis

WHAT THE REFERRING PHYSICIAN NEEDS TO KNOW
- Radiologic differential diagnosis for inflammatory pseudotumor occurring as solitary pulmonary nodule includes primary or secondary neoplasm and granuloma.
- Treatment of choice is complete surgical resection.
- Inflammatory pseudotumors consist of variable proportions of inflammatory cells, myofibroblastic spindle cells, and plasma cells.
- Pseudotumors with predominance of plasma cells are commonly referred to as plasma cell granulomas.
- Pseudotumors with approximately equal numbers of fibroblasts and histiocytes are referred to as fibrous histiocytomas.
- Most common presentation is as a smoothly marginated or spiculated lung nodule.
- Inflammatory pseudotumors tend to have high intensity on PET.

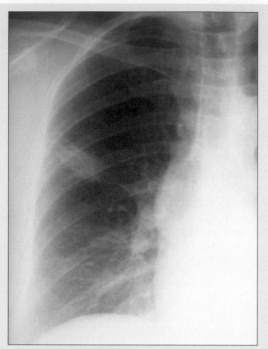

Figure 1. Inflammatory pseudotumor. View of the right lung from a chest radiograph shows right upper lobe nodule with spiculated margins. The patient was a 79-year-old smoker with inflammatory pseudotumor confirmed after surgical resection of the lesion.

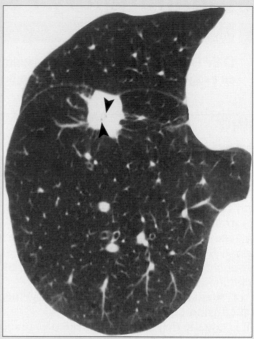

Figure 2. Inflammatory pseudotumor. High-resolution CT scan of the right lung shows minimal emphysema and lower lobe nodule with spiculated margins and containing two small areas of increased lucency (bubble lucencies) (*arrowheads*). Histologically, the nodule was shown to be an inflammatory pseudotumor containing several patent small bronchi.

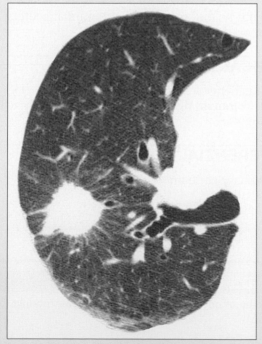

Figure 3. Inflammatory pseudotumor: CT findings. CT scan photographed at lung windows settings shows spiculated right upper lobe nodule. Note mild emphysema. The patient was a 79-year-old smoker with inflammatory pseudotumor confirmed after surgical resection of the lesion.

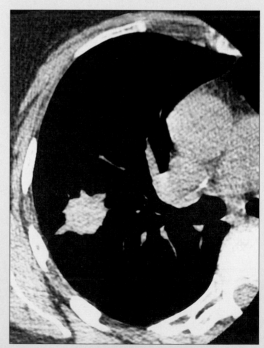

Figure 4. Inflammatory pseudotumor: CT findings. Soft tissue windows shows spiculated right upper lobe nodule. The patient was a 79-year-old smoker with inflammatory pseudotumor confirmed after surgical resection of the lesion.

PATHOLOGY

- Histologically consists of mixture of inflammatory cells, myofibroblastic spindle cells, and plasma cells.
- Fibroinflammatory lesions that are believed to result from an exaggerated response to tissue injury.
- Progenitor cell: myofibroblast.
- Focal organizing pneumonia pattern: small airways and adjacent parenchyma filled with fibroblasts and foamy histiocytes.
- Fibrous histiocytic pattern: spindle-shaped myofibroblasts in whorls.
- Lymphohistiocytic pattern: mixture of lymphocytes and plasma cells with only minimal fibrous connective tissue.

INCIDENCE/PREVALENCE AND EPIDEMIOLOGY

- Rare
- Affects individuals of any age but has a predilection for children and young adults
- Most common primary lung mass seen in children
- Multiple lesions in 5% of cases
- Manifest as endobronchial masses in approximately 10%

Suggested Readings

Kovach SJ, Fischer AC, Katzman PJ, et al: Inflammatory myofibroblastic tumors. *J Surg Oncol* 94:385-391, 2006.

Melloni G, Carretta A, Ciriaco P, et al: Inflammatory pseudotumor of the lung in adults. *Ann Thorac Surg* 79(2):426-432, 2005.

Narla LD, Newman B, Spottswood SS, et al: Inflammatory pseudotumor. *RadioGraphics* 23:719-729, 2003.

Slosman DO, Spiliopoulos A, Keller A, et al: Quantitative metabolic PET imaging of a plasma cell granuloma. *J Thorac Imaging* 9(2):116-119, 1994.

Yao X, Alvarado Y, Brackeen J, et al: Plasma cell granuloma: A case report of multiple lesions in the lung and review of the literature. *Am J Med Sci* 334(5):402-406, 2007.

Pulmonary Metastases: Lymphangitic Carcinomatosis

DEFINITION: Lymphangitic carcinomatosis develops either from invasion of adjacent interstitial space and lymphatics by intravascular tumor emboli or from retrograde spread from infiltrated mediastinal and hilar lymph nodes.

IMAGING

Radiography
Findings
- Normal findings in 30%-50% of cases
- Reticulonodular pattern
- Kerley B (septal) lines
- Thickening of peribronchovascular interstitium
- Hilar and mediastinal lymphadenopathy in 20%-40%
- Pleural effusion in 30%-50%

CT
Findings
- Smooth or nodular thickening of interlobular septa and polygonal arcades
- Smooth or nodular thickening of peribronchovascular interstitium
- Smooth or nodular thickening of interlobar fissures
- Preservation of normal lung architecture
- Bilateral involvement
- Unilateral or markedly asymmetric in 50% of cases
- Ground-glass opacities (usually representing pulmonary edema)
- Nodules separate from interlobular septa uncommon
- Pleural effusion in 30% of cases
- Hilar or mediastinal lymphadenopathy in 40%

Utility
- High-resolution CT useful in detection of disease in patients with normal or nonspecific radiographic findings.
- CT, particularly volumetric thin-section CT, superior to radiography in the detection of lymphatic spread of tumor.

CLINICAL PRESENTATION

- Most common presentation is dyspnea, which is insidious in onset but progresses rapidly.

DIAGNOSTIC PEARLS

- Pulmonary lymphatic spread of tumor occurs most commonly with carcinoma of the breast, stomach, pancreas, and prostate.
- Characteristic radiologic findings of lymphatic spread of tumor consist of septal lines (Kerley B lines) and thickening of the peribronchovascular interstitium, simulating interstitial pulmonary edema.
- Lymphatic spread is usually bilateral except in pulmonary carcinoma.
- Pleural effusion is present in 30%-50% of cases; hilar or mediastinal lymphadenopathy is present in 20%-40% of cases.
- Most common presentation is dyspnea, which is insidious in onset but progresses rapidly.

DIFFERENTIAL DIAGNOSIS

- Hydrostatic pulmonary edema
- Niemann-Pick disease
- Amyloidosis
- Sarcoidosis
- Lymphoma

PATHOLOGY

- Most common etiology is invasion of interstitial space and lymphatics by hematogenously spreading tumor cells.
- Less commonly there is retrograde lymphangitic spread from infiltrated mediastinal or hilar lymph nodes.
- Neoplastic cells can be present within the lymphatic spaces and/or in adjacent peribronchovascular and interlobular interstitial tissue.

WHAT THE REFERRING PHYSICIAN NEEDS TO KNOW

- Most common clinical manifestation of lymphatic spread of tumor is dyspnea.
- Pulmonary lymphatic spread of tumor occurs most commonly with carcinoma of breast, stomach, pancreas, and prostate.
- Characteristic radiologic findings of lymphatic spread are septal lines (Kerley B lines) and peribronchovascular interstitial thickening. Findings resemble those of interstitial pulmonary edema.
- CT, particularly volumetric thin-section CT, is superior to radiography in detection of lymphatic spread of tumor.
- Lymphatic spread is usually bilateral except in pulmonary carcinoma.
- Virtually any metastatic neoplasm can result in lymphatic spread.

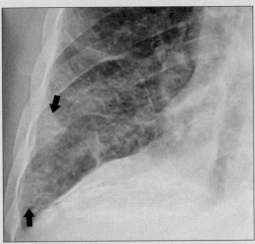

Figure 1. Lymphangitic carcinomatosis. Magnified view of right lower lung zone shows septal lines (*arrows*) (Kerley B lines). The patient was an 80-year-old man with lymphangitic carcinomatosis.

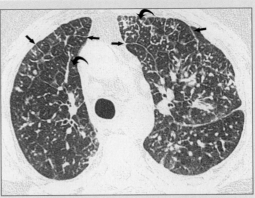

Figure 2. Lymphangitic carcinomatosis: characteristic high-resolution CT findings. High-resolution CT image shows 0.5- to 2.0-cm long lines (*straight arrows*) and polygonal arcades outlining one or more pulmonary lobules. These linear opacities (*septal lines*) reflect the presence of thickening of the interlobular septa. The vast majority of thickened septa have smooth margins. Also noted are prominent centrilobular dots (*curved arrows*), which represent thickening of the interstitium along the centrilobular bronchovascular bundle. Also noted is a small left pleural effusion.

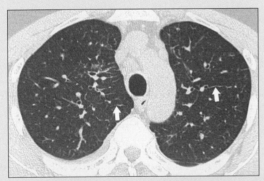

Figure 3. Lymphangitic carcinomatosis: mild abnormalities. High-resolution CT image demonstrates mild smooth bilateral septal thickening (*arrow*). Also noted is a small right pleural effusion. The patient was a 53-year-old man with pulmonary lymphatic spread of metastatic carcinoma of the colon.

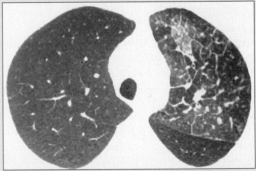

Figure 4. Lymphangitic carcinomatosis: unilateral distribution. High-resolution CT image demonstrates septal thickening and ground-glass opacities in the left upper lobe due to lymphangitic carcinomatosis of adenocarcinoma of the lung and associated interstitial pulmonary edema.

INCIDENCE/PREVALENCE AND EPIDEMIOLOGY

- Pulmonary metastases are very common, being seen at autopsy in 20%-50% of cases with extrapulmonary malignancy.
- Most common associated primary sites include breast, colon, kidney, uterus, and head and neck.
- Virtually any metastatic neoplasm can result in lymphatic spread.
- Usually involvement is bilateral.
- Unilateral disease is particularly common in pulmonary carcinoma.

Suggested Readings

Janower ML, Blennerhassett JB: Lymphangitic spread of metastatic cancer to the lung: A radiologic-pathologic classification. *Radiology* 101:267-273, 1971.

Johkoh T, Ikezoe J, Tomiyama N, et al: CT findings in lymphangitic carcinomatosis of the lung: Correlation with histologic findings and pulmonary function tests. *AJR Am J Roentgenol* 158: 1217-1222, 1992.

Munk PL, Müller NL, Miller RR, Ostrow DN: Pulmonary lymphangitic carcinomatosis: CT and pathologic findings. *Radiology* 166: 705-709, 1988.

Stein MG, Mayo J, Müller N, et al: Pulmonary lymphangitic spread of carcinoma: Appearance on CT scans. *Radiology* 162:371-375, 1987.

Pulmonary Metastases: Multiple Lung Nodules and Masses

DEFINITION: Pulmonary metastatic nodules are formed from parenchymal extension of an intravascular tumor that developed from tumor emboli lodged in arterioles and capillaries.

IMAGING

Radiography

Findings
- Most commonly, multiple nodules of various sizes (few millimeters to several centimeters in diameter)
- Most numerous in lower lung zones
- Less often, solitary pulmonary nodule
- Pulmonary masses
- Pleural effusion

Utility
- Chest radiographs are less sensitive than CT in detecting pulmonary metastases.

CT

Findings
- Most commonly, multiple nodules of various sizes (few millimeters to several centimeters in diameter) in outer third of lungs, particularly in subpleural regions of lower zones.
- Pulmonary masses.
- Nodules in random distribution within secondary pulmonary lobules that are round or lobulated.
- CT halo sign or perilesional halo of ground-glass attenuation (seen in highly vascular or hemorrhagic tumors).
- Cavitations, usually irregular and thick walled, seen in 4% of cases and common in squamous cell carcinoma.
- Calcifications are uncommon, usually seen in sarcomas, metastatic adenocarcinoma of the colon, and in post-chemotherapy lesions.
- Pneumothorax.

Utility
- CT is almost routinely used for suspected pulmonary metastases.
- CT has greater sensitivity than chest radiography for identification of pulmonary metastases.
- Sensitivity is affected by technique employed or by computer-aided diagnosis.

DIAGNOSTIC PEARLS

- The most common radiologic manifestation consists of multiple nodules that are typically of varying sizes and most numerous in the lower lobes.
- Single nodule is most common in carcinoma of colon or kidneys and osteosarcoma.
- Involvement of lower lobe and peripheral regions is predominant.
- Calcification is uncommon but may be seen in osteogenic sarcoma, chondrosarcoma, synovial sarcoma, and carcinoma of the colon, ovary, breast, and thyroid.
- Cavitation occurs in 4% of cases and is most common in metastases from carcinoma of head and neck and cervix.

- Detection increases with thinner sections (≤1.5 mm) and workstation viewing.
- Nodules < 3 mm in diameter are frequently missed.
- Findings are not specific (low specificity).

MRI

Findings
- Multiple lung nodules
- Lower lobe predominance

Utility
- MRI sensitivity has increased with improvement of image quality and specialized sequences.
- Sliding, rolling table concepts and rapid fat-saturated 3D gradient-echo sequences have reduced time, allowing image acquisition during single breath-hold.
- MRI has a potential role in whole-body screening for the detection of metastases.

Nuclear Medicine

Findings
- Increased uptake on FDG-PET imaging

WHAT THE REFERRING PHYSICIAN NEEDS TO KNOW

- Most pulmonary metastases presenting as single or multiple nodules are asymptomatic.
- Common radiologic manifestation includes multiple nodules, typically of varying sizes, most numerous in lower lobes and periphery.
- CT, particularly volumetric thin-section CT, is superior to radiography in detection of pulmonary metastases.
- Single metastatic pulmonary nodule is most common in carcinoma of colon or kidneys and osteosarcoma.
- Occurrence of spontaneous pneumothorax in association with metastatic pulmonary disease should suggest sarcoma as a primary neoplasm.

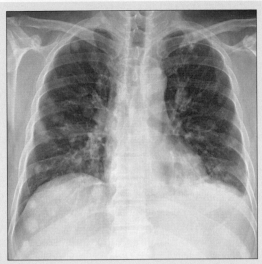

Figure 1. Pulmonary metastases: radiographic findings. Chest radiograph demonstrates multiple bilateral pulmonary nodules ranging from a few millimeters to 2 cm in diameter. The nodules have smooth margins and involve mainly the lower lung zones. A small left pleural effusion is also present. The patient was a 53-year-old man with metastatic sarcoma.

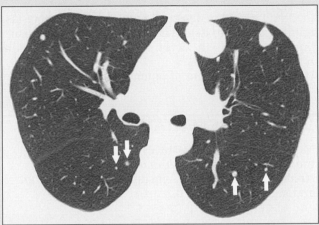

Figure 2. Small and large lung metastases. CT image shows several large nodules in the anterior aspects of the right and left lungs and several small nodules (*arrows*) in the lower lobes. The nodules have well-defined smooth margins and range from 2 to 35 mm in diameter. The patient was a 40-year-old man with lung metastases from synovial sarcoma.

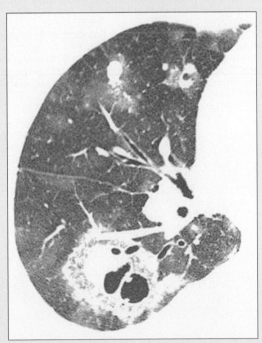

Figure 3. Hemorrhagic and cavitating metastases. View of the right lung from a CT scan demonstrates several nodules of various sizes surrounded by a halo of ground-glass attenuation. Also noted is cavitation of some of the nodules. The patient was a 55-year-old man with metastatic angiosarcoma.

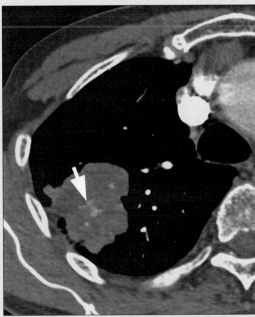

Figure 4. Foci of calcification in metastatic adenocarcinoma. CT image shows foci of calcification (*arrow*). The extent of calcification increased on a subsequent CT. The patient was a 79-year-old man with metastatic adenocarcinoma of the rectum.

Utility

- FDG-PET useful in detection of intrathoracic metastases
- Limited ability to detect nodules < 1 cm in diameter
- Superior to CT in detecting hilar and mediastinal lymph node metastases
- Useful for assessment of potentially resectable lesions

CLINICAL PRESENTATION

- Most pulmonary metastases presenting as single or multiple nodules are asymptomatic.
- Nonspecific symptoms include cough, hemoptysis, and shortness of breath.

DIFFERENTIAL DIAGNOSIS

- Histoplasmosis
- Tuberculosis
- Wegener granulomatosis
- Amyloidosis
- Septic embolism
- Lymphoma

PATHOLOGY

- Hematogenous spread is the most common route.
- Tumor cells lodge within small pulmonary arteries and arterioles.
- Extension of intravascular tumor into surrounding lung parenchyma forms well-defined nodules.
- Nodules have more peripheral lung distribution and a random distribution in the secondary lobule.

INCIDENCE/PREVALENCE AND EPIDEMIOLOGY

- Pulmonary metastases are very common, seen in autopsies in 20%-50% of cases with extrapulmonary malignancy.
- Most common associated primary site includes breast, colon, kidney, uterus, and head and neck.
- Multiple nodules of varying size are the most common radiologic presentations of pulmonary metastases.
- Only 2%-10% of solitary pulmonary nodules are metastatic in origin.
- Cavitation in 4% of cases and is most common in carcinoma of head and neck or cervix.
- Identification of concomitant primary neoplasm elsewhere or prior history of neoplasia does not indicate that solitary pulmonary nodule is metastatic.

Suggested Readings

Awai K, Murao K, Ozawa A, et al: Pulmonary nodules at chest CT: Effect of computer-aided diagnosis on radiologists' detection performance. *Radiology* 230:347-352, 2004.

Diederich S, Semik M, Lentschig MG, et al: Helical CT of pulmonary nodules in patients with extrathoracic malignancy: CT-surgical correlation. *AJR Am J Roentgenol* 172:353-360, 1999.

Fischbach F, Knollmann F, Griesshaber V, et al: Detection of pulmonary nodules by multislice computed tomography: Improved detection rate with reduced slice thickness. *Eur Radiol* 13: 2378-2383, 2003.

Maile CW, Rodan BA, Godwin JD, et al: Calcification in pulmonary metastases. *Br J Radiol* 55:108-113, 1982.

Murata K, Takahashi M, Mori M, et al: Pulmonary metastatic nodules: CT-pathologic correlation. *Radiology* 182:331-335, 1992.

Primack SL, Hartman TE, Lee KS, Müller NL: Pulmonary nodules and the CT halo sign. *Radiology* 190:513-515, 1994.

Pulmonary Metastases: Unusual Manifestations

DEFINITION: Unusual manifestations of metastatic disease include intravascular tumor emboli and endotracheal and endobronchial metastases.

IMAGING

Radiography
Findings
- May be normal
- Dilatation of central pulmonary arteries and right ventricle (pulmonary arterial hypertension)
- Endotracheal and bronchial focal opacity
- Lobar or segmental atelectasis

Utility
- Chest radiographs are less sensitive than CT in detecting pulmonary metastases.
- Limited value in the diagnosis of intravascular and endobronchial metastases.

CT
Findings
- Intravascular tumor emboli
- Polypoid or glove-finger enhancing mass
- Filling defects in central pulmonary arteries
- Nodular contour (beading) of peripheral pulmonary arteries
- Nodular and branching centrilobular opacities representing enlarged centrilobular arteries ("tree-in-bud" pattern)
- Endotracheal and endobronchial metastases
- Bronchial dilatation
- Bronchial obstruction
- Endoluminal soft tissue densities

Utility
- Almost routinely used for suspected pulmonary metastases.
- CT has greater sensitivity than chest radiography for identification of pulmonary metastases.

Nuclear Medicine
Findings
- Increased uptake on FDG-PET

Utility
- FDG-PET useful diagnostic tool for detection of intrathoracic metastases.

DIAGNOSTIC PEARLS

- Endotracheal and endobronchial metastases usually are secondary to carcinoma of the breast, colorectum, kidney, and cervix or to melanoma or sarcoma.
- Volumetric thin-section CT with multiplanar reformatted imaging is required for optimal imaging assessment of endobronchial metastases.
- Intravascular metastases may result in filling defects in central pulmonary arteries or, more commonly, nodular contour (beading) of peripheral arteries and a "tree-in-bud" pattern.

CLINICAL PRESENTATION

- Most common symptom of endobronchial metastases is dyspnea.
- Other common symptoms include cough and hemoptysis.

PATHOLOGY

- Intravascular tumor emboli develop when tumor grows within the vessel lumen without extension into extravascular tissue.
- Tracheobronchial spread may occur with primary pulmonary tumors (especially bronchoalveolar carcinoma) or upper airway tumors.
- Endotracheal and endobronchial metastases occur most commonly from hematogenous spread of carcinoma of the breast, colorectum, kidney, and cervix, or melanoma.

INCIDENCE/PREVALENCE AND EPIDEMIOLOGY

- Pulmonary metastases are very common, being seen in autopsies in 20%-50% of cases with extrapulmonary malignancy.

WHAT THE REFERRING PHYSICIAN NEEDS TO KNOW

- CT, particularly volumetric thin-section CT, is superior to radiography in the detection of pulmonary metastases.
- The most common symptoms of endobronchial metastases are dyspnea, cough, and hemoptysis.
- Endobronchial metastases usually are secondary to carcinoma of the breast, colorectum, kidney, and cervix or to melanoma or sarcoma.
- Volumetric thin-section CT with multiplanar reformatted imaging is required for optimal imaging assessment of endobronchial metastases.

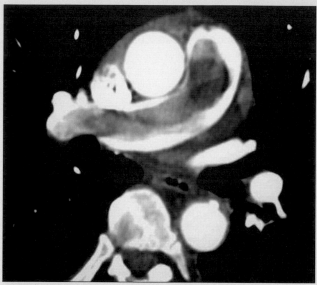

Figure 1. Intravascular metastases. Contrast-enhanced CT image shows large filling defect in the main and right pulmonary arteries. The patient was a 57-year-old man with proven intraventricular and pulmonary artery metastases from leiomyosarcoma of the left arm. (*Courtesy of Dr. Marcos Manzini, Department of Radiology, Heart Institute, São Paulo, Brazil.*)

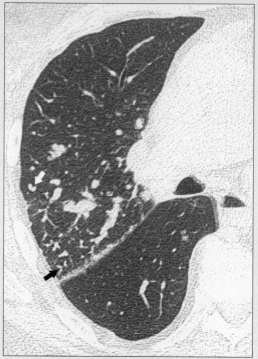

Figure 2. Intravascular metastases. View of the right lung at the level of the bronchus intermedius demonstrates nodular thickening of the pulmonary vessels and centrilobular nodular and branching opacities ("tree-in-bud" pattern) (*arrow*). The patient was a 78-year-old man with metastatic renal cell carcinoma.

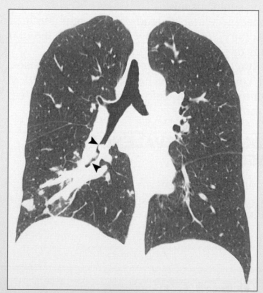

Figure 3. Endobronchial metastases. Coronal reformatted image from a spiral CT shows endoluminal polypoid lesions (*arrowheads*) in the intermediate and right lower lobe bronchi and distal branching opacities. The polypoid lesions were due to endobronchial metastatic carcinoma of the cervix and the branching opacities due to mucoid impaction of the obstructed bronchi. The patient was a 53-year-old woman.

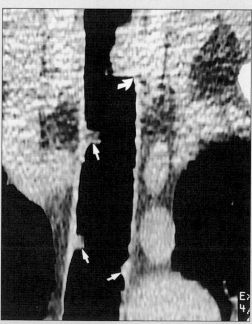

Figure 4. Tracheal metastases from squamous cell carcinoma of the oropharynx. Coronal reconstruction from spiral CT scan shows several endotracheal polypoid lesions (*straight arrows*). The largest nodule extends beyond the tracheal wall (*curved arrow*). The patient developed tracheal metastases 2 years after surgical resection of a squamous cell carcinoma of the oropharynx.

- Endobronchial metastases usually are secondary to carcinoma of breast, colorectum, kidney, or cervix or to melanoma or sarcoma.
- Intravascular metastases are most commonly due to carcinoma of the breast, kidney, or liver.

Suggested Readings

Han D, Lee KS, Franquet T, et al: Thrombotic and nonthrombotic pulmonary arterial embolism: Spectrum of imaging findings. *RadioGraphics* 23:1521-1539, 2003.

Seo JB, Im JG, Goo JM, et al: Atypical pulmonary metastases: Spectrum of radiologic findings. *RadioGraphics* 21:403-417, 2001.

Sorensen JB: Endobronchial metastases from extrapulmonary solid tumors. *Acta Oncol* 43:73-79, 2004.

Lymphoproliferative Disorders and Leukemia

Part 26

LYMPHOID HYPERPLASIA AND LYMPHOID INTERSTITIAL PNEUMONIA

Lymphoid Hyperplasia and Follicular Bronchiolitis

DEFINITION: Benign lung disease that is characterized by the presence of hyperplastic lymphoid tissue mainly along the bronchioles and pulmonary lymphatics.

IMAGING

Radiography
Findings
- Bilateral reticular or reticulonodular opacities
Utility
- Chest radiograph may be normal.
- Radiography usually first imaging modality performed in suspected interstitial lung disease.

CT
Findings
- Bilateral diffuse or lower lung centrilobular and peribronchial nodules
- Nodules usually < 3 mm in diameter; occasionally 3-10 mm in diameter
- Patchy ground-glass opacities and small foci of consolidation
Utility
- High-resolution CT is used routinely for further characterization.

CLINICAL PRESENTATION

- Usually asymptomatic
- Symptoms include cough and dyspnea

DIFFERENTIAL DIAGNOSIS

- Hypersensitivity pneumonitis
- Respiratory bronchiolitis
- Infectious bronchiolitis
- Lymphoid interstitial pneumonia
- Sarcoidosis

DIAGNOSTIC PEARLS

- Most commonly seen in patients with collagen vascular disease or immunodefiency
- Diffuse or lower lung centrilobular and peribronchial nodules
- Patchy ground-glass opacities and small foci of consolidation
- Radiologic findings to not allow a specific diagnosis

PATHOLOGY

- Discrete foci of hyperplastic lymphoid tissue, often with germinal centers, along bronchovascular bundles.
- Hyperplastic lymphoid tissue in interlobular septa and visceral pleura.
- Associated with collagen vascular disease, immunodeficiency, hypersensitivity disorders, nonspecific response in patients with airway infection, obstruction, and bronchiectasis.

INCIDENCE/PREVALENCE AND EPIDEMIOLOGY

- Uncommon cause of radiologically and clinically evident parenchymal lung disease.
- Most commonly seen in association with collagen vascular disease and immunodeficiency.
- Occurs in children and adults (age range: 1.5 to 77 years).

WHAT THE REFERRING PHYSICIAN NEEDS TO KNOW

- Symptomatic disease occurs most commonly in patients with rheumatoid arthritis and immunodeficiency.
- Radiologic findings are nonspecific; definitive diagnosis requires surgical lung biopsy.
- Prognosis usually favorable.

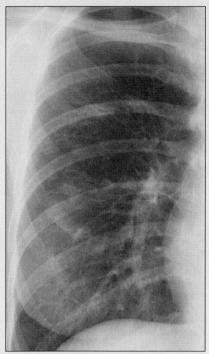

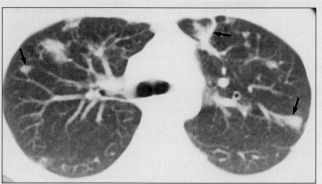

Figure 2. Pulmonary lymphoid hyperplasia in rheumatoid arthritis. Conventional 10-mm collimation CT scan shows focal nodular areas of consolidation in both lungs in a predominantly peribronchovascular distribution (*arrows*). The patient was a 24-year-old woman who had rheumatoid disease and biopsy-proven pulmonary lymphoid hyperplasia (follicular bronchiolitis). (*From Müller NL, Fraser RS, Colman NC, et al: Radiologic Diagnosis of Diseases of the Chest, Philadelphia, Saunders, 2001.*)

Figure 1. Pulmonary lymphoid hyperplasia in rheumatoid arthritis. View of the right lung from posteroanterior chest radiograph shows ill-defined nodular opacities. A similar pattern was present in the left lung. The patient was a 24-year-old woman who had rheumatoid disease and biopsy-proven pulmonary lymphoid hyperplasia (follicular bronchiolitis). (*From Müller NL, Fraser RS, Colman NC, et al: Radiologic Diagnosis of Diseases of the Chest, Philadelphia, Saunders, 2001.*)

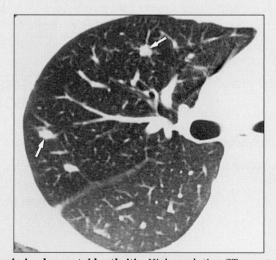

Figure 3. Pulmonary lymphoid hyperplasia in rheumatoid arthritis. High-resolution CT scan targeted to the right lung shows sharply defined peribronchovascular nodular infiltrates in the right upper lobe (*arrows*). The patient was a 24-year-old woman who had rheumatoid disease and biopsy-proven pulmonary lymphoid hyperplasia (follicular bronchiolitis). (*From Müller NL, Fraser RS, Colman NC, et al: Radiologic Diagnosis of Diseases of the Chest, Philadelphia, Saunders, 2001.*)

Suggested Readings

Aerni MR, Vassallo R, Myers JL, et al: Follicular bronchiolitis in surgical lung biopsies: Clinical implications in 12 patients. *Respir Med* 102(2):307-312, 2008.

Howling SJ, Hansell DM, Wells AU, et al: Follicular bronchiolitis: Thin-section CT and histologic findings. *Radiology* 212:637-642, 1999.

Nicholson AG: Lymphocytic interstitial pneumonia and other lymphoproliferative disorders in the lung. *Semin Respir Crit Care Med* 22(4):409-422, 2001.

Travis WD, Galvin JR: Non-neoplastic pulmonary lymphoid lesions. *Thorax* 56:964-971, 2001.

Lymphoid Interstitial Pneumonia

DEFINITION: Interstitial lung disease that is characterized by extensive infiltration of the alveolar septa with polyclonal lymphocytes and variable numbers of plasma cells.

IMAGING

Radiography
Findings
- Lower lung reticular or reticulonodular pattern
- Less common: nodular pattern, ground-glass opacities, airspace consolidation
- Cystic lesions occasionally

Utility
- Chest radiograph first imaging modality used in suspected interstitial lung disease
- Radiographic findings nonspecific

CT
Findings
- Characteristic: extensive bilateral ground-glass opacities, several cystic airspaces, and poorly defined centrilobular nodules
- Common: subpleural nodules, thickened bronchovascular bundles
- Uncommon: large nodules, consolidation, bronchiectasis, and honeycombing
- Slightly enlarged mediastinal lymph nodes
- Occasional predominantly cystic pattern
- Lower lobe predominance

Utility
- High-resolution CT is routinely used for further characterization.
- Parenchymal changes may resolve, but cystic and fibrotic changes persist or worsen.

CLINICAL PRESENTATION

- Typical insidious onset over several years
- Cough, dyspnea, and fatigue
- Approximately 80% with serum dysproteinemia (polyclonal hypergammaglobulinemia)
- Bronchial alveolar lavage fluid lymphocytosis (30%)

DIFFERENTIAL DIAGNOSIS

- Lymphoid hyperplasia
- Hypersensitivity pneumonitis

DIAGNOSTIC PEARLS

- Usually occurs in patients with autoimmune disease or immunodeficiency, most commonly Sjögren syndrome.
- Bilateral ground-glass opacities with several associated thin-walled cystic spaces, lower lobe predominance.

- Respiratory bronchiolitis/interstitial lung disease
- Pulmonary Langerhans histiocytosis
- Nonspecific interstitial pneumonia (NSIP)
- Lymphangioleiomyomatosis
- Lymphoma

PATHOLOGY

- Extensive infiltration of alveolar septa with polyclonal lymphocytes and variable numbers of plasma cells.
- Occurs in patients with underlying autoimmune disease or immunodeficiency (e.g., Sjögren syndrome, autoimmune disorders, dysproteinemia, AIDS).
- Small nodular foci as a result of localized proliferation or formation of germinal centers.
- Peribronchiolar infiltration with obstruction and cystic airspace enlargement.
- Fibrosis and remodeling with honeycombing.
- Amyloid deposition.

INCIDENCE/PREVALENCE AND EPIDEMIOLOGY

- Rare condition
- Occurs in patients with underlying autoimmune disease or immunodeficiency (e.g., Sjögren syndrome, autoimmune disorders, dysproteinemia, AIDS); idiopathic type rare
- Average clinical presentation at age 50-60 years
- Women affected twice as often as men

WHAT THE REFERRING PHYSICIAN NEEDS TO KNOW
- Lymphoid interstitial pneumonia usually occurs in association with underlying immunologic disorder, most commonly Sjögren syndrome.
- Approximately 80% of patients have serum dysproteinemia, most commonly polyclonal hypergammaglobulinemia.
- Radiographic findings are nonspecific.
- Presumptive diagnosis can be made in proper clinical context based on high-resolution CT.
- Definitive diagnosis requires surgical lung biopsy.

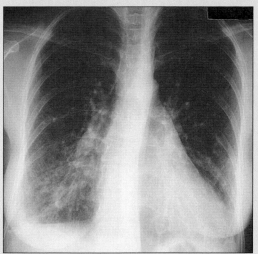

Figure 1. Lymphoid interstitial pneumonia. Posteroanterior chest radiograph shows bilateral areas of hazy increased opacity and consolidation involving the lower lung zones. The patient was a 26-year-old woman with juvenile rheumatoid arthritis and Sjögren syndrome. The diagnosis was proven at video-assisted thoracoscopic biopsy.

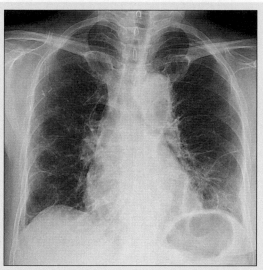

Figure 2. Lymphoid interstitial pneumonia. Posteroanterior chest radiograph demonstrates numerous cystic lesions throughout the lungs involving predominantly the mid and lower lung zones. Also noted are hazy increased opacities in the left lower lobe and previous right mastectomy.

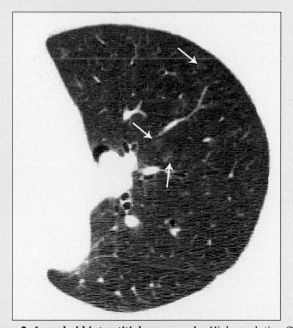

Figure 3. Lymphoid interstitial pneumonia. High-resolution CT image targeted to the left lung shows mild ground-glass opacities and a few poorly defined centrilobular nodules (*arrows*). The patient was a 42-year-old woman with mixed connective tissue disease and lymphoid interstitial pneumonia.

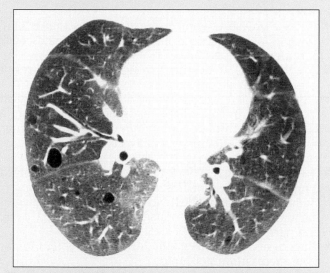

Figure 4. Lymphoid interstitial pneumonia: classic CT findings. High-resolution CT image shows extensive ground-glass opacities and a few bilateral cysts. The patient was a 50-year-old woman with lymphoid interstitial pneumonia and Sjögren syndrome. The diagnosis of lymphoid interstitial pneumonia was proven at biopsy.

Suggested Readings

Cha SI, Fessler MB, Cool CD, et al: Lymphoid interstitial pneumonia: Clinical features, associations and prognosis. *Eur Respir J* 28(2):364-369, 2006.

Honda O, Johkoh T, Ichikado K, et al: Differential diagnosis of lymphocytic interstitial pneumonia and malignant lymphoma on high-resolution CT. *AJR Am J Roentgenol* 173:71-74, 1999.

Ichikawa Y, Kinoshita M, Koga T, et al: Lung cyst formation in lymphocytic interstitial pneumonia: CT features. *J Comput Assist Tomogr* 18:745-748, 1994.

Johkoh T, Müller NL, Pickford HA, et al: Lymphocytic interstitial pneumonia: Thin-section CT findings in 22 patients. *Radiology* 212:567-572, 1999.

Silva CI, Flint JD, Levy RD, Müller NL: Diffuse lung cysts in lymphoid interstitial pneumonia: High-resolution CT and pathologic findings. *J Thorac Imaging* 21:241-244, 2006.

Swigris JJ, Berry GJ, Raffin TA, Kuschner WG: Lymphoid interstitial pneumonia: A narrative review. *Chest* 122:2150-2164, 2002.

Hodgkin Lymphoma of the Mediastinum

DEFINITION: Hodgkin lymphoma is a neoplasm of B lymphocytes characterized by the presence of Reed-Sternberg cells.

IMAGING

Radiography

Findings

- Widening of superior mediastinum by lobulated mass is evident.
- Destruction of ribs, vertebrae, or sternum typically results in focal lytic areas.
- Vertebral involvement other than by direct extension often is purely osteoblastic (ivory vertebra).

Utility

- Usually first imaging modality used in the evaluation of these patients
- Of limited value in the differential diagnosis

CT

Findings

- Discrete anterosuperior mediastinal mass that is usually lobulated represents enlargement and coalescence of multiple lymph nodes.
- The thymus is frequently involved, which may result in diffuse thymic enlargement.
- Thymic involvement may be difficult to distinguish from anterior mediastinal lymph node involvement.
- Enlarged lymph nodes commonly have homogeneous soft tissue attenuation but may contain areas of low attenuation.
- Dystrophic calcification may develop in involved lymph nodes after mediastinal irradiation.
- Hodgkin disease may extend into mediastinal interstitial tissue to invade esophagus, superior vena cava, and pericardium.
- The chest wall is affected by direct extension of tumor from mediastinum or lungs.
- Concomitant pulmonary involvement appears as multiple, irregularly marginated pulmonary nodules or masses.

Utility

- Superior to the radiograph in demonstrating the extent of disease.

DIAGNOSTIC PEARLS

- Typically presents as a large lobulated anterior mediastinal mass and some have low-attenuation areas of necrosis.
- Lymphadenopathy most commonly involves anterior mediastinal and paratracheal lympy nodes but may extend to involve all nodal stations.
- In approximately 40% of cases, the intrathoracic disease is confined to the anterior mediastinum.
- Dystrophic calcification develops in some cases after mediastinal radiation.
- Pleuropulmonary involvement findings show multiple pulmonary nodules, often with irregular margins.

Positron Emission Tomography

Findings

- Increased FDG uptake in involved nodes.

Utility

- FDG-PET provides whole-body images that give comprehensive assessment of disease extent during staging and follow-up.
- PET mostly upstages disease when compared with findings of CT alone.
- In majority of patients, PET/CT performed with low-dose nonenhanced CT is satisfactory for staging of lymphoma.
- PET has high diagnostic accuracy for restaging lymphoma after initial treatment.
- Integrated PET/CT is more sensitive and specific for evaluation of lymph node and organ involvement than contrast-enhanced CT.

CLINICAL PRESENTATION

- Incidental finding of mediastinal mass on chest radiograph is common presentation.

WHAT THE REFERRING PHYSICIAN NEEDS TO KNOW

- Hodgkin disease typically involves predominantly or exclusively the anterior mediastinum or paratracheal regions.
- PET mostly upstages disease when compared with findings of CT alone, which has bearing on treatment strategy.
- Integrated PET/CT is more sensitive and specific for evaluation of lymph node and organ involvement than is contrast-enhanced CT.

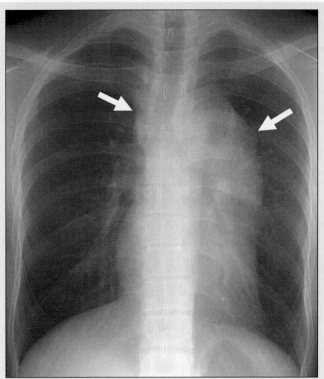

Figure 1. Nodular sclerosing Hodgkin disease in a 23-year-old man. Chest radiograph shows bilateral superior mediastinal widening (*arrows*). (*Courtesy of Dr. Kyung Soo Lee, Seoul, Korea*)

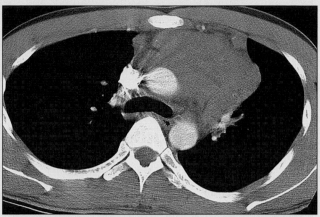

Figure 2. Nodular sclerosing Hodgkin disease in a 23-year-old man. Contrast-enhanced CT image at level of main bronchi shows large left anterior mediastinal soft tissue mass with lobulated contour. (*Courtesy of Dr. Kyung Soo Lee, Seoul, Korea*)

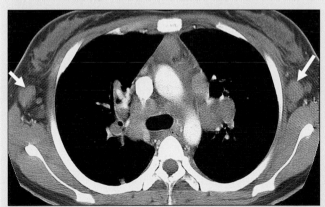

Figure 3. Mixed cellularity Hodgkin disease in a 20-year-old woman. Contrast-enhanced CT image obtained at level of main bronchi demonstrates enlarged lymph nodes in hila, axillae (*arrows*), right paratracheal region, aortopulmonary window, and anterior mediastinum. (*Courtesy of Dr. Kyung Soo Lee, Seoul, Korea*)

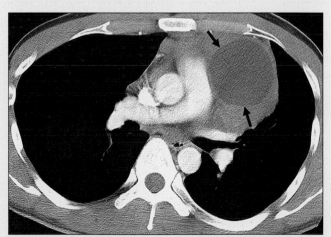

Figure 4. Nodular sclerosing Hodgkin disease with cystic area. Contrast-enhanced CT image at level of the bronchus intermedius demonstrates left anterior mediastinal mass containing large round area of low attenuation (*arrows*). (*Courtesy of Dr. Kyung Soo Lee, Seoul, Korea*)

- Systemic symptoms such as unexplained and persistent fever, night sweats, and weight loss may be present.
- More localized complaints such as cough and chest pain may also be present.
- Pruritus is another characteristic systemic symptom of Hodgkin disease.

DIFFERENTIAL DIAGNOSIS

- Non-Hodgkin lymphoma
- Thymoma
- Thymic carcinoma
- Germ cell tumor
- Pulmonary carcinoma

PATHOLOGY

- Histologic diagnosis requires presence of characteristic Reed-Sternberg giant cells in association with appropriate stromal or cellular background.
- Reed-Sternberg cell is large, bilobed cell with prominent eosinophilic nucleoli, perinucleolar clearing, thickened nuclear membrane, and abundant cytoplasm.
- Hodgkin disease is classified histopathologically into four subtypes: lymphocyte predominance, nodular sclerosis, mixed cellularity, and lymphocyte depletion types.

INCIDENCE/PREVALENCE AND EPIDEMIOLOGY

- Hodgkin disease is uncommon, having annual incidence of 2 to 3 per 100,000 in Europe and United States.
- Hodgkin disease accounts for 25%-30% of all cases of lymphoma and is slightly more common in men.
- Peak ages are during the third decade and in those older than age 50 years.
- In approximately 40% of cases, the intrathoracic disease is confined to the anterior mediastinum.
- Primary pulmonary Hodgkin disease (not associated with evidence of disease in lymph nodes or other tissues) is uncommon.
- Most cases of Hodgkin disease in the mediastinum are of the nodular sclerosis subtype, usually occurring in young women.
- The mixed cellularity type occurs in middle-aged patients.

Suggested Readings

Gossmann A, Eich HT, Engert A, et al: CT and MR imaging in Hodgkin's disease—present and future. *Eur J Haematol Suppl* 66:83-89, 2005.

Guermazi A, Brice P, de Kerviler EE, et al: Extranodal Hodgkin disease: Spectrum of disease. *RadioGraphics* 21:161-179, 2001.

Jhanwar YS, Straus DJ: The role of PET in lymphoma. *J Nucl Med* 47:1326-1334, 2006.

Thomas RK, Re D, Zander T, et al: Epidemiology and etiology of Hodgkin's lymphoma. *Ann Oncol* 13(Suppl 4):147-152, 2002.

Pulmonary Hodgkin Lymphoma

DEFINITION: Pulmonary involvement in Hodgkin lymphoma may occur in isolation (primary pulmonary Hodgkin lumphoma) or in association with current or previous mediastinal involvement (secondary pulmonary Hodgkin lymphoma).

IMAGING

Radiography

Findings

- Disease appears as single/multiple pulmonary nodules, lobar/segmental consolidation, and reticular pattern with bronchovascular bundle and interlobular septal thickening.
- Consolidation of lung parenchyma remote from mediastinum is common.
- Other findings include disseminated small nodules, cavitating masses, and endobronchial nodules.

Utility

- Helpful in demonstrating presence of parenchymal disease

CT

Findings

- Multiple, irregularly marginated pulmonary nodules or masses are noted.
- Individual foci may coalesce to form a large homogeneous nonsegmental mass, with shaggy, ill-defined borders.
- Such masses can undergo necrosis, forming thick- or thin-walled cavities; in many cases, they are multiple.
- Areas of consolidation may occur.
- Thoracic Hodgkin disease typically presents as lymphadenopathy.
- Primary pulmonary Hodgkin disease usually presents as single or multiple nodules, frequently showing cavitation.

Utility

- Superior to radiography in the staging of Hodgkin lymphoma.

Positron Emission Tomography

Findings

- FDG uptake in lung nodules is variable; thus, PET may show false-negative results in lung involvement of Hodgkin disease.

Utility

- PET particularly when integrated with CT (PET/CT) is superior to CT in the staging of Hodgkin lymphoma and in the assessment of tumor recurrence.

DIAGNOSTIC PEARLS

- Primary pulmonary Hodgkin lymphoma is rare.
- Pulmonary Hodgkin lymphoma is almost always associated with hilar and/or mediastinal lymphadenopathy.
- Secondary pulmonary Hodgkin lymphoma may manifest as nodules, masses, areas of consolidation, or endobronchial lesions.
- Pulmonary involvement occurs in about 10% at presentation and eventually in 30%-40% of patients.

CLINICAL PRESENTATION

- Most common clinical manifestation of pulmonary involvement is a dry cough.
- Patients also often have systemic symptoms, including fever, night sweats, and weight loss.

DIFFERENTIAL DIAGNOSIS

- Non-Hodgkin lymphoma
- Lymphangitic carcinomatosis
- Metastases

PATHOLOGY

- Hodgkin disease is neoplasm of B lymphocytes characterized by Reed-Sternberg cells.
- Pulmonary involvement results most commonly by direct extension from involved mediastinal and hilar lymph nodes.
- The most common histologic feature is infiltration and thickening of peribronchovascular interstitium by Hodgkin lymphoma.

INCIDENCE/PREVALENCE AND EPIDEMIOLOGY

- Hodgkin disease is uncommon, with an annual incidence of 2 to 3 per 100,000 in Europe and United States.

WHAT THE REFERRING PHYSICIAN NEEDS TO KNOW

- Pulmonary involvement occurs at presentation in about 10% of patients with Hodgkin disease and eventually in 30%-40% of cases.
- It is almost always associated with hilar or mediastinal lymphadenopathy.
- Pleural effusion is seen at presentation in 10% of patients and eventually develops in approximately 30% of patients.

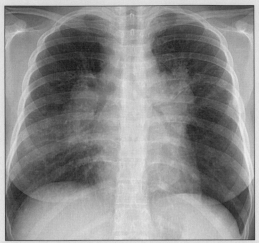

Figure 1. Mixed cellularity Hodgkin disease in a 20-year-old woman. Chest radiograph shows enlarged bilateral hila, widened mediastinum, and multiple pulmonary nodules in both lungs. (*Courtesy of Kyung Soo Lee, Seoul, Korea*)

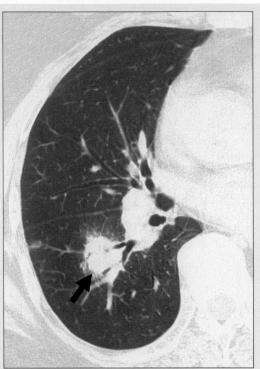

Figure 2. Hodgkin disease with pulmonary involvement. Target CT image of right lung at the level of basal trunk demonstrates poorly defined nodule (*arrow*) containing air bronchograms. The patient was a 70-year-old woman with diagnosis of mixed cellularity Hodgkin disease. (*Courtesy of Kyung Soo Lee, Seoul, Korea*)

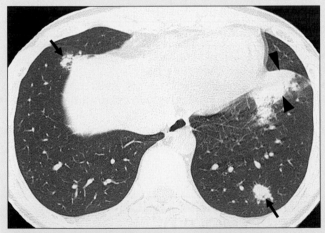

Figure 3. Recurrent Hodgkin disease with pulmonary involvement. CT scan at the level of the right hemidiaphragm shows nodules (*arrows*) and airspace consolidation (*arrowheads*) in both lower lobes. The patient was a 23-year-old man with recurrent nodular sclerosing Hodgkin disease. (*Courtesy of Kyung Soo Lee, Seoul, Korea*)

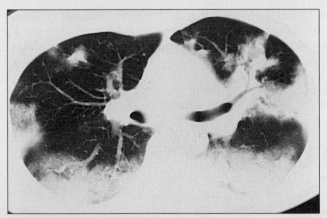

Figure 4. Recurrent Hodgkin disease with extensive parenchymal consolidation. Parenchymal consolidation in Hodgkin disease. Lung window reveals peribronchial and peripheral areas of consolidation. Surgical lung biopsy demonstrated Hodgkin disease. (*From Müller NL, Fraser RS, Colman NC, et al: Radiologic Diagnosis of Diseases of the Chest, Philadelphia, Saunders, 2001.*)

- Hodgkin disease occurs in two age groups, with the first peak in third decade and the second peak after the age of 50.
- Pulmonary involvement occurs in about 12% at presentation and eventually in 30%-40% of patients.
- Hilar or mediastinal lymphadenopathy is almost always associated.
- Primary pulmonary Hodgkin disease (not associated with evidence of disease in lymph nodes or other tissues) is uncommon.
- The disease is slightly more common in men than in women.

Suggested Readings

Gossmann A, Eich HT, Engert A, et al: CT and MR imaging in Hodgkin's disease—present and future. *Eur J Haematol Suppl* 66:83-89, 2005.

Guermazi A, Brice P, de Kerviler EE, et al: Extranodal Hodgkin disease: Spectrum of disease. *RadioGraphics* 21:161-179, 2001.

Jhanwar YS, Straus DJ: The role of PET in lymphoma. *J Nucl Med* 47:1326-1334, 2006.

Thomas RK, Re D, Zander T, et al: Epidemiology and etiology of Hodgkin's lymphoma. *Ann Oncol* 13(Suppl 4):147-152, 2002.

Mediastinal Non-Hodgkin Lymphoma

DEFINITION: Mediastinal non-Hodgkin lymphoma is a neoplastic proliferation of lymphocytes not classified under the Hodgkin type of lymphoma in medistinal lymph nodes or thymus.

IMAGING

Radiography

Findings

- Mediastinal large cell lymphomas present as a thymic mass with or without lymph node involvement and with grossly invasive features.
- Lymphoma confined to thymus results in a rounded, homogeneous, soft tissue mass in the anterior mediastinum.
- Mediastinal borders with adjacent lung are typically sharp until invasion has occurred.

Utility

- Chest radiography usually is the first imaging modality used in the assessment of these patients.

CT

Findings

- Most tumors have homogeneous soft tissue attenuation; large tumors contain areas of low attenuation due to hemorrhage or necrosis.
- In secondary or recurrent mediastinal non-Hodgkin lymphoma, involvement of the paratracheal or prevascular nodal groups is the most common, followed by hilar, subcarinal, cardiophrenic angle, internal mammary, and posterior mediastinal lymph nodes.
- Enlarged nodes in contiguous lymph node groups are frequently present.
- Enlarged nodes may be discrete or matted together, with edges well or ill defined; they show minor enhancement.
- Dystrophic calcification may develop in involved lymph nodes after mediastinal irradiation.
- Pleural and pericardial effusion occurs in about one third of patients.

Utility

- CT is superior to radiography in the diagnosis and staging of lymphoma.

DIAGNOSTIC PEARLS

- Mediastinal lymphomas most commonly present as a large lobulated anterior mediastinal mass; some have low-attenuation areas of necrosis.
- Mediastinal lymphomas tend to involve mainly the thymus and the prevascular and paratracheal lymph nodes.
- Non-Hodgkin lymphoma accounts for 70%-75% of all cases of lymphoma.
- The mediastinum is the sole site of involvement in only 5% of cases.

Positron Emission Tomography

Findings

- Increased FDG uptake

Utility

- FDG-PET is more accurate for detecting nodal lymphoma than contrast-enhanced CT.
- In integrated PET/CT, the CT component provides anatomic mapping images and attenuation correction data for PET.
- Whole-body PET or integrated PET/CT is the initial and follow-up study of choice in patients with biopsy-proved non-Hodgkin lymphoma.

CLINICAL PRESENTATION

- Patients with mediastinal lymphoma commonly present with systemic symptoms or more localized complaints.
- Less common symptoms include stridor secondary to tracheal obstruction and signs of superior vena cava obstruction.
- Occasionally non-Hodgkin lymphoma may be first recognized as an incidental finding of a mediastinal mass on a chest radiograph.

WHAT THE REFERRING PHYSICIAN NEEDS TO KNOW

- Mediastinal lymphomas present as a large lobulated anterior mediastinal mass; some have low-attenuation areas consistent with necrosis.
- Symptomatic patients may be treated with local radiation therapy or a combination of chemotherapy and radiation therapy.
- Advanced-stage lymphomas are treated with chemotherapy.
- FDG-PET is helpful in diagnosis and staging and for follow-up after treatment.

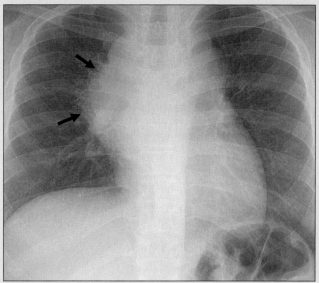

Figure 1. Primary mediastinal lymphoma of large B-cell type. Chest radiograph shows bilateral superior mediastinal widening. Also note poorly defined interface (*arrows*) between right lung and mediastinal lesion, suggestive of pulmonary parenchymal infiltration by lymphoma. Right hemidiaphragm is elevated, suggesting involvement of the phrenic nerve. (*Courtesy of Dr. Kyung Soo Lee, Seoul, Korea*)

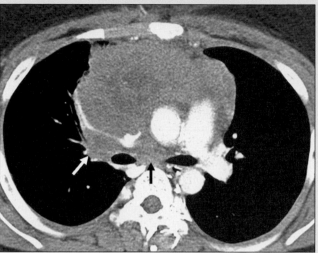

Figure 2. Primary mediastinal lymphoma of large B-cell type. Contrast-enhanced CT image obtained at level of main bronchi shows slightly inhomogeneous anterior mediastinal mass. Also note retrovascular components (*arrows*) of tumor. (*Courtesy of Dr. Kyung Soo Lee, Seoul, Korea*)

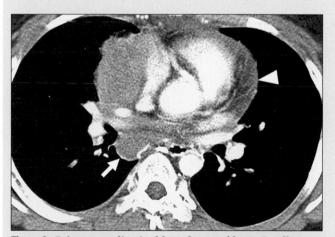

Figure 3. Primary mediastinal lymphoma of large B-cell type. CT image at level of right middle lobe bronchus demonstrates anterior mediastinal tumor, subcarinal lymph node enlargement (*arrow*), and pericardial effusion (*arrowhead*). (*Courtesy of Dr. Kyung Soo Lee, Seoul, Korea*)

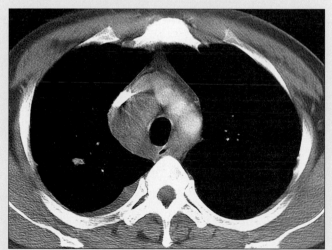

Figure 4. Primary mediastinal lymphoma of large B-cell type manifesting as mediastinal lymph node enlargement. Contrast-enhanced CT image at level of azygos arch shows extensive right paratracheal lymphadenopathy. Also note small right pleural effusion. (*Courtesy of Dr. Kyung Soo Lee, Seoul, Korea*)

DIFFERENTIAL DIAGNOSIS

- Thymoma
- Thymic carcinoma
- Germ cell tumor
- Small cell carcinoma
- Sarcoidosis

PATHOLOGY

- Revised European-American Lymphoma Classification separates lymphomas into categories by histology, immunophenotyping, and certain other characteristics.
- Current recommendations are that histologic finding of monomorphous, particularly monoclonal, infiltrates are indicative of lymphoma.
- The majority are B-cell lymphomas, but T-cell lymphomas are also seen.

INCIDENCE/PREVALENCE AND EPIDEMIOLOGY

- Non-Hodgkin lymphoma accounts for 70%-75% of all cases of lymphoma, with men and women equally affected.

- Forty to 50% of these patients have intrathoracic disease at initial presentation.
- There are 55,000 to 60,000 new cases of non-Hodgkin lymphoma diagnosed annually in the United States.
- Lymphoma constitutes about 20% of all mediastinal neoplasms in adults and 50% in children.
- The mediastinum is the sole site of involvement in about 5% of cases.

Suggested Readings

Harris NL, Jaffe ES, Stein H, et al: A revised European-American classification of lymphoid neoplasms: A proposal from the International Lymphoma Study Group. *Blood* 84:1361-1392, 1994.

Hoh CK, Glaspy J, Rosen P, et al: Whole-body FDG-PET imaging for staging of Hodgkin's disease and lymphoma. *J Nucl Med* 38:343-348, 1997.

Koss MN: Pulmonary lymphoid disorders. *Semin Diagn Pathol* 12:158-171, 1995.

Lee KS, Kim Y, Primack SL: Imaging of pulmonary lymphomas. *AJR Am J Roentgenol* 168:339-345, 1997.

Moog F, Bangerter M, Diederichs CG, et al: Lymphoma: Role of whole-body 2-deoxy-2-[F-18]fluoro-d-glucose (FDG) PET in nodal staging. *Radiology* 203:795-800, 1997.

Tatsumi M, Cohade C, Nakamoto Y, et al: Direct comparison of FDG PET and CT findings in patients with lymphoma: Initial experience. *Radiology* 237:1038-1045, 2005.

Pulmonary Non-Hodgkin Lymphoma

DEFINITION: Pulmonary involvement with Non-Hodgkin lymphoma may occur in isolation (primary pulmonary lymphoma) or in association with current or previous mediastinal lymphoma (secondary pulmonary lymphoma).

IMAGING

Radiography
Findings
- Primary low-grade marginal zone B-cell lymphoma appears as nodules or area of opacification with air bronchogram and with poorly defined margins.
- High-grade primary pulmonary lymphoma pattern is most commonly nodules or masses; less common patterns include nodules, bilateral airspace consolidation, and segmental or lobar atelectasis.
- Secondary pulmonary lymphoma may present as various patterns: bronchovascular or lymphangitic, nodular, pneumonic or alveolar, or miliary or hematogenous; less common findings include focal areas of consolidation or diffuse reticulonodular pattern.
- Lymphadenopathy, pleural effusions, and cavitated and endobronchial masses can also be present in secondary pulmonary lymphoma.

Utility
- Helpful in demonstrating presence of parenchymal disease.

CT
Findings
- Primary pulmonary lymphoma usually manifests as airspace consolidation or nodules with internal air bronchograms or adjacent ground-glass opacities.
- Thickening of interlobular septa and interlobar fissures may be seen in primary pulmonary lymphoma; lymph node enlargement is typically initially absent.
- Pleural effusion is relatively uncommon in primary pulmonary lymphoma.
- In two thirds of patients with primary pulmonary lymphoma, lesions are multiple and bilateral.
- Single nodule or mass is uncommon; nodules have well-defined margins but may have rim of ground-glass opacity (CT halo sign).
- Most common findings of secondary pulmonary lymphoma are nodules or areas of consolidation; other manifestations include ground-glass opacities, thickening of interlobular septa, and endobronchial lesions.

DIAGNOSTIC PEARLS

- Primary pulmonary lymphoma shows single or multiple nodules with irregular margins or focal areas of consolidation, usually with air bronchograms.
- Lymphadenopathy is initially absent in primary pulmonary lymphoma and usually present in secondary pulmonary lymphoma.
- Imaging findings in secondary pulmonary lymphoma include thickening of interlobular septa, discrete pulmonary nodules, and areas of consolidation.
- Primary pulmonary lymphoma should be suspected in patients with focal area of consolidation that progresses slowly over several months.

- Lymphadenopathy is initially absent in primary pulmonary lymphoma and usually present in secondary pulmonary lymphoma.

Utility
- Superior to radiography in the diagnosis and staging of lymphoma.

Positron Emission Tomography
Findings
- Positive PET results have been reported to be uncommon for low-grade primary pulmonary lymphoma.
- Anecdotal cases of increased fluorodeoxyglucose (FDG) accumulation in marginal zone B-cell lymphoma of lung have been described.
- Uptake on PET may be slight or intense in primary pulmonary lymphoma.
- High-grade primary and secondary pulmonary lymphomas show avid FDG uptake.

Utility
- PET particularly when integrated with CT (PET/CT) is superior to CT in the staging of lymphoma and in the assessment of tumor recurrence.

WHAT THE REFERRING PHYSICIAN NEEDS TO KNOW
- Primary pulmonary lymphoma is usually non-Hodgkin type.
- Secondary pulmonary lymphoma is more common in patients with recurrent disease.
- Recurrent or secondary pulmonary involvement may result from direct mediastinal nodal extension, from lymphatic or hematogenous dissemination from distant sites, or from foci of parenchymal lymphoid tissue.
- Imaging findings in primary pulmonary lymphoma include nodules with irregular margins or focal areas of consolidation with air bronchograms.
- Imaging findings in secondary pulmonary lymphoma include thickening of interlobular septa, discrete pulmonary nodules, and areas of consolidation.

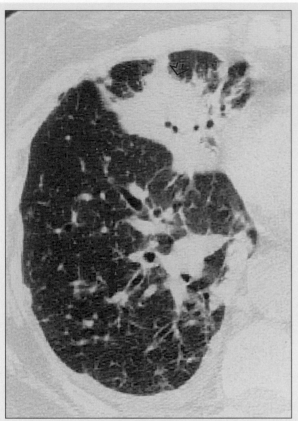

Figure 1. Primary pulmonary low-grade B-cell lymphoma. Magnified view of the right lung from high CT scan shows a focal area of consolidation with air bronchograms in the right middle lobe and a small right pleural effusion. The patient was a 73-year-old woman who presented with a 6-month history of dry cough and progressive shortness of breath.

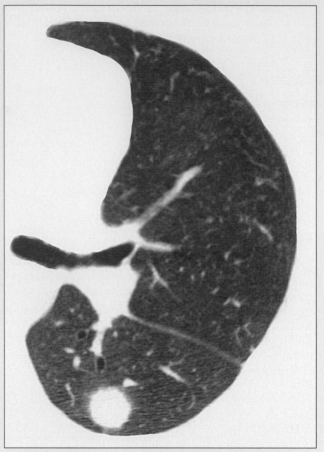

Figure 2. Post-transplantation lymphoproliferative disease after double-lung transplantation presenting with lung nodules. View of the left lung shows nodule with CT halo sign in left lower lobe.

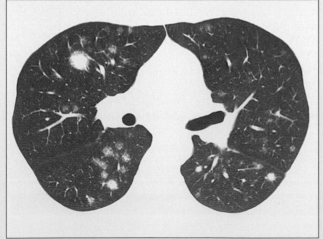

Figure 3. Secondary lung involvement of peripheral T-cell lymphoma. CT image at level of bronchus intermedius shows solid and semisolid nodules and masses in both lungs. (*Courtesy of Dr. Kyung Soo Lee, Seoul, Korea*)

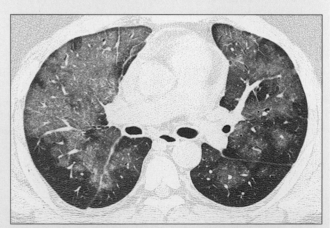

Figure 4. Recurrent lung involvement of NK/T-cell lymphoma 1 month after autologous stem cell transplantation. CT image at level of bronchus intermedius show extensive bilateral ground-glass opacities. (*Courtesy of Dr. Kyung Soo Lee, Seoul, Korea*)

CLINICAL PRESENTATION

- Solitary nodule or mass may occur without symptoms.
- Patients with diffuse lung involvement may have cough, dyspnea, or chest pain.
- Airway involvement may result in cough, hemoptysis, and obstructive symptoms, including pneumonia.
- Patients with MALT lymphoma rarely have systemic symptoms.
- Secondary pulmonary lymphoma frequently causes no symptoms.

DIFFERENTIAL DIAGNOSIS

- Pulmonary carcinoma
- Multicentric adenocarcinoma
- Focal infection
- Pulmonary metastases
- Organizing pneumonia

PATHOLOGY

- Primary pulmonary lymphoma is lymphoma developing primarily in the lung, which may be low grade or high grade.
- Most cases of primary high-grade pulmonary lymphoma are of B-cell type.
- Primary pulmonary lymphoma is usually non-Hodgkin type: MALT or low grade B-cell lymphoma.
- In MALT lymphoma, tumor infiltration develops in multiple extranodal mucosal sites throughout lung.
- Secondary pulmonary lymphoma may present as various patterns: bronchovascular or lymphangitic, nodular, pneumonic or alveolar, or miliary or hematogenous.

- Immunochemical techniques are the most accurate methods of differentiating benign from malignant lymphoproliferative disorders.
- Monomorphous, particularly monoclonal, infiltrates are indicative of lymphoma.
- Occasional cases of anaplastic (Ki-1) or peripheral T-cell lymphoma or derivation from low-grade B-cell lymphoma have been reported.

INCIDENCE/PREVALENCE AND EPIDEMIOLOGY

- Frequency of primary lymphoma is estimated to be less than 1% of all lymphomas.
- Primary low-grade B-cell lymphomas of the lung occur most commonly in adults; mean age at diagnosis is 55 to 60 years.
- High-grade primary pulmonary lymphoma occurs in patients with organ transplants or in association with AIDS.
- Secondary pulmonary lymphoma has been reported to occur in 4% of patients with non-Hodgkin lymphoma.

Suggested Readings

Ansell SM, Armitage J: Non-Hodgkin lymphoma: Diagnosis and treatment. *Mayo Clin Proc* 80:1087-1097, 2005.

Brown LR, Aughenbaugh GL: Masses of the anterior mediastinum: CT and MR imaging. *AJR Am J Roentgenol* 157:1171-1180, 1991.

Jhanwar YS, Straus DJ: The role of PET in lymphoma. *J Nucl Med* 47:1326-1334, 2006.

Lee KS, Kim Y, Primack SL: Imaging of pulmonary lymphomas. *AJR Am J Roentgenol* 168:339-345, 1997.

Angiocentric Immunoproliferative Lesions (Lymphomatoid Granulomatosis)

DEFINITION: This group of abnormalities is characterized histologically by a polymorphic lymphoid infiltrate with a variable degree of cytologic atypia and prominent vascular infiltration.

IMAGING

Radiography
Findings
- Multiple nodules or masses measuring 0.5-8.0 cm in diameter are usually seen.
- In some, initial abnormality consists of poorly defined opacities that progress over many weeks to form nodules or masses.
- Other findings include areas of consolidation (in 50% of patients) and reticulonodular pattern (in approximately 25%).
- Hilar lymph node enlargement is uncommon.

Utility
- Radiographic findings are nonspecific.
- Neoplastic process should be suspected in patients with multiple nodules or masses that progress over weeks or months.

CT
Findings
- Peribronchovascular distribution of nodules
- Coarse irregular opacities
- Conglomerating small nodules
- Large masses and occlusion of large vessels possible

Utility
- CT findings are nonspecific.
- Diagnosis should be suspected by a combination of radiologic features together with clinical manifestations of associated skin and/or central nervous system involvement.

Positron Emission Tomography
Findings
- Strong uptake of FDG in parenchymal lung lesions

Utility
- Information about PET findings of lymphomatoid granulomatosis is limited.
- Strong uptake of FDG on PET is highly suggestive of a malignant process.

DIAGNOSTIC PEARLS

- Multiple nodules or masses that are 0.5-8.0 cm in diameter
- Peribronchovascular distribution of nodules
- Areas of consolidation in 50% of patients

CLINICAL PRESENTATION

- Clinical symptoms may be related to lung parenchymal, skin, and/or central nervous system involvement.
- Patients commonly present with cough, dyspnea, fever, and malaise.
- Skin involvement occurs in approximately 50% of patients and results in patchy erythematous macular or papular lesions.
- Central nervous system manifestations occur in 25% of patients and range from mild to very severe disease.
- Patients with grade II or III lesions have involvement of extrathoracic tissues, particularly skin and central nervous system.

DIFFERENTIAL DIAGNOSIS

- Lymphoma
- Wegener granulomatosis
- Pulmonary metastases

PATHOLOGY

- Group of abnormalities characterized histologically by polymorphic lymphoid infiltrate with variable degree of cytologic atypia and prominent vascular infiltration.
- Destructive, inflammatory granulomatous angiitis.
- Lymphoid infiltrate composed of atypical and immature cells with abundant mitoses and a paucity of polymorphonuclear or eosinophilic leukocytes.

WHAT THE REFERRING PHYSICIAN NEEDS TO KNOW
- Disease progression is rapid.
- Symptoms are related to pulmonary, skin, or central nervous system involvement.
- Peribronchovascular distribution of nodules occurs.
- Patients with symptoms may be treated with corticosteroids and antineoplastic drugs such as cyclophosphamide.
- Disease has a poor prognosis, with half or more of patients succumbing within 5 years.

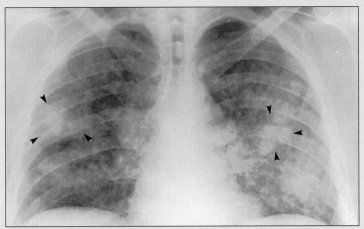

Figure 1. Angiocentric immunoproliferative lesion (lymphomatoid granulomatosis). Posteroanterior chest radiograph shows bilateral confluent and isolated nodular opacities; some of the larger opacities (*arrowheads*) possess features of airspace consolidation. Bilateral hilar lymph node enlargement is present, and the aortopulmonary window is prominent, suggesting mediastinal node involvement. (*From Müller NL, Fraser RS, Colman NC, et al: Radiologic Diagnosis of Diseases of the Chest. Philadelphia, Saunders, 2001.*)

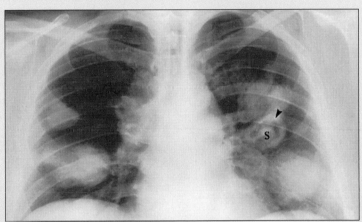

Figure 2. Angiocentric immunoproliferative lesion (lymphomatoid granulomatosis). Two months later after initial radiograph (see Fig. 1), a repeat chest radiograph shows that the diffuse disease has resolved but has been replaced by large cavitary and noncavitary nodules. One cavitary lesion on the left (*arrowhead*) contains a central loose body (S) that could represent infarcted tissue or a blood clot. Several of the nodules relate to the more confluent areas of consolidation identified in the first radiograph in Figure 1. Open-lung biopsy revealed infarcts caused by involvement of peripheral vessels by lymphomatoid granulomatosis. The patient was a 52-year-old man. (*From Müller NL, Fraser RS, Colman NC, et al: Radiologic Diagnosis of Diseases of the Chest. Philadelphia, Saunders, 2001.*)

- Varied tumors ranging from those composed predominantly of benign-appearing cells (grade I) to frankly malignant (grade III).
- Neoplastic cells with either T-cell or B-cell phenotype.

INCIDENCE/PREVALENCE AND EPIDEMIOLOGY

- Uncommon

Suggested Readings

Donnelly TJ, Tuder RM, Vendegna TR: A 48-year-old woman with peripheral neuropathy, hypercalcemia, and pulmonary infiltrates. *Chest* 114:1205-1209, 1998.

Fauci AS, Haynes BF, Costa J, et al: Lymphomatoid granulomatosis: Prospective clinical and therapeutic experience over 10 years. *N Engl J Med* 306:68-74, 1982.

Katzenstein AL, Carrington CB, Liebow AA: Lymphomatoid granulomatosis: A clinicopathologic study of 152 cases. *Cancer* 43:360-373, 1979.

Lee JS, Tuder R, Lynch DA: Lymphomatoid granulomatosis: Radiologic features and pathologic correlations. *AJR Am J Roentgenol* 175:1335-1339, 2000.

Liebow AA, Carrington CR, Friedman PJ: Lymphomatoid granulomatosis. *Hum Pathol* 3:457-558, 1972.

Prenovault JM, Weisbrod GL, Herman SJ: Lymphomatoid granulomatosis: A review of 12 cases. *Can Assoc Radiol J* 39:263-266, 1988.

Wechsler RJ, Steiner RM, Israel HL, Patchefsky AS: Chest radiograph in lymphomatoid granulomatosis: Comparison with Wegener granulomatosis. *AJR Am J Roentgenol* 42:79-83, 1984.

Leukemia

DEFINITION: In leukemia, chest involvement may include lymphadenopathy, lung parenchyma infiltration, and pleural and chest wall abnormalities.

IMAGING

Radiography
Findings
- Mediastinal widening
- Mediastinal and hilar lymphadenopathy
- Septal lines
- Focal consolidative process to diffuse, bilateral reticular or reticulonodular opacities

Utility
- Initial modality for suspected cases
- Used in follow-up

CT
Findings
- Mediastinal lymphadenopathy is relatively common in lymphocytic leukemia and less common in myelogenous leukemia.
- High-resolution CT findings of pulmonary leukemic infiltration include smooth or nodular thickening of interlobular septa, thickening of bronchovascular bundles, nodules, and ground-glass opacities.

Utility
- CT gives more accurate assessment of presence, pattern, and extent of mediastinal and parenchymal disease.

CLINICAL PRESENTATION

- Anemia, fever, weight loss, cough

DIFFERENTIAL DIAGNOSIS

- Lymphoma
- Lymphangitic carcinomatosis
- Pulmonary edema
- Pneumonia

DIAGNOSTIC PEARLS

- Mediastinal and hilar lymphadenopathy is relatively common
- Pulmonary involvement is uncommon
- Pulmonary abnormalities are usually due to complications related to leukemia or its treatment
- Most common pulmonary complications: infection, hemorrhage, and edema

PATHOLOGY

- Involvement of thoracic lymph nodes: seen in lymphocytic leukemia and myelogenous leukemia.
- Granulocytic sarcoma (previously known as chloroma): extramedullary masses of malignant myeloid precursor cells that may be seen in lungs, mediastinum, pleura, pericardium, and chest wall.
- Pulmonary involvement with leukemia uncommon; has perilymphatic distribution.

INCIDENCE/PREVALENCE AND EPIDEMIOLOGY

- Mediastinal lymph node enlargement is relatively common, particularly in acute and chronic lymphocytic leukemia.
- Clinically significant leukemic infiltration of lungs is a rare diagnosis.
- Involvement of thoracic lymph nodes is present at autopsy in up to 67% of patients with lymphocytic leukemia and in up to 36% of patients with myelogenous leukemia.
- Pulmonary abnormalities seen in patients with leukemia are most commonly due to infection, edema, or hemorrhage.

WHAT THE REFERRING PHYSICIAN NEEDS TO KNOW

- Mediastinal lymph node enlargement is relatively common, particularly in acute and chronic lymphocytic leukemia.
- Clinically significant leukemic infiltration of lungs is a rare diagnosis.
- When present, it is usually seen in association with uncontrolled leukemia.
- Most common pulmonary complications in patients with leukemia are infection, hemorrhage, and edema.

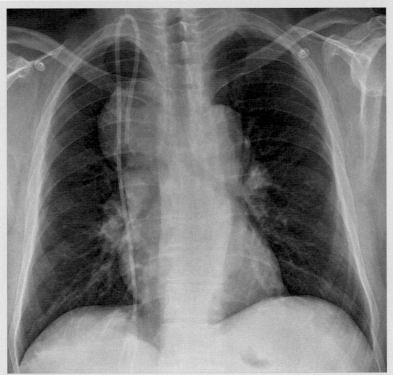

Figure 1. Leukemia. Chest radiograph in a 66-year-old man with chronic lymphocytic leukemia shows extensive right paratracheal and bilateral hilar lymphadenopathy. Also noted is a central venous line in place.

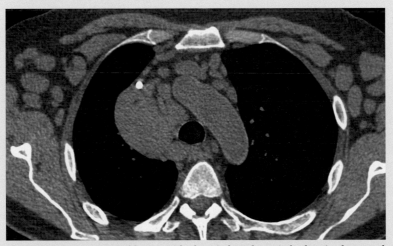

Figure 2. Leukemia. CT scan of the chest in a 66-year-old man with chronic lymphocytic leukemia shows enlarged axillary, prevascular, internal mammary, paratracheal, and paraesophageal lymph nodes. Also noted is a central veneous line in place.

Suggested Readings

Fritz J, Vogel W, Bares R, Horger M: Radiologic spectrum of extramedullary relapse of myelogenous leukemia in adults. *AJR Am J Roentgenol* 189:209-218, 2007.

Heyneman LE, Johkoh T, Ward S, et al: Pulmonary leukemic infiltrates: High-resolution CT findings in 10 patients. *AJR Am J Roentgenol* 174:517-521, 2000.

Koh TT, Colby TV, Müller NL: Myeloid leukemias and lung involvement. *Semin Respir Crit Care Med* 26:514-519, 2005.

Maile CW, Moore AV, Ulreich S, Putman CE: Chest radiographic-pathologic correlation in adult leukemia patients. *Invest Radiol* 18:495-499, 1983.

Interstitial Lung Diseases

Part 30

IDIOPATHIC INTERSTITIAL PNEUMONIAS

Idiopathic Pulmonary Fibrosis

DEFINITION: Idiopathic pulmonary fibrosis is defined as a chronic fibrosing interstitial pneumonia of unknown cause, limited to the lung and associated with a histologic appearance of usual interstitial pneumonia.

IMAGING

Radiography

Findings

- Symmetric, predominantly basal, small to medium-sized irregular linear opacities form a reticular pattern.
- These opacities may be diffuse throughout both lungs or distributed in lower lung zones or peripherally.
- As disease progresses, abnormalities become more diffuse, assuming a coarser reticular or reticulonodular pattern associated with loss of volume.
- Advanced disease is characterized by presence of honeycomb cysts usually measuring 0.5-1.0 cm in diameter.
- Decreased lung volumes are radiographically evident at initial evaluation in 50%-60% of cases.
- Chest radiograph is normal in about 10% of patients.
- Evidence of pleural disease (effusion, pneumothorax, or diffuse thickening) is uncommon.

Utility

- Radiographic findings of idiopathic pulmonary fibrosis often are sufficient to suggest the diagnosis, but the degree of confidence in the specific diagnosis is usually low.

CT

Findings

- Patchy irregular intralobular lines with reticular pattern involving mainly subpleural regions and lower lung zones.
- Architectural distortion, dilation of bronchi and bronchioles (traction bronchiectasis, bronchiolectasis), and irregular pleural, vascular, and bronchial interfaces.
- Air-containing cysts measuring 2 to 20 mm in diameter (honeycombing).
- Predominantly subpleural or lower lung zone distribution of reticular pattern and honeycombing.

DIAGNOSTIC PEARLS

- Chest radiograph typically shows reticular pattern mainly in lower lobes, but normal radiograph does not exclude diagnosis.
- High-resolution CT typically shows reticular pattern and honeycombing in a subpleural and basal distribution.
- Serial high-resolution CT scans typically show progressive increase in extent and severity of fibrosis over several months or years.
- In the proper clinical context, a confident diagnosis can be made on high-resolution CT in 50% to 60% of cases based on predominantly peripheral and basal reticulation and honeycombing.

- Mild ground-glass opacities present in majority and emphysema evident in 30%; extensive ground-glass opacities more common in acute exacerbation of idiopathic pulmonary fibrosis or superimposed opportunistic infection.
- Mild mediastinal lymph node enlargement evident on CT in 70%, involving only one or two nodal stations.
- Progressive increase in extent and severity of fibrosis over several months or years, typically shown by serial high-resolution CT.

Utility

- High-resolution CT findings are highly specific.
- Diagnostic accuracy based on high-resolution CT findings increases with severity of disease.
- In the appropriate clinical setting the diagnosis of idiopathic pulmonary fibrosis can be made on high-resolution CT provided that the findings are classic.

WHAT THE REFERRING PHYSICIAN NEEDS TO KNOW

- Chest radiograph typically shows a reticular pattern mainly in lower lobes, but normal radiograph does not exclude the diagnosis.
- High-resolution CT typically shows a reticular pattern and honeycombing in a subpleural and basal distribution.
- In 50%-60% of patients, confident diagnosis can be made based on characteristic clinical and high-resolution CT findings.
- Pulmonary carcinoma develops in approximately 10% of patients with idiopathic pulmonary fibrosis.

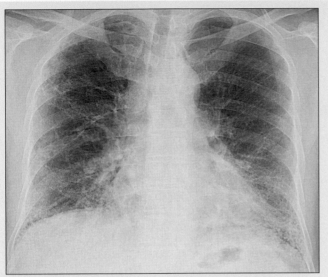

Figure 1. **Idiopathic pulmonary fibrosis: radiographic manifestations.** Posteroanterior chest radiograph in a 58-year-old man with idiopathic pulmonary fibrosis shows extensive bilateral reticular pattern worse in the lower lung zones.

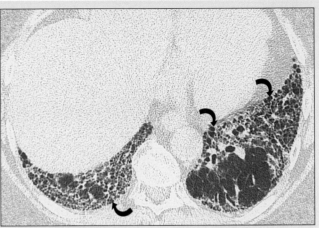

Figure 2. **Idiopathic pulmonary fibrosis with mild honeycombing.** High-resolution CT image at the level of the lung bases shows more extensive reticulation and mild subpleural honeycombing (*arrows*).

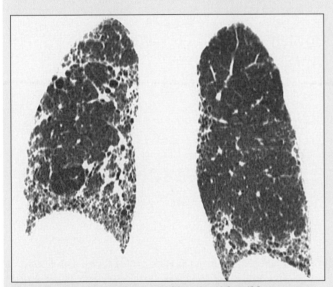

Figure 3. **Idiopathic pulmonary fibrosis with mild honeycombing.** Coronal reformatted image demonstrates reticulation in all lobes but most severe involvement in the subpleural lung regions and lung bases. The patient was a 70-year-old man with idiopathic pulmonary fibrosis.

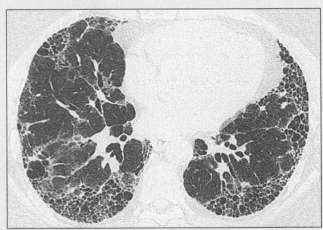

Figure 4. **Idiopathic pulmonary fibrosis with extensive honeycombing.** High-resolution CT images at the level of the lower lung zone show extensive subpleural honeycombing mainly in the lower lobes. Note patchy distribution of the subpleural fibrosis alternating with areas of relatively normal lung parenchyma.

CLINICAL PRESENTATION

- Progressive dyspnea, nonproductive cough, weight loss, and fatigue occur.
- Clinical course of idiopathic pulmonary fibrosis is one of relentless progressive increase in extent of fibrosis and severity of clinical manifestations.
- Acute deterioration with abrupt, unexpected worsening of symptoms may occur secondary to infection, pulmonary embolism, pneumothorax, or heart failure.
- If no cause for acute decline is identified, these episodes are called "acute exacerbation" or "accelerated phase" of idiopathic pulmonary fibrosis.
- Deterioration is gradual and inexorable in most patients, with increasing shortness of breath and eventually respiratory failure.
- Mean survival after time of diagnosis ranges from 2 to 4 years.

DIFFERENTIAL DIAGNOSIS

- Chronic hypersensitivity pneumonitis
- Asbestos-related parenchymal disease
- Nonspecific interstitial pneumonia (NSIP)
- Usual interstitial pneumonia in collagen vascular disease

PATHOLOGY

- Idiopathic pulmonary fibrosis is a form of chronic fibrosing interstitial pneumonia limited to the lung.
- Pathogenesis is unclear.
- Epithelial injury and activation of fibroblast foci are currently considered main early events that trigger a cascade of changes.
- Idiopathic pulmonary fibrosis by definition is idiopathic usual interstitial pneumonia.
- Key histologic features are temporal and geographic heterogeneity, fibroblastic foci, and predilection for periphery of lobule and subpleural regions.
- However, the histologic pattern of usual interstitial pneumonia is not diagnostic of idiopathic pulmonary fibrosis—it may also be seen in asbestosis, collagen vascular disease, chronic hypersensitivity pneumonitis, and, occasionally, drug reaction.

INCIDENCE/PREVALENCE AND EPIDEMIOLOGY

- Idiopathic pulmonary fibrosis is the most common idiopathic interstitial lung disease.
- Prevalence is 20 per 100,000 for males and 13 per 100,000 for females.
- Incidence is 11 per 100,000 per year in males and 7 per 100,000 per year in females.
- Majority of patients with idiopathic pulmonary fibrosis are older than 50 years of age, and approximately 80% are age 65 years and older.
- Idiopathic pulmonary fibrosis has been reported worldwide, in both rural and urban settings, and has no racial predominance.
- It is more common in smokers.
- Occasionally, clusters of idiopathic pulmonary fibrosis may occur in families.

Suggested Readings

American Thoracic Society: Idiopathic pulmonary fibrosis: Diagnosis and treatment. International consensus statement. American Thoracic society (ATS) and the European Respiratory Society (ERS). *Am J Respir Crit Care Med* 161:646-664, 2000.

American Thoracic Society, European Respiratory Society: American Thoracic Society/European Respiratory Society International Multidisciplinary Consensus Classification of the idiopathic interstitial pneumonias. *Am J Respir Crit Care Med* 165:277-304, 2002.

Churg A, Müller NL: Cellular vs fibrosing interstitial pneumonias and prognosis: A practical classification of the idiopathic interstitial pneumonias and pathologically/radiologically similar conditions. *Chest* 130:1566-1570, 2006.

Kim DS, Collard HR, King T Jr: Classification and natural history of the idiopathic interstitial pneumonias. *Proc Am Thorac Soc* 3:285-292, 2006.

Kim DS, Park JH, Park BK, et al: Acute exacerbation of idiopathic pulmonary fibrosis: Frequency and clinical features. *Eur Respir J* 27:143-150, 2006.

Lynch DA, Godwin J, Safrin S, et al: High-resolution computed tomography in idiopathic pulmonary fibrosis: Diagnosis and prognosis. *Am J Respir Crit Care Med* 172:488-493, 2005.

Lynch DA, Travis WD, Müller NL, et al: Idiopathic interstitial pneumonias: CT features. *Radiology* 236:10-21, 2005.

Silva CIS, Müller NL, Lynch DA, et al: Chronic hypersensitivity pneumonitis: Differentiation from idiopathic pulmonary fibrosis and nonspecific interstitial pneumonia by using thin-section CT. *Radiology* 246:288-297, 2008.

Silva CIS, Müller NL, Fujimoto K, et al: Acute exacerbation of chronic interstitial pneumonia: High-resolution computed tomography and pathologic findings. *J Thorac Imaging* 22:221-229, 2007.

Nonspecific Interstitial Pneumonia

DEFINITION: Nonspecific interstitial pneumonia is a chronic interstitial lung disease characterized by relatively homogenous expansion of the alveolar walls by inflammation and/or fibrosis.

IMAGING

Radiography
Findings
- Bilateral patchy or confluent ground-glass opacities involving mainly middle and lower lung zones.
- Reticular pattern or combination of reticular opacities and ground-glass opacities.

Utility
- In up to 15% of patients with nonspecific interstitial pneumonia and abnormal high-resolution CT findings, chest radiograph is normal.

CT
Findings
- Bilateral symmetric ground-glass opacities.
- Fine reticular pattern and traction bronchiectasis, and traction bronchiolectasis superimposed on ground-glass opacities.
- Honeycombing in 10%-30% of patients but usually mild and only at lung bases.
- Mainly involves lower lung zones (60%-90% of patients), predominantly peripheral lung regions (50%-70% of patients).
- Fibrosis often spares the lung immediately adjacent to the pleura in the lower dorsal regions.
- Mediastinal lymph node enlargement common but mild and involving only one or two nodal stations.

Utility
- High-resolution CT is superior to radiography in demonstrating the presence, pattern, and distribution of parenchymal findings.
- High-resolution CT is recommended almost routinely in the initial evaluation of patients with suspected chronic interstitial lung disease.

CLINICAL PRESENTATION

- Progressive dyspnea and dry cough with duration ranging from 6 months to 3 years before diagnosis are noted.
- Finger clubbing occurs in 10%-35% of patients.

DIAGNOSTIC PEARLS

- Bilateral symmetric ground-glass opacities are seen.
- Fine reticular pattern and traction bronchiectasis superimposed on ground-glass opacities are evident.
- Fibrotic nonspecific interstitial pneumonia often spares lung immediately adjacent to pleura at two or more levels in the lower lobe dorsal regions.
- Usually involves mainly the lung bases.
- Honeycombing uncommon at presentation.

- Auscultation reveals basal or widespread crackles.
- Lung function is restricted (decreased total lung capacity and vital capacity).
- Gas exchange is impaired.
- Patients may develop acute deterioration with abrupt worsening of symptoms due to infections, pulmonary embolism, pneumothorax, or heart failure.

DIFFERENTIAL DIAGNOSIS

- Cryptogenic organizing pneumonia (idiopathic bronchiolitis obliterans organizing pneumonia)
- Hypersensitivity pneumonitis
- Idiopathic pulmonary fibrosis
- Acute interstitial pneumonia
- Lymphoid interstitial pneumonia

PATHOLOGY

- There is relative homogeneous expansion of alveolar walls by inflammation and/or fibrosis.
- Pathogenesis is unknown (hence, idiopathic).
- Histologic findings may range from inflammation to predominant fibrosis.
- Cellular nonspecific interstitial pneumonia: alveolar septa are thickened by infiltrates of lymphocytes and plasma cells.

WHAT THE REFERRING PHYSICIAN NEEDS TO KNOW

- Patients tend to be younger than patients with idiopathic pulmonary fibrosis.
- Clinical, functional manifestations resemble those of idiopathic pulmonary fibrosis.
- Nonspecific interstitial pneumonia has better prognosis than idiopathic pulmonary fibrosis.
- Prognosis is better in cellular type than in fibrotic type.
- Drug reaction, collagen vascular diseases, and hypersensitivity pneumonitis should be excluded before making a diagnosis of idiopathic nonspecific interstitial pneumonia.
- Diagnosis of nonspecific interstitial pneumonia requires a team approach, including clinician, radiologist, and pathologist.

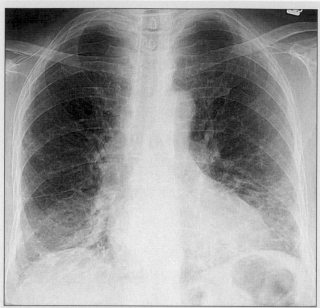

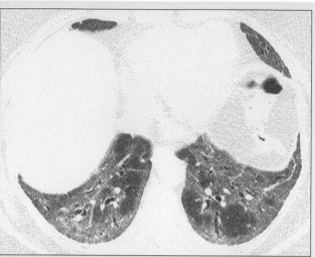

Figure 2. Nonspecific interstitial pneumonia: high-resolution CT findings. High-resolution CT in a 48-year-old woman with nonspecific interstitial pneumonia shows extensive bilateral ground-glass opacities. The findings are consistent with the cellular type of disease.

Figure 1. Nonspecific interstitial pneumonia: radiographic findings. Posteroanterior chest radiograph in a woman with nonspecific interstitial pneumonia shows hazy increased opacity (ground-glass opacity) and irregular linear opacities in the middle and lower lung zones.

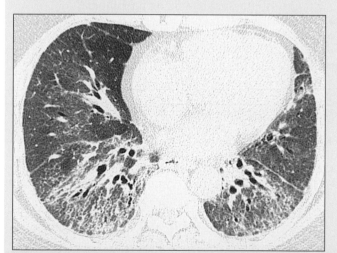

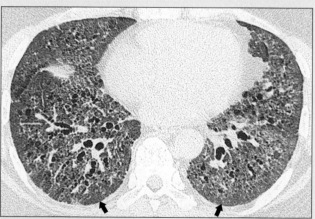

Figure 3. Fibrotic nonspecific interstitial pneumonia: high-resolution CT findings. High-resolution CT in a 62-year-old man with nonspecific interstitial pneumonia shows extensive bilateral ground-glass opacities. A reticular pattern is present mainly in the lower lobes and is associated with lower lobe volume loss with posterior displacement of the major fissures due to lower lobe fibrosis.

Figure 4. Nonspecific interstitial pneumonia: relative subpleural sparing. High-resolution CT in a 60-year-old man with nonspecific interstitial pneumonia shows extensive bilateral ground-glass opacities, traction bronchiectasis and bronchiolectasis, and reticulation. The reticulation is less severe in the lung immediately adjacent to the pleura (*arrows*) than in the lung 1 cm away from the pleura (relative subpleural sparing), a characteristic finding seen in approximately 50% of patients with the fibrotic form of the disease.

- Fibrotic nonspecific interstitial pneumonia: thickening is mainly due to collagen accumulation.
- Fibrosis may involve alveolar septa, peribronchiolar interstitium, interlobular septa, and visceral pleura.
- Fibroblastic foci (aggregates of proliferating fibroblasts, myofibroblasts) are absent or inconspicuous.

INCIDENCE/PREVALENCE AND EPIDEMIOLOGY

- This second most common interstitial pneumonia accounts for 14%-35% of cases.
- It may be idiopathic but it is also a common reaction pattern seen in collagen vascular diseases, hypersensitivity pneumonitis, and drug toxicity.
- Median age of onset at symptoms is 40 to 50 years.
- It may occur in childhood or the elderly and has been reported in patients ranging from 9 to 75 years of age.

Suggested Readings

American Thoracic Society, European Respiratory Society: American Thoracic Society/European Respiratory Society International Multidisciplinary Consensus Classification of the Idiopathic Interstitial Pneumonias. *Am J Respir Crit Care Med* 165:277-304, 2002.

Churg A, Müller NL: Cellular vs fibrosing interstitial pneumonias and prognosis: A practical classification of the idiopathic interstitial pneumonias and pathologically/radiologically similar conditions. *Chest* 130:1566-1570, 2006.

Kim DS, Collard HR, King T Jr: Classification and natural history of the idiopathic interstitial pneumonias. *Proc Am Thorac Soc* 3:285-292, 2006.

Lynch DA, Travis WD, Müller NL, et al: Idiopathic interstitial pneumonias: CT features. *Radiology* 236:10-21, 2005.

Silva CIS, Müller NL, Hansell DM, et al: Nonspecific interstitial pneumonia and idiopathic pulmonary fibrosis: Changes in pattern and distribution of disease over time. *Radiology* 247:251-259, 2008.

Silva CIS, Müller NL, Lynch DA, et al: Chronic hypersensitivity pneumonitis: Differentiation from idiopathic pulmonary fibrosis and nonspecific interstitial pneumonia by using thin-section CT. *Radiology* 246:288-297, 2008.

Cryptogenic Organizing Pneumonia (Idiopathic Bronchiolitis Obliterans Organizing Pneumonia)

DEFINITION: Organizing pneumonia is a histologic pattern characterized by the presence of intraluminal granulation tissue polyps within alveolar ducts and surrounding alveoli associated with chronic inflammation of the surrounding lung parenchyma.

IMAGING

Radiography

Findings

- Bilateral symmetric or asymmetric areas of consolidation.
- Consolidation usually has a patchy distribution but may involve mainly the subpleural regions with indistinct margins and contain air bronchograms.
- Lung volume may appear preserved or decreased.
- Occasionally areas of consolidation may be round, resulting in multiple large nodular opacities or masses.
- A pattern of small nodular, reticular, or reticulonodular opacities may be seen in association with airspace opacities or as an isolated finding.
- Small unilateral or bilateral pleural effusions occur in about 20% of patients.

Utility

- Chest radiograph is the first and commonly the only imaging modality used in the assessment of patients with organizing pneumonia.

CT

Findings

- Bilateral patchy areas of consolidation most commonly involving mainly middle and lower lung zones in a predominantly peribronchial and/or subpleural distribution.
- Perilobular pattern.
- Crescentic or ring-shaped opacities surrounding areas of ground-glass opacification (atoll sign or reversed halo sign).
- Ground-glass opacities, small centrilobular nodules, and large nodules or mass-like areas of consolidation.
- Smooth septal thickening superimposed on the ground-glass opacities ("crazy-paving" pattern) may occur but is uncommon.
- Nodular opacities measuring 1-10 mm, usually in association with areas of consolidation.

DIAGNOSTIC PEARLS

- Bilateral patchy areas of consolidation most commonly involving mainly the middle and lower lung zones in a predominately peribronchial and/or subpleural distribution
- Atoll sign or reversed halo sign
- Progressive increase in bilateral consolidation over several weeks in spite of antibiotic therapy

- Large nodules or mass-like areas of consolidation, bronchial wall thickening and dilatation, and small unilateral or bilateral pleural effusions.

Utility

- High-resolution CT can be helpful in patients with suspected diagnosis and nonspecific radiographic findings.
- CT is superior to radiography in demonstrating characteristic and common peribronchial and subpleural distribution of organizing pneumonia and perilobular opacities.

CLINICAL PRESENTATION

- Cough that is dry or productive of clear sputum and progressive dyspnea of relatively short duration (median, < 3 months).
- Weight loss, chills, and intermittent fever.
- Clinical presentation similar to that of community-acquired pneumonia.
- Auscultation: localized or widespread crackles.
- Finger clubbing absent.
- Pulmonary function tests: mild to moderate restrictive ventilatory pattern with decrease in total lung capacity and vital capacity.
- Patients often hypoxemic.

WHAT THE REFERRING PHYSICIAN NEEDS TO KNOW

- The most common radiographic manifestation of cryptogenic organizing pneumonia consists of bilateral symmetric or asymmetric areas of consolidation resembling bronchopneumonia.
- Bilateral areas of consolidation increasing in extent over several weeks in spite of antibiotic therapy are suggestive of the disease.
- Cryptogenic organizing pneumonia is readily distinguished from the majority of other chronic interstitial and airspace lung diseases on high-resolution CT.
- CT findings frequently resemble those of chronic eosinophilic pneumonia.

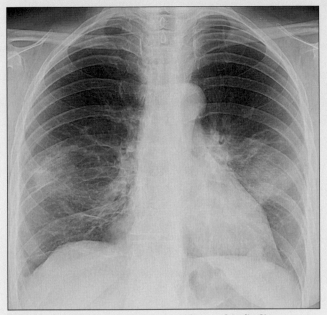

Figure 1. Organizing pneumonia: radiographic findings.
Posteroanterior chest radiograph shows patchy bilateral areas of consolidation and ground-glass opacities. The patient was a 50-year-old woman with cryptogenic organizing pneumonia.

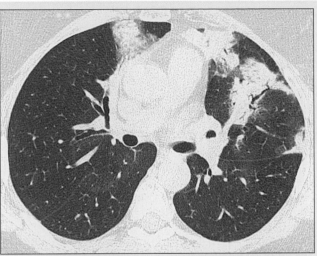

Figure 2. Organizing pneumonia: high-resolution CT findings.
High-resolution CT image shows bilateral peripheral and peribronchial areas of consolidation in the upper lobes. The patient was a 55-year-old woman with cryptogenic organizing pneumonia.

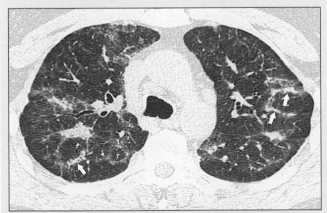

Figure 3. Organizing pneumonia with perilobular opacities.
High-resolution CT shows bilateral ground-glass opacities and polygonal linear opacities (*arrows*) marginating the secondary lobules. These polygonal arcades reflect the presence of consolidation in the alveoli adjacent to the interlobular septa and are referred to as perilobular opacities.

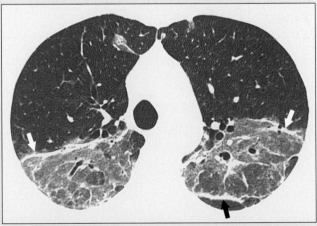

Figure 4. Organizing pneumonia: ground-glass opacity and reversed halo sign. High-resolution CT image in a 58-year-old immunocompromised woman with organizing pneumonia shows extensive bilateral ground-glass opacities, a few small nodular opacities, and bilateral crescentic and ring-like consolidation (*arrows*) surrounding areas of ground-glass opacification (reversed halo sign).

DIFFERENTIAL DIAGNOSIS

- Organizing pneumonia of known etiology
- Lymphoma
- Sarcoidosis
- Chronic eosinophilic pneumonia
- Wegener granuomatosis
- Bacterial, fungal, or viral pneumonia

PATHOLOGY

- Histologically, intraluminal plugs of granulation tissue within alveolar ducts and surrounding alveoli with or without concomitant granulation tissue polyps within the respiratory bronchioles.
- No underlying cause.
- Distribution typically patchy and involving connective tissue of same age.
- Mild associated interstitial inflammation typically presents as type II cell metaplasia and an increase in alveolar macrophages.

INCIDENCE/PREVALENCE AND EPIDEMIOLOGY

- Cryptogenic organizing pneumonia accounts for 4%-12% of cases of idiopathic interstitial pneumonias.
- Mean annual incidence is 1 to 2 cases per 100,000 population.

- Cryptogenic organizing pneumonia has an equal sex distribution and is approximately twice more common in nonsmokers than in smokers.
- The average age at presentation is 50 to 60 years (range: 20-80 years).
- Occasionally, cryptogenic organizing pneumonia may have seasonal recurrence.

Suggested Readings

American Thoracic Society, European Respiratory Society: American Thoracic Society/European Respiratory Society International Multidisciplinary Consensus Classification of the Idiopathic Interstitial Pneumonias. *Am J Respir Crit Care Med* 165:277-304, 2002.

Cordier JF: Cryptogenic organising pneumonia. *Eur Respir J* 28: 422-446, 2006.

Lynch DA, Travis WD, Müller NL, et al: Idiopathic interstitial pneumonias: CT features. *Radiology* 236:10-21, 2005.

Ryu JH: Classification and approach to bronchiolar diseases. *Curr Opin Pulm Med* 12:145-151, 2006.

Organizing Pneumonia of Known Etiology

DEFINITION: Organizing pneumonia can be secondary to underlying conditions such as infection, connective tissue disease (particularly rheumatoid arthritis and polymyositis), inflammatory bowel disease, inhalational injury, hypersensitivity pneumonitis, drug reaction, radiation therapy, and aspiration.

IMAGING

Radiography

Findings
- Patchy unilateral or bilateral consolidation
- Symmetric or asymmetric distribution

Utility
- First and commonly the only imaging modality used in the assessment of patients with organizing pneumonia

CT

Findings
- Patchy unilateral or bilateral areas of consolidation are often in a peribronchial or subpleural distribution and frequently associated with perilobular opacities.
- Ground-glass opacities, small centrilobular nodules, and large nodules or mass-like areas of consolidation may occur.
- Bronchial wall thickening and dilatation and small unilateral or bilateral pleural effusions are seen.
- Underlying cause (e.g., lung tumor, lymphoma) may be apparent on CT.
- High attenuation within areas of consolidation is characteristic of organizing pneumonia reaction to amiodarone.

Utility
- High-resolution CT can be helpful in patients with suspected diagnosis and nonspecific radiographic findings.
- CT is superior to radiography in demonstrating characteristic and common peribronchial and subpleural distribution of organizing pneumonia and perilobular opacities.
- Findings are similar to those of cryptogenic organizing pneumonia.

CLINICAL PRESENTATION

- Cough, dry or productive of clear sputum, and progressive dyspnea of relatively short duration (median, < 3 months) present.

DIAGNOSTIC PEARLS

- Bilateral areas of consolidation in peribronchial or subpleural distribution and frequently associated with perilobular opacities.
- Organizing pneumonia is commonly secondary to connective tissue disease, drug reaction, inhalational injury, and pulmonary infection.

- Weight loss, chills, and intermittent fever occur.
- Clinical presentation mimics that of community-acquired pneumonia.

DIFFERENTIAL DIAGNOSIS

- Cryptogenic organizing pneumonia (idiopathic bronchiolitis obliterans organizing pneumonia)
- Bronchioloalveolar cell carcinoma
- Lymphoma
- Sarcoidosis
- Wegener granulomatosis

PATHOLOGY

- Intraluminal granulation tissue polyps within alveolar ducts and surrounding alveoli associated with chronic inflammation of surrounding lung parenchyma
- Underlying conditions: infection, connective tissue disease, inflammatory bowel disease, inhalational injury, hypersensitivity pneumonitis, drug reaction, radiation therapy, and aspiration

INCIDENCE/PREVALENCE AND EPIDEMIOLOGY

- Organizing pneumonia is a common reaction pattern.

WHAT THE REFERRING PHYSICIAN NEEDS TO KNOW

- Organizing pneumonia is a common histologic reaction pattern.
- Conditions associated with organizing pneumonia include infection, drug reaction, collagen vascular disease, hypersensitivity pneumonitis, vasculitis (particularly Wegener granulomatosis), hemorrhage, cocaine abuse, and neoplasms (lymphoma, lung cancer).
- Clinical presentation of organizing pneumonia mimics that of community-acquired pneumonia.
- The radiographic findings consist of patchy unilateral or bilateral areas of consolidation.
- The characteristic CT manifestations consist of bilateral areas of consolidation in peribronchial or subpleural distribution and frequently associated with perilobular opacities.

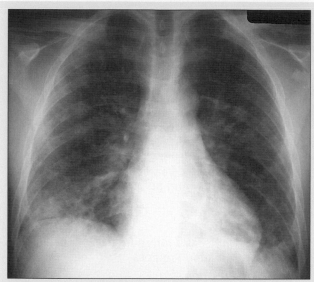

Figure 1. Organizing pneumonia in polymyositis. Chest radiograph shows bilateral areas of consolidation involving mainly the lower lung zones.

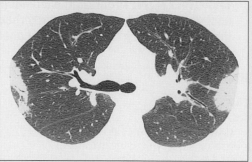

Figure 2. Organizing pneumonia secondary to drug reaction. High-resolution CT image shows patchy bilateral air space consolidation in a peripheral distribution with associated air bronchograms. The patient was a 20-year-old woman who developed organizing pneumonia secondary to a 5-aminosalicylic acid derivate (mesalamine) for treatment of ulcerative colitis. (*From Silva CI, Müller NL: Drug-induced lung diseases: Most common reaction patterns and corresponding high-resolution CT manifestations. Semin Ultrasound CT MRI 27:111-116, 2006, with permission.*)

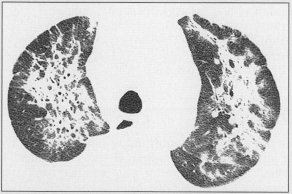

Figure 3. Organizing pneumonia (broncholitis obliterans organizing pneumonia–like reaction) due to amiodarone. High-resolution CT image at the level of the upper lobes shows extensive bilateral areas of consolidation in a peribronchial distribution. (*From Silva CI, Müller NL: Drug-induced lung diseases: Most common reaction patterns and corresponding high-resolution CT manifestations. Semin Ultrasound CT MRI 27:111-116, 2006 with permission.*)

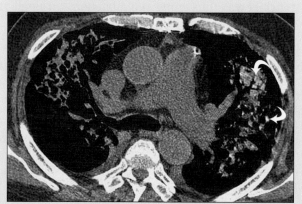

Figure 4. Organizing pneumonia (broncholitis obliterans organizing pneumonia–like reaction) due to amiodarone. Soft tissue window image at the level of the upper lobes shows areas of high attenuation (*arrows*) characteristic of amiodarone toxicity. Also noted are small bilateral pleural effusions secondary to left-sided heart failure. (*From Silva CI, Müller NL: Drug-induced lung diseases: Most common reaction patterns and corresponding high-resolution CT manifestations. Semin Ultrasound CT MRI 27:111-116, 2006 with permission.*)

■ Conditions commonly associated with organizing pneumonia include infection, drug reaction, collagen vascular disease, hypersensitivity pneumonitis, vasculitis (particularly Wegener granulomatosis), hemorrhage, cocaine abuse, and neoplasms (lymphoma, lung cancer).

Suggested Readings

American Thoracic Society, European Respiratory Society: American Thoracic Society/European Respiratory Society International Multidisciplinary Consensus Classification of the Idiopathic Interstitial Pneumonias. *Am J Respir Crit Care Med* 165:277-304, 2002.

Epler GR: Bronchiolitis obliterans organizing pneumonia. *Arch Intern Med* 161(2):158-164, 2001.

Lynch DA, Travis WD, Müller NL, et al: Idiopathic interstitial pneumonias: CT features. *Radiology* 236:10-21, 2005.

Oikonomou A, Hansell DM: Organizing pneumonia: The many morphological faces. *Eur Radiol* 12(6):1486-1496, 2002.

Ryu JH: Classification and approach to bronchiolar diseases. *Curr Opin Pulm Med* 12:145-151, 2006.

Silva CI, Müller NL: Drug-induced lung diseases: Most common reaction patterns and corresponding high-resolution CT manifestations. *Semin Ultrasound CT MR* 27(2):111-116, 2006.

Acute Interstitial Pneumonia

DEFINITION: Acute interstitial pneumonia is a severe acute disease of unknown etiology that usually occurs in a previously healthy person and produces histologic findings of diffuse alveolar damage.

IMAGING

Radiography
Findings
- Bilateral airspace consolidation with air bronchograms
- Often initially patchy but tends to become rapidly confluent and diffuse
- Upper or lower lung zone predominance

Utility
- Usually first imaging modality used to assess patients who present with clinical findings of acute respiratory distress syndrome (ARDS).

CT
Findings
- Patchy or diffuse bilateral ground-glass opacities are noted.
- Smooth interlobular septal thickening and intralobular lines are superimposed on ground-glass opacities ("crazy-paving" pattern).
- Sparing of lung lobules frequently results in geographic appearance.
- More diffuse ground-glass opacities, extensive areas of consolidation, architectural distortion, and traction bronchiectasis are seen with progression of disease.
- Consolidation tends to involve mainly dependent lung regions.

Utility
- Helpful in evaluation of patients with questionable or nonspecific radiographic findings.
- Used for assessment of suspected complications.

CLINICAL PRESENTATION

- Prodromal illness of fever, chills, myalgias, and arthralgias is commonly present.
- Dry cough and rapidly progressive and severe dyspnea occur.
- Approximately two thirds of patients have symptoms for less than 1 week.
- One third have symptoms for up to 60 days before diagnosis.
- There is a restrictive ventilatory defect (decrease in total lung capacity and vital capacity).

DIAGNOSTIC PEARLS

- Upper or lower lung zone predominance
- Patchy or diffuse ground-glass opacities or consolidation on radiograph or high-resolution CT
- "Crazy-paving" pattern without or with dependent consolidation on CT
- Indistinguishable from acute respiratory distress syndrome (ARDS) except for lack of etiology
- Acute interstitial pneumonia is an uncommon condition. Diagnosis can only be made after exclusion of all known causes of ARDS

- Impaired gas exchange leads to progressive hypoxemic respiratory failure.

DIFFERENTIAL DIAGNOSIS

- Acute respiratory distress syndrome
- Pneumonia
- Diffuse pulmonary hemorrhage

PATHOLOGY

- Idiopathic diffuse alveolar damage
- Acute, exudative phase: edema, hyaline membranes, acute interstitial inflammation, and intra-alveolar hemorrhage
- Organizing phase: loose organizing fibrosis and type II pneumocyte hyperplasia
- Chronic phase: fibrosis that may be associated with extensive architectural remodeling resulting in honeycomb formation or cystic changes

INCIDENCE/PREVALENCE AND EPIDEMIOLOGY

- Uncommon
- No sex predominance
- No association with cigarette smoking
- Average age at presentation: 50 to 60 years (range: 7 to 83 years)

WHAT THE REFERRING PHYSICIAN NEEDS TO KNOW

- Clinical, radiologic, and pathologic manifestations of acute interstitial pneumonia are identical to those of ARDS.
- Diagnosis can only be made after exclusion of all known causes of ARDS, particularly infection, aspiration, and drug reaction.

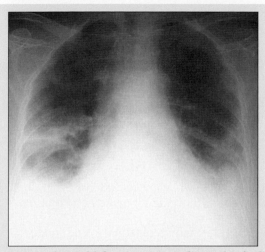

Figure 1. Acute interstitial pneumonia: radiographic findings. Chest radiograph in an 81-year-old woman with acute interstitial pneumonia shows extensive bilateral areas of consolidation involving mainly the lower lung zones.

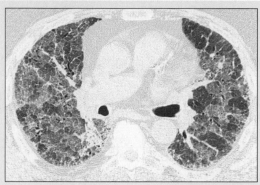

Figure 2. Acute interstitial pneumonia: high-resolution CT findings. High-resolution CT in an 80-year-old man with acute interstitial pneumonia shows extensive bilateral ground-glass opacities. Smooth septal thickening and intralobular lines are seen superimposed on the ground-glass opacities ("crazy-paving" pattern) mainly in the right lung. Relative sparing of some of the secondary lobules results in a geographic appearance.

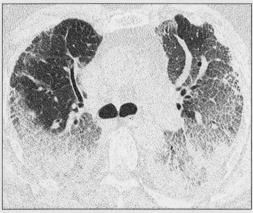

Figure 3. Acute interstitial pneumonia: "crazy-paving" pattern. High-resolution CT image in a 78-year-old man with acute interstitial pneumonia shows bilateral ground-glass opacities with superimposed smooth linear opacities ("crazy-paving" pattern) and dependent areas of consolidation.

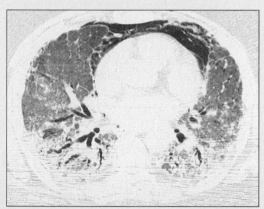

Figure 4. Acute interstitial pneumonia: high-resolution CT findings on follow-up. High-resolution CT performed a few days after hospital admission in a 65-year-old man with acute interstitial pneumonia shows extensive bilateral ground-glass opacities, dependent areas of consolidation, pneumomediastinum, and traction bronchiectasis and bronchiolectasis.

Suggested Readings

American Thoracic Society, European Respiratory Society: American Thoracic Society/European Respiratory Society International Multidisciplinary Consensus Classification of the Idiopathic Interstitial Pneumonias. *Am J Respir Crit Care Med* 165:277-304, 2002.

Ichikado K, Suga M, Müller NL, et al: Acute interstitial pneumonia: Comparison of high-resolution computed tomography findings between survivors and nonsurvivors. *Am J Respir Crit Care Med* 165(11):1551-1556, 2002.

Johkoh T, Müller NL, Taniguchi II, et al: Acute interstitial pneumonia: Thin-section CT findings in 36 patients. *Radiology* 211(3):859-863, 1999.

Lynch DA, Travis WD, Müller NL, et al: Idiopathic interstitial pneumonias: CT features. *Radiology* 236:10-21, 2005.

Tomiyama N, Müller NL, Johkoh T, et al: Acute respiratory distress syndrome and acute interstitial pneumonia: Comparison of thin-section CT findings. *J Comput Assist Tomogr* 25(1):28-33, 2001.

Hilar and Mediastinal Manifestations

DEFINITION: Sarcoidosis is a systemic inflammatory disorder of unknown etiology that affects multiple organs and is characterized by formation of noncaseating granulomas.

IMAGING

Radiography

Findings

- Bilateral hilar and right paratracheal lymph node enlargement is characteristic and common manifestation.
- *Stage 0:* no demonstrable abnormality on radiograph.
- *Stage I:* Hilar and mediastinal lymph node enlargement without parenchymal abnormality.
- *Stage II:* Hilar and mediastinal lymph node enlargement plus parenchymal abnormality.
- *Stage III:* Parenchymal abnormality alone.
- *Stage IV:* Advanced fibrosis with reticulation, architectural distortion, hilar retraction, and occasional honeycombing.
- Hilar and mediastinal nodes may calcify.
- Eggshell calcification of hilar and mediastinal nodes may occur but is uncommon.

Utility

- Chest radiograph remains the first and foremost imaging modality used in initial evaluation and follow-up of patients with sarcoidosis.
- Radiographic abnormalities are classified into five stages and apply only to chest radiograph.
- Main utility of staging system is predicting outcome.

CT

Findings

- Most commonly enlarged lymph nodes include the paratracheal and hilar lymph nodes.
- Lymphadenopathy is frequently present in aorto-pulmonary window and subcarinal, anterior mediastinal and posterior mediastinal lymph node groups.
- Calcification of lymph nodes is initially focal and soft ("icing sugar" calcification).
- Over time, calcification becomes dense.

DIAGNOSTIC PEARLS

- Bilateral hilar and right paratracheal lymph node enlargement is a characteristic and common manifestation.
- Stage I: Hilar and mediastinal lymph node enlargement without parenchymal abnormality.
- Stage II: Hilar and mediastinal lymph node enlargement plus parenchymal abnormality.
- Calcification of lymph nodes is common on long-term follow-up.

- Pattern of calcification is most commonly focal but may be diffuse or eggshell.
- Expiratory high-resolution CT shows air trapping.

Utility

- More sensitive than radiography in detecting lymph node enlargement.
- Used when radiographic findings are negative, nonspecific, or atypical and for detection of complications.

Nuclear Medicine

Findings

- Increased uptake in areas of active inflammation.

Utility

- Gallium-67 scintigraphy plays a limited role in the assessment of patients with sarcoidosis.

PET

Findings

- Increased FDG-PET uptake in lung parenchyma and lymph nodes.

Utility

- FDG-PET is comparable to gallium-67 scintigraphy in detection of pulmonary sarcoidosis.
- It is superior to gallium-67 scintigraphy in assessment of extrapulmonary involvement.

WHAT THE REFERRING PHYSICIAN NEEDS TO KNOW

- In the majority of patients confident diagnosis of sarcoidosis can be made based on clinical findings and chest radiography.
- CT is indicated when radiographic findings are nonspecific, atypical, or negative but suspicion is high and for detection of complications.
- CT is indicated for assessment of stage II or III sarcoidosis to differentiate active inflammation from irreversible fibrosis.

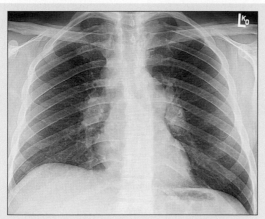

Figure 1. Stage I sarcoidosis: radiographic findings. Posteroanterior chest radiograph in a 33-year-old man with sarcoidosis shows right paratracheal, aortopulmonary window, and symmetric bilateral hilar lymph node enlargement.

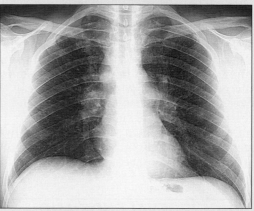

Figure 2. Stage II sarcoidosis: radiographic findings. Posteroanterior chest radiograph in a 35-year-old man with sarcoidosis demonstrates right paratracheal, aortopulmonary window, and symmetric bilateral hilar lymph node enlargement and small round and irregular opacities in the upper zones. Note medial deviation of the gastric bubble due to splenomegaly.

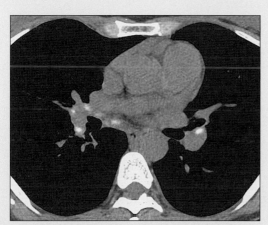

Figure 3. Sarcoidosis: characteristic focal calcification of lymph nodes. CT image in a 40-year-old woman with sarcoidosis shows soft ("icing sugar") calcification of bilateral hilar and subcarinal lymph nodes.

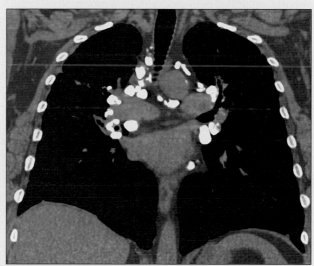

Figure 4. Sarcoidosis: extensive nodal calcification on CT. Coronal reformatted CT image demonstrates numerous densely calcified mediastinal and bilateral hilar lymph nodes. The patient was a 53-year-old man with a 20-year history of sarcoidosis.

CLINICAL PRESENTATION

- About half of patients are asymptomatic.
- Constitutional symptoms are common and include weight loss, fatigue, weakness, and malaise.
- Löfgren syndrome is the acute presentation of sarcoidosis with fever, symmetric bilateral hilar lymphadenopathy, and erythema nodosum (tender red nodules, usually on the shins).

DIFFERENTIAL DIAGNOSIS

- Non-Hodgkin lymphoma
- Hodgkin lymphoma
- Metastases

PATHOLOGY

- Etiology of initial stimulus and reason why granuloma formation is persistent are unknown.
- Exposure of genetically susceptible individuals to specific environmental agents triggers an exaggerated cellular immune response leading to granuloma formation.
- Accumulation of numerous activated macrophages and T lymphocytes releasing TH1-predominant cytokines results in granuloma formation.

- Pathologic hallmark is granuloma with a central core of clustered epithelioid histiocytes and occasional multinucleated giant cells surrounded by fibroblasts and collagen.
- Vast majority of granulomas are non-necrotizing; some may show small amount of central fibrinoid necrosis.
- Initially granulomas are discrete and appear "active"; however, they tend to become confluent and undergo progressive fibrosis over time.
- Lymph node involvement is characterized by diffuse replacement of node by granulomas, often with variable histologic appearance.

INCIDENCE/PREVALENCE AND EPIDEMIOLOGY

- Etiology is unknown; familial clustering suggests important genetic contribution, and environmental influences also have important effect.
- It occurs at any age but is most common between the ages of 20 and 40 years and slightly more common in women.
- Second peak incidence occurs in women older than 50.

- It is common in African-Americans (2.4% in United States), Scandinavian countries (Sweden: 64/100,000; Finland: 11/100,000), and Ireland.
- It is more prevalent in Irish living in London than native Londoners and in natives of Martinique living in France than indigenous French.
- Approximately 1/100,000 new cases have been reported in Japan.
- Overall mortality is 1%-5%.

Suggested Readings

American Thoracic Society (ATS), the European Respiratory Society (ERS), the World Association of Sarcoidosis and Other Granulomatous Disorders (WASOG): Statement on Sarcoidosis. Joint Statement of the American Thoracic Society (ATS) the European Respiratory Society (ERS), the World Association of Sarcoidosis and Other Granulomatous Disorders (WASOG) adopted by the ATS Board of Directors and by the ERS Executive Committee, February 1999. *Am J Respir Crit Care Med* 160:736-755, 1999.

Hennebicque AS, Nunes H, Brillet PY, et al: CT findings in severe thoracic sarcoidosis. *Eur Radiol* 15:23-30, 2005.

Koyama T, Ueda H, Togashi K, et al: Radiologic manifestations of sarcoidosis in various organs. *RadioGraphics* 24:87-104, 2004.

Nunes H, Brillet PY, Valeyre D, et al: Imaging in sarcoidosis. *Semin Respir Crit Care Med* 28(1):102-120, 2007.

Pulmonary Parenchymal Manifestations

DEFINITION: Sarcoidosis is a systemic inflammatory disorder of unknown etiology that frequently involves the lung parenchyma.

IMAGING

Radiography

Findings

- Nodular pattern: nodules from 1 to 10 mm in diameter, with irregular margins, mainly in middle and upper lung zones.
- Reticulonodular pattern: combination of nodules and thickening of interlobular septa or combination of nodules and intralobular linear opacities.
- Parenchymal consolidation: typically bilateral and symmetric; involves mainly middle and upper lung zones.
- Fibrosis: typically in perihilar regions of middle and upper lung zones.
- Fibrosis associated with superior retraction of hila, distortion of bronchovascular bundles, bulla formation, traction bronchiectasis, and compensatory lower lobe overinflation.
- Cavitation and aspergilloma formation in advanced sarcoidosis.

Utility

- Radiographic findings are basis of staging, which is useful for predicting outcome.
- *Stage 0:* No demonstrable abnormality on radiograph.
- *Stage I:* Hilar and mediastinal lymph node enlargement without parenchymal abnormality.
- *Stage II:* Hilar and mediastinal lymph node enlargement plus parenchymal abnormality.
- *Stage III:* Parenchymal abnormality alone.
- *Stage IV:* Advanced fibrosis with reticulation, architectural distortion, hilar retraction, and occasional honeycombing.

CT

Findings

- Characteristic pattern is of small nodules in a perilymphatic distribution.

DIAGNOSTIC PEARLS

- Characteristic pattern is of small nodules in a perilymphatic distribution.
- Frequent patterns are nodular and reticulonodular; less commonly, reticular pattern, air space consolidation, or, rarely, ground-glass opacities predominate.
- Consolidation has bilateral and symmetric distribution involving mainly the middle and upper lung zones.
- Fibrosis typically involves perihilar regions of the middle and upper lung zones.
- Frequently associated bilateral symmetric hilar and mediastinal lymphadenopathy.

<hr/>

- Nodules are seen adjacent to bronchi, pulmonary arteries and veins, along interlobular septa, and in interlobar fissures and costal subpleural regions.
- Occasionally, nodules may be small and form miliary pattern or involve predominantly subpleural lung regions and resemble pleural plaques (pseudoplaques).
- Sarcoid granulomas along peribronchovascular interstitium extend to peribronchiolar interstitium resulting in prominence of centrilobular core and centrilobular nodules.
- Air trapping is often seen on expiratory high-resolution CT due to endoluminal or submucosal sarcoid granulomas or fibrotic obstruction.
- Extensive microscopic interstitial granulomas may also result in ground-glass opacities, large nodules, or consolidation superimposed on interstitial nodules or fibrosis.
- Fibrosis results in irregular linear opacities, irregular septal thickening, traction bronchiectasis and bronchiolectasis, and, occasionally, honeycombing.

WHAT THE REFERRING PHYSICIAN NEEDS TO KNOW

- In the majority of patients, a confident diagnosis of sarcoidosis can be made based on clinical findings and chest radiography.
- The prognosis correlates with radiographic stage at presentation.
- CT indications include normal/nonspecific chest radiographs with high clinical suspicion, complication detection, and discrimination between active inflammation and irreversible fibrosis.
- Pulmonary fibrosis is seen at presentation in approximately 5% of patients and eventually develops in 20%-25% of patients.
- Frequent patterns are nodular and reticulonodular; less commonly, reticular pattern, air space consolidation, or, rarely, ground-glass opacities predominate.
- Nodules, interlobular septal thickening, ground-glass opacities, and consolidation represent potentially reversible disease.
- Architectural distortion and honeycombing represent irreversible disease.

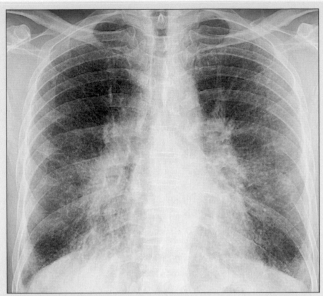

Figure 1. Sarcoidosis: reticulonodular pattern. Posteroanterior chest radiograph shows diffuse reticulonodular pattern. Also noted is paratracheal, aortopulmonary window, and symmetric bilateral hilar lymph node enlargement.

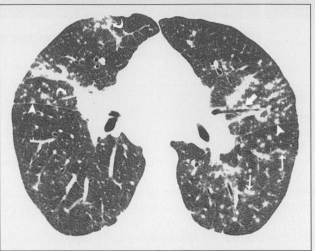

Figure 2. Sarcoidosis: characteristic perilymphatic distribution on high-resolution CT. High-resolution CT image at the level of the right middle lobe bronchus shows numerous small nodules located mainly along the bronchi (*broad straight arrows*), vessels (*narrow straight arrows*), and interlobar fissures (*arrowheads*). Also evident are small nodules along the subpleural regions (pseudoplaques) and interlobular septa (*curved arrows*). This distribution is characteristic of sarcoidosis and consistent with the perilymphatic distribution of sarcoid granulomas. Note subcarinal and bilateral hilar lymph node enlargement.

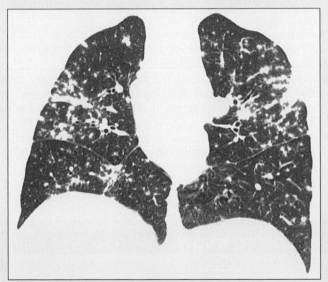

Figure 3. Sarcoidosis: characteristic perilymphatic distribution on high-resolution CT. Coronal maximum intensity projection (MIP) image demonstrates that the nodules involve mainly the upper lobe and have a perilymphatic distribution.

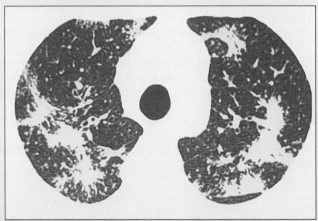

Figure 4. Sarcoidosis: large nodules on high-resolution CT. High-resolution CT image in a 30-year-old woman demonstrates bilateral irregular nodular opacities in a perilymphatic and subpleural distribution with adjacent small nodules. The large opacities result from the confluence of numerous small nodules.

Utility

- CT may demonstrate parenchymal abnormalities in patients with normal radiographs (stage 0) or with only lymphadenopathy evident on the radiograph (stage I).
- CT is superior to radiography in demonstrating the pattern and distribution of abnormalities.

PET
Findings

- Increased FDG-PET uptake seen in lung lesions

Utility

- FDG-PET is comparable to gallium-67 scintigraphy in detection of pulmonary sarcoidosis.
- PET and gallium-67 scintigraphy are of limited value in the assessment of pulmonary parenchymal abnormalities in sarcoidosis.

CLINICAL PRESENTATION

- Thirty percent to 50% of patients are asymptomatic.
- Most common pulmonary complaints are dyspnea, cough, and chest pain.
- Constitutional symptoms are common and include weight loss, fatigue, weakness, and malaise.

DIFFERENTIAL DIAGNOSIS

- Lymphoma
- Lymphangitic carcinomatosis
- Silicosis
- Coal workers' pneumoconiosis

PATHOLOGY

- Pathologic hallmark is granuloma: central core of tightly clustered epithelioid histiocytes and multinucleated giant cells surrounded by fibroblasts and collagen.
- Sarcoid granulomas have perilymphatic distribution, with pulmonary involvement being most prominent in peribronchovascular, interlobular septal, and pleural interstitial tissue.

- Gross appearance of pulmonary sarcoidosis depends on stage and severity of disease.
- Early, milder forms include inflammation; appearance can resemble lymphangitic carcinomatosis.
- As disease progresses, entire lobules can be replaced by granulomas and fibrous tissue.
- Disease is most severe in upper lobes, occurring in solid areas of fibrous tissue associated with bronchiectasis.

INCIDENCE/PREVALENCE AND EPIDEMIOLOGY

- Etiology is unknown; familial clustering suggests important genetic contribution, and environmental influences also have important effect.
- It occurs at any age but is most common between the ages of 20 and 40 years and is slightly more common in women.
- Second peak incidence occurs in women older than 50.
- It is common in African-Americans (2.4% in United States), Scandinavian countries (Sweden: 64/100,000; Finland: 11/100,000), and Ireland.
- It is more prevalent in Irish living in London than native Londoners and in natives of Martinique living in France than indigenous French.
- Approximately 1/100,000 new cases have been reported in Japan.
- Overall mortality is 1%-5%.

Suggested Readings

American Thoracic Society (ATS), the European Respiratory Society (ERS), the World Association of Sarcoidosis and Other Granulomatous Disorders (WASOG): Statement on Sarcoidosis. Joint Statement of the American Thoracic Society (ATS), the European Respiratory Society (ERS), and the World Association of Sarcoidosis and Other Granulomatous Disorders (WASOG) adopted by the ATS Board of Directors and by the ERS Executive Committee, February 1999. *Am J Respir Crit Care Med* 160:736-755, 1999.
Hennebicque AS, Nunes H, Brillet PY, et al: CT findings in severe thoracic sarcoidosis. *Eur Radiol* 15:23-30, 2005.
Koyama T, Ueda H, Togashi K, et al: Radiologic manifestations of sarcoidosis in various organs. *RadioGraphics* 24:87-104, 2004.
Nunes H, Brillet PY, Valeyre D, et al: Imaging in sarcoidosis. *Semin Respir Crit Care Med* 28(1):102-120, 2007.

Acute and Subacute Hypersensitivity Pneumonitis

DEFINITION: Hypersensitivity pneumonitis is an immune-mediated inflammatory form of diffuse interstitial pulmonary disease caused by inhalation of various antigens that affect susceptible patients.

IMAGING

Radiography

Findings

- Acute: diffuse airspace opacities with similar pattern and distribution to pulmonary edema, ill-defined nodular opacities
- May be normal in patients with mild symptoms and, rarely, in patients with severe symptoms
- Subacute: hazy areas of increased opacity (ground-glass opacities) and poorly defined nodular opacities
- Diffuse consolidation possible in patients with subacute disease but rare
- Pneumomediastinum, pneumothorax, and subcutaneous emphysema (air-leak syndrome) uncommon.
- Findings may be diffuse but tendency for mainly involvement of lower lung zones

Utility

- Usually first imaging modality
- Limited value in diagnosis

CT

Findings

- Most common high-resolution CT findings of acute form consist of diffuse ground-glass opacities and consolidation.
- Centrilobular nodules and diffuse airspace opacification may also be seen in acute disease.
- In subacute form there are poorly defined small centrilobular nodules and symmetric patchy or diffuse bilateral ground-glass opacities.
- There may be a combination of ground-glass opacities, areas of normal lung, and lobular areas of decreased attenuation and vascularity.

DIAGNOSTIC PEARLS

- A combination of bilateral ground-glass opacities, centrilobular nodules, and lobular areas of air trapping on high-resolution CT are highly suggestive of subacute hypersensitivity pneumonitis.
- The abnormalities are usually diffuse throughout the lungs or involve mainly the middle and lower lung zones.
- The prevalance of hypersensitivity pneumonitis is lower in smokers.
- Only approximately 5% of patients with hypersensitivity pneumonitis are cigarette smokers.

- Lobular areas of decreased attenuation and vascularity are noted on inspiratory images, and air trapping is seen on expiratory CT.
- Focal areas of consolidation are seen occasionally in subacute disease.
- A few thin-walled cysts are present in the areas of ground-glass opacity in a small percentage of cases.

Utility

- High-resolution CT is important in diagnosis of hypersensitivity pneumonitis and frequently demonstrates characteristic findings in patients with nonspecific or normal chest radiographs.
- Because of clinical manifestations and the rapid resolution of symptoms, high-resolution CT is uncommonly performed in patients with acute disease.
- Expiratory CT scans can be helpful when there is a clinical suspicion of hypersensitivity pneumonitis.

WHAT THE REFERRING PHYSICIAN NEEDS TO KNOW

- Radiologic findings of acute hypersensitivity pneumonitis mimic those of acute pulmonary edema or may be normal.
- High-resolution CT findings of subacute hypersensitivity pneumonitis are often characteristic enough to strongly suggest the diagnosis.
- Characteristic high-resolution CT manifestations of subacute hypersensitivity pneumonitis include bilateral ground-glass opacities, poorly defined centrilobular nodules, and lobular areas of decreased attenuation and air trapping on expiratory scans.
- Diagnosis can often be made based on history, antibodies to offending antigen, and high-resolution CT findings without bronchoscopy or biopsy.
- Immunologic tests, lung function tests, and bronchoalveolar lavage may also be done; definitive diagnosis may require lung biopsy.

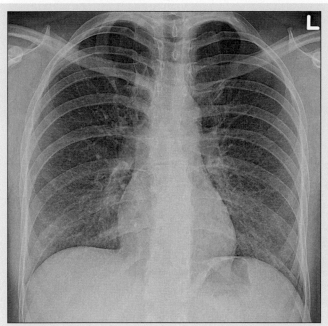

Figure 1. Subacute hypersensitivity pneumonitis on chest radiography. Posteroanterior chest radiograph shows bilateral hazy areas of increased opacity (ground-glass opacities) involving mainly the lower lung zones. Incidental note is made of azygos fissure. The patient was a 31-year-old woman (bird fancier) with biopsy-proven hypersensitivity pneumonitis who presented with clinical findings of asthma.

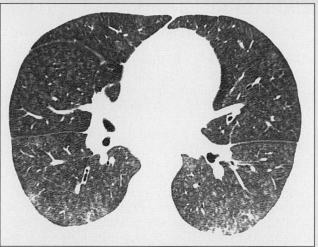

Figure 2. Subacute hypersensitivity pneumonitis (bird fancier's lung): high-resolution CT findings. High-resolution CT image shows diffuse ground-glass opacities and bilateral poorly defined small nodules in a characteristic centrilobular distribution.

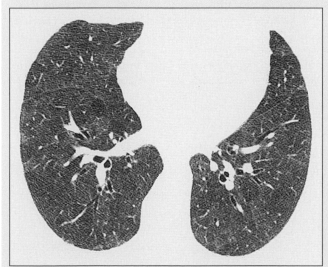

Figure 3. Subacute hypersensitivity pneumonitis. High-resolution CT image at the level of inferior pulmonary vein shows diffuse ground-glass opacity interposed with areas of normal lung and lobular areas of decreased attenuation and vascularity. The combination of ground-glass opacity, normal lung, and areas of increased attenuation gives the lung a heterogeneous geographic appearance denominated the "head-cheese sign."

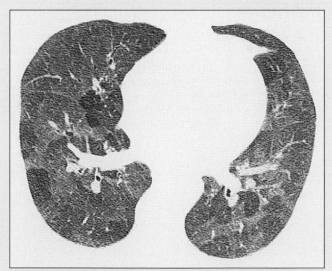

Figure 4. Subacute hypersensitivity pneumonitis. Expiratory CT image at the same level as Figure 3 shows focal areas of air trapping reflecting cellular bronchiolitis or, less commonly, bronchiolitis obliterans.

CLINICAL PRESENTATION

- Acute hypersensitivity pneumonitis is characterized by abrupt onset of symptoms after heavy antigen exposure in a previously sensitized patient.
- Symptoms begin hours after exposure, last from hours to days, and gradually decrease when patient is removed from offending antigen.
- Influenza-like symptoms often predominate, including chills, fever, myalgia, lassitude, headache, and nausea.
- Respiratory symptoms range from mild cough to severe dyspnea and, occasionally, respiratory failure.
- Subacute hypersensitivity pneumonitis is caused by intermittent or continuous exposure to low doses of antigen; symptoms appear gradually.
- Patients with subacute disease usually present with exertional dyspnea, cough, and fever; pneumothorax, pneumomediastinum, and subcutaneous emphysema are rare.
- Numerous exacerbations and remissions of subacute disease may be seen in affected patients who have frequent and recurrent exposure.

DIFFERENTIAL DIAGNOSIS

- Nonspecific interstitial pneumonia
- Respiratory bronchiolitis/interstitial lung disease
- Collagen vascular disease
- Drug reaction

PATHOLOGY

- Wide spectrum of antigens may cause hypersensitivity pneumonitis, including thermophilic bacteria, fungi, mycobacteria, animal proteins, and small-molecular-weight chemical compounds.
- Development is influenced by size, immunogenicity, number of inhaled particles, duration of exposure, and immune response of affected individual.

- Exact pathogenesis is incompletely understood; however, it is well known that hypersensitivity pneumonitis results from non–IgE-mediated hypersensitivity reaction.
- Subacute features include temporally uniform cellular bronchiolitis, chronic bronchiolocentric cellular interstitial pneumonia composed predominantly of lymphocytes, scattered, small, poorly formed noncaseating granulomas.

INCIDENCE/PREVALENCE AND EPIDEMIOLOGY

- Prevalence and incidence of hypersensitivity pneumonitis in the general population are unknown.
- Hypersensitivity pneumonitis occurs most commonly in adult patients, mainly middle-aged individuals.
- Reported prevalence in selected groups of patients varies considerably between countries.
- Farmer's lung is one of most common types, estimated to occur in 9%-12% of exposed farmers.
- Bird fancier's lung occurs in up to 15% of bird keepers.
- Clinical diagnosis is difficult; therefore, prevalence is probably higher than recognized in clinical practice.
- The prevalence of hypersensitivity pneumonitis is lower in smokers.

Suggested Readings

Ismail T, McSharry C, Boyd G: Extrinsic allergic alveolitis. *Respirology* 11:262-268, 2006.

Mohr LC: Hypersensitivity pneumonitis. *Curr Opin Pulm Med* 10: 401-411, 2004.

Selman M: Hypersensitivity pneumonitis: A multifaceted deceiving disorder. *Clin Chest Med* 25:531-547, 2004.

Silva CIS, Müller NL, Churg A: Hypersensitivity pneumonitis: Spectrum of high-resolution CT and pathologic findings. *AJR Am J Roentgenol* 188:334-344, 2007.

Chronic Hypersensitivity Pneumonitis

DEFINITION: This chronic immune-mediated inflammatory form of diffuse interstitial pulmonary disease is caused by inhalation of various antigens that affect susceptible patients and is associated with fibrosis.

IMAGING

Radiography
Findings
- Irregular linear opacities (reticular pattern), honeycombing, and volume loss

Utility
- Often first imaging modality
- Helpful in follow-up of patients

CT
Findings
- Reticulation in chronic disease can be patchy, random, or peribronchovascular or have predominantly subpleural distribution.
- May have upper, middle or lower lung zone predominance and may spare the lung bases.
- Ground-glass opacities, centrilobular nodules, and lobular areas of air trapping due to subacute disease superimposed on findings of fibrosis.
- Cystic changes are noted in approximately 40% of cases.
- Occasionally, findings may mimic those of idiopathic pulmonary fibrosis.
- Mild lymph node enlargement is common; usually only one or two nodes are enlarged and their short-axis diameter is <15 mm.

Utility
- High-resolution CT is important in diagnosis of hypersensitivity pneumonitis and frequently demonstrates findings in patients with nonspecific chest radiographs.
- High-resolution CT findings are often characteristic and highly suggestive of the diagnosis.
- In some patients, CT findings may mimic those of idiopathic pulmonary fibrosis or nonspecific interstitial pneumonia.

CLINICAL PRESENTATION

- Exertional dyspnea and cough occur over several months or years.

DIAGNOSTIC PEARLS

- Classically, chronic hypersensitivity pneumonitis presents as fibrosis with reticulation, architectural distortion, traction bronchiectasis and bronchiolectasis, and honeycombing.
- Fibrosis may have upper, middle or lower lung zone predominance and may spare the lung bases.
- CT features that distinguish chronic hypersensitivity pneumonitis are presence of lobular areas of decreased attenuation and vascularity and centrilobular nodules.

- Increasing cough and exertional dyspnea are common, and fatigue and weight loss may be prominent symptoms.
- Bilateral crackles are commonly present on auscultation, and digital clubbing may occur.

DIFFERENTIAL DIAGNOSIS

- Idiopathic pulmonary fibrosis
- Nonspecific interstitial pneumonia
- Respiratory bronchiolitis/interstitial lung disease
- Sarcoidosis

PATHOLOGY

- Development is influenced by size, immunogenicity, number of inhaled particles, exposure duration, and immune response of affected individual.
- Exact pathogenesis is incompletely understood; however, it is well known that the disease results from a non–IgE-mediated hypersensitivity reaction.
- Reaction results from a very low-level persistent or recurrent exposure to an antigen.
- Repeated exposure determines progression of inflammation to irreversible pulmonary fibrosis.
- Histologically, the chronic stage shows fibrosis and, frequently, findings of subacute disease.

WHAT THE REFERRING PHYSICIAN NEEDS TO KNOW

- Radiographic findings are nonspecific.
- High-resolution CT shows reticulation and commonly superimposed characteristic findings of subacute disease.
- Diagnosis can be made based on history, presence of antibodies to antigen, and CT findings.
- Pattern and distribution of high-resolution CT findings of chronic hypersensitivity pneumonitis allow confident distinction versus interstitial pulmonary fibrosis and nonspecific interstitial pneumonitis in approximately 50% of cases.
- Diagnosis can often be made or rejected with confidence based on clinical history, precipitating antibodies to an offending antigen, and high-resolution CT findings.

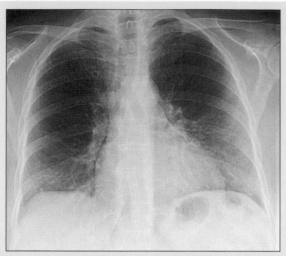

Figure 1. Chronic hypersensitivity pneumonitis: radiographic findings. Posteroanterior chest radiograph shows mild bilateral reticular pattern in the lower lung zones in a 58-year-old woman with symptoms of dyspnea over 2 years.

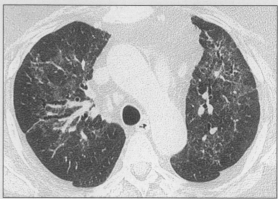

Figure 2. Chronic hypersensitivity pneumonitis in a bird breeder. High-resolution CT image at the level of aortic arch shows mild ground-glass opacities with superimposed reticulation in a peribronchovascular/perihilar distribution. Note bilateral traction bronchiectasis suggesting fibrosis.

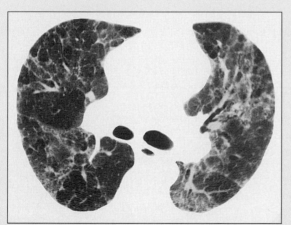

Figure 3. Chronic hypersensitivity pneumonitis in a 47-year-old man exposed to red cedar. High-resolution CT at the level of left main-stem bronchus shows patchy ground-glass opacities, minimal reticulation, and lobular areas of decreased attenuation.

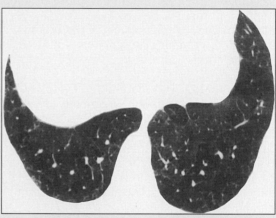

Figure 4. Chronic hypersensitivity pneumonitis in a 47-year-old man exposed to red cedar. High-resolution CT at the level of the lung bases shows ground-glass opacities but only minimal fibrosis.

■ Nonspecific interstitial pneumonia pattern and a usual interstitial pneumonia pattern may be the only findings of chronic hypersensitivity pneumonitis.

INCIDENCE/PREVALENCE AND EPIDEMIOLOGY

■ Prevalence and incidence in the general population are unknown.

■ Hypersensitivity pneumonitis occurs most commonly in adult patients, mainly middle-aged individuals; it is less common in smokers.
■ Reported prevalence in selected groups of patients varies considerably between countries.
■ Farmer's lung is one of most common types, estimated to occur in 9%-12% of exposed farmers.
■ Bird fancier's lung occurs in up to 15% of bird keepers.
■ Clinical diagnosis of chronic hypersensitivity pneumonitis is difficult; its prevalence is probably higher than recognized in clinical practice.

Suggested Readings

Ismail T, McSharry C, Boyd G: Extrinsic allergic alveolitis. *Respirology* 11:262-268, 2006.

Mohr LC: Hypersensitivity pneumonitis. *Curr Opin Pulm Med* 10:401-411, 2004.

Selman M: Hypersensitivity pneumonitis: A multifaceted deceiving disorder. *Clin Chest Med* 25:531-547, 2004.

Silva CIS, Müller NL, Churg A: Hypersensitivity pneumonitis: Spectrum of high-resolution CT and pathologic findings. *AJR Am J Roentgenol* 188:334-344, 2007.

Silva CI, Müller NL, Lynch DA, et al: Chronic hypersensitivity pneumonitis: Differentiation from idiopathic pulmonary fibrosis and nonspecific interstitial pneumonia by using thin-section CT. *Radiology* 246(1):288-297, 2008.

Pulmonary Langerhans Cell Histiocytosis

DEFINITION: Pulmonary Langerhans cell histiocytosis (PLCH) is a clonal proliferation of histiocytes due to an abnormal inflammatory immunologic response.

IMAGING

Radiography

Findings

- Nodular or reticulonodular pattern has an upper and mid-zone distribution that spares the costophrenic angles.
- Distribution of nodules and curvilinear or reticular opacities is symmetric without central or peripheral predilection.
- Reticular pattern is a result of composite of superimposed multiple cysts.
- Lung volumes are preserved or enlarged.
- Pneumothorax commonly occurs.
- Advanced disease involves large areas of destroyed lung with parenchymal distortion and hyperinflation.
- Pulmonary arterial hypertension results in pulmonary artery enlargement.

Utility

- Initial investigation
- Useful for follow-up or demonstration of complicating pneumothoraces

CT

Findings

- In early disease there are multiple ill-defined micronodules (1-5 mm in diameter) with bronchiolocentric (centrilobular) distribution.
- Nodules may be profuse and predominate in upper and mid lungs.
- Sparing of costophrenic angles and tips of lingula and right middle lobe occurs.
- As disease progresses, nodules tend to cavitate and combination of cysts and nodules is characteristic.
- Cysts, which are initially thick-walled and spherical, become thinner walled and more eccentric with coalescence.
- Centrilobular opacities, reticular pattern, and thickening of interlobular septa are noted.

DIAGNOSTIC PEARLS

- Reticulonodular pattern with upper and mid lung zone distribution.
- Sparing of costophrenic angles.
- Combination of cysts and nodules in the middle and upper lung zones on high-resolution CT.
- Vast majority of patients are smokers.
- Presence of multiple cysts and nodules in the upper and middle lung zones with relative sparing of the lung bases is highly suggestive of the diagnosis.

- Commonly associated ground-glass opacities due to respiratory bronchiolitis.

Utility

- High-resolution CT is imaging modality of choice for diagnosis.
- Diagnostic accuracy of high-resolution CT is high.
- CT may provide information about disease reversibility.

CLINICAL PRESENTATION

- Cough
- Dyspnea
- Fever
- Malaise
- Chest pain
- May present with pneumothorax
- Bone lesions: may cause chest wall pain and tenderness

DIFFERENTIAL DIAGNOSIS

- Emphysema
- Respiratory bronchiolitis/interstitial lung disease
- Lymphangioleiomyomatosis
- Pneumocystis pneumonia

WHAT THE REFERRING PHYSICIAN NEEDS TO KNOW

- Pulmonary Langerhans cell histiocytosis in an adult is found almost exclusively in current smokers or ex-smokers.
- In the majority of cases, confident diagnosis is made based on characteristic pattern and distribution findings on high-resolution CT.
- Pneumothoraces are a frequent complication and may require surgical pleurodesis.

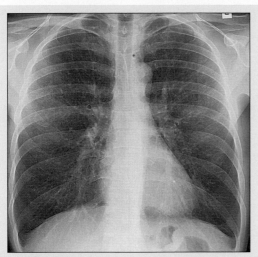

Figure 1. Pulmonary Langerhans' cell histiocytosis: early radiographic findings. Chest radiograph shows subtle nodularity in the upper zones. (*Courtesy of Dr. Susan J. Copley, London, UK*)

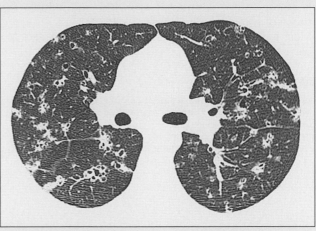

Figure 2. Pulmonary Langerhans' cell histiocytosis: characteristic thick-walled cysts. High-resolution CT image shows widespread thick-walled spherical cysts and a few irregular nodules. (*Courtesy of Dr. Susan J. Copley, London, UK*)

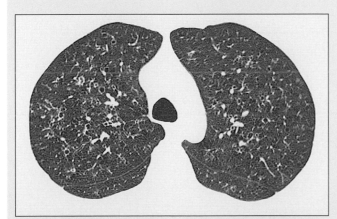

Figure 3. Pulmonary Langerhans' cell histiocytosis: progression of characteristic CT findings. High-resolution CT image shows the characteristic combination of micronodules and spherical cysts. (*Courtesy of Dr. Susan J. Copley, London, UK*)

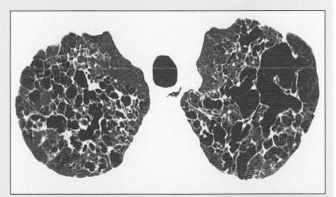

Figure 4. Pulmonary Langerhans' cell histiocytosis: nodules, cysts, and reticular pattern. High-resolution CT image at the level of the lung apices shows numerous bilateral thin-walled cysts. Conglomeration of cysts in the left upper lobe has led to the formation of large cysts with bizarre shapes. (*Courtesy of Dr. Susan J. Copley, London, UK*)

PATHOLOGY

- Pulmonary involvement of adult cases in Langerhans cell histiocytosis usually occurs in isolation.
- The histiocytic cells have features suggestive of "activated" Langerhans cells and contain an increased number of Birbeck granules.
- Multiple nodular cellular infiltrates centered around the membranous bronchioles and extending into surrounding interstitium result in a stellate appearance.
- The bronchiolocentric cellular inflammation results in destruction of the bronchiolar walls and cyst formation.
- Macroscopically, the findings consist of multiple nodules with varying degrees of cavitation, fibrosis, and cysts in the upper and middle lung zones, with relative sparing of the lung bases.

- Vast majority of adults have other findings related to cigarette smoking, mainly respiratory bronchiolitis and emphysema.

INCIDENCE/PREVALENCE AND EPIDEMIOLOGY

- This disease is uncommon.
- Isolated pulmonary Langerhans cell histiocytosis in adults is almost exclusively encountered in smokers.
- In children it often occurs as part of a systemic disorder and is not associated with smoking.
- It has been reported in 6.6% of 1382 cases of diffuse interstitial lung disease.
- There is an equal sex incidence.

■ It occurs more commonly in white individuals than those of other ethnic groups.
■ Most individuals are in the third or the fourth decade of life.

Suggested Readings

Abbott GF, Rosado-de-Christenson ML, Franks TJ, et al: From the archives of the AFIP: Pulmonary Langerhans' cell histiocytosis. *RadioGraphics* 24:821-841, 2004.

Bonelli FS, Hartman TE, Swensen SJ, Sherrick A: Accuracy of high-resolution CT in diagnosing lung diseases. *AJR Am J Roentgenol* 170(6):1507-1512, 1998.

Hansell DM, Nicholson AG: Smoking-related diffuse parenchymal lung disease: HRCT-pathologic correlation. *Sem Respir Crit Care Med* 24:377-392, 2003.

Koyama M, Johkoh T, Honda O, et al: Chronic cystic lung disease: Diagnostic accuracy of high-resolution CT in 92 patients. *AJR Am J Roentgenol* 180(3):827-835, 2003.

Sundar KM, Gosselin MV, Chung HL, Cahill BC: Pulmonary Langerhans cell histiocytosis: Emerging concepts in pathobiology, radiology, and clinical evolution of disease. *Chest* 123:1673-1683, 2003.

Tazi A: Adult pulmonary Langerhans' cell histiocytosis. *Eur Respir J* 27(6):1272-1285, 2006.

Vassallo R, Ryu JH: Pulmonary Langerhans' cell histiocytosis. *Clin Chest Med* 25:561-571, 2004.

Part 34

SMOKING-RELATED INTERSTITIAL LUNG DISEASE

Respiratory Bronchiolitis/Interstitial Lung Disease

DEFINITION: Respiratory bronchiolitis/interstitial lung disease is a smoking-related condition characterized by accumulation of pigmented macrophages mainly in the bronchioles and peribronchiolar airspaces and associated with clinical symptoms.

IMAGING

Radiography
Findings
- Variable and nonspecific; often normal
- Fine, diffuse reticulonodular pattern with normal lung volumes
- Ill-defined small nodules with lower zone predominance
- Ground-glass opacities
- Bronchial wall thickening

Utility
- Often normal
- Limited value in the diagnosis

CT
Findings
- Moderate to extensive bilateral ground-glass opacity.
- Poorly defined centrilobular nodules of ground-glass attenuation.
- Diffuse or mainly upper or lower lobes.
- Occasional thickening of interlobular septa and intralobular lines resulting in reticular pattern.
- Areas of decreased attenuation and vascularity on inspiratory high-resolution CT present mainly in lower lobes; areas of air trapping common on expiratory CT.
- Paraseptal or centrilobular emphysema.
- Bronchial wall thickening.

Utility
- High-resolution CT is the imaging modality of choice.
- End-expiratory CT may emphasize regional differences in lung density.

DIAGNOSTIC PEARLS
- Seen almost exclusively in smokers and ex-smokers
- Poorly defined centrilobular nodules and ground-glass opacities
- Upper or lower lobe predominance
- Emphysema and air trapping commonly present
- Finding resemble those of hypersensitivity pneumonitis but only 5% of patients with hypersensitivity pneumonitis are cigarette smokers

- Diagnosis on high-resolution CT requires presence of characteristic findings in the clinical context of a heavy smoker of cigarettes.
- CT findings often resemble those of hypersensitivity pneumonitis; however, only approximately 5% of patients with hypersensitivity pneumonitis are cigarette smokers.

CLINICAL PRESENTATION
- Dyspnea, insidious onset, progressive
- Cough, sometimes severe
- Chest pain
- Bilateral end-inspiratory crackles, predominantly basal
- Finger clubbing, rare
- Lung function: mixed obstructive-restrictive defect; reduced carbon monoxide diffusing capacity; normal, reduced, or slightly increased total lung capacity

---

WHAT THE REFERRING PHYSICIAN NEEDS TO KNOW
- Seen almost exclusively in smokers and ex-smokers
- Chest radiograph often normal or shows findings of chronic obstructive pulmonary disease
- High-resolution CT findings similar to those of hypersensitivity pneumonitis
- Surgical biopsy required for confident diagnosis
- Prognosis improved in individuals who stop smoking, although persisting radiologic/functional abnormalities seen
- Improvement in symptoms and of lung function indices with corticosteroids in majority of patients
- Differential diagnosis: desquamative interstitial pneumonia and hypersensitivity pneumonitis

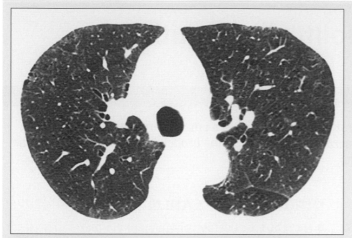

Figure 1. **Respiratory bronchiolitis/interstitial lung disease.** High-resolution CT image in a patient with biopsy-proven disease demonstrates bilateral centrilobular nodules, ground-glass opacities, and mild paraseptal emphysema. Note a few poorly defined micronodules. (*Courtesy of Dr. Susan J. Copley, London, UK*)

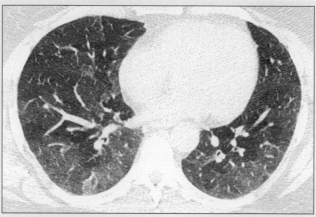

Figure 2. **Respiratory bronchiolitis/interstitial lung disease.** High-resolution CT image shows bilateral lower lobe ground-glass opacities and localized lobular areas of decreased attenuation and vascularity consistent with small airway obstruction. (*Courtesy of Dr. Susan J. Copley, London, UK*)

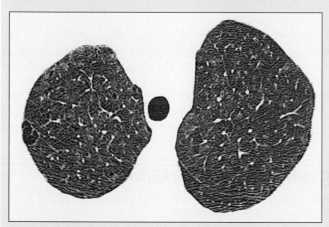

Figure 3. **Respiratory bronchiolitis/interstitial lung disease.** High-resolution CT images show patchy ground-glass opacities, ill-defined centrilobular micronodules, and a few thickened interlobular septa. Note mild paraseptal and centrilobular emphysema. (*Courtesy of Dr. Susan J. Copley, London, UK*)

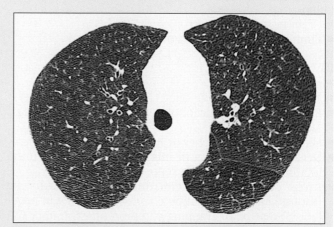

Figure 4. **Respiratory bronchiolitis/interstitial lung disease.** High-resolution CT images show patchy ground-glass opacities, ill-defined centrilobular micronodules, and a few thickened interlobular septa. Note mild paraseptal and centrilobular emphysema. (*Courtesy of Dr. Susan J. Copley, London, UK*)

DIFFERENTIAL DIAGNOSIS

- Respiratory bronchiolitis
- Desquamative interstitial pneumonia
- Hypersensitivity pneumonitis
- Nonspecific interstitial pneumonia

PATHOLOGY

- Intraluminal and peribronchiolar airspace accumulation of pigmented macrophages (smoker's macrophage).
- Ongoing inflammatory process denoted by mild peribronchiolar mononuclear inflammatory submucosal infiltrate associated with fibroblast/collagen deposition causing stellate fibrous scarring.
- Peribronchiolar fibrosis, thickening of peribronchiolar alveolar septa and alveolar ducts, histiocytes within peribronchiolar fibrous tissue displaying anthracotic pigment.
- Foci of goblet cell metaplasia and metaplastic cuboidal epithelium in airway epithelium.
- Emphysema.

INCIDENCE/PREVALENCE AND EPIDEMIOLOGY

- Rare clinicopathologic entity
- Seen almost exclusively in cigarette smokers
- Occurs in fourth and fifth decades of life
- Males and females almost equally affected, with slight male predominance

Suggested Readings

Desai SR, Ryan SM, Colby TV: Smoking-related interstitial lung diseases: Histopathological and imaging perspectives. *Clin Radiol* 58:259-268, 2003.

Heyneman LE, Ward S, Lynch DA, et al: Respiratory bronchiolitis, respiratory bronchiolitis-associated interstitial lung disease, and desquamative interstitial pneumonia: Different entities or part of the spectrum of the same disease process? *AJR Am J Roentgenol* 173:1622, 1999.

Holt RM, Schmidt RA, Godwin JD, Raghu G: High resolution CT in respiratory bronchiolitis-associated interstitial lung disease. *J Comput Assist Tomogr* 17:46-50, 1993.

Nakanishi M, Demura Y, Mizuno S, et al: Changes in HRCT findings in patients with respiratory bronchiolitis-associated interstitial lung disease after smoking cessation. *Eur Respir J* 29(3):453-461, 2007.

Park JS, Brown KK, Tuder RM, et al: Respiratory bronchiolitis-associated interstitial lung disease: Radiologic features with clinical and pathologic correlation. *J Comput Assist Tomogr* 26(1):13-20, 2002.

Wells AU, Nicholson AG, Hansell DM: Challenges in pulmonary fibrosis: 4. Smoking-induced diffuse interstitial lung diseases. *Thorax* 62(10):904-910, 2007.

Desquamative Interstitial Pneumonia

DEFINITION: Desquamative interstitial pneumonia is a rare interstitial lung disease characterized by widespread filling of alveoli with macrophages.

IMAGING

Radiography
Findings
- Bilateral, basal, hazy increased opacification with reduction in lung volumes
- Nonspecific reticular or reticulonodular pattern with basal distribution

Utility
- Findings may be subtle or even normal.
- Radiography is initial imaging investigation used for these patients.

CT
Findings
- Diffuse ground-glass opacity with subpleural and lower lung predominance
- Mild reticular pattern
- Architectural distortion of lung parenchyma and traction bronchiectasis (uncommon)
- Small cystic changes within areas of ground-glass opacification
- Occasionally mild honeycombing

Utility
- High-resolution CT is the imaging modality of choice for assessment of presence and extent of disease.
- CT findings are relatively nonspecific.

CLINICAL PRESENTATION

- Insidious onset of dyspnea and nonproductive cough
- Crepitations
- Finger clubbing (50%)
- Lung function: restrictive defect with reduction in diffusing capacity and lung volumes

DIFFERENTIAL DIAGNOSIS

- Respiratory bronchiolitis/interstitial lung disease
- Nonspecific interstitial pneumonia
- Hypersensitivity pneumonitis

DIAGNOSTIC PEARLS

- Diffuse ground-glass opacity with subpleural and lower lung predominance
- Vast majority of cases occur in cigarette smokers
- It is rare
- Confident diagnosis requires surgical lung biopsy

PATHOLOGY

- Pigmented macrophage accumulation is seen in alveolar spaces.
- Extent of involvement is uniform and diffuse and recognized at low magnification.
- Background architecture of alveoli is generally well-maintained; alveolar septa may be minimally thickened due to inflammatory cells and fibrosis.

INCIDENCE/PREVALENCE AND EPIDEMIOLOGY

- This disorder is rare.
- Male-to-female ratio is 2:1.
- Over 90% of patients are smokers.
- Occasionally the disorder may result from inhalational exposure (beryllium, aluminum, diesel fumes) or drugs (nitrofurantoin, busulfan).
- It presents in the third to fifth decades, with average age at presentation of about 40 years.

Suggested Readings

Akira M, Yamamoto S, Hara H, et al: Serial computed tomographic evaluation in desquamative interstitial pneumonia. *Thorax* 52: 333-337, 1997.

Desai SR, Ryan SM, Colby TV: Smoking-related interstitial lung diseases: Histopathological and imaging perspectives. *Clin Radiol* 58:259-268, 2003.

Hartman TE, Primack SL, Swensen SJ, et al: Desquamative interstitial pneumonia: Thin-section CT findings in 22 patients. *Radiology* 187(3):787-790, 1993.

WHAT THE REFERRING PHYSICIAN NEEDS TO KNOW

- High-resolution CT findings are relatively nonspecific.
- Confident diagnosis requires surgical biopsy.
- Spontaneous improvement may occur in untreated patients.
- Most patients are advised to stop smoking because the prognosis seems to be improved in individuals who do so.
- Roughly 25% of cases will worsen despite treatment with corticosteroids.
- No accepted surgical treatment exists, but lung transplant has been performed in selected patients.
- Differential diagnosis includes interstitial lung diseases (nonspecific interstitial pneumonia, respiratory bronchiolitis/interstitial lung disease, hypersensitivity pneumonitis).

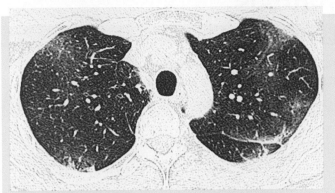

Figure 1. Desquamative interstitial pneumonia: high-resolution CT findings. High-resolution CT image in a patient with biopsy-proven desquamative interstitial pneumonia shows bilateral ground-glass opacities and minimal irregular linear opacities. Note the predominantly subpleural distribution of the abnormalities. (*Courtesy of Dr. Susan J. Copley, London, UK*)

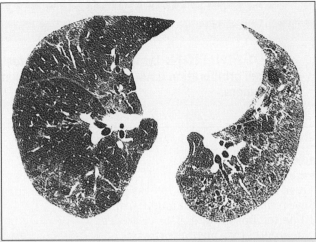

Figure 2. Desquamative interstitial pneumonia: ground-glass opacities, small cysts, and reticulation. High-resolution CT image in a patient with desquamative interstitial pneumonia shows a mixed ground-glass and fine reticular pattern. Note presence of microcysts. These are within areas of ground-glass opacity, are not associated with architectural distortion, have very thin walls, and are not contiguous, all features that distinguish this pattern from honeycombing. (*Courtesy of Dr. Susan J. Copley, London, UK*)

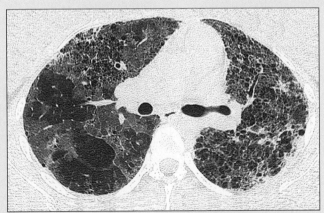

Figure 3. Desquamative interstitial pneumonia and emphysema. High-resolution CT image in a patient with a combination of ground-glass opacity and emphysema. Note that there is some distortion of the lung parenchyma, an unusual feature in this patient with histopathologically proven desquamative interstitial pneumonia. (*Courtesy of Dr. Susan J. Copley, London, UK*)

Heyneman LE, Ward S, Lynch DA, et al: Respiratory bronchiolitis, respiratory bronchiolitis-associated interstitial lung disease, and desquamative interstitial pneumonia: Different entities or part of the spectrum of the same disease process? *AJR Am J Roentgenol* 173(6):1617-1622, 1999.

Kanne JP, Bilawich AM, Lee CH, et al: Smoking-related emphysema and interstitial lung diseases. *J Thorac Imaging* 22(3):286-291, 2007.

Lynch DA, Travis WD, Müller NL, et al: Idiopathic interstitial pneumonias: CT features. *Radiology* 236(1):10-21, 2005.

Wells AU, Nicholson AG, Hansell DM: Challenges in pulmonary fibrosis: 4. Smoking-induced diffuse interstitial lung diseases. *Thorax* 62(10):904-910, 2007.

Lymphangioleiomyomatosis

DEFINITION: Lymphangioleiomyomatosis (LAM) is characterized by idiosyncratic smooth muscle cell proliferation (LAM cells) that leads to lung cysts, systemic lymphatic abnormalities, and abdominal tumors.

IMAGING

Radiography
Findings
- Overlapping of outlines of cyst resulting in widespread fine reticular or reticulonodular pattern
- Ill-defined or ground-glass opacities
- Pneumothorax, pleural effusion
- Combination of delicate reticular opacities and normal or expanded lungs

Utility
- Findings are often normal in early disease.
- In general, radiographic abnormalities correlate roughly with disease severity.

CT
Findings
- Bilateral thin-walled cysts are scattered throughout both lungs with no zonal predominance.
- Cysts may coalesce.
- Surrounding parenchyma is normal, but occasionally there are ground-glass opacities generally secondary to hemorrhage.
- Spontaneous pneumothorax occurs in up to half of patients and is often recurrent.
- Pleural effusion is nearly always chylous.

Utility
- High-resolution CT is more sensitive and useful to assess severity and complications.
- High-resolution CT is usually characteristic enough to allow diagnosis in proper clinical context (i.e., woman of childbearing age).

CLINICAL PRESENTATION

- Common clinical features are dyspnea, fatigue, and pneumothorax.
- Pleural effusion/chylothorax occurs.
- Ascites or abdominal masses are noted.
- Main manifestation is progressive destructive process of lungs, which may result in respiratory failure.

DIAGNOSTIC PEARLS

- Bilateral thin-walled cysts scattered through lungs with no zonal predominance.
- Normal surrounding parenchyma but occasionally ground-glass opacities and/or interlobular septal thickening.
- Pneumothorax, chylothorax.
- Seen almost exclusively in women of childbearing age.
- The pulmonary manifestations of tuberous sclerosis are identical to those of lymphangioleiomyomatosis.

DIFFERENTIAL DIAGNOSIS

- Emphysema
- Pulmonary Langerhans cell histiocytosis
- Birt-Hogg-Dubé syndrome
- Lymphoid interstital pneumonia

PATHOLOGY

- Two key microscopic features characterize LAM: cyst formation and proliferation of LAM cells that express actin, desmin, and vimentin consistent with smooth muscle lineage.
- LAM cells tend to proliferate to form microscopic nodules.
- Nodule center contains predominantly spindle-shaped LAM cells, with immunoreactivity for actin and focal positivity for melanoma-associated antigens; periphery comprises larger epithelioid LAM cells.

INCIDENCE/PREVALENCE AND EPIDEMIOLOGY

- Sporadic LAM occurs in about 1 per 1 million persons.
- Pulmonary involvement with sporadic LAM is seen only in females of childbearing age with average age of 40 years.

WHAT THE REFERRING PHYSICIAN NEEDS TO KNOW

- Diagnosis is usually made clinically, with pivotal role of imaging to detect pulmonary or extrapulmonary pathologic processes.
- Gold standard for diagnosis of LAM is thoracoscopic lung biopsy.
- Biopsy is not required with classic high-resolution CT appearance.

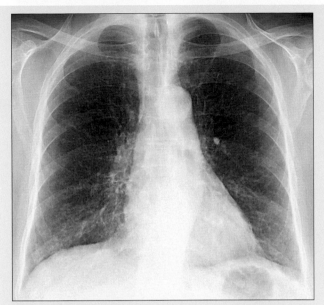

Figure 1. Lymphangioleiomyomatosis in a 78-year-old woman with cough and dyspnea. Posteroanterior chest radiograph shows a diffuse reticular pattern.

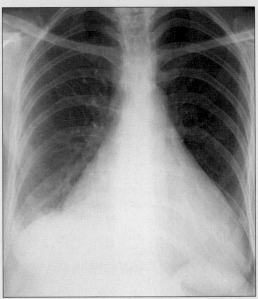

Figure 2. Chylous pleuropericardial effusion in a 40-year-old woman with lymphangioleiomyomatosis. Posteroanterior chest radiograph shows an enlarged cardiac silhouette and a moderate-sized right pleural effusion. Several small cysts were identified on an accompanying high-resolution CT scan. (*Courtesy of Drs. Nicola Sverzellati and David M. Hansell, London, UK*)

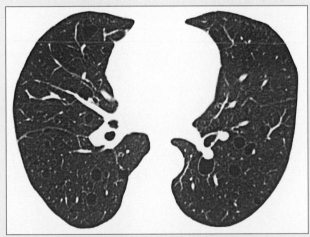

Figure 3. Lymphangioleiomyomatosis in a 38-year-old woman with dyspnea. High-resolution CT through the lower lobes demonstrates scattered thin-walled cysts of relatively uniform size. (*Courtesy of Drs. Nicola Sverzellati and David M. Hansell, London, UK*)

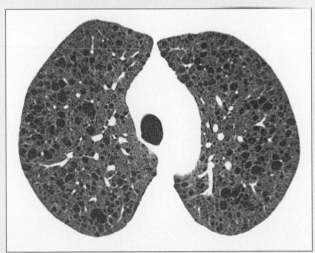

Figure 4. Lymphangioleiomyomatosis in a 75-year-old woman with dyspnea. High-resolution CT through the upper lobes demonstrates diffuse thin-walled cysts of relatively uniform size. (*Courtesy of Drs. Nicola Sverzellati and David M. Hansell, London, UK*)

- There are increasing reports of women developing LAM after menopause, including women in their eighth decade.
- LAM complicates 25%-35% of patients with tuberous sclerosis complex.

Suggested Readings

Abbott GF, Rosado-de-Christenson ML, Frazier AA, et al: From the archives of the AFIP: Lymphangioleiomyomatosis: Radiologic-pathologic correlation. *RadioGraphics* 25:803-828, 2005.

Johnson SR: Lymphangioleiomyomatosis. *Eur Respir J* 27(5):1056-1065, 2006.

Lenoir S, Grenier P, Brauner MW, et al: Pulmonary lymphangiomyomatosis and tuberous sclerosis: Comparison of radiographic and thin-section CT findings. *Radiology* 175:329-334, 1990.

Connective Tissue Diseases

Rheumatoid Arthritis: Pulmonary Parenchymal and Pleural Manifestations

DEFINITION: Rheumatoid arthritis may be associated with abnormalities of the lung parenchyma and pleura.

IMAGING

Radiography

Findings

- Cavitating necrobiotic nodules: readily recognizable on chest radiography
- Pulmonary fibrosis: reticular or reticulonodular pattern, usually symmetric and basal
- Subpleural distribution: may be appreciated in upper and mid lungs with overall lung volume reduction
- Organizing pneumonia: patches of changing, bilateral, peripheral consolidation
- Unilateral or bilateral pleural effusion or thickening

Utility

- Many interstitial lung diseases encountered in rheumatoid arthritis are nonspecific, and some may not be readily detected by chest radiography.

CT

Findings

- Usual interstitial pneumonia and nonspecific interstitial pneumonia patterns: reticulation and honeycombing with or without ground-glass opacities, with basal predominance.
- Organizing pneumonia: focal areas of consolidation, perilobular pattern, bands of consolidation, and centrilobular nodules.
- Lymphoid interstitial pneumonia: ground-glass opacities, poorly defined centrilobular nodules, interlobular septal thickening, and cysts.
- Rheumatoid nodules: peripheral, predominantly basal nodules.
- Unilateral or bilateral pleural effusion or thickening; pericardial effusion.

Utility

- Superior to the radiograph in demonstrating pattern and distribution of lung disease in rheumatoid arthritis.

DIAGNOSTIC PEARLS

- Honeycombing and reticulation with or without ground-glass opacities and lower lobe predominance in usual interstital pneumonia.
- Focal areas of consolidation, perilobular pattern, bands of consolidation, acinar opacities, and nodules in organizing pneumonia.
- Ground-glass opacities, poorly defined centrilobular nodules, and cysts in lymphoid interstitial pneumonia.
- Pleural and pericardial effusion typically occur during episodes of active arthritis.

- Evidence of interstitial lung disease eventually seen in 20%-30% of patients compared with 5% on radiograph.

CLINICAL PRESENTATION

- Most common respiratory symptoms in rheumatoid arthritis are exertional dyspnea and cough.

DIFFERENTIAL DIAGNOSIS

- Systemic lupus erythematosus
- Dermatomyositis
- Polymyositis
- Methotrexate lung toxicity
- Idiopathic pulmonary fibrosis
- Pneumonia

PATHOLOGY

- Rheumatoid arthritis is an autoimmune disorder of unknown cause with variable clinical manifestations.
- Most common interstitial lung diseases associated with rheumatoid arthritis are usual interstitial pneumonia and nonspecific interstitial pneumonia.

WHAT THE REFERRING PHYSICIAN NEEDS TO KNOW

- Rheumatoid factor positivity is associated with more severe pulmonary disease, with extra-articular manifestations and increased mortality.
- Chest radiograph is useful first-line investigation for symptomatic thoracic disease.
- Evidence of interstitial lung disease is evident on high-resolution CT in 20%-30% of patients compared with 5% on chest radiograph.
- Echocardiography should be performed to investigate for pulmonary hypertension even in the presence of normal high-resolution CT.
- Decreased diffusing capacity (DLCO) may alert clinician to presence of subtle pulmonary vasculopathy.
- Although nodules are generally asymptomatic, they can cavitate and result in catastrophic hemoptysis or pneumothorax.
- Solitary lung nodules in patients with rheumatoid arthritis are more likely to be lung cancer than necrobiotic nodules.

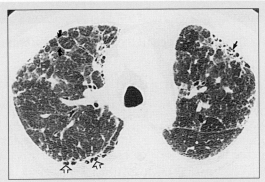

Figure 1. Usual interstitial pneumonia in rheumatoid arthritis. High-resolution CT image shows reticular pattern involving mainly the peripheral lung. The reticular pattern is due to a combination of intralobular linear opacities (*straight arrows*) and thickening of the interlobular septa (*curved arrows*). Honeycombing is evident, particularly in the right lower lobe (*open arrows*). The patient was a 73-year-old man who had long-standing rheumatoid disease. (*Courtesy of Drs. Maureen Quigley and David M. Hansell, London, UK*)

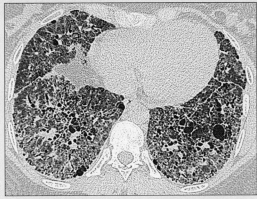

Figure 2. Nonspecific interstitial pneumonia in rheumatoid arthritis. High-resolution CT image shows extensive ground-glass opacities and reticulation reflecting severe fibrosis. The patient was a 30-year-old woman with rheumatoid arthritis and nonspecific interstitial pneumonia at lung biopsy. (*Courtesy of Drs. Maureen Quigley and David M. Hansell, London, UK*)

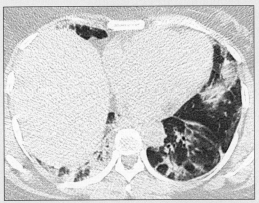

Figure 3. Organizing pneumonia in rheumatoid arthritis. High-resolution CT image shows patchy peripheral and perilobular consolidation, typical of organizing pneumonia. The patient was a 74-year old woman with rheumatoid arthritis. (*Courtesy of Drs. Maureen Quigley and David M. Hansell, London, UK*)

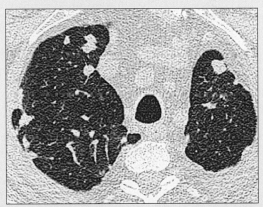

Figure 4. Necrobiotic nodules. High-resolution CT image shows bilateral nodules and pleural effusions. This 59-year-old man with rheumatoid arthritis had multiple histologically proven necrobiotic nodules and died when one of the nodules eroded an adjacent bronchial vessel. (*Courtesy of Drs. Maureen Quigley and David M. Hansell, London, UK*)

- Organizing pneumonia and lymphoid interstitial pneumonia are seen in some patients.
- Pulmonary rheumatoid nodules are uncommon: they range from 0.5-7.0 cm in diameter, with a necrotic center surrounded by palisaded histiocytes and leukocytes (like subcutaneous nodules).
- Pleural manifestations include pleurisy, effusion, and pleural thickening

INCIDENCE/PREVALENCE AND EPIDEMIOLOGY

- Rheumatoid arthritis is estimated to affect 1% of the adult population worldwide and occurs in women two to three times more often than men.
- Some manifestations of rheumatoid arthritis, such as pleural effusions, necrobiotic nodules, and idiopathic pulmonary fibrosis, are more frequent in men.

- Pulmonary complications are the second most common cause of death in patients with rheumatoid arthritis after infection.
- Pleural effusions are usually small and typically occur during episodes of active arthritis.

Suggested Readings

Anaya JM, Diethelm L, Ortiz LA, et al: Pulmonary involvement in rheumatoid arthritis. *Semin Arthritis Rheum* 24(4):242-254, 1995.

Gabbay E, Tarala R, Will R, et al: Interstitial lung disease in recent-onset rheumatoid arthritis. *Am J Respir Crit Care Med* 156(2 Pt 1): 528-535, 1997.

Remy-Jardin M, Remy J, Cortet B, et al: B: Lung changes in rheumatoid arthritis: CT findings. *Radiology* 193(2):375-382, 1994.

Tanaka N, Kim JS, Newell JD, et al: Rheumatoid arthritis–related lung diseases: CT findings. *Radiology* 232(1):81-91, 2004.

Tansey D, Wells AU, Colby TV, et al: Variations in histological patterns of interstitial pneumonia between connective tissue disorders and their relationship to prognosis. *Histopathology* 44(6): 585-596, 2004.

Rheumatoid Arthritis: Bronchial and Bronchiolar Manifestations

DEFINITION: Rheumatoid arthritis may be associated with abnormalities of the bronchi and bronchioles.

IMAGING

Radiography

Findings

- Follicular bronchiolitis (lymphoid hyperlasia) may be seen as ill-defined nodular opacities.
- Obliterative bronchiolitis commonly manifests as a normal radiograph.
- Severe obliterative bronchiolitis results in hyperinflation and attenuation of the peripheral vascular markings.
- Mild to moderate bronchiectasis is difficult to detect on the radiograph.
- Severe bronchiectasis results in tram-tracking and cystic changes.

Utility

- Some bronchial and bronchiolar manifestations may not be readily detected by chest radiography even with functionally severe air flow limitation.

CT

Findings

- Follicular bronchiolitis (lymphoid hyperlasia) is commonly seen on high-resolution CT as small centrilobular nodular opacities in the subpleural lung regions.
- Other features of follicular bronchiolitis include centrilobular and peribronchovascular nodules (1-12 mm diameter) and patchy areas of ground-glass opacity.
- Characteristic findings of obliterative bronchiolitis on high-resolution CT are areas of decreased attenuation and vascularity on inspiratory images and air trapping on images obtained at the end of maximal expiration.
- Ancillary findings of obliterative bronchiolitis include central and peripheral bronchial dilatation (bronchiectasis), bronchiolectasis, and bronchial wall thickening.
- On high-resolution CT, bronchiectasis has been reported in 15% of asymptomatic rheumatoid arthritis patients.

Utility

- High-resolution CT is imaging modality of choice in the assessment of presence and extent of bronchiolitis and bronchiectasis in patients with rheumatoid arthritis.
- Expiratory CT is superior to inspiratory CT in demonstrating the presence of findings consistent with obliterative bronchiolitis.

DIAGNOSTIC PEARLS

- Bronchiectasis.
- Areas of decreased attenuation and vascularity on inpiratory CT and air trapping an expiratory CT in patients with obliterative bronchiolitis.
- Bronchiectasis and obliterative bronchiolitis frequently coexist.
- Centrilobular and peribronchovascular nodules and patchy areas of ground-glass opacity in follicular bronchiolitis (lymphoid hyperplasia).

CLINICAL PRESENTATION

- Common respiratory symptoms in rheumatoid arthritis are exertional dyspnea or cough.
- Airways disease may present as wheeze but can be asymptomatic.
- Obliterative bronchiolitis is probably subclinical in many patients with rheumatoid arthritis.

DIFFERENTIAL DIAGNOSIS

- Infectious bronchiolitis
- Bronchopneumonia
- Drug reaction

PATHOLOGY

- Follicular bronchiolitis is characterized by lymphoid hyperplasia of bronchus-associated lymphoid tissue (BALT) with follicles distributed along bronchioles.
- Obliterative bronchiolitis, also known as constrictive bronchiolitis or bronchiolitis obliterans, is a condition characterized histologically by submucosal and peribronchiolar fibrosis with resulting bronchiolar narrowing or obliteration of the bronchiolar lumen.
- Bronchiectasis is defined as permanent, abnormal dilation of the bronchi.

INCIDENCE/PREVALENCE AND EPIDEMIOLOGY

- There is a strong association between rheumatoid arthritis and airway disease, with bronchiectasis and obliterative bronchiolitis frequently coexisting.

WHAT THE REFERRING PHYSICIAN NEEDS TO KNOW

- Rheumatoid factor positivity is associated with more severe pulmonary disease, with extra-articular manifestations and increased mortality.
- Pulmonary manifestations include interstitial lung diseases, pulmonary arterial hypertension, bronchiectasis, obliterative bronchiolitis, and follicular bronchiolitis.

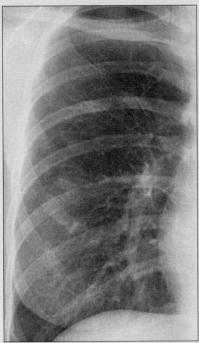

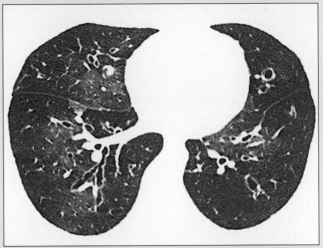

Figure 2. **Bronchiolitis obliterans in rheumatoid arthritis.** High-resolution CT shows bilateral areas of decreased attenuation and vascularity and extensive bronchiectasis. The patient was a 33-year-old woman with rheumatoid arthritis and severe air flow limitation. (*Courtesy of Drs. Maureen Quigley and David M. Hansell, London, UK*)

Figure 1. **Follicular bronchiolitis in rheumatoid arthritis.** View of the right lung from posterior chest radiograph shows ill-defined nodular opacities. A similar pattern was present in the left lung. The patient was a 24-year-old woman who had rheumatoid disease and biopsy-proven pulmonary lymphoid hyperplasia (follicular bronchiolitis). (*From Müller NL, Fraser RS, Colman N, et al: Radiologic Diagnosis of Diseases of the Chest. Philadelphia, WB Saunders, 2001.*)

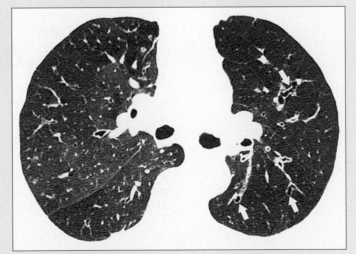

Figure 3. **Bronchiectasis in rheumatoid arthritis.** High-resolution CT image shows bronchiectasis (*arrows*), bronchial wall thickening, and areas of decreased attenuation and vascularity mainly in the left lung.

Suggested Readings

Franquet T, Müller NL: Disorders of the small airways: High-resolution computed tomographic features. *Semin Respir Crit Care Med* 24(4):437-444, 2003.

Hansell DM: Small airways diseases: Detection and insights with computed tomography. *Eur Respir J* 17(6):1294-1313, 2001.

Howling SJ, Hansell DM, Wells AU, et al: Follicular bronchiolitis: Thin-section CT and histologic findings. *Radiology* 212(3):637-642, 1999.

Tanaka N, Kim JS, Newell JD, et al: Rheumatoid arthritis–related lung diseases: CT findings. *Radiology* 232:81-91, 2004.

Scleroderma

DEFINITION: Scleroderma can result in pulmonary interstitial lung disease, pulmonary arterial hypertension, and pleural and esophageal abnormalities.

IMAGING

Radiography

Findings
- Widespread symmetric basal reticulonodular pattern
- Association with dilated air-filled esophagus
- Signs of pulmonary hypertension

Utility
- Chest radiograph is the first requested modality but lacks sensitivity.
- Findings may be normal.

CT

Findings
- Ground-glass opacities in lower lung zones and subpleural regions with reticulation, architectural distortion, and honeycombing.
- Progressive reticulation, traction bronchiectasis, traction bronchiolectasis, and, less commonly, honeycombing
- Increased diameter of main pulmonary artery (>3 cm)
- Dilated esophagus in majority of patients
- Pleural effusions occur in 5%-10%
- Slightly enlarged mediastinal nodes common

Utility
- High-resolution CT is more sensitive.
- Rule out coexisting carcinoma.
- Consolidation may occur owing to superimposed or coexistent pathologic process.

Nuclear Medicine

Findings
- Clearance of inhaled technetium 99m-labeled diethylenetriamine pentaacetic acid (^{99m}Tc-DTPA) is index of lung epithelial permeability.

Utility
- ^{99m}Tc-DTPA scanning can be used to evaluate potential longitudinal behavior of fibrotic lung disease.
- Modality is seldom used in clinical practice.

CLINICAL PRESENTATION

- Shortness of breath on exertion
- Dry cough

DIAGNOSTIC PEARLS

- Ground-glass opacities in lower lung and subpleural region
- Progressive reticulation and architectural distortion with little honeycombing
- Dilated esophagus
- Signs of pulmonary arterial hypertension
- Increased incidence of lung cancer

DIFFERENTIAL DIAGNOSIS

- Idiopathic nonspecific interstitial pneumonia
- Hypersensitivity pneumonitis
- Infection
- Drug reaction

PATHOLOGY

- Autoimmune process involves cellular microchimerism
- Fibrosis and vascular obliteration of skin, gastrointestinal tract, lungs, heart, and kidneys occur.
- Histologic type of pulmonary fibrosis is usually nonspecific interstitial pneumonia rather than usual interstitial pneumonia.
- Few cases of diffuse alveolar damage have been reported.
- Patients with systemic sclerosis have increased incidence of lung cancer.

INCIDENCE/PREVALENCE AND EPIDEMIOLOGY

- Uncommon
- Annual incidence of approximately 20 per million population per year
- Estimated prevalence of 500 cases per million population
- Affects mainly women in their childbearing years
- Pulmonary fibrosis in 80% of patients
- Increased risk of pulmonary carcinoma

WHAT THE REFERRING PHYSICIAN NEEDS TO KNOW

- Positive anti–Scl-70 antibody patients are more likely to develop fibrotic lung disease.
- Patients have increased incidence of lung cancer.
- Chest radiography is first imaging modality; if normal, confirmatory high-resolution CT is often performed.
- High-resolution CT pattern is most commonly of nonspecific interstitial pneumonia.
- Interstitial lung disease may precede other manifestations of systemic sclerosis by several years.
- Lung function is most sensitively monitored by measurements of diffusing capacity (DLco).

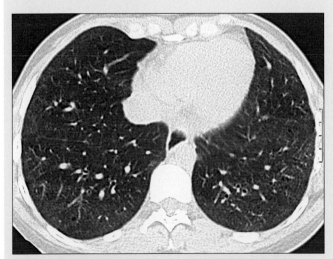

Figure 1. Systemic sclerosis: radiograph. Chest radiograph shows a reticular pattern mainly in the lower lung zones and decreased lung volumes. Also note the air-filled lucency in the left paratracheal region due to a dilated esophagus. The patient was a 73-year-old woman with diffuse systemic sclerosis. (*Courtesy of Drs. Maureen Quigley and David M. Hansell, London, UK*)

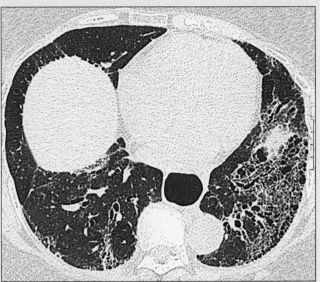

Figure 2. Systemic sclerosis: high-resolution CT findings. High-resolution CT demonstrates ground-glass opacities, extensive reticulation, and traction bronchiectasis and bronchiolectasis in the left lower lobe. Mild fibrosis is seen in the right lower and middle lobes and lingula. Note minimal bilateral subpleural honeycombing. The parenchymal findings were confirmed to be nonspecific interstitial pneumonia. Note dilated esophagus. The patient was a 73-year-old woman with diffuse systemic sclerosis.(*Courtesy of Drs. Maureen Quigley and David M. Hansell, London, UK*)

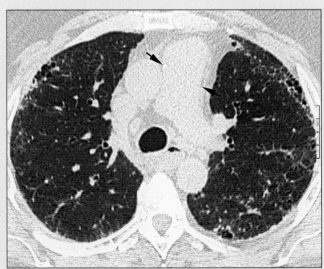

Figure 3. Nonspecific interstitial pneumonia in systemic sclerosis. High-resolution CT shows diffuse bilateral ground-glass opacities. Note minimal bilateral peripheral reticulation and dilated esophagus. The patient was a 31-year-old man with diffuse systemic sclerosis.(*Courtesy of Drs. Maureen Quigley and David M. Hansell, London, UK*)

Figure 4. Pulmonary hypertension and fibrotic lung disease in systemic sclerosis. CT image shows bilateral ground-glass opacities and predominantly peripheral reticulation and minimal honeycombing consistent with interstitial fibrosis. The diameter of the pulmonary artery (*arrows*) is greater than that of the adjacent ascending aorta. The patient was a 62-year-old man with diffuse systemic sclerosis, fibrotic lung disease, and pulmonary hypertension confirmed by right-sided heart catheterization. (*Courtesy of Drs. Maureen Quigley and David M. Hansell, London, UK*)

Suggested Readings

Desai SR, Veeraraghavan S, Hansell DM, et al: CT features of lung disease in patients with systemic sclerosis: Comparison with idiopathic pulmonary fibrosis and nonspecific interstitial pneumonia. *Radiology* 232(2):560-567, 2004.

Devaraj A, Wells AU, Hansell DM: Computed tomographic imaging in connective tissue diseases. *Semin Respir Crit Care Med* 28(4):389-397, 2007.

Highland KB, Garin MC, Brown KK: The spectrum of scleroderma lung disease. *Semin Respir Crit Care Med* 28(4):418-429, 2007.

Orlandi I, Camiciottoli G, Diciotti S, et al: Thin-section and low-dose volumetric computed tomographic densitometry of the lung in systemic sclerosis. *J Comput Assist Tomogr* 30(5):823-827, 2006.

Systemic Lupus Erythematosus

DEFINITION: Systemic lupus erythematosus may result in pulmonary, pleural, cardiac, and pericardial abnormalities.

IMAGING

Radiography

Findings

- Bilateral pleural effusions or pleural thickening
- Enlargement of the cardiopericardial silhouette due to pericardial effusion or cardiomegaly
- Most common pulmonary manifestation: consolidation due to infection
- Acute lupus pneumonitis: nonspecific but characteristically shows unilateral or bilateral patchy ground-glass opacities or consolidation, predominantly in lower zones
- Pulmonary hemorrhage: bilateral ground-glass opacities or consolidation that may be patchy or diffuse
- "Shrinking lung" syndrome: elevated hemidiaphragms, adjacent atelectasis, and, rarely, small pleural effusions
- Interstitial disease: a reticular pattern in a predominantly basal distribution

Utility

- First and often only imaging modality utilized in the diagnosis and follow-up of patients

CT

Findings

- "Shrinking lung" syndrome: elevated hemidiaphragms, adjacent atelectasis, and, rarely, small pleural effusions
- Interstitial disease: ground-glass opacities, and reticular pattern in a predominantly basal distribution
- Diffuse alveolar hemorrhage: patchy or widespread ground-glass opacity and airspace consolidation
- Acute lupus pneumonitis: extensive ground-glass opacities or confluent consolidation and air bronchograms evident on high-resolution CT
- Consolidation often accompanied by pleural effusions
- Antiphospholipid syndrome and tendency to develop pulmonary embolism in > 50%

Utility

- Any clinical suspicion of pulmonary embolism should be investigated by CT, pulmonary angiography, or radionuclide ventilation-perfusion scanning.
- High-resolution CT is the test of choice for the investigation of known or suspected interstitial lung disease.

DIAGNOSTIC PEARLS

- Acute lupus pneumonitis: nonspecific but characteristically shows unilateral or bilateral patchy ground-glass opacities or consolidation predominantly in lower zones
- "Shrinking lung" syndrome: elevated hemidiaphragms, adjacent atelectasis, and, rarely, small pleural effusions
- Small pleural and pericardial effusions
- Most common pulmonary manifestation: consolidation due to pneumonia
- Increased prevalence of pulmonary embolism
- Interstitial fibrosis is uncommon

Nuclear Medicine

Findings

- Positive ventilation-perfusion scan in patients with pulmonary embolism.

Utility

- Ventilation-perfusion scanning has role in the investigation of pulmonary embolus.

CLINICAL PRESENTATION

- May be asymptomatic.
- Most frequent symptoms: arthritis, malar rash, photosensitivity, and neurologic involvement.
- Recurrent pleuritic chest pain, cough, dyspnea.
- "Shrinking lung" syndrome, diaphragmatic weakness, and chest wall restriction; unexplained dyspnea, initially on exertion, that progresses over several months.
- Lupus pneumonitis: can present as fulminant respiratory failure, secondary to opportunistic infections, drugs, or impaired renal or cardiac function.
- Diffuse alveolar hemorrhage: can be clinically silent but usually manifests as hemoptysis, hypoxemia, cough, anemia, and blood on bronchoalveolar lavage.

DIFFERENTIAL DIAGNOSIS

- Pneumonia
- Diffuse pulmonary hemorrhage
- Drug reaction
- Diffuse alveolar damage

WHAT THE REFERRING PHYSICIAN NEEDS TO KNOW

- Serologic positivity for antinuclear antibodies is a sensitive test and is found in nearly all patients.
- Anti-DNA antibodies are far more specific.
- Diagnosis is often elusive and may take up to 2 years from first manifestations to be definitive.
- There is a wide spectrum of clinical presentations.
- Death results from acute exacerbations of the disease, infections, or thrombotic events.

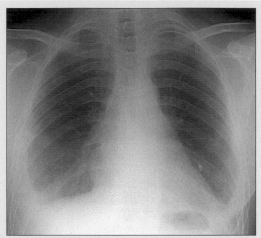

Figure 1. Bilateral pleural effusions in systemic lupus erythematosus. Chest radiograph in a 30-year-old woman shows bilateral, small pleural effusions (left-sided chest drain is in situ). (*Courtesy of Drs. Maureen Quigley and David M. Hansell, London, UK*)

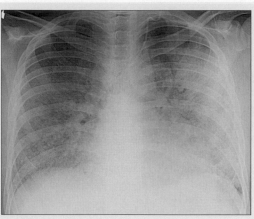

Figure 2. Diffuse pulmonary hemorrhage in systemic lupus erythematosus. Chest radiograph shows diffuse bilateral consolidation. The patient was an 18-year-old male who presented with hemoptysis.

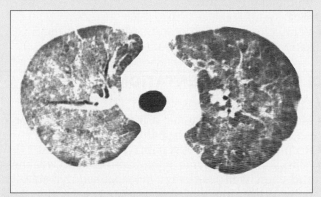

Figure 3. Diffuse pulmonary hemorrhage in systemic lupus erythematosus: CT findings. High-resolution CT at the level of the upper lobes shows bilateral ground-glass opacities, areas of consolidation, mild septal thickening, and poorly defined nodular opacities more severe on the right.

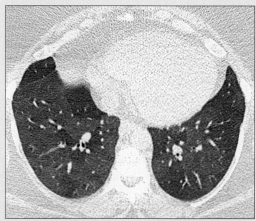

Figure 4. Acute lupus pneumonitis. A 37-year-old woman presented with acute respiratory compromise and systemic lupus erythematosus. High-resolution CT shows widespread ground-glass opacities. The patient went on to develop a subtle fibrosis in the same distribution as the ground-glass opacity. (*Courtesy of Drs. Maureen Quigley and David M. Hansell, London, UK*)

PATHOLOGY

- Diffuse alveolar damage or acute lupus pneumonitis results in healing and fibrinolysis or parenchymal fibrosis (permanent scarring).
- Pure small airways disease (e.g., such as constrictive obliterative bronchiolitis) is rare.
- Myopathy can affect the diaphragm, resulting in a raised diaphragm and basal atelectasis, the so-called shrinking lung syndrome.

INCIDENCE/PREVALENCE AND EPIDEMIOLOGY

- Prevalence rate ranges from 17 to 48/100,000 of the population.
- Most patients are female (F:M ratio, 8:1) between the ages of 15 and 45 years.
- During childhood and after the menopause the female-to-male ratio is closer to 2:1.

- Highest mortality occurs in patients with infections, renal disease, non-Hodgkin lymphoma, and lung cancer.
- Mortality risk is greatest with female gender, younger age, disease duration of <1 year, and African-American ethnicity.
- The frequency of acute lupus pneumonitis in hospitalized patients with lupus is up to 6%.

Suggested Readings

Devaraj A, Wells AU, Hansell DM: Computed tomographic imaging in connective tissue diseases. *Semin Respir Crit Care Med* 28(4):389-397, 2007.

Kim JS, Lee KS, Koh EM, et al: Thoracic involvement of systemic lupus erythematosus: Clinical, pathologic, and radiologic findings. *J Comput Assist Tomogr* 24:9-18, 2000.

Mackillop LH, Germain SJ, Nelson-Piercy C: Systemic lupus erythematosus. *BMJ* 335:933-936, 2007.

Memet B, Ginzler EM: Pulmonary manifestations of systemic lupus erythematosus. *Semin Respir Crit Care Med* 28:441-450, 2007.

Wiedemann HP, Matthay RA: Pulmonary manifestations of systemic lupus erythematosus. *J Thorac Imaging* 7:1-18, 1992.

Polymyositis/Dermatomyositis

DEFINITION: Polymyositis (PM)/dermatomyositis (DM) may result in pulmonary parenchymal and vascular abnormalities, and may affect the pleura, diaphragm, heart, and chest wall muscles.

IMAGING

Radiography

Findings
- Bibasal irregular linear opacities (reticulation) or consolidation.
- Nonspecific interstitial pneumonia: lower lung reticulation and hazy increased opacity (ground-glass).
- Organizing pneumonia: bilateral patchy, mainly peribronchial or subpleural consolidation.
- Diffuse alveolar damage: sudden-onset ground-glass opacities with rapid progression to extensive bilateral consolidation.
- Dependent consolidation due to aspiration.

Utility
- Chest radiography is main imaging modality to exclude clinically occult disease or respiratory infection.

CT

Findings
- Linear opacities, consolidation, ground-glass opacity, rarely honeycombing
- Nonspecific interstitial pneumonia: lower lung ground-glass opacities with variable superimposed intralobular reticulation
- Fibrotic nonspecific interstitial pneumonia: later stage of predominant reticulation, architectural distortion, traction bronchiectasis, and bronchiolectasis
- Organizing pneumonia: patchy or random predominately subpleural or peribronchovascular consolidation
- Mixed nonspecific interstitial pneumonia and organizing pneumonia
- Diffuse alveolar damage: patchy consolidation and ground-glass attenuation with or without interstitial fibrosis
- Consolidation in the dependent lung regions due to aspiration
- Pleural effusion may occur
- Signs of pulmonary arterial hypertension

DIAGNOSTIC PEARLS

- Chronic diffuse lung disease usually with pattern of nonspecific interstitial pneumonia or organizing pneumonia.
- Nonspecific interstitial pneumonia: lower lung ground-glass opacities with superimposed reticulation.
- Organizing pneumonia pattern: bilateral peribronchial and peripheral consolidation.
- Recurrent aspiration: consolidation and centrilobular nodules in the dependent lung regions.

Utility
- High-resolution CT is used to further characterize diffuse lung disease.
- Consolidation may be due to superimposed pneumonia.

CLINICAL PRESENTATION

- Wide range of pulmonary symptoms include acute/fulminant (diffuse alveolar damage, pneumonia) to chronic/insidious (interstitial lung disease), sometimes occult disease.
- Pulmonary symptoms may precede inflammatory myopathy.
- PM hallmark is proximal muscle weakness with muscle tenderness and myalgia.
- Dyspnea and aspiration pneumonia are common.
- Respiratory failure is secondary to weakness of respiratory muscles.
- DM hallmark is heliotrope periorbital edema and scaly erythematous dermatitis.

DIFFERENTIAL DIAGNOSIS

- Idiopathic nonspecific interstitial pneumonia
- Cryptogenic organizing pneumonia

WHAT THE REFERRING PHYSICIAN NEEDS TO KNOW

- A wide range of pulmonary symptoms are present; onset can be acute/fulminant/fatal or chronic and progressive.
- Presence of occult pulmonary disease should always be considered.
- Most common cause of mortality is sepsis; patients are immunosuppressed and susceptible to many pathogens.
- Acute symptoms include pneumonia, aspiration, diffuse alveolar damage, diffuse hemorrhage, and left-sided heart failure due to cardiac involvement.
- Chronic symptoms include recurrent aspiration, nonspecific interstitial pneumonia, and organizing pneumonia.
- Patients with anti-synthetase antibodies are more likely to have interstitial lung disease.
- Patients without anti-synthetase antibodies with acute interstitial pneumonitis have poor prognosis.
- An increased risk of malignancy is associated; screening should be performed in adults.

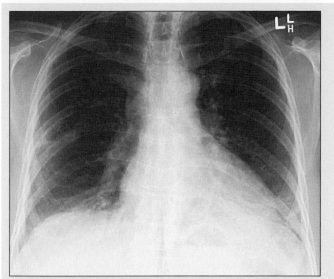

Figure 1. **Nonspecific interstitial pneumonia in polymyositis.** Chest radiograph shows low lung volumes, hazy increased opacity (ground-glass opacities) in the lower lung zones, and mild basal reticular pattern. The patient was a 55-year-old woman with polymyositis and biopsy-proven nonspecific interstitial pneumonia.

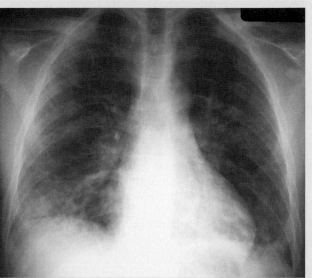

Figure 2. **Organizing pneumonia in polymyositis.** Chest radiograph shows bilateral areas of consolidation involving mainly the lower lung zones. The patient was a 27-year-old man with polymyositis. The diagnosis of organizing pneumonia was proven at surgical biopsy.

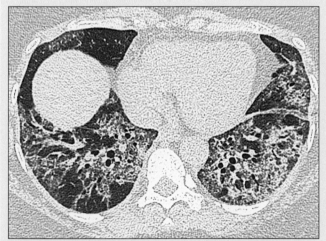

Figure 3. **Nonspecific interstitial pneumonia in polymyositis.** High-resolution CT image shows bilateral ground-glass opacities and mild reticulation. The patient was a 58-year-old woman with polymyositis and fibrotic nonspecific interstitial pneumonia. (*Courtesy of Drs. Maureen Quigley and David M. Hansell, London, UK*)

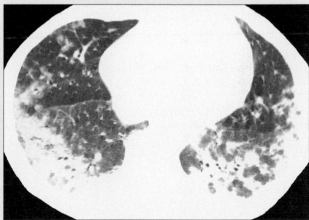

Figure 4. **Organizing pneumonia in polymyositis.** High-resolution CT image demonstrate areas of consolidation mainly in the subpleural regions. The patient was a 27-year-old man with polymyositis. The diagnosis of organizing pneumonia was proven at surgical biopsy.

- Drug reaction
- Bacterial bronchopneumonia
- Aspiration

PATHOLOGY

- Immune-mediated muscle inflammation and vascular damage.
- Acute epithelial injury, then organization with intra-alveolar buds of granulation tissue.
- Associated parenchymal lung disease: nonspecific interstitial pneumonia, organizing pneumonia, diffuse alveolar damage, usual interstitial pneumonia, and alveolar hemorrhage.
- Immunosuppressed patients prone to opportunistic infections.

INCIDENCE/PREVALENCE AND EPIDEMIOLOGY

- Incidence of 5-10 cases of DM/PM per million per year
- DM peaks: children and young to middle-aged adults
- PM: female-to-male ratio 2:1; more prevalent in African-Americans
- Interstitial lung disease in 39%-65% of patients

Suggested Readings

Akira M, Hara H, Sakatani M: Interstitial lung disease in association with polymyositis-dermatomyositis: Long-term follow-up CT evaluation in seven patients. *Radiology* 210(2):333-338, 1999.

Arakawa H, Yamada H, Kurihara Y, et al: Nonspecific interstitial pneumonia associated with polymyositis and dermatomyositis: Serial high-resolution CT findings and functional correlation. *Chest* 123(4):1096-1103, 2003.

Dalakas MC, Hohlfeld R: Polymyositis and dermatomyositis. *Lancet* 362(9388):971-982, 2003.

Devaraj A, Wells AU, Hansell DM: Computed tomographic imaging in connective tissue diseases. *Semin Respir Crit Care Med* 28(4):389-397, 2007.

Ikezoe J, Johkoh T, Kohno N, et al: High-resolution CT findings of lung disease in patients with polymyositis and dermatomyositis. *J Thorac Imaging* 11(4):250-259, 1996.

Mino M, Noma S, Taguchi Y, et al: Pulmonary involvement in polymyositis and dermatomyositis: Sequential evaluation with CT. *AJR Am J Roentgenol* 169(1):83-87, 1997.

Sjögren Syndrome

DEFINITION: Sjögren syndrome is a disorder of the immune system that is largely defined by its two most common symptoms: dry eyes and a dry mouth.

IMAGING

Radiography

Findings
- Reticular or reticulonodular pattern and ground-glass opacities usually involving mainly the lower lung zones.
- Bilateral consolidation and reticulonodular opacities or multiple cysts.
- Abnormal mediastinal and hilar contours if supervening lymphoma is associated.
- Lymphoma: indolent, or indeed static, areas of consolidation on serial radiographs.

Utility
- Radiography is the main imaging modality in the initial assessment and follow-up.
- Normal chest radiograph does not preclude parenchymal or nodal disease.

CT

Findings
- Nonspecific interstitial pneumonia: ground-glass opacities associated with superimposed reticulation, traction bronchiectasis, and bronchiolectasis, involving mainly lower lung zones.
- More extensive reticulation with/without associated honeycombing evident in usual interstitial pneumonia.
- Lymphocytic interstitial pneumonia: ground-glass opacities, poorly defined centrilobular nodules and, sometimes, areas of consolidation and interlobular septal thickening.
- Cysts superimposed on ground-glass opacities in 50% to 60% of patients with lymphocytic interstitial pneumonia; isolated cysts possible.
- Organizing pneumonia: bilateral areas of consolidation, predominantly in a peribronchial, perilobular, or subpleural distribution.
- Airway abnormalities including bronchiectasis, bronchiolectasis, areas of decreased attenuation and vascularity, and air trapping on expiratory CT in approximately 30% of patients.

DIAGNOSTIC PEARLS

- Chronic interstitial lung diseases include nonspecific interstitial pneumonia, usual interstitial pneumonia, lymphocytic interstitial pneumonia, and organizing pneumonia.
- Nonspecific interstitial pneumonia: ground-glass opacities and reticulation mainly in lower lung zones.
- Lymphocytic interstitial pneumonia: ground-glass opacities and cysts mainly in lower lung zones.
- Organizing pneumonia: peribronchial and peripheral areas of consolidation; perilobular pattern.
- Bronchiectasis and air trapping are common.
- Malignant lymphoma is major cause of morbidity and mortality.
- Lymphoma: slowly progressive focal or multifocal consolidation; lymphadenopathy.

Utility
- High-resolution CT is the investigation of choice to assess the presence and extent of interstitial and airway disease.
- The presence of thin-walled cysts superimposed on ground-glass opacities in patients with Sjögren syndrome is virtually diagnostic of lymphocytic interstitial pneumonia.

CLINICAL PRESENTATION

- Dry eyes and a dry mouth
- Arthralgia
- Dry cough and progressive shortness of breath

DIFFERENTIAL DIAGNOSIS

- Drug reaction
- Bacterial pneumonia
- Lymphoma

WHAT THE REFERRING PHYSICIAN NEEDS TO KNOW

- Malignant lymphoma is a major cause of morbidity and mortality in patients with primary Sjögren syndrome.
- Common pulmonary manifestations include interstitial fibrosis, most commonly nonspecific interstitial pneumonia, lymphocytic interstitial pneumonia, bronchiectasis, obliterative bronchiolitis, and lymphoma.
- The radiographic findings are nonspecific.
- Persistent or slowly progressive focal areas of consolidation or lymphadenopathy should raise concern for lymphoma.
- Nonspecific, usual, and lymphocytic forms of interstitial pneumonia frequently have characteristic findings on high-resolution CT.

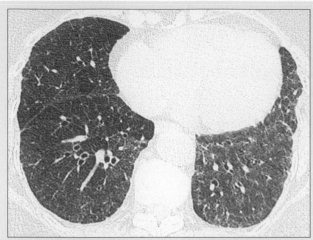

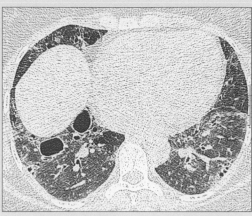

Figure 2. **Lymphoid interstitial pneumonia in Sjögren syndrome.** High-resolution CT image in a 50-year-old woman with lymphoid interstitial pneumonia shows cystic airspaces, ground-glass opacities, and small nodules. (*Courtesy of Drs. Maureen Quigley and David M. Hansell, London, UK*)

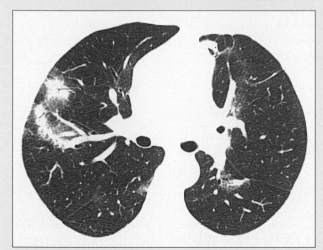

Figure 1. **Nonspecific interstitial pneumonia in Sjögren syndrome.** High-resolution CT image demonstrates extensive bilateral ground-glass opacities and minimal reticulation. The patient was a 77-year-old woman with Sjögren syndrome and nonspecific interstitial pneumonia.

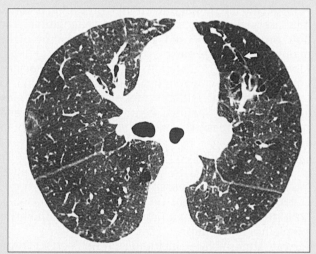

Figure 3. **Organizing pneumonia in Sjögren syndrome.** High-resolution CT image shows bilateral areas of consolidation in a predominantly peribronchial distribution surrounded by a halo of ground-glass attenuation. Also noted is perilobular distribution in the right upper lobe and patchy bilateral ground-glass opacities. The patient was a 52-year-old woman with Sjögren syndrome and organizing pneumonia.

Figure 4. **Bronchiectasis in Sjögren syndrome.** High-resolution CT in a 70-year-old woman with Sjögren syndrome shows left upper lobe bronchiectasis (*arrow*) and focal areas of decreased attenuation and vascularity consistent with obliterative bronchiolitis. Also evident is minimal bilateral ground-glass opacities.

PATHOLOGY

- Primary Sjögren syndrome: occurs in the absence of an accompanying connective tissue disease.
- Secondary Sjögren syndrome: accompanied by another connective tissue disease.
- Major histologic lung disease patterns found on biopsy: nonspecific interstitial pneumonia, lymphocytic interstitial pneumonia, bronchiolitis, malignant lymphoma, amyloidosis, atelectatic fibrosis, honeycombing.
- Lymphocytic interstitial pneumonia: diffuse interstitial proliferation of mature small lymphocytes and plasma cells; commonly occurs in patients with Sjögren syndrome.

INCIDENCE/PREVALENCE AND EPIDEMIOLOGY

- The disorder can develop at any age, but 59 years of age is the average age at presentation (range: age 43-75 years).
- Two age peaks for primary disease include after menarche (in the third decade) and after menopause.

- Worldwide prevalence is 14.4 per 100,000 population.
- It is nine times more frequent in women than in men.
- Prevalence of clinically significant lung disease in the population of patients with Sjögren syndrome is low.
- Malignant lymphoma is a major cause of morbidity and mortality in patients with primary Sjögren syndrome.

Suggested Readings

Devaraj A, Wells AU, Hansell DM: Computed tomographic imaging in connective tissue diseases. *Semin Respir Crit Care Med* 28(4):389-397, 2007.

Fox RI: Sjogren's syndrome. *Lancet* 366(9482):321-331, 2005.

Franquet T, Giménez A, Monill JM, et al: Primary Sjögren's syndrome and associated lung disease: CT findings in 50 patients. *AJR Am J Roentgenol* 169(3):655-658, 1997.

Ito I, Nagai S, Kitaichi M, et al: Pulmonary manifestations of primary Sjogren's syndrome: A clinical, radiologic, and pathologic study. *Am J Respir Crit Care Med* 171(6):632-638, 2005.

Lohrmann C, Uhl M, Warnatz K, et al: High-resolution CT imaging of the lung for patients with primary Sjogren's syndrome. *Eur J Radiol* 52(2):137-143, 2004.

Papiris SA, Tsonis IA, Moutsopoulos HM: Sjögren's syndrome. *Semin Respir Crit Care Med* 28(4):459-471, 2007.

Mixed Connective Tissue Disease

DEFINITION: Pulmonary manifestations of mixed connective tissue disease include chronic interstitial lung disease, diffuse pulmonary hemorrhage, and pulmonary hypertension.

IMAGING

Radiography
Findings
- Reticular or reticulonodular pattern in lower zones
- Ill-defined hazy opacities (ground-glass opacities) or consolidation
- Enlarged central pulmonary arteries
- Pleural effusion

Utility
- Less sensitive than high-resolution CT for detection of interstitial lung disease

CT
Findings
- Enlarged central pulmonary arteries due to pulmonary artery hypertension with or without associated interstitial lung disease.
- Interstitial lung disease with ground-glass opacities, intralobular linear opacities (reticulation) predominantly in lower lung zones, and sometimes honeycombing.
- Peribronchial and peripheral consolidation in patients with organizing pneumonia.
- Micronodules (lymphoid hyperplasia).
- Occasionally diffuse ground-glass opacities or consolidation due to diffuse pulmonary hemorrhage.
- Pleural effusion.

Utility
- Interstitial lung disease should be investigated with high-resolution CT.
- Echocardiography is superior to CT in demonstrating the presence of pulmonary hypertension.

Nuclear Medicine
Findings
- Active interstitial disease: abnormal clearance time for technetium-99m–labeled diethylenetriamine pentaacetic acid (^{99m}Tc-DTPA).

DIAGNOSTIC PEARLS

- Nonspecific interstitial pneumonia, organizing pneumonia, or less commonly, usual interstitial pneumonia pattern.
- Pulmonary hypertension with or without associated interstitial lung disease.
- Diffuse pulmonary hemorrhage may occur.
- Key diagnostic criteria component: positive anti–U1-RNP antibodies at hemagglutination titer of 1:1600 or greater.
- Clinical criteria (at least three): edema of hands, synovitis, myositis, Raynaud's phenomenon, acrosclerosis.

Utility
- Limited utility in diagnosis and management

Echocardiography
Findings
- Pulmonary artery hypertension
- Pericardial effusion

Utility
- Imaging modality of choice for assessment of pulmonary artery hypertension

CLINICAL PRESENTATION

- Dyspnea on exertion is common presentation of pulmonary hypertension; other pulmonary clinical manifestations are pleuritic chest pain and bibasilar rales.
- Raynaud's phenomenon, arthralgia, arthritis, swollen hands, sclerodactyly or acrosclerosis, and frank myositis may occur.
- Esophageal dysmotility and reflux, generalized lymphadenopathy, and secondary Sjögren syndrome can occur.

WHAT THE REFERRING PHYSICIAN NEEDS TO KNOW

- Mixed connective tissue disease is a distinct entity characterized by features of systemic sclerosis, systemic lupus erythematosus, and polymyositis/dermatomyositis, with respiratory involvement occurring in up to 80% of patients.
- Key diagnostic criteria include clinical manifestations and positive anti–U1-RNP antibodies at hemagglutination titer of 1:1600 or greater.
- Normal radiography does not rule out pulmonary disease.
- Rule out infective process in presence of nonspecific pulmonary abnormalities because these patients are immunosuppressed.
- Echocardiography, clinical history, and decreased diffusing capacity (DLco) can assist in identifying pulmonary hypertension.
- Large proportion of patients with early mixed connective tissue disease appear to have steroid-responsive interstitial lung disease.

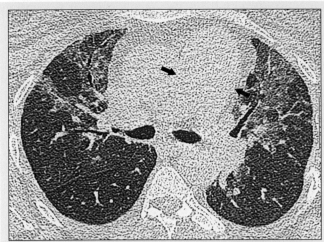

Figure 1. Pulmonary hypertension and fibrotic lung disease in mixed connective tissue disease. High-resolution CT shows bilateral ground-glass opacities and mild reticulation and traction bronchiectasis in a bronchovascular distribution. Also note dilatation of the pulmonary artery (*arrows*). (*Courtesy of Drs. Maureen Quigley and David M. Hansell, London, UK*)

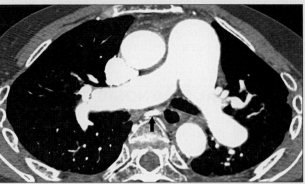

Figure 2. Pulmonary hypertension in mixed connective tissue disease. Contrast-enhanced CT shows marked dilatation of the main, right, and left pulmonary arteries. Also note enlarged bronchial arteries (*arrow*). The patient was a 44-year-old woman with mixed connective tissue disease and severe pulmonary artery hypertension.

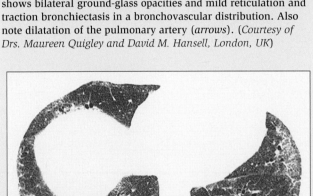

Figure 3. Nonspecific interstitial pneumonia in mixed connective tissue disease. High-resolution CT shows bilateral ground-glass opacities, fine reticulation, traction bronchiectasis, and traction bronchiolectasis mainly in the peripheral lung regions. Note the relative sparing of the subpleural lung in the dorsal regions, a feature characteristic of nonspecific interstitial pneumonia. The patient was a 43-year-old woman with mixed connective tissue disease and a pattern of nonspecific interstitial pneumonia on CT.

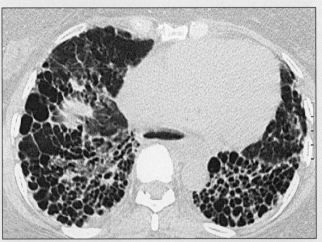

Figure 4. Honeycombing in mixed connective tissue disease. High-resolution CT shows marked honeycombing and a dilated esophagus. The patient was a 55-year-old woman with mixed connective tissue disease. The histologic subtype of the fibrosis was not established, but the pattern is suggestive of usual interstitial pneumonia. (*Courtesy of Drs. Maureen Quigley and David M. Hansell, London, UK*)

- Pericarditis, myocarditis, and complete heart block can occur.
- Cutaneous manifestations of mixed connective tissue disease include photosensitivity, livedo reticularis, and calcinosis.

DIFFERENTIAL DIAGNOSIS

- Systemic lupus erythematosus
- Rheumatoid arthritis
- Progressive systemic sclerosis
- Idiopathic pulmonary hypertension
- Idiopathic nonspecific interstitial pneumonia
- Drug reaction

INCIDENCE/PREVALENCE AND EPIDEMIOLOGY

- Pulmonary disease has been reported in 73% of patients with mixed connective tissue disease.
- Pulmonary hypertension may be associated with interstitial lung disease or may be the sole intrathoracic manifestation of mixed connective tissue disease.

- It is estimated to have the same incidence as systemic sclerosis.
- Majority of patients are women, and average age at diagnosis is 37 years (range: 4-80 years).
- Pulmonary hypertension and severe infection secondary to immunosuppression are common causes of death.

Suggested Readings

Devaraj A, Wells AU, Hansell DM: Computed tomographic imaging in connective tissue diseases. *Semin Respir Crit Care Med* 28(4):389-397, 2007.

Kozuka T, Johkoh T, Honda O, et al: Pulmonary involvement in mixed connective tissue disease: High-resolution CT findings in 41 patients. *J Thorac Imaging* 16(2):94-98, 2001.

Pope JE: Other manifestations of mixed connective tissue disease. *Rheum Dis Clin North Am* 31(3):519-533, 2005:VII.

Prakash UB: Respiratory complications in mixed connective tissue disease. *Clin Chest Med* 19:733-746, 1998.

Saito Y, Terada M, Takada T, et al: Pulmonary involvement in mixed connective tissue disease: Comparison with other collagen vascular diseases using high resolution CT. *J Comput Assist Tomogr* 26(3):349-357, 2002.

Venables PJ: Mixed connective tissue disease. *Lupus* 15(3):132-137, 2006.

Relapsing Polychondritis

DEFINITION: Relapsing polychondritis is a rare autoimmune disease characterized by episodic inflammation of cartilaginous structures anywhere in the body but predominantly of the major airways.

IMAGING

Radiography
Findings
- Gross tracheal narrowing or focal tracheal stenosis may be evident on chest radiography.
- Consolidation secondary to lower respiratory tract infection is an important finding.
- Arthropathy associated with relapsing polychondritis is characterized by joint space narrowing without erosions.

Utility
- Chest radiography has a role in identification of lower respiratory tract infection, which can occur secondary to upper airway obstruction.

CT
Findings
- Smoothly thickened tracheal wall with sparing of posterior membranous wall.
- Increased tracheal and bronchial wall thickness secondary to inflammation typically involves the cartilaginous portion.
- Increased airway wall attenuation occurs (range: from subtle to frankly calcified).
- Luminal narrowing of trachea or bronchi is evident.
- Tracheal stenoses or tracheal collapse due to cartilaginous destruction may be evident.
- Airway malacia with airway wall collapse and air trapping can be seen on expiratory scans.
- Parenchymal appearances are in keeping with lower respiratory tract infection.

Utility
- CT is the preferred method for accurate delineation of extent and degree of airway obstruction.

Ultrasonography
Utility
- Echocardiography is used for investigation of cardiac, aortic, and valvular disease.
- Endobronchial ultrasound evaluation has been used to identify cartilaginous fragmentation and edema.

DIAGNOSTIC PEARLS
- Smoothly thickened tracheal wall with sparing of the posterior membranous wall is virtually pathognomonic of relapsing polychondritis.
- Increased tracheal and bronchial wall thickness secondary to inflammation is evident typically involving the cartilaginous portion.
- Airway malacia with airway wall collapse and air trapping can be seen on expiratory scans.

CLINICAL PRESENTATION
- Auricular chondritis in a third of cases; pinna affected in majority of patients.
- Upper airway obstruction: hoarseness, breathlessness, cough, stridor, wheeze, and tenderness over laryngo-tracheal cartilage.
- Episodic painful chondritis of nose, ribs, and small and large articular joints.
- Hearing impairment.
- Inflammation of ocular structures: conjunctivitis, keratitis, scleritis/episcleritis, and/or uveitis.
- Vasculitis in aorta, renal vessels, neurologic system, and skin.
- Skin lesions: livedo reticularis, urticaria, erythema multiforme, and angioedema.

DIFFERENTIAL DIAGNOSIS
- Tracheobronchial amyloidosis
- Wegener granulomatosis
- Adenoid cystic carcinoma
- Tracheobronchopathia osteochondroplastica

PATHOLOGY
- Presence of autoantibodies against cartilaginous collagen
- Unknown cause
- Histologic features: loss of basophilic staining of cartilage matrix; perichondral inflammation and destruction of cartilage, replaced by fibrous tissue

---

WHAT THE REFERRING PHYSICIAN NEEDS TO KNOW
- Airway obstruction in relapsing polychondritis can be sudden and catastrophic.
- Relapsing polychondritis can be diffuse or localized and is usually progressive.
- CT may suggest diagnosis and is useful in estimating disease severity.

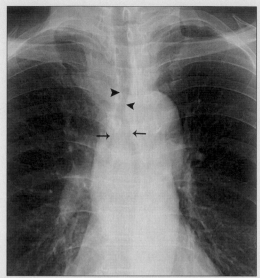

Figure 1. Tracheal and bronchial involvement in relapsing polychondritis. Magnified view from a frontal chest radiograph shows narrowing of the distal trachea (*arrowheads*) and main bronchi (*arrows*).

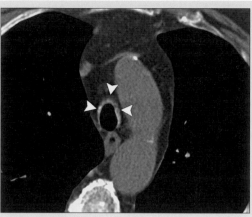

Figure 2. Tracheal involvement in relapsing polychondritis. Middle-aged man with relapsing polychondritis. CT shows thickening of the slightly narrowed trachea. Note that the anterior and lateral tracheal walls (i.e., the cartilaginous portions) are thickened (*arrowheads*). (*Courtesy of Dr. N. Sverzellati, Parma, Italy.*)

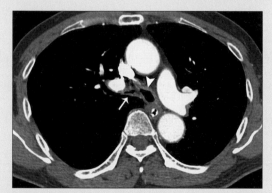

Figure 3. Tracheal and bronchial involvement in relapsing polychondritis. Soft tissue window settings demonstrate thickening of the wall of the right (*straight arrow*) and left (*arrowhead*) main bronchi.

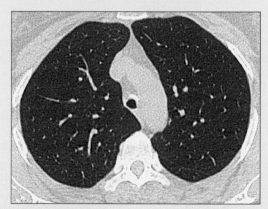

Figure 4. Tracheal narrowing in relapsing polychondritis. High-resolution CT image in a middle-aged woman with relapsing polychondritis shows marked concentric narrowing of the trachea. Note the heavy calcification of the thickened anterior wall of the trachea. (*Courtesy of Drs. Maureen Quigley and David M. Hansell, London, UK*)

INCIDENCE/PREVALENCE AND EPIDEMIOLOGY

- Estimated incidence is 3.5 cases per million population per year.
- Mean age at diagnosis is 44 years, and there is an almost equal sex ratio.
- Five-year survival is approximately 75%.
- Prognosis of patients who have both systemic vasculitis and relapsing polychondritis is worse than those with relapsing polychondritis alone.
- Five-year survival rate for patients with both relapsing polychondritis and vasculitis is reported to be 45%.
- In those with serious airway complications the female-to-male ratio in this group is near 3:1.

Suggested Readings

Behar JV, Choi YW, Hartman TA, et al: Relapsing polychondritis affecting the lower respiratory tract. *AJR Am J Roentgenol* 178(1):173-177, 2002.

Lee KS, Ernst A, Trentham DE, et al: Relapsing polychondritis: Prevalence of expiratory CT airway abnormalities. *Radiology* 240(2):565-573, 2006.

Marom EM, Goodman PC, McAdams HP: Diffuse abnormalities of the trachea and main bronchi. *AJR Am J Roentgenol* 176(3):713-717, 2001.

Marom EM, Goodman PC, McAdams HP: Focal abnormalities of the trachea and main bronchi. *AJR Am J Roentgenol* 176(3):707-711, 2001.

Nakajima T, Sekine Y, Yasuda M, et al: Long-term management of polychondritis with serial tracheobronchial stents. *Ann Thorac Surg* 81(6):e24-e26, 2006.

Prince JS, Duhamel DR, Levin DL, et al: Nonneoplastic lesions of the tracheobronchial wall: Radiologic findings with bronchoscopic correlation. *RadioGraphics* 22(Spec No):S215-S230, 2002.

Webb EM, Elicker BM, Webb WR: Using CT to diagnose nonneoplastic tracheal abnormalities: Appearance of the tracheal wall. *AJR Am J Roentgenol* 174(5):1315-1321, 2000.

Vasculitis and Granulomatosis

Vasculitis (Overview)

DEFINITION: Vasculitis is inflammation of blood vessels.

IMAGING

Radiography

Findings

- Diffuse pulmonary hemorrhage: findings ranging from normal to patchy bilateral ground-glass opacities to confluent consolidation can occur in Goodpasture syndrome, microscopic polyangiitis, and Wegener granulomatosis.
- Wegener granulomatosis: multiple, often cavitated lung nodules or masses (often <10) of a few millimeters to 10 cm in diameter are evident.
- Pulmonary artery aneurysms in Behçet disease present as round perihilar opacities, measure 1 to 3 cm in diameter, or rapidly develop unilateral hilar enlargement.
- Churg-Strauss syndrome: transient or migratory opacities are noted.

Utility

- Usually the initial imaging modality used in the evaluation of these patients
- Limited value in differential diagnosis

CT

Findings

- Acute diffuse pulmonary hemorrhage can occur in Goodpasture syndrome, microscopic polyangiitis, and Wegener granulomatosis and manifests as bilateral ground-glass opacities and consolidation that may be patchy or diffuse.
- Wegener granulomatosis: nodules or masses are usually multiple and bilateral, involve mainly subpleural regions, have smooth or irregular margins, and frequently cavitate.
- Churg-Strauss syndrome: bilateral ground-glass opacities or consolidation often shows a peripheral predominance with thickening of the interlobular septa.
- Contrast-enhanced CT (CT angiography) in Behçet disease: pulmonary artery aneurysms are seen as saccular or fusiform dilatations of 1 to 7 cm in diameter that show homogeneous contrast filling simultaneously with the pulmonary artery.

DIAGNOSTIC PEARLS

- Small vessel vasculitis (microscopic polyangiitis, Goodpasture syndrome, Wegener granulomatosis) manifests as pulmonary hemorrhage and glomerulonephritis.
- Large vessel vasculitis (Takayasu arteritis, Behçet disease) manifests as stenosis or aneurysm.
- Churg-Strauss syndrome: eosinophilic lung disease and vasculitis in patient with asthma.

- Behçet disease: wall of involved pulmonary artery is often thickened and enhances after intravenous administration of a contrast agent.
- Takayasu arteritis: usually involves aorta and great vessels and may involve pulmonary arteries. Contrast CT usually shows arterial wall thickening and stenosis and occasionally aneurysm formation.
- Active Takayasu arteritis: delayed-phase CT images obtained 20 to 40 minutes after intravenous injection show circumferential enhancement of vessel wall.

Utility

- High-resolution CT is recommended in patients with clinically suspected diffuse pulmonary hemorrhage and normal or questionable radiographic abnormalities.
- Contrast-enhanced CT (CT angiography) is imaging of choice for evaluation of patients with Behçet disease and suspected pulmonary artery aneurysms and assessment of patients with Takayasu arteritis.

MRI

Findings

- Takayasu arteritis: concentric wall thickening of involved vessels, signal alterations within and surrounding inflamed vessels, mural thrombi, multifocal stenoses, and occasional aneurysm formation.
- Behçet disease: presence, size, and location of pulmonary aneurysms and superior vena caval thrombosis.

WHAT THE REFERRING PHYSICIAN NEEDS TO KNOW

- Wegener granulomatosis, Churg-Strauss syndrome, and microscopic polyangiitis: diagnosis can often be made by combination of clinical and radiologic findings and the presence of positive serum c- or p-ANCA antibodies.
- Goodpasture syndrome is usually diagnosed by demonstration of circulating or tissue-bound anti-GBM antibodies.
- Criteria for diagnosis of Behçet disease include recurrent oral ulcerations plus two of following: recurrent genital ulcerations, eye lesions (uveitis and retinal vasculitis), skin lesions (folliculitis, erythema nodosum), and positive skin pathergy test (pustule formation 24-48 hours after a skin prick).
- Alveolar hemorrhage and capillaritis may be seen in microscopic polyangitis, Wegener granulomatosis, systemic lupus erythematosus, antiphospholipid syndrome, and drug hypersensitivity.

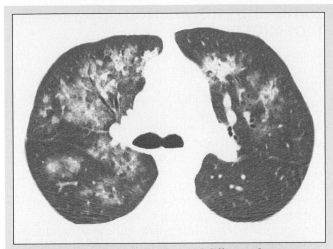

Figure 1. Microscopic polyangiitis and diffuse pulmonary hemorrhage. High-resolution CT performed on a multidetector scanner in a 34-year-old man shows asymmetric bilateral ground-glass opacities and small areas of consolidation.

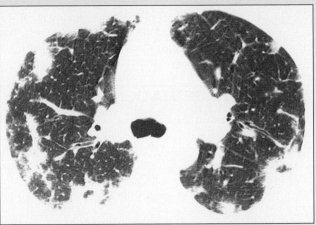

Figure 2. Churg-Strauss syndrome: chronic eosinophilic pneumonia pattern. High-resolution CT image shows bilateral areas of consolidation in a predominantly subpleural distribution. The patient was a 52-year-old man with the diagnosis of Churg-Strauss syndrome proved by surgical lung biopsy.

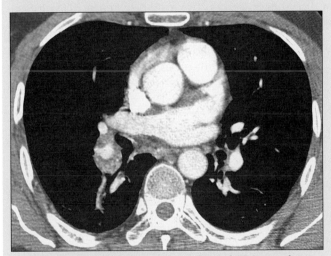

Figure 3. Behçet's disease. Contrast-enhanced CT image shows partially thrombosed aneurysm of the right interlobar pulmonary artery. The patient was a 50-year-old man with Behçet disease, pulmonary artery aneurysm, and pulmonary hemorrhage.

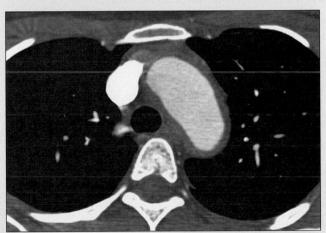

Figure 4. Takayasu arteritis: CT findings. Contrast-enhanced CT at the level of the aortic arch shows circumferential thickening of the wall of aortic arch. The patient was a 32-year-old woman with Takayasu arteritis.

Utility

- Limited value in assessment of pulmonary vasculitis.
- Gadolinium-enhanced MRI (MR angiography) is modality of choice for assessment of patients with suspected or proven Takayasu arteritis.

CLINICAL PRESENTATION

- Wegener granulomatosis: epistaxis, sinusitis, cough, hemoptysis.
- Churg-Strauss syndrome: asthma, allergic rhinitis, cough, dyspnea, rash, peripheral neuropathy; peripheral blood eosinophilia >10%.
- Goodpasture syndrome: hemoptysis, dyspnea, proteinuria, and hematuria.
- Microscopic polyangiitis: glomerulonephritis, hemoptysis, dyspnea.
- Behçet disease: recurrent oral, genital ulcers, hemoptysis, uveitis.
- Takayasu arteritis: fever, weight loss, diminished or absent pulses, and limb claudication.

DIFFERENTIAL DIAGNOSIS

- Systemic lupus erythematosus
- Pneumonia
- Drug reaction
- Lymphoma

PATHOLOGY

- Wegener granulomatosis: vessels show focal or extensive inflammation, manifested by fibrinoid necrosis of media, or infiltration of vessel wall by inflammatory cell infiltrate.
- Churg-Strauss syndrome: findings in lungs consist of parenchymal eosinophilic infiltration, vasculitis, and necrotizing extravascular granulomatous inflammation.
- Goodpasture syndrome: pulmonary alveolar capillaritis and necrotizing glomerulonephritis.
- Capillaritis in Goodpasture syndrome is identical to that of Wegener granulomatosis and microscopic polyangiitis.
- ANCA-positive vasculitides: included are microscopic polyangiitis (c- and p-ANCA), Wegener granulomatosis (c-ANCA), and Churg-Strauss syndrome (p-ANCA).
- Behçet disease: there is transmural vascular inflammation by lymphocytes, plasma cells, and polymorphonuclear leukocytes with thinning of muscular and elastic layers.

INCIDENCE/PREVALENCE AND EPIDEMIOLOGY

- Wegener granulomatosis typically affects adults between 40 and 60 years of age; 50%-80% have glomerulonephritis.
- Churg-Strauss syndrome occurs almost exclusively in patients with asthma.
- The incidence of Goodpasture syndrome is approximately 1 per million population per year; peaks occur at 20-30 and 60-70 years of age, and male-to-female ratio is approximately 3:2.
- Microscopic polyangiitis is the most common cause of the pulmonary-renal syndrome (coexistence of pulmonary hemorrhage and glomerulonephritis).
- Incidence of microscopic polyangiitis is approximately 1:100,000 per year, with slight predominance in men; mean age at onset is approximately 50 years.
- Prevalence of Behçet disease in Europe and United States is <1 case per 100,000 population; male-to-female ratio is 10:1, and mean age at presentation is 30 years; it is much more common in Turkey, the Middle East, and Southeast Asia.
- Vasculitis is seen in 20% to 40% of Behçet disease cases.
- Takayasu arteritis is seen most commonly in Japan, South East Asia, India, Mexico, and Brazil; the incidence in North America is 2.6 cases per million population per year, with an age at diagnosis between 10 and 40 years.

Suggested Readings

Brown KK: Pulmonary vasculitis. *Proc Am Thorac Soc* 3:48-57, 2006.

Gotway MB, Araoz PA, Macedo TA, et al: Imaging findings in Takayasu's arteritis. *AJR Am J Roentgenol* 184:1945-1950, 2005.

Hiller N, Lieberman S, Chajek-Shaul T, et al: Thoracic manifestations of Behcet disease at CT. *RadioGraphics* 24:801-808, 2004.

Keogh KA, Specks U: Churg-Strauss syndrome. *Semin Respir Crit Care Med* 27:148-157, 2006.

Marten K, Schnyder P, Schirg E, et al: Pattern-based differential diagnosis in pulmonary vasculitis using volumetric CT. *AJR Am J Roentgenol* 184:720-733, 2005.

Noth I, Strek ME, Leff AR: Churg-Strauss syndrome. *Lancet* 361:587-594, 2003.

Ravenel JG, McAdams HP: Pulmonary vasculitis: CT features. *Semin Respir Crit Care Med* 24:427-436, 2003.

Silva CI, Müller NL, Fujimoto K, et al: Churg-Strauss syndrome: High resolution CT and pathologic findings. *J Thorac Imaging* 20(2):74-80, 2005.

Diffuse Pulmonary Hemorrhage

DEFINITION: Diffuse alveolar hemorrhage is a manifestation of various diseases such as microscopic polyangiitis, Goodpasture syndrome, Wegener granulomatosis, and systemic lupus erythematosus.

IMAGING

Radiography

Findings
- Patchy, bilateral hazy increased opacity (ground-glass opacities) or consolidation.
- May be patchy or confluent but tends to involve mainly perihilar regions and mid and lower lung zones.

Utility
- Usually the initial and only imaging modality used in evaluation of these patients.

CT

Findings
- Patchy or diffuse bilateral ground-glass opacities and consolidation are seen.
- Smooth septal thickening and intralobular lines may be present superimposed on ground-glass opacities, resulting in crazy-paving pattern.

Utility
- Recommended in patients with clinically suspected diffuse pulmonary hemorrhage and normal or questionable radiographic abnormalities.
- Helpful to rule out other causes of hemoptysis such as bronchiectasis and bronchogenic carcinoma.

CLINICAL PRESENTATION

- Hemoptysis, cough, dyspnea

DIFFERENTIAL DIAGNOSIS

- Microscopic polyangiitis
- Goodpasture syndrome
- Wegener granulomatosis
- Systemic lupus erythematosus
- Bronchiectasis

PATHOLOGY

- Pulmonary and systemic vasculitis: microscopic polyangiitis, Goodpasture syndrome, Wegener granulomatosis, systemic lupus erythematosus.

DIAGNOSTIC PEARLS

- Patchy, bilateral airspace opacities, more prominent in perihilar areas and mid and lower lung zones.
- CT: patchy or diffuse bilateral ground-glass opacities and consolidation.
- Hemoptysis.

- Impaired platelet function: leukemia, chemotherapy, bone marrow transplantation.
- Bleeding disorders: antiphospholipid antibody syndrome, anticoagulant therapy.

INCIDENCE/PREVALENCE AND EPIDEMIOLOGY

- Diffuse alveolar hemorrhage is a common manifestation of autoimmune diseases associated with pulmonary vasculitis.
- Common causes include microscopic polyangiitis, Goodpasture syndrome, Wegener granulomatosis, and systemic lupus erythematosus.
- Diffuse alveolar hemorrhage may also result from a decreased number or impaired function of platelets, as seen in leukemia and in patients undergoing chemotherapy and bone marrow transplantation.

Suggested Readings

Heeringa P, Schreiber A, Falk RJ, Jennette JC: Pathogenesis of pulmonary vasculitis. *Semin Respir Crit Care Med* 25:465-474, 2004.

Primack SL, Miller RR, Müller NL: Diffuse pulmonary hemorrhage: Clinical, pathologic, and imaging features. *AJR Am J Roentgenol* 164:295-300, 1995.

Seo JB, Im JG, Chung JW, et al: Pulmonary vasculitis: The spectrum of radiological findings. *Br J Radiol* 73(875):1224-1231, 2000.

Travis WD, Colby TV, Lombard C, Carpenter HA: A clinicopathologic study of 34 cases of diffuse pulmonary hemorrhage with lung biopsy confirmation. *Am J Surg Pathol* 14:1112-1125, 1990.

WHAT THE REFERRING PHYSICIAN NEEDS TO KNOW

- Radiologic manifestations of diffuse pulmonary hemorrhage are indistinguishable from other causes of acute interstitial or airspace disease.
- CT is indicated in patients with hemoptysis and atypical clinical presentation to rule out other causes of hemoptysis, such as bronchiectasis and bronchogenic carcinoma.

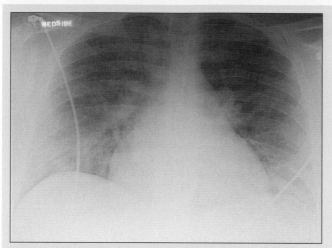

Figure 1. **Microscopic polyangiitis and diffuse pulmonary hemorrhage.** Chest radiograph in a 34-year-old man shows bilateral subtle hazy increased opacity (ground-glass pattern). Also noted are small areas of consolidation in the lower lung zones.

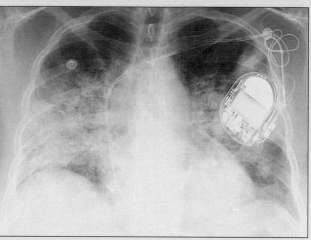

Figure 2. **Microscopic polyangiitis and severe pulmonary hemorrhage.** Chest radiograph in a 36-year-old man shows extensive bilateral areas of consolidation. Incidental note is made of a permanent pacemaker with atrioventricular leads in place.

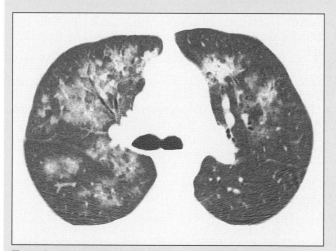

Figure 3. **Microscopic polyangiitis and diffuse pulmonary hemorrhage.** High-resolution CT performed on a multidetector scanner shows asymmetric bilateral ground-glass opacities and small areas of consolidation.

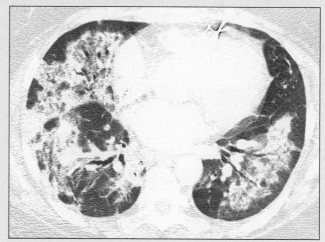

Figure 4. **Microscopic polyangiitis and severe pulmonary hemorrhage.** High-resolution CT image at the level of the lower lobe demonstrates extensive bilateral areas of consolidation in a predominantly central peribronchial distribution.

Wegener Granulomatosis

DEFINITION: Wegener granulomatosis is a multisystem disease characterized by necrotizing granulomatous inflammation of the upper and lower respiratory tract, glomerulonephritis, and necrotizing vasculitis of the lungs and of a variety of other organs and tissues.

IMAGING

Radiography
Findings
- Multiple (often < 10) lung nodules or masses a few millimeters to 10 cm in diameter are evident.
- A solitary nodule may be present.
- Nodules tend to be bilateral but without predilection for any lung zone.
- Cavities are thick walled and tend to have an irregular, shaggy inner lining; they may become large and sometimes involve the whole lobe.
- Areas of airspace consolidation or ground-glass opacities can be diffuse, wedge-shaped, pleural based, peribronchial, and patchy.
- Involvement of the lower airways may result in areas of air trapping due to partial airway obstruction or atelectasis.
- Focal airway stenosis most commonly in the subglottic trachea.

Utility
- Main imaging modality used in initial assessment and follow-up of patients.

CT
Findings
- Nodules or masses are usually multiple, bilateral, and involve mainly subpleural regions; they have smooth or irregular margins and range in diameter from a few millimeters to >6 cm.
- Cavitating masses that can have a thick or thin wall and irregular inner lining.
- Nodules/masses may be surrounded by a rim of ground-glass attenuation (CT halo sign); reversed CT halo sign may occur due to organizing pneumonia reaction.
- Ground-glass opacities and consolidation are seen particularly in patients with hemoptysis.

DIAGNOSTIC PEARLS
- Multiple pulmonary nodules and masses often cavitated
- Patchy, confluent, or peribronchial consolidation
- Diffuse ground-glass opacities and consolidation
- Focal airway stenosis most commonly in the subglottic trachea
- Commonly associated with sinusitis and glomerulonephritis
- Positive antineutrophil cytoplasmic (c-ANCA) antibodies

- Areas of consolidation may have a random distribution and present as peripheral wedge-shaped lesions abutting pleura and mimicking pulmonary infarcts or have a peribronchial distribution.
- Patchy air trapping.
- Tracheal or bronchial wall thickening and focal stenosis.

Utility
- CT may show nodules that are not apparent on radiography and is superior in showing the presence of cavitation.

CLINICAL PRESENTATION
- Epistaxis, sinusitis, cough, hemoptysis, dyspnea are noted.
- Hemoptysis occurs in 30%-40% of patients, and diffuse alveolar hemorrhage occurs in 10%.
- Dyspnea occurs most commonly with diffuse alveolar hemorrhage and, occasionally, as a result of tracheal involvement.
- Other symptoms include fever, malaise, weight loss, and fatigue.

WHAT THE REFERRING PHYSICIAN NEEDS TO KNOW
- Majority of patients present with upper and lower respiratory symptoms: epistaxis, sinusitis, cough, hemoptysis, dyspnea, and pleuritic chest pain.
- Most common radiologic findings are lung nodules or masses, which are seen in up to 90% of patients.
- Cavitation occurs eventually in approximately 50% of cases.
- Chest radiography is the main imaging modality used in the initial assessment and follow-up.
- CT may show nodules and cavitation that are not apparent on the radiograph.
- Diagnosis is made by the combination of clinical and radiologic findings and presence of positive serum c-ANCA.
- Current aims of therapy include rapidly control disease, limit extent and severity of permanent organ damage, and minimize short- and long-term morbidity.

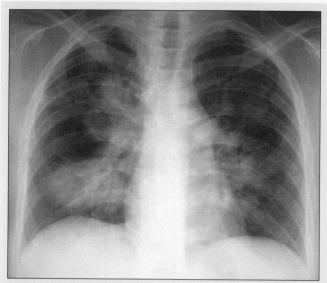

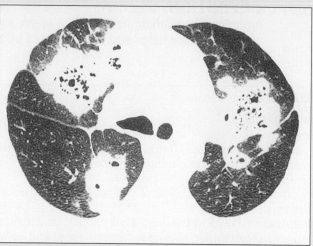

Figure 2. Wegener granulomatosis: cavitating masses. High-resolution CT image shows bilateral masses with foci of cavitation. Also noted are patchy ground-glass opacities. (*Courtesy of Dr. Jorge Kavakama, São Paulo, Brazil.*)

Figure 1. Wegener granulomatosis: bilateral nodules and masses. Chest radiograph demonstrates bilateral nodules, masses, and focal areas of consolidation in a central distribution.

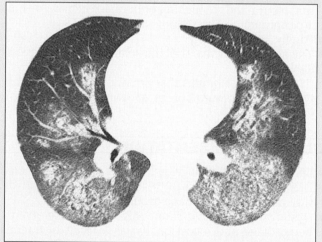

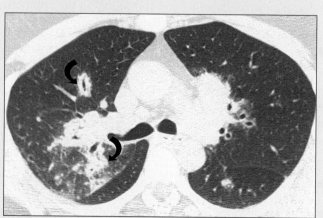

Figure 4. Wegener granulomatosis: peribronchial consolidation. High-resolution CT image at the level of the right upper lobe bronchus shows asymmetric bilateral consolidation in a predominantly peribronchial (*arrows*) distribution. The patient was a 48-year-old woman with Wegener granulomatosis.

Figure 3. Wegener granulomatosis: ground-glass opacities and consolidation. High-resolution CT image shows extensive bilateral ground-glass opacities and small areas of consolidation. The patient was a 52-year-old man with Wegener granulomatosis and diffuse pulmonary hemorrhage.

DIFFERENTIAL DIAGNOSIS

- Lymphoma
- Septic embolism
- Metastases

PATHOLOGY

- Multisystem disease characterized by necrotizing granulomatous upper and lower respiratory tract inflammation, glomerulonephritis, and necrotizing vasculitis of lungs.
- May manifest as full-blown systemic disease or involve primarily or exclusively the respiratory tract.
- Characteristic findings: well-circumscribed pulmonary nodules or masses of inflammation and necrosis.
- Histologic findings: parenchymal necrosis, vasculitis, granulomatous inflammation accompanied by mixed cellular infiltrate of neutrophils, lymphocytes, plasma cells, histiocytes, eosinophils.

INCIDENCE/PREVALENCE AND EPIDEMIOLOGY

- Wegener granulomatosis is rare, having an estimated annual incidence of 10 cases per million.

- It affects adults in their fifth decade, men slightly more often than women.
- Antineutrophil cytoplasmic (c-ANCA) antibodies are highly sensitive in active systemic disease but less sensitive in organ-limited disease.

Suggested Readings

Frazier AA, Rosado-de-Christenson ML, Galvin JR, Fleming MV: Pulmonary angiitis and granulomatosis: Radiologic-pathologic correlation. *RadioGraphics* 18:687-710, 1998;quiz 727.

Lee KS, Kim TS, Fujimoto K, et al: Thoracic manifestation of Wegener's granulomatosis: CT findings in 30 patients. *Eur Radiol* 13:43-51, 2003.

Lohrmann C, Uhl M, Kotter E, et al: Pulmonary manifestations of Wegener granulomatosis: CT findings in 57 patients and a review of the literature. *Eur J Radiol* 53:471-477, 2005.

Lohrmann C, Uhl M, Schaefer O, et al: Serial high-resolution computed tomography imaging in patients with Wegener granulomatosis: Differentiation between active inflammatory and chronic fibrotic lesions. *Acta Radiol* 46:484-491, 2005.

Sheehan RE, Flint JD, Müller NL: Computed tomography features of the thoracic manifestations of Wegener granulomatosis. *J Thorac Imaging* 18:34-41, 2003.

Churg-Strauss Syndrome

DEFINITION: Churg-Strauss syndrome is an antineutrophil cytoplasmic antibody (ANCA)-associated small-vessel vasculitis seen almost exclusively in patients with asthma.

IMAGING

Radiography
Findings
- Transient, patchy nonsegmental areas of consolidation occur without predilection for any lung zone and often with a peripheral distribution.
- Less commonly, ground-glass opacities may have a random distribution or central predominance.
- Bilateral small and large nodular opacities are noted that may become confluent.
- Cardiomegaly may occur.
- Pleural effusion.

Utility
- Abnormal in approximately 70% of patients
- Initial imaging modality used in suspected pulmonary complications of asthma
- Findings may be indistinguishable from those of simple pulmonary eosinophilia (Löffler syndrome) and chronic eosinophilic pneumonia

CT
Findings
- Bilateral areas of ground-glass opacities or consolidation, usually with symmetric distribution; often with peripheral predominance; less commonly, patchy, random distribution
- Septal lines
- Small centrilobular nodules and multiple nodules or masses measuring 0.5-3.5 cm in diameter
- Bronchial wall thickening
- Pleural effusion

Utility
- CT is superior to radiography in showing predominantly peripheral distribution of eosinophilic lung disease.

DIAGNOSTIC PEARLS
- Radiographic findings: transient, patchy nonsegmental areas of consolidation, pleural effusions.
- CT findings: bilateral ground-glass opacities, presence of septal lines, small centrilobular nodules, bronchial wall thickening or dilation.
- American College of Rheumatology criteria (four or more): asthma, eosinophilia, neuropathy, migratory pulmonary opacities, paranasal sinus abnormalities, extravascular eosinophils.

- It is indicated in patients with clinically suspected parenchymal abnormalities and normal or nonspecific radiographic findings.

CLINICAL PRESENTATION
- Asthma is disease-defining feature that usually precedes onset of vasculitis by several years.
- Allergic rhinitis, systemic vasculitis, and peripheral eosinophilia (>10% on differential count) are usually present.
- Cough and shortness of breath and, occasionally, hemoptysis occur.

DIFFERENTIAL DIAGNOSIS
- Cryptogenic organizing pneumonia (idiopathic bronchiolitis obliterans organizing pneumonia)
- Acute eosinophilic pneumonia

WHAT THE REFERRING PHYSICIAN NEEDS TO KNOW
- Most common clinical manifestations of Churg-Strauss syndrome are asthma, allergic rhinitis, vasculitis, and peripheral eosinophilia.
- Diagnosis often can be made from a combination of clinical and radiologic findings, peripheral eosinophilia, and positive serum p-ANCA.
- Approximately 70% of patients have positive serum p-ANCA.
- Cardiac involvement occurs in 13%-47% of cases and may result in angina, myocardial infarction, myocarditis, left-sided heart failure, and pericarditis.
- Differential diagnosis in asthmatics with areas of consolidation involving peripheral third of lung includes chronic eosinophilic pneumonia and organizing pneumonia.
- Other considerations include allergic bronchopulmonary aspergillosis, simple pulmonary eosinophilia, and bacterial, fungal, and viral pneumonia.
- Opportunistic infections such as *Pneumocystis jiroveci* and cytomegalovirus should be suspected in asthmatic patients being treated with corticosteroids.

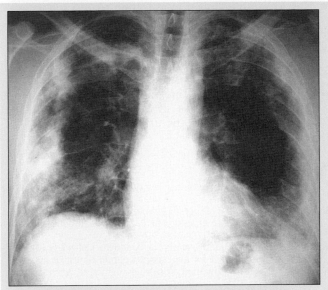

Figure 1. Churg-Strauss syndrome: chronic eosinophilic pneumonia pattern. Posteroanterior chest radiograph shows patchy bilateral areas of consolidation in a predominantly subpleural distribution. The patient was a 71-year-old woman with diagnosis of Churg-Strauss syndrome proved by surgical lung biopsy.

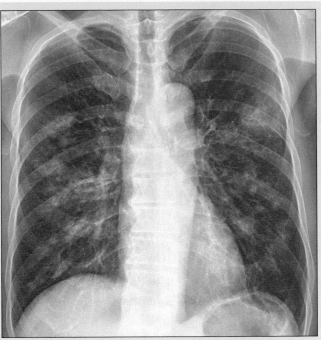

Figure 2. Churg-Strauss syndrome: patchy distribution. Posteroanterior chest radiograph shows patchy bilateral areas of consolidation and ground-glass opacities. The patient was a 67-year-old man with diagnosis of Churg-Strauss syndrome based on history of asthma, peripheral eosinophilia, positive serum p-ANCA, and renal biopsy.

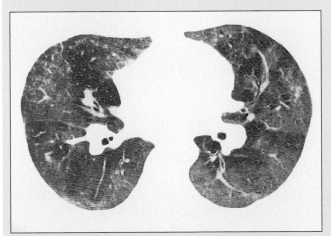

Figure 3. Churg-Strauss syndrome: extensive ground-glass opacities. High-resolution CT image shows extensive bilateral ground-glass opacities and a few centrilobular nodules. The patient was a 21-year-old man with the diagnosis of Churg-Strauss syndrome proved by skin and lung biopsy.

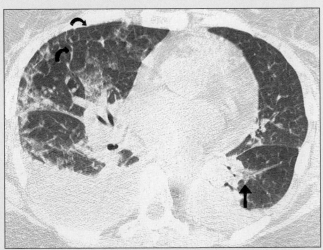

Figure 4. Churg-Strauss syndrome: septal lines. High-resolution CT shows ground-glass opacities mainly in the peripheral regions of the right middle and lower lobes. Airspace consolidation and a small area of ground-glass attenuation (*straight arrow*) are seen in the left lower lobe. Also noted are thickening of the interlobular septa (*curved arrows*) mainly in the right middle lobe and bilateral pleural effusions. The patient was a 54-year-old woman with Churg-Strauss syndrome proved at autopsy. (*From Silva CIS, et al: Churg-Strauss syndrome: High-resolution CT and pathologic findings. J Thorac Imaging 20:74-80, 2005 with permission.*)

- Chronic eosinophilic pneumonia
- Bacterial, fungal, or viral pneumonia
- Drug reaction
- Allergic bronchopulmonary aspergillosis

PATHOLOGY

- Classic histologic findings of Churg-Strauss syndrome in lungs consist of parenchymal eosinophilic infiltration, vasculitis, and necrotizing extravascular granulomatous inflammation.
- It is currently believed to be an autoimmune process involving mainly eosinophils, endothelial cells, and lymphocytes.
- ANCA has a pathogenic role, which seems to modulate disease phenotype.
- Interstitial pulmonary edema is secondary to cardiac involvement or eosinophilic infiltration of septa.
- Cardiomegaly may result from myocarditis or ischemic cardiomyopathy.

INCIDENCE/PREVALENCE AND EPIDEMIOLOGY

- This disease is rare.
- Estimated annual incidence is 1 to 3 per million in general population and 67 per million in patients with asthma.
- It typically occurs in middle-aged patients and affects men slightly more often than women.

- Most common clinical manifestations include asthma, allergic rhinitis, vasculitis, and peripheral eosinophilia, which are present in virtually all patients.
- Serum perinuclear antineutrophil cytoplasmic antibodies (p-ANCA) are present in 40%-75% of patients with active disease.
- Clinical remission is achieved in over 90% of patients; 5-year survival is 60% to 80%; 25% have relapse; mortality in treated patients who relapse is approximately 3%.

Suggested Readings

Keogh KA, Specks U: Churg-Strauss syndrome. *Semin Respir Crit Care Med* 27:148-157, 2006.

Kim YK, Lee KS, Chung MP, et al: Pulmonary involvement in Churg-Strauss syndrome: An analysis of CT, clinical, and pathologic findings. *Eur Radiol* 17(12):3157-3165, 2007.

Masi AT, Hunder GG, Lie JT, et al: The American College of Rheumatology 1990 criteria for the classification of Churg-Strauss syndrome (allergic granulomatosis and angiitis). *Arthritis Rheum* 33:1094-1100, 1990.

Silva CI, Müller NL, Fujimoto K, et al: Churg-Strauss syndrome: High resolution CT and pathologic findings. *J Thorac Imaging* 20(2): 74-80, 2005.

Worthy SA, Müller NL, Hansell DM, Flower CD: Churg-Strauss syndrome: The spectrum of pulmonary CT findings in 17 patients. *AJR Am J Roentgenol* 170(2):297-300, 1998.

Goodpasture Syndrome

DEFINITION: Goodpasture syndrome is an autoimmune disorder characterized by repeated episodes of pulmonary hemorrhage, usually associated with glomerulonephritis and the presence of anti–glomerular basement membrane (anti-GBM) antibodies.

IMAGING

Radiography
Findings
- Radiographic pattern is one of patchy hazy areas of increased opacity (ground-glass opacities) scattered fairly evenly throughout lungs.
- With more severe hemorrhage, pattern may progress to focal or confluent areas of consolidation often associated with air bronchograms.
- Opacities are widespread but may be more prominent in perihilar areas and in mid and lower lung zones.
- Areas of consolidation are gradually replaced by reticular/reticulonodular pattern within 2-3 days and gradually return to normal after 10-12 days.
- With repeated hemorrhage there is persistence of fine reticulonodular pattern, indicative of irreversible interstitial disease.

Utility
- Chest radiograph may be normal in patients with diffuse pulmonary hemorrhage.
- Chest radiography is the initial imaging modality used in the evaluation of patients with diffuse pulmonary hemorrhage and Goodpasture syndrome.

CT
Findings
- Bilateral ground-glass opacities and, less commonly, areas of consolidation.
- Ground-glass opacities that may have patchy distribution or be diffuse.
- Decrease in ground-glass opacities and consolidation, presence of small poorly defined centrilobular nodules, and interlobular septal thickening 2-3 days later.

Utility
- CT is helpful to rule out other causes of hemoptysis, such as bronchiectasis and bronchogenic carcinoma.

DIAGNOSTIC PEARLS
- Bilateral patchy or diffuse ground-glass opacities or consolidation is noted.
- Reticulonodular pattern develops as hemorrhage resolves.
- Interlobular septal thickening and centrilobular nodules superimposed on ground-glass opacities occur as hemorrhage resolves.
- Hemoptysis.
- Anti–glomerular basement membrane (anti-GBM) antibodies.

CLINICAL PRESENTATION
- Hemoptysis may range from mild to copious and life threatening.
- Dyspnea, fatigue, weakness, pallor, cough, and (occasionally) frank hematuria are noted.
- Although initial urinalysis results may be normal, proteinuria, hematuria, and cellular and granular casts almost invariably develop at some stage.
- More than 90% of patients have anti-GBM antibodies, and approximately 80% have crescentic glomerulonephritis on renal biopsy.
- Over 90% of patients have iron-deficiency anemia due to blood loss from pulmonary hemorrhage.

DIFFERENTIAL DIAGNOSIS
- Systemic lupus erythematosus
- Wegener granulomatosis
- Microscopic polyangiitis

WHAT THE REFERRING PHYSICIAN NEEDS TO KNOW
- Most common presenting symptom of Goodpasture syndrome is hemoptysis, which occurs in 80%-95% of patients.
- Findings of initial urinalysis may be normal, but proteinuria and hematuria almost invariably develop at some stage.
- Serum anti-GBM antibodies are present in 90% of patients.
- Diagnosis of Goodpasture syndrome is suspected in an adult with hemoptysis and bilateral airspace consolidation with manifestations of renal disease.
- Radiologic findings are those of diffuse pulmonary hemorrhage and range from patchy bilateral ground-glass opacities to confluent consolidation.

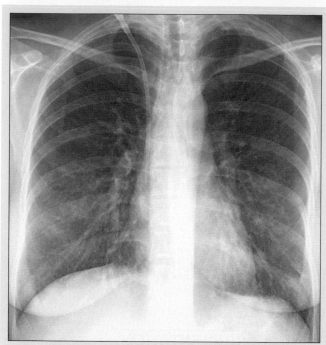

Figure 1. **Goodpasture syndrome with mild diffuse pulmonary hemorrhage: radiographic findings.** Chest radiograph in a 41-year-old man with Goodpasture syndrome, diffuse pulmonary hemorrhage, and renal failure shows bilateral subtle hazy increased opacity (ground-glass pattern). A hemodialysis catheter is evident.

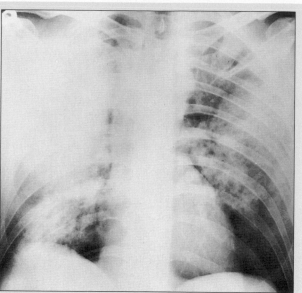

Figure 2. **Acute massive pulmonary hemorrhage in a 49-year-old patient with Goodpasture syndrome.** Posteroanterior radiograph shows extensive consolidation of both lungs. A well-defined air bronchogram is visualized. (*From Müller NL, Fraser RS, Colman NC, et al: Radiologic Diagnosis of Diseases of the Chest. Philadelphia, WB Saunders, 2001.*)

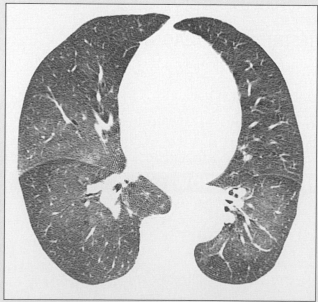

Figure 3. **Goodpasture syndrome with severe diffuse pulmonary hemorrhage: CT findings.** High-resolution CT at the level of the middle and lower lobes in a 78-year-old woman with Goodpasture syndrome and severe acute pulmonary hemorrhage shows diffuse bilateral ground-glass opacities.

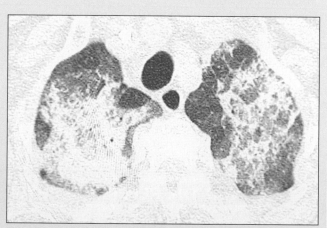

Figure 4. **Goodpasture syndrome with severe diffuse pulmonary hemorrhage: CT findings.** High-resolution CT at the level of the upper lobes in a 78-year-old woman with Goodpasture syndrome and severe acute pulmonary hemorrhage demonstrates extensive ground-glass opacities and areas of consolidation.

PATHOLOGY

- This autoimmune disorder is characterized by the presence of autoantibodies against the glomerular and alveolar basement membranes.
- In the kidney, complement activation and inflammatory cell enzymes are responsible for glomerular damage.
- Pulmonary alveolar capillaritis results in diffuse pulmonary hemorrhage.
- Segmental necrotizing glomerulonephritis progresses to crescentic glomerulonephritis.
- Hemosiderin-laden macrophages in alveolar airspaces and interstitial tissue and mild to moderate interstitial fibrosis are noted.
- Immunofluorescence studies show characteristic linear staining most readily recognized in glomerulus but also frequently evident in alveolar capillary walls.
- IgG is the usual antibody detected, although IgA and IgM are occasionally present as well.

INCIDENCE/PREVALENCE AND EPIDEMIOLOGY

- Goodpasture syndrome is rare, with an incidence of approximately 1 patient per million population per year.
- Bimodal distribution with respect to age shows peaks at 20-30 and 60-70 years of age.
- Male to female ratio is approximately 3:2.

Suggested Readings

Erlich JH, Sevastos J, Pussell BA: Goodpasture's disease: Antiglomerular basement membrane disease. *Nephrology (Carlton)* 9:49–51, 2004.

Frankel SK, Cosgrove GP, Fischer A, et al: Update in the diagnosis and management of pulmonary vasculitis. *Chest* 129:452-465, 2006.

Hansell DM: Small-vessel diseases of the lung: CT-pathologic correlates. *Radiology* 225:639-653, 2002.

Mayberry JP, Primack SL, Müller NL: Thoracic manifestations of systemic autoimmune diseases: Radiographic and high-resolution CT findings. *RadioGraphics* 20:1623-1635, 2000.

Shah MK, Hugghins SY: Characteristics and outcomes of patients with Goodpasture's syndrome. *South Med J* 95:1411-1418, 2002.

Microscopic Polyangiitis

DEFINITION: Microscopic polyangiitis is a necrotizing vasculitis of small vessels (arterioles, venules, and capillaries) characterized by the coexistence of pulmonary hemorrhage and glomerulonephritis.

IMAGING

Radiography
Findings
- Patchy, bilateral airspace opacities, more prominent in perihilar areas and mid and lower lung zones.

Utility
- Usually the initial and only imaging modality used in evaluation of these patients.

CT
Findings
- Patchy or diffuse bilateral ground-glass opacities representing alveolar hemorrhage.
- Consolidation representing diffuse alveolar hemorrhage.

Utility
- High-resolution CT recommended in patients with clinically suspected diffuse pulmonary hemorrhage and normal or questionable radiographic abnormalities.
- Indicated in patients with hemoptysis in whom clinical presentation is not characteristic of microscopic polyangiitis.
- Helpful to rule out other causes of hemoptysis, such as bronchiectasis and bronchogenic carcinoma.

CLINICAL PRESENTATION

- Main pulmonary manifestation: hemoptysis.
- Constitutional symptoms: fever, chills, weight loss, arthralgias, myalgia.
- Relatively common manifestations: hemoptysis, skin lesions, peripheral neuritis (mononeuritis multiplex), and gastrointestinal hemorrhage.

DIAGNOSTIC PEARLS

- Diffuse pulmonary hemorrhage: patchy or diffuse bilateral ground-glass opacities and consolidation
- Coexistence of pulmonary hemorrhage and glomerulonephritis
- Majority of patients have serum antineutrophil cytoplasmic antibodies, most commonly perinuclear (p-ANCA)
- Microscopic polyangiitis is the most common cause of pulmonary-renal syndrome.

- Five-year survival is approximately 70%, with main causes of death being severe vasculitis and side effects of treatment.

DIFFERENTIAL DIAGNOSIS

- Wegener granulomatosis
- Goodpasture syndrome
- Systemic lupus erythematosus

PATHOLOGY

- ANCA have been shown to induce glomerulonephritis and vasculitis but not all patients are ANCA positive.
- Renal disease is due to pauci-immune necrotizing and crescentic glomerulonephritis.
- Pulmonary histologic findings are neutrophilic capillaritis and alveolar hemorrhage.
- Sometimes lesions of capillaritis are associated with alveolar fibrin, which may show polypoid morphology.

WHAT THE REFERRING PHYSICIAN NEEDS TO KNOW

- Microscopic polyangiitis is the most common cause of pulmonary-renal syndrome and is characterized by the coexistence of pulmonary hemorrhage and glomerulonephritis.
- Clinical manifestations are usually renal and, less commonly, pulmonary.
- Majority of patients have serum antineutrophil cytoplasmic antibodies, most commonly p-ANCA.
- CT is indicated in patients with hemoptysis and an atypical clinical presentation; rule out other causes of hemoptysis.
- The diagnosis is suggested in patients with rapidly progressive glomerulonephritis, positive p-ANCA, and clinical and radiologic findings of diffuse pulmonary hemorrhage.
- Positive p-ANCA is also found in Churg-Strauss syndrome, rheumatoid arthritis, and Goodpasture syndrome.
- Main differential diagnosis clinically is with conditions with pulmonary and renal manifestations (Goodpasture syndrome, Wegener granulomatosis, systemic lupus erythematosus).

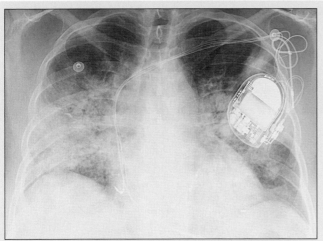

Figure 1. Microscopic polyangiitis and severe pulmonary hemorrhage. Chest radiograph in a 36-year-old man shows extensive bilateral areas of consolidation. Incidental note is made of a permanent pacemaker with atrioventricular leads in place.

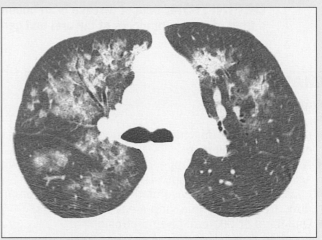

Figure 2. Microscopic polyangiitis and diffuse pulmonary hemorrhage. High-resolution CT performed on a multidetector scanner shows asymmetric bilateral ground-glass opacities and small areas of consolidation.

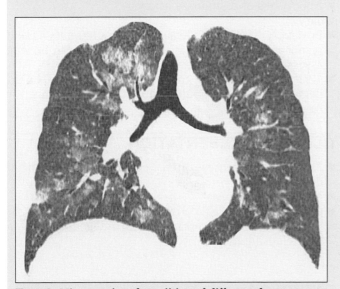

Figure 3. Microscopic polyangiitis and diffuse pulmonary hemorrhage. Coronal reformatted image demonstrates the overall distribution of the findings.

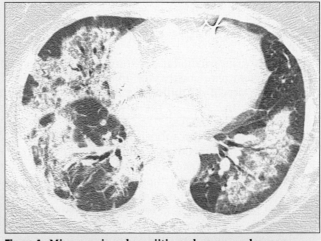

Figure 4. Microscopic polyangiitis and severe pulmonary hemorrhage. High-resolution CT image at the level of the lower lobes demonstrates extensive bilateral areas of consolidation and ground-glass opacities in a predominantly central peribronchial distribution.

INCIDENCE/PREVALENCE AND EPIDEMIOLOGY

- Most common cause of pulmonary-renal syndrome: rapidly progressive glomerulonephritis in more than 90%, with pulmonary hemorrhage in 10%-30%.
- Incidence: approximately 1:100,000 per year.
- Slight predominance in men, with mean age at onset approximately 50 years.
- Positive perinuclear-ANCA in 50%-75% of patients; positive cytoplasmic-ANCA in 10%-15% of patients.

Suggested Readings

Bosch X, Guilabert A, Font J: Antineutrophil cytoplasmic antibodies. *Lancet* 368:404-418, 2006.
Brown KK: Pulmonary vasculitis. *Proc Am Thorac Soc* 3:48-57, 2006.
Collins CE, Quismorio FP Jr: Pulmonary involvement in microscopic polyangiitis. *Curr Opin Pulm Med* 11:447-451, 2005.
Guillevin L, Durand-Gasselin B, Cevallos R, et al: Microscopic poly-angiitis: Clinical and laboratory findings in eighty-five patients. *Arthritis Rheum* 42:421-430, 1999.
Heeringa P, Schreiber A, Falk RJ, Jennette JC: Pathogenesis of pulmo-nary vasculitis. *Semin Respir Crit Care Med* 25:465-474, 2004.
Lauque D, Cadranel J, Lazor R, et al: Microscopic polyangiitis with alveolar hemorrhage: A study of 29 cases and review of the literature. Groupe d'Etudes et de Recherche sur les Maladies "Orphelines" Pulmonaires (GERM"O"P). *Medicine (Baltimore)* 79:222-233, 2000.

Behçet Disease

DEFINITION: Behçet disease is an uncommon systemic disorder characterized by vasculitis and a triad of recurrent ulcers of the oral and genital mucosa with relapsing uveitis.

IMAGING

Radiography
Findings
- Round perihilar opacities or rapidly developing unilateral hilar enlargement.
- A poorly marginated appearance when associated with acute episode of hemoptysis.
- Localized areas of consolidation as a result of infarction, areas of oligemia, and areas of atelectasis.
- Unilateral or bilateral pleural effusions.
- Focal, multifocal, or diffuse airspace consolidation representing pulmonary hemorrhage.
- Mediastinal widening due to thrombosis of the superior vena cava or brachiocephalic veins and associated collateral circulation and mediastinal edema.

Utility
- Findings are nonspecific.

CT
Findings
- Saccular or fusiform dilatations show homogeneous contrast filling simultaneously with the pulmonary artery.
- Aneurysms are often multiple and range from 1-7 cm in diameter; the wall of the involved artery is often thickened and enhances.
- Partial or complete thrombosis of aneurysm may occur and result in localized areas of consolidation.
- Pulmonary hemorrhage is seen as focal, multifocal, or diffuse ground-glass opacities or consolidation.
- Bilateral areas of consolidation involving mainly peripheral lung regions represent organizing pneumonia.
- Thrombosis of the superior vena cava appearing as partial or complete obstruction with collateral circulation and mediastinal edema.
- Thrombosis of the brachiocephalic and subclavian veins.

Utility
- Presence, size, and location of pulmonary aneurysms are best assessed on contrast-enhanced CT.
- CT is the imaging modality of choice.

DIAGNOSTIC PEARLS
- Saccular or fusiform dilatations that show homogeneous contrast filling simultaneously with the pulmonary artery
- Pulmonary hemorrhage seen as focal, multifocal, or diffuse ground-glass opacities or consolidation
- Partial or complete thrombosis of aneurysm
- Vasculitis and triad of recurrent ulcers of the oral and genital mucosa and relapsing uveitis

MRI
Findings
- Aneurysms of pulmonary artery

Utility
- Presence, size, and location of pulmonary aneurysms and superior vena cava thrombosis can be well assessed on MR angiography.
- MRI is less sensitive than contrast-enhanced CT in demonstrating small pulmonary artery aneurysms.

CLINICAL PRESENTATION
- Pulmonary features often initial manifestation of disease
- Massive hemoptysis
- Chest pain, dyspnea, cough
- Triad of recurrent ulcers of the oral and genital mucosa and relapsing uveitis

PATHOLOGY
- Etiology is unknown.
- Earliest pulmonary vascular abnormality is transmural vascular inflammation by lymphocytes, plasma cells, and polymorphonuclear leukocytes.

WHAT THE REFERRING PHYSICIAN NEEDS TO KNOW
- Behçet disease is characterized by vasculitis and a triad of recurrent ulcers of the oral and genital mucosa and relapsing uveitis.
- Vascular complications develop in 20%-40% of patients and include subcutaneous thrombophlebitis, deep vein thrombosis, and pulmonary and systemic arterial aneurysms and occlusions.
- Pulmonary artery aneurysms present radiographically as round perihilar opacities or as unilateral hilar enlargement.
- The presence, size, and location of the pulmonary aneurysms are best assessed on contrast-enhanced CT.

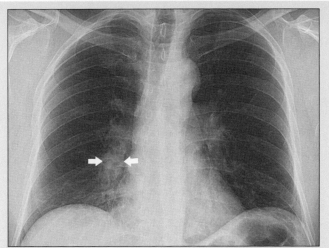

Figure 1. Behçet disease. Chest radiograph reveals increased size and opacity of the right interlobar and lower lobe pulmonary arteries (*arrows*). The patient was a 50-year-old man with Behçet disease, pulmonary artery aneurysm, and pulmonary hemorrhage.

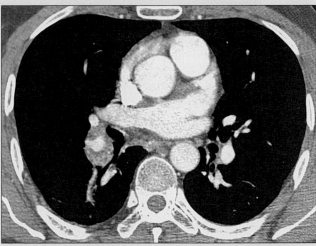

Figure 2. Behçet disease. Contrast-enhanced CT image shows partially thrombosed aneurysm of right interlobar pulmonary artery. The patient was a 50-year-old man with Behçet disease, pulmonary artery aneurysm, and pulmonary hemorrhage.

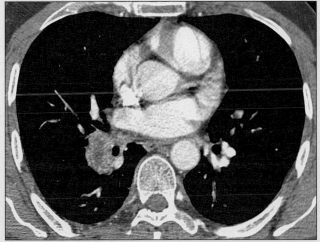

Figure 3. Behçet disease. CT image at slightly lower level than in Figure 2 demonstrates thrombosis of right lower lobe pulmonary artery. The patient was a 50-year-old man with Behçet disease, pulmonary artery aneurysm, and pulmonary hemorrhage.

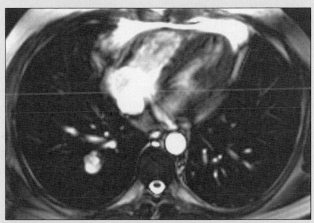

Figure 4. Behçet disease: MR findings. Cross-sectional MR image shows right lower lobe pulmonary artery aneurysm. (*Courtesy of Dr. Erkan Yilmaz, Turkey.*)

■ Extension into adjacent airways causes bronchial and or pulmonary artery erosion and hemoptysis.

■ Thinning of muscular and elastic layers results in aneurysm formation, with partial or complete thrombus formation.

INCIDENCE/PREVALENCE AND EPIDEMIOLOGY

■ Frequency of pulmonary complications is highly variable, ranging from 1% to 18% of patients.

■ Men are much more commonly affected than women (ratio: 10:1).

■ Mean age at presentation is 30 years (range: 10 to 59 years).

■ Highest prevalence rate is in Turkey (4 cases per 1000 population).

■ Approximately 80% of patients with pulmonary artery aneurysms have concomitant extrapulmonary venous thrombi or thrombophlebitis.

Suggested Readings

Alpagut U, Ugurlucan M, Dayioglu E: Major arterial involvement and review of Behçet's disease. *Ann Vasc Surg* 21:232-239, 2007.

Erkan F, Gul A, Tasali E: Pulmonary manifestations of Behçet's disease. *Thorax* 56:572-578, 2001.

Hiller N, Lieberman S, Chajek-Shaul T, et al: Thoracic manifestations of Behçet disease at CT. *RadioGraphics* 24:801-808, 2004.

International Study Group for Behçet's Disease: Criteria for diagnosis of Behçet's disease. *Lancet* 335:1078-1080, 1990.

Takayasu Arteritis: Aorta and Systemic Vessels

DEFINITION: Takayasu arteritis is an inflammatory disease of unknown etiology affecting the aorta and its main branches.

IMAGING

Radiography
Findings
- Wavy or scalloped contour of descending thoracic aorta
- Ectasia of aortic arch

Utility
- Limited value in the diagnosis

CT Angiography
Findings
- Luminal stenosis or aneurysm formation, inflammation, wall thickening, mural calcification.
- Circumferential enhancement of vessel wall on delayed-phase CT images obtained 20-40 minutes after intravenous injection of a contrast agent.
- Most commonly aortic arch, descending aorta, left subclavian, and left carotid arteries.
- May involve pulmonary arteries, most commonly segmental and subsegmental branches.

Utility
- Helical CT angiography has high sensitivity and specificity in diagnosis of Takayasu arteritis.
- Main limitations of CT are radiation dose and need for iodinated contrast material.

MRI
Findings
- Concentric wall thickening of aorta and signal alterations within and surrounding inflamed vessels
- Mural thrombi, multifocal stenoses, vascular dilation, and aneurysm formation

Utility
- MRI is imaging modality of choice for assessment of patients with suspected or proven Takayasu arteritis.
- T2-weighted fat-suppressed multiplanar sequences detect vessel wall edema.

DIAGNOSTIC PEARLS

- CT: luminal stenosis or aneurysm formation, wall thickening, mural calcification.
- MRI: concentric wall thickening of aorta, signal alterations in inflamed vessels.
- Involvement mainly of aorta and its branches.
- Usually occurs in patients between 10 and 40 years of age; more common in women.
- Occurs most commonly in Japan, Southeast Asia, India, Mexico, and Brazil.

- Precontrast, postcontrast T1-weighted fast spoiled gradient-echo, fast spin-echo double inversion recovery multiplanar sequences detect vessel wall thickening.
- MRI avoids radiation exposure and risks of iodinated contrast load.
- Limitations of MRI include low sensitivity in detection of abnormalities in small branches of aorta and overestimation of moderate stenosis.

Conventional Angiography
Findings
- Long, smooth, tapered stenoses ranging from mild to severe, occlusions, and collateral circulation.

Utility
- Angiography does not depict vessel wall and cannot distinguish stenoses due to acute inflammation from stenoses due to chronic fibrosis.
- Angiography is invasive, associated with substantial radiation dose, and difficult to perform in patients with long-segment stenoses and extensive arterial calcification.
- Angiography is being replaced by MRI or contrast-enhanced CT in initial evaluation of patients with Takayasu arteritis.

WHAT THE REFERRING PHYSICIAN NEEDS TO KNOW

- Marked inflammation and more acute progression may lead to aneurysm formation or rupture of involved arteries.
- MRI is imaging modality of choice for assessment of patients with suspected or proven Takayasu arteritis.
- Diminished, absent pulses are present in up to 96% of patients and typically associated with limb claudication and blood pressure discrepancies.
- Medical treatment is aimed at controlling active inflammation and preventing further vascular damage.

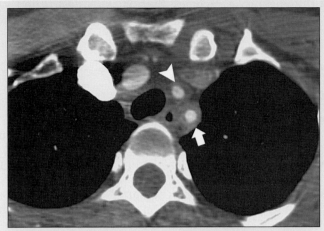

Figure 1. Takayasu arteritis: CT findings. Contrast-enhanced CT at the level of the proximal great vessels demonstrates circumferential thickening of the wall of the left carotid artery (*arrowhead*) and left subclavian artery (*straight arrow*). The patient was a 32-year-old woman with Takayasu arteritis.

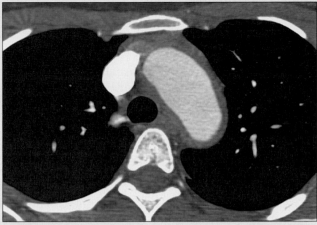

Figure 2. Takayasu arteritis: CT findings. Contrast-enhanced CT at the level of the aortic arch, demonstrates circumferential thickening of the wall of the aortic arch. The patient was a 32-year-old woman with Takayasu arteritis.

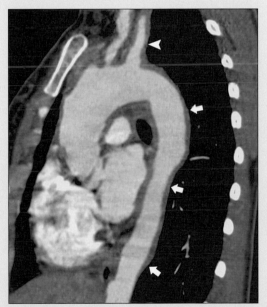

Figure 3. Takayasu arteritis: CT findings. Contrast-enhanced CT sagittal reformatted image demonstrates thickening of the thoracic aorta (*straight arrows*) and great vessels (*arrowhead*). The patient was a 32-year-old woman with Takayasu arteritis.

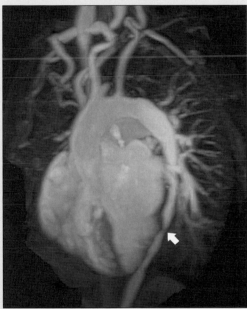

Figure 4. Takayasu arteritis: MRI findings. 3D-fast gradient-echo contrast-enhanced MR angiogram shows tapered narrowing of the descending aorta with focal area of severe stenosis (*arrow*). Note marked collateral circulation with hypertrophy of the internal mammary arteries. Poor visualization of the distal left common carotid artery suggests severe stenosis. (*Courtesy of Dr. Kiminori Fujimoto, Department of Radiology, Kurume University School of Medicine, Kurume, Japan.*)

Positron Emission Tomography

Findings

- High uptake of FDG reflects the presence of active inflammation.

Utility

- FDG-PET may identify more vascular regions involved in inflammatory process than MRI.
- Although promising, these results need to be confirmed in prospective studies done in a large number of patients.

CLINICAL PRESENTATION

- Fever, myalgias, arthralgias, and weight loss are typically present for months to years before more specific features of disease become evident.
- Most common vascular manifestation is diminished or absent pulses, associated with limb claudication and blood pressure discrepancies.

PATHOLOGY

- Main histologic finding consists of patchy panarteritis involving large elastic vessels.
- Inflammation tends to be most marked in adventitia, with infiltration of B and T lymphocytes.
- Acute phase includes vasculitis of vasa vasorum in adventitia, media infiltration by lymphocytes, and intimal thickening.
- Chronic phase includes fibrosis with destruction of elastic tissue and narrowing of arterial lumen in patchy distribution.

INCIDENCE/PREVALENCE AND EPIDEMIOLOGY

- Takayasu arteritis occurs most commonly in Japan, Southeast Asia, India, Mexico, and Brazil, usually in persons between 10 and 40 years of age.
- Female-to-male ratio ranges from 10:1 in Japan to 3:1 in South Africa.
- Abdominal aorta and renal artery involvement are considerably more common in other South Asian countries.

Suggested Readings

Frankel SK, Cosgrove GP, Fischer A, et al: Update in the diagnosis and management of pulmonary vasculitis. *Chest* 129:452-465, 2006.

Gotway MB, Araoz PA, Macedo TA, et al: Imaging findings in Takayasu's arteritis. *AJR Am J Roentgenol* 184:1945-1950, 2005.

Johnston SL, Lock RJ, Gompels MM: Takayasu arteritis: A review. *J Clin Pathol* 55:481-486, 2002.

Steeds RP, Mohiaddin R: Takayasu arteritis: Role of cardiovascular magnetic imaging. *Int J Cardiol* 109:1-6, 2006.

Eosinophilic Lung Diseases

Simple Pulmonary Eosinophilia (Löffler Syndrome)

DEFINITION: Simple pulmonary eosinophilia, also known as Löffler syndrome, is characterized by blood eosinophilia and migratory, usually transient, areas of consolidation visible on chest radiographs.

IMAGING

Radiography
Findings
- Transient and migratory areas of consolidation typically clear spontaneously within 1 month.
- Foci of consolidation may be single or multiple and usually have ill-defined margins.
- Distribution is typically patchy, although peripheral predominance may be seen.

Utility
- Chest radiography is the main and usually the only modality required in initial assessment and follow-up of patients.

CT
Findings
- Ground-glass opacities (100%), airspace consolidation (58%), bronchial wall thickening (50%), and small nodules (42%) are found.
- Abnormalities may involve mainly upper lung zones and have a peripheral distribution but also often have a random distribution.
- Focal areas of consolidation and nodules may be surrounded by a rim of ground-glass attenuation (CT halo sign).

Utility
- CT is seldom performed.
- It is helpful in patients with more severe symptoms or with suspected underlying abnormalities.

CLINICAL PRESENTATION
- This mild, self-limited condition resolves spontaneously in less than 1 month.
- Patients are frequently asymptomatic or have only mild symptoms, most commonly fever and cough.

DIAGNOSTIC PEARLS
- Typical transient and migratory areas of consolidation are seen on the chest radiograph.
- Patchy bilateral ground-glass opacities and consolidation appear on CT.

DIFFERENTIAL DIAGNOSIS
- Bronchopneumonia
- Chronic eosinophilic pneumonia
- Drug-induced eosinophilic pneumonia
- Parasitic infections
- Allergic bronchopulmonary aspergillosis
- Organizing pneumonia

PATHOLOGY
- Diagnosis of simple pulmonary eosinophilia should be reserved for cases with unknown etiology.
- Eosinophils accumulate in the alveolar spaces and alveolar walls.

INCIDENCE/PREVALENCE AND EPIDEMIOLOGY
- The disease is uncommon.
- Most patients with eosinophilic lung disease have an underlying cause, including parasitic infection, allergic bronchopulmonary aspergillosis, or drug reaction.
- Parasitic infection is the main cause of eosinophilic lung disease worldwide, with most common organisms being nematodes, particularly *Ascaris lumbricoides* and *Strongyloides stercoralis*.

WHAT THE REFERRING PHYSICIAN NEEDS TO KNOW
- Diagnostic features of simple pulmonary eosinophilia are blood eosinophilia and transient migratory areas of consolidation on chest radiographs.
- Differential diagnosis includes parasitic infestation, allergic bronchopulmonary aspergillosis, drug-induced lung disease, and chronic eosinophilic pneumonia.
- Patients are frequently asymptomatic or have only mild symptoms, most commonly fever and cough.

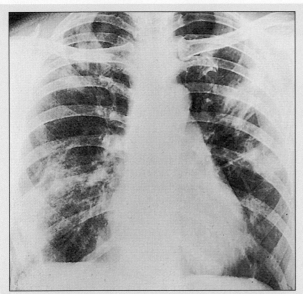

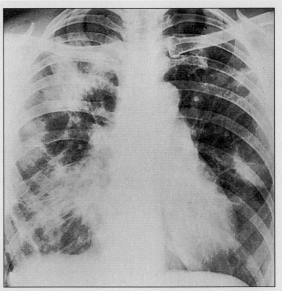

Figure 1. Simple pulmonary eosinophilia. Posteroanterior chest radiograph in a 61-year-old woman shows bilateral areas of consolidation occupying no precise segmental distribution; in particular, there is a broad shadow of increased density along the lower axillary zone of the right lung. At this time her total white blood cell count was 11,000/mL with 1700 (15%) eosinophils. (*From Müller NL, Fraser RS, Colman NC, Paré PD: Radiologic Diagnosis of Diseases of the Chest. Philadelphia, WB Saunders, 2001.*)

Figure 2. Simple pulmonary eosinophilia. In same patient as in Figure 1, radiograph 1 week later shows the anatomic distribution of the areas of consolidation had changed considerably, being more extensive in the right upper and both lower lobes and less extensive in the left upper lobe; at this time, the total white blood cell count was 14,000/mL with 20% eosinophils. A diagnosis of simple pulmonary eosinophilia was made; treatment resulted in prompt remission of symptoms and complete resolution of the radiographic abnormalities. (*From Müller NL, Fraser RS, Colman NC, Paré PD: Radiologic Diagnosis of Diseases of the Chest. Philadelphia, WB Saunders, 2001.*)

Suggested Readings

Alberts WM: Eosinophilic interstitial lung disease. *Curr Opin Pulm Med* 10:419-424, 2004.

Allen JN, Davis WB: Eosinophilic lung diseases. *Am J Respir Crit Care Med* 150:1423-1438, 1994.

Bain GA, Flower CD: Pulmonary eosinophilia. *Eur J Radiol* 23:3-8, 1996.

Cottin V, Cordier JF: Eosinophilic pneumonias. *Allergy* 60:841-857, 2005.

Johkoh T, Müller NL, Akira M, et al: Eosinophilic lung diseases: Diagnostic accuracy of thin-section CT in 111 patients. *Radiology* 216:773-780, 2000.

Kim Y, Lee KS, Choi DC, et al: The spectrum of eosinophilic lung disease: Radiologic findings. *J Comput Assist Tomogr* 21:920-930, 1997.

Chronic Eosinophilic Pneumonia

DEFINITION: Chronic eosinophilic pneumonia is an idiopathic condition characterized by extensive filling of alveoli by a mixed inflammatory infiltrate consisting primarily of eosinophils.

IMAGING

Radiography
Findings
- Characteristic pattern is bilateral, nonsegmental consolidation involving predominately or exclusively the outer two thirds of the lungs.
- Peripheral distribution, involving mainly upper lobes, is apparent on approximately 60% of radiographs.
- Areas of consolidation are usually bilateral but may be asymmetric.
- Occasionally, pleural effusions and, rarely, hilar lymphadenopathy may be apparent.

Utility
- Radiography is main imaging modality used in initial assessment and follow-up of patients with chronic eosinophilic pneumonia.

CT
Findings
- Bilateral peripheral nonsegmental areas of consolidation and ground-glass opacities often involving upper lobes are seen.
- Small centrilobular nodules and smooth intralobular lines superimposed on ground-glass opacities, "crazy-paving" pattern, may occur.
- Airspace nodules and perilobular opacities are seen most commonly in patients who are improving.
- Consolidation and ground-glass opacities sometimes may have lower lobe predominance.
- Small unilateral or bilateral pleural effusions are seen in 10% of patients, and mediastinal lymphadenopathy occurs in 10%-15%.

Utility
- CT is superior to chest radiography in showing characteristic peripheral distribution of chronic eosinophilic pneumonia.

DIAGNOSTIC PEARLS
- Peripheral consolidation ("photographic negative of pulmonary edema pattern") in approximately 50% on radiograph and 90% on CT.
- Increased number of eosinophils in bronchoalveolar fluid and peripheral blood.
- Approximately 50% of patients have asthma or atopy.
- Insidious onset with progressive cough, dyspnea, and fever.
- Rapid improvement with corticosteroids.

- Peripheral distribution is apparent on chest radiography in approximately 60% of cases and on CT in 85%-100% of cases.

CLINICAL PRESENTATION
- Symptoms are present for a least 1 month before diagnosis.
- Dry cough, shortness of breath, and, frequently, fever, weight loss, and malaise occur.
- Laboratory investigation reveals blood eosinophilia in most patients but its absence does not exclude the diagnosis.
- Chronic eosinophilic pneumonia typically has a protracted course: areas of consolidation remain unchanged over weeks or months.

DIFFERENTIAL DIAGNOSIS
- Simple pulmonary eosinophilia (Löffler syndrome)
- Organizing pneumonia of known etiology
- Cryptogenic organizing pneumonia (idiopathic bronchiolitis obliterans organizing pneumonia)
- Churg-Strauss syndrome

WHAT THE REFERRING PHYSICIAN NEEDS TO KNOW
- It is almost always associated with increased number of eosinophils in bronchoalveolar lavage fluid and in peripheral blood.
- Approximately 50% of patients have a history of asthma or atopy.
- Symptoms are usually present for at least 1 month before diagnosis.
- A combination of chronic symptoms, blood eosinophilia, peripheral consolidation on radiograph, and a rapid response to corticosteroid therapy is often sufficiently characteristic.
- Main differential diagnosis radiologically is with Churg-Strauss syndrome and with cryptogenic organizing pneumonia (idiopathic bronchiolitis obliterans organizing pneumonia).

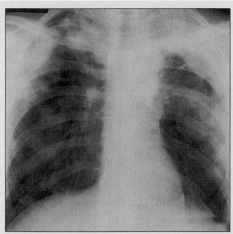

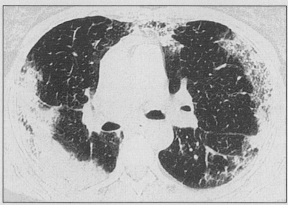

Figure 1. Chronic eosinophilic pneumonia. Posteroanterior chest radiograph reveals bilateral airspace consolidation, predominantly in the upper lobe; the peripheral (cortical) distribution is highly characteristic of the disease. The patient was a middle-aged woman who presented with wheezing, cough, nocturnal fever, and blood eosinophilia. (*From Müller NL, Fraser RS, Colman NC, et al:. Radiologic Diagnosis of Diseases of the Chest. Philadelphia, WB Saunders, 2001.*)

Figure 2. Chronic eosinophilic pneumonia. High-resolution CT at the level of the bronchus intermedius in a 49-year-old woman with chronic eosinophilic pneumonia shows extensive bilateral consolidation in a peripheral distribution.

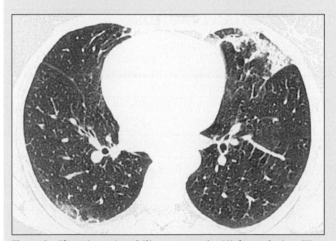

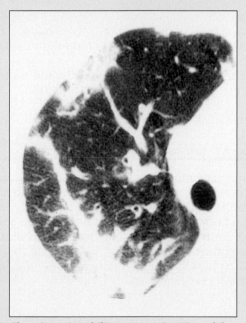

Figure 3. Chronic eosinophilic pneumonia. High-resolution CT at the level of the inferior pulmonary veins shows mild patchy peripheral ground-glass opacities and consolidation.

Figure 4. Chronic eosinophilic pneumonia. View of the right upper lobe from a high-resolution CT shows peripheral consolidation and perilobular bandlike opacity.

PATHOLOGY

- Idiopathic condition is characterized by extensive filling of alveoli by mixed inflammatory infiltrate consisting primarily of eosinophils.
- It is almost always associated with increased number of eosinophils in bronchoalveolar lavage fluid and in peripheral blood.

INCIDENCE/PREVALENCE AND EPIDEMIOLOGY

- Approximately 50% of patients have a history of asthma or atopy.
- Females are affected approximately twice as often as males.
- Peak incidence is in fifth decade, but age range is from 18 to 80 years.

Suggested Readings

Al Jederlinic PJ, Sicilian L, Gaensler EA: Chronic eosinophilic pneumonia: A report of 19 cases and a review of the literature. *Medicine* 67:154-162, 1988.

Bain GA, Flower CD: Pulmonary eosinophilia. *Eur J Radiol* 23:3-8, 1996.

Ebara H, Ikezoe J, Johkoh T, et al: Chronic eosinophilic pneumonia: Evolution of chest radiograms and CT features. *J Comput Assist Tomogr* 18:737-744, 1994.

Fox B, Seed WA: Chronic eosinophilic pneumonia. *Thorax* 35: 570-580, 1980.

Gaensler EA, Carrington CB: Peripheral opacities in chronic eosinophilic pneumonia: The photographic negative of pulmonary edema. *AJR Am J Roentgenol* 128:1-13, 1977.

Mayo JR, Müller NL, Road J, et al: Chronic eosinophilic pneumonia: CT findings in six cases. *AJR Am J Roentgenol* 153:727-730, 1989.

Naughton M, Fahy J, FitzGerald MX: Chronic eosinophilic pneumonia: A long-term follow-up of 12 patients. *Chest* 103:162-165, 1993.

Acute Eosinophilic Pneumonia

DEFINITION: Acute eosinophilic pneumonia is a severe acute febrile illness associated with rapidly increasing shortness of breath and hypoxemic respiratory failure and characterized histologically by the presence of a large number of interstitial and airspace eosinophils.

IMAGING

Radiography
Findings
- Earliest findings consist of reticular opacities and septal (Kerley B) lines.
- Over a few hours or days, there are extensive bilateral interstitial opacities and confluent consolidation; most patients have small bilateral pleural effusions.

Utility
- Findings mimic those of left-sided heart failure.

CT
Findings
- Smooth interlobular septal thickening, bilateral ground-glass opacities, consolidation, and small pleural effusions are seen.
- Combination of ground-glass opacity and septal thickening may result in "crazy-paving" pattern.

Utility
- Findings mimic those of left-sided heart failure.

CLINICAL PRESENTATION

- This severe acute febrile illness is associated with rapidly increasing shortness of breath and hypoxemic respiratory failure.
- Clinical findings of acute respiratory failure and markedly elevated eosinophils in bronchoalveolar lavage fluid are diagnostic.
- Pleuritic chest pain is present in 75% of cases, and myalgia occurs in 50%.

DIAGNOSTIC PEARLS

- Radiologic findings: septal lines, ground-glass opacities, consolidation, and small pleural effusions.
- Rapidly progressive dyspnea, fever, and acute respiratory failure.
- Numerous eosinophils in bronchoalveolar lavage fluid.
- Histologic findings of diffuse alveolar damage with numerous eosinophils.

- Majority of patients have symptoms for <7 days before diagnosis.
- Peripheral eosinophilia is usually absent.

DIFFERENTIAL DIAGNOSIS

- Acute interstitial pneumonia
- Acute respiratory distress syndrome
- Drug-induced eosinophilic pneumonia
- Hydrostatic pulmonary edema
- Bacterial, fungal, or viral pneumonia

PATHOLOGY

- Histologic findings are those of diffuse alveolar damage associated with a large number of interstitial and airspace eosinophils.

WHAT THE REFERRING PHYSICIAN NEEDS TO KNOW

- Acute eosinophilic pneumonia is a severe acute febrile illness associated with rapidly increasing shortness of breath and hypoxemic respiratory failure.
- Diagnosis is based on findings of acute respiratory failure and presence of markedly elevated eosinophils in bronchoalveolar lavage fluid.
- Majority of cases are idiopathic; occasionally it may result from infection, drug reaction, or inhalational exposure to smoke, particularly cigarette smoke.
- Radiologic findings are those of acute interstitial and airspace pulmonary edema.
- Two-thirds of patients require mechanical ventilation.
- Patients respond rapidly to corticosteroid therapy.

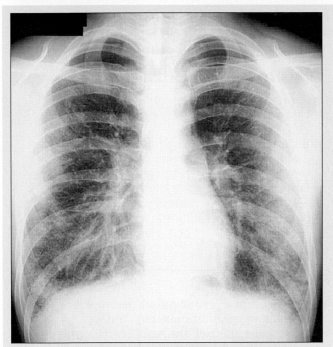

Figure 1. Acute eosinophilic pneumonia. Chest radiograph shows prominence of the vascular markings, poorly defined opacities, and septal lines. The findings are similar to those of interstitial pulmonary edema. (*Courtesy of Dr. Takeshi Johkoh, Osaka, Japan.*)

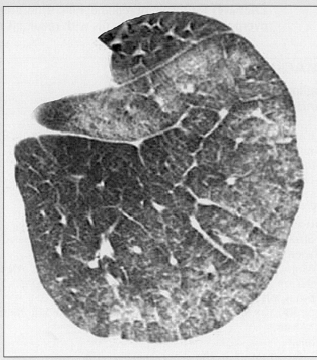

Figure 2. Acute eosinophilic pneumonia. View of the left lung from a high-resolution CT shows ground-glass opacities and smooth thickening of the interlobular septa. (*Courtesy of Dr. Takeshi Johkoh, Osaka, Japan.*)

- Majority of cases are idiopathic; occasionally it may result from infection, drug reaction, or inhalational exposure to smoke, particularly cigarette smoke.
- Tobacco smoke has been shown to be a trigger for acute eosinophilic pneumonia, especially in new smokers.

INCIDENCE/PREVALENCE AND EPIDEMIOLOGY

- No sex predominance is noted.
- It is more common in young adults (average age 29 years) but can affect all ages.

- In a study of acute eosinophilic pneumonia in U.S. military personnel, 18 cases occurred among 183,000 personnel, mostly smokers.
- The disease commonly occurs in smokers; especially new smokers (78%).

Suggested Readings

Alberts WM: Eosinophilic interstitial lung disease. *Curr Opin Pulm Med* 10:419-424, 2004.
Allen J: Acute eosinophilic pneumonia. *Semin Respir Crit Care Med* 27:142-147, 2006.
Bain GA, Flower CD: Pulmonary eosinophilia. *Eur J Radiol* 23:3-8, 1996.
Cottin V, Cordier JF: Eosinophilic pneumonias. *Allergy* 60:841-857, 2005.

Hypereosinophilic Syndrome

DEFINITION: Hypereosinophilic syndrome is a rare idiopathic condition characterized by overproduction of eosinophils with resultant multiorgan infiltration and damage.

IMAGING

Radiography
Findings
- Transient hazy opacities or areas of consolidation.
- Cardiac involvement eventually resulting in cardiomegaly, pulmonary edema, and pleural effusion.
Utility
- Nonspecific radiographic manifestations

CT
Findings
- Small nodules and patchy ground-glass opacities are seen.
- Majority of nodules have a halo of ground-glass attenuation and involve mainly peripheral lung regions.
- Small pleural effusions can occur.
- Septal thickening is noted in patients with left heart failure.
Utility
- Limited value in the diagnosis

CLINICAL PRESENTATION

- Chronic cough, wheezing, and shortness of breath occur.
- Initial symptoms are nonspecific.
- Diagnostic criteria include sustained eosinophilia (eosinophil count >1500 cells/µL) for at least 6 months, evidence of end-organ damage, and exclusion of other causes of eosinophilia.

DIFFERENTIAL DIAGNOSIS

- Acute eosinophilic pneumonia
- Drug-induced eosinophilic pneumonia
- Simple pulmonary eosinophilia (Löffler syndrome)
- Parasitic infection

DIAGNOSTIC PEARLS

- Cardiac involvement eventually leads to cardiomegaly, pulmonary edema, and pleural effusion.
- Bilateral pulmonary small nodules, patchy ground-glass opacities and consolidation, and septal thickening are present.
- Eosinophilia lasts for at least 6 months.
- All other causes of eosinophilia are excluded.
- Rare idiopathic condition.

PATHOLOGY

- There is an overproduction of eosinophils with resultant multiorgan infiltration and damage.
- Main organs affected are heart (valvular fibrosis with regurgitation) and nervous system (meningitis, peripheral neuropathies).

INCIDENCE/PREVALENCE AND EPIDEMIOLOGY

- This is a rare idiopathic condition.
- Majority of patients are between 20 and 50 years of age (mean, 33 years).
- Pulmonary and pleural involvement occurs in approximately 40% of cases.

Suggested Readings

Alberts WM: Eosinophilic interstitial lung disease. *Curr Opin Pulm Med* 10:419-424, 2004.
Bain GA, Flower CD: Pulmonary eosinophilia. *Eur J Radiol* 23:3-8, 1996.
Cottin V, Cordier JF: Eosinophilic pneumonias. *Allergy* 60:841-857, 2005.

WHAT THE REFERRING PHYSICIAN NEEDS TO KNOW

- Diagnostic criteria include sustained eosinophilia (eosinophil count >1500 cells/µL) for at least 6 months, evidence of end-organ damage, and exclusion of other causes of eosinophilia.
- Radiologic findings are nonspecific.
- Cardiac disease is the main cause of morbidity and mortality and includes endocardial fibrosis, restrictive cardiomyopathy, and valvular damage.
- Patients are usually treated with corticosteroids.
- Prognosis is poor.

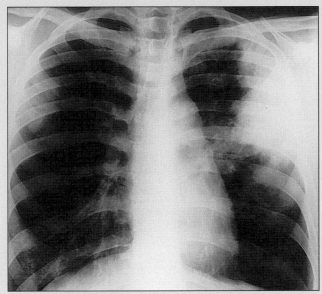

Figure 1. Hypereosinophilic syndrome. Posteroanterior chest radiograph shows asymmetric bilateral areas of consolidation involving predominantly the peripheral regions of the upper lobes. The patient was a 20-year-old man who recently had developed asthma and had marked eosinophilia. The parenchymal abnormalities resolved after treatment with corticosteroids. The patient subsequently developed myocarditis. (*Case courtesy of Dr. Christopher Flower, Addenbrooke's Hospital, Cambridge, England. From Müller NL, Fraser RS, Colman NC, Paré PD: Radiologic Diagnosis of Diseases of the Chest. Philadelphia, WB Saunders, 2001.*)

Metabolic Lung Diseases

Tracheobronchial and Pulmonary Amyloidosis

DEFINITION: Amyloidosis is a heterogeneous group of disorders characterized by accumulation of various insoluble fibrillar proteins.

IMAGING

Radiography
Findings
- Focal or diffuse thickening of airway wall with associated airway lumen narrowing (tracheobronchial amyloidosis).
- Solitary or multiple nodules, usually peripherally located (nodular primary parenchymal amyloidosis).
- Reticular, nodular, or reticulonodular pattern that may be diffuse or involve mainly lower lobes (diffuse interstitial amyloidosis).
- Pleural effusion.

CT
Findings
- Thickened airway wall, narrowing of lumen, and foci of calcification (tracheobronchial amyloidosis).
- The thickening of the tracheal wall is circumferential.
- Solitary or multiple nodules ranging from 0.5-5.0 cm (nodular primary parenchymal amyloidosis).
- Reticular opacities and interlobular septal thickening (diffuse interstitial amyloidosis).
- Multiple subpleural micronodules (diffuse interstitial amyloidosis).
- Ground-glass opacities, areas of consolidation, traction bronchiectasis, honeycombing (diffuse interstitial amyloidosis).

CLINICAL PRESENTATION

- In tracheobronchial amyloidosis, dyspnea, cough, and, occasionally, hemoptysis, may cause symptoms that simulate asthma.
- Discrete tracheal and endobronchial nodules are usually asymptomatic but occasionally may result in airway obstruction with distal atelectasis or bronchiectasis.
- Nodular parenchymal form of amyloidosis usually is asymptomatic with no evidence of extrathoracic disease.

DIAGNOSTIC PEARLS

- Focal or diffuse thickening of airway wall with associated airway lumen narrowing (tracheobronchial amyloidosis)
- The thickening of the tracheal wall is typically circumferential whereas the thickening in relapsing polychondritis typically spares the posterior membrane
- Solitary or multiple nodules, usually peripherally located (nodular primary parenchymal amyloidosis)
- Multiple subpleural micronodules and interlobular septal thickening (diffuse interstitial amyloidosis)

- Diffuse interstitial amyloidosis frequently results in progressive dyspnea and respiratory insufficiency.

DIFFERENTIAL DIAGNOSIS

- Adenoid cystic carcinoma of the trachea and bronchi
- Relapsing polychondritis
- Multiple lung nodules
- Lymphangitic carcinomatosis

PATHOLOGY

- Amyloidosis can be hereditary or acquired and localized or systemic.
- Amyloidosis is a disorder of protein folding rather than amino acid sequence.
- Abnormal proteins are deposited in extracellular space and cause disease by compression of adjacent cells and tissues.
- Histologically it is characterized by amorphous, eosinophilic, extracellular material that shows apple-green birefringence when stained with Congo red.
- Diffuse interstitial amyloidosis involves the parenchymal interstitium and the media of small blood vessels.

WHAT THE REFERRING PHYSICIAN NEEDS TO KNOW
- Amyloidosis typically causes circumferential tracheal thickening whereas relapsing polychondritis typically spares the posterior membrane.
- Most important proteins associated with respiratory tract disease are amyloid L and amyloid A.
- Amyloid L is derived from immunoglobulin light chains and is therefore usually associated with abnormal plasma cell function.

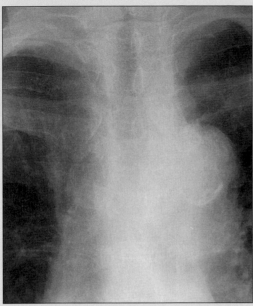

Figure 1. **Diffuse tracheal amyloidosis.** Magnified view from a chest radiograph shows irregular narrowing of the trachea. (*From Müller NL, Fraser RS, Colman NC, Paré PD: Radiologic Diagnosis of Diseases of the Chest. Philadelphia, WB Saunders, 2001.*)

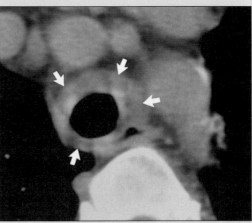

Figure 2. **Diffuse tracheal amyloidosis.** CT scan immediately above the level of the aortic arch shows marked circumferential thickening of the trachea (*arrows*). On CT and at bronchoscopy, the entire trachea was abnormal. The diagnosis of diffuse tracheal amyloidosis was proved by endoscopic biopsy. (*From Müller NL, Fraser RS, Colman NC, Paré PD: Radiologic Diagnosis of Diseases of the Chest. Philadelphia, WB Saunders, 2001.*)

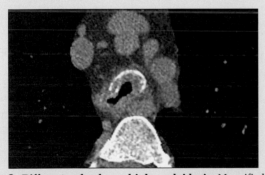

Figure 3. **Diffuse tracheobronchial amyloidosis.** Magnified view of the trachea shows circumferential thickening and foci of calcification.

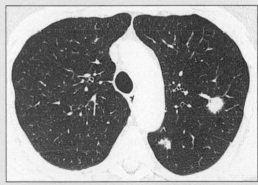

Figure 4. **Nodular parenchymal amyloidosis.** High-resolution CT image at the level of the aortic arch shows bilateral nodules with irregular margins. Diagnosis of amyloidosis was proved at surgical resection of left upper lobe nodules.

INCIDENCE/PREVALENCE AND EPIDEMIOLOGY

- Amyloidosis is uncommon.
- Tracheobronchial amyloidosis typically manifests after the fifth decade.
- Airway involvement occurs most commonly in the trachea and proximal bronchi.
- The nodular parenchymal form is usually of the amyloid L type and localized to the lung.

Suggested Readings

Aylwin AC, Gishen P, Copley SJ: Imaging appearance of thoracic amyloidosis. *J Thorac Imaging* 20:41-46, 2005.
Gillmore JD, Hawkins PN: Amyloidosis and the respiratory tract. *Thorax* 54:444-451, 1999.
Hui AN, Koss MN, Hochholzer L, Wehnut WD: Amyloidosis presenting in the lower respiratory tract: clinicopathologic, radiologic, immunohistochemical and histochemical studies on 48 cases. *Arch Pathol Lab Med* 110:212-218, 1986.
O'Regan A, Fenlon HM, Beamis JF Jr, et al: Tracheobronchial amyloidosis. The Boston University experience from 1984 to 1999. *Medicine (Baltimore)* 79:69-79, 2000.
Travis WD, Colby TV, Koss MN, et al: Miscellaneous diseases of uncertain etiology. In Travis WD, Colby TV, Koss MN, et al: *Non-Neoplastic Disorders of the Lower Respiratory Tract*, Washington, DC, 2002, Armed Forces Institute of Pathology, pp 857-900.
Utz JP, Swensen SJ, Gertz MA: Pulmonary amyloidosis: The Mayo Clinic experience from 1980 to 1993. *Ann Intern Med* 124:407-413, 1996.

Metastatic Pulmonary Calcification

DEFINITION: Metastatic calcification is pulmonary calcification that develops secondary to hypercalcemia.

IMAGING

Radiography

Findings
- Numerous 3-10 mm in diameter fluffy, poorly defined nodular opacities mimicking airspace nodules or patchy areas of parenchymal opacification.

Utility
- Nodules tend to involve mainly upper lobes
- Calcification of nodules is seldom evident on radiograph

CT

Findings
- Fluffy poorly defined nodular opacities measuring 3-10 mm in diameter
- Nodules are centrilobular in distribution and most numerous in upper lung zones
- Nodule calcification may be stippled, diffuse, or, occasionally, ring-like
- Calcified vessels seen between pectoralis major and minor
- Extensive ground-glass opacities
- Patchy consolidation
- Calcification of pulmonary arteries and left atrial wall

Utility
- Thin-section CT often demonstrates parenchymal calcification not evident on the radiograph.

Nuclear Medicine

Findings
- Increased uptake with bone-imaging agents such as ^{99m}Tc-diphosphonate.

Utility
- Calcific nature of pulmonary opacities can be confirmed by scanning with bone-imaging agents.

CLINICAL PRESENTATION

- Usually asymptomatic
- Most common symptom: progressive shortness of breath

DIFFERENTIAL DIAGNOSIS

- Bronchopneumonia
- Sarcoidosis
- Amyloidosis
- Tuberculosis

DIAGNOSTIC PEARLS

- Fluffy, poorly defined nodular opacities are seen.
- Nodules are centrilobular in distribution and most numerous in upper lung zones.
- Nodule calcification may or may not be evident on thin-section CT.
- Calcific nature of pulmonary opacities can be confirmed by scintigraphy using bone-imaging agents such as ^{99m}Tc-diphosphonate.
- Calcified vessels are seen between the pectoralis major and minor.
- The calcification is located mainly in the alveolar septa (interstitium) in previously normal lung.
- Patients with chronic renal failure.

PATHOLOGY

- The disorder occurs when there is release of excess calcium salts from bone and after their transport through circulation.
- Histologically the calcification is located mainly in the alveolar septa (interstitium) and bronchial walls and, to a lesser extent, in bronchioles and pulmonary arterioles.

INCIDENCE/PREVALENCE AND EPIDEMIOLOGY

- Seen most commonly as a complication of end-stage renal failure with secondary hyperparathyroidism
- Particularly common in patients undergoing maintenance hemodialysis

Suggested Readings

Chan ED, Morales DV, Welsh CH, et al: Calcium deposition with or without bone formation in the lung. *Am J Respir Crit Care Med* 165:1654-1669, 2002.

Faubert PF, Shapiro WB, Porush JG, et al: Pulmonary calcification in hemodialyzed patients detected by technetium-99m diphosphonate scanning. *Kidney Int* 18:95-102, 1980.

Hartman TE, Müller NL, Primack SL, et al: Metastatic pulmonary calcification in patients with hypercalcemia: Findings on chest radiographs and CT scans. *AJR Am J Roentgenol* 162:799-802, 1994.

Marchiori E, Müller NL, Souza AS Jr, et al: Unusual manifestations of metastatic pulmonary calcification: High-resolution CT and pathological findings. *J Thorac Imaging* 20:66-70, 2005.

WHAT THE REFERRING PHYSICIAN NEEDS TO KNOW

- Metastatic pulmonary calcification has a predilection for upper lung zones.
- Diagnosis can be confirmed with thin-section CT or scintigraphy.
- Treatment is aimed at primary disease, usually chronic renal failure, and normalization of calcium, phosphate, and parathyroid hormone levels.

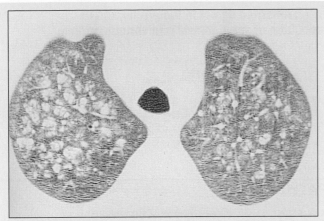

Figure 1. **Metastatic pulmonary calcification.** High-resolution CT scan through the lung apices shows nodular areas of increased attenuation. *(From Müller NL, Fraser RS, Colman NC, Paré PD: Radiologic Diagnosis of Diseases of the Chest. Philadelphia, WB Saunders, 2001.)*

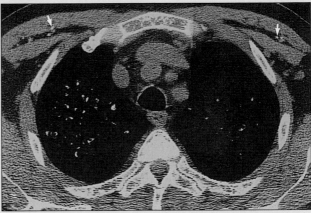

Figure 2. **Metastatic pulmonary calcification.** Same patient as in Figure 1. Soft tissue windows show the presence of calcification within the opacities. Vascular calcification in the chest wall also is evident *(arrows)*. *(From Müller NL, Fraser RS, Colman NC, Paré PD: Radiologic Diagnosis of Diseases of the Chest. Philadelphia, WB Saunders, 2001.)*

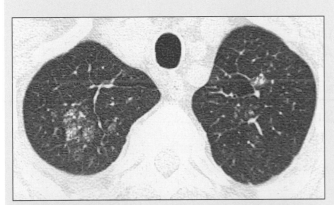

Figure 3. **Metastatic pulmonary calcification.** High-resolution CT image at the level of the upper lobes show poorly defined centrilobular nodular opacities and septal lines. The patient was a 60-year-old man with chronic renal failure. The septal lines were due to fluid overload, and the nodular opacities were due to metastatic pulmonary calcification.

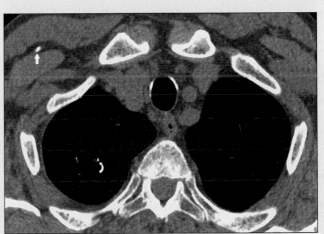

Figure 4. **Metastatic pulmonary calcification.** Same patient as in Figure 3. Soft tissue windows demonstrate foci of calcification within the nodular opacities *(curved arrow)* and in chest wall vessels *(straight arrow)*.

Niemann-Pick Disease

DEFINITION: Niemann-Pick disease is caused by an inherited defect in the production of sphingomyelinase, a deficiency that results in the deposition of sphingomyelin in various organs.

IMAGING

Radiography
Findings
- Reticular or reticulonodular pattern involving mainly the lower lung zones
- Hepatomegaly and splenomegaly

Utility
- Usually the first imaging modality used in the evaluation of these patients

CT
Findings
- Patchy bilateral ground-glass opacities
- Smooth thickening of interlobular septa
- Smooth intralobular lines
- "Crazy paving" pattern
- Hepatomegaly and splenomegaly

Utility
- CT provides excellent depiction of the extent of parenchymal abnormalities.

CLINICAL PRESENTATION

- Pulmonary involvement can be asymptomatic or (rarely) severe enough to cause respiratory failure.
- Hepatomegaly and splenomegaly are common.

DIFFERENTIAL DIAGNOSIS

- Nonspecific interstitial pneumonia
- Lymphangitic carcinomatosis
- Sarcoidosis
- Amyloidosis
- Alveolar proteinosis

DIAGNOSTIC PEARLS

- Bilateral ground-glass opacities
- Smooth thickening of the interlobular septa
- Hepatomegaly and splenomegaly
- Patients commonly asymptomatic

PATHOLOGY

- An inherited defect in production of sphingomyelinase results in deposition of sphingomyelin mainly in cells of the reticuloendothelial system.
- Vast majority of patients with type A die in infancy whereas most of those with type B survive into adulthood.
- Virtually all patients with Niemann-Pick disease type B develop interstitial lung disease.

INCIDENCE/PREVALENCE AND EPIDEMIOLOGY

- This autosomal recessive disorder is uncommon.
- The adult form (type B) occurs in all populations.

Suggested Readings

Duchateau F, Dechambre S, Coche E: Imaging of pulmonary manifestations in subtype B of Niemann-Pick disease. *Br J Radiol* 74: 1059-1061, 2001.
Mendelson DS, Wasserstein MP, Desnick RJ, et al: Type B Niemann-Pick disease: Findings at chest radiography, thin-section CT, and pulmonary function testing. *Radiology* 238:339-345, 2006.
Nicholson AG, Florio R, Hansell DM, et al: Pulmonary involvement by Niemann-Pick disease: A report of six cases. *Histopathology* 48:596-603, 2006.
Niggemann B, Rebien W, Rahn W, Wahn U: Asymptomatic pulmonary involvement in 2 children with Niemann-Pick disease type B. *Respiration* 61:55-57, 1994.

WHAT THE REFERRING PHYSICIAN NEEDS TO KNOW
- Pulmonary involvement is often asymptomatic.

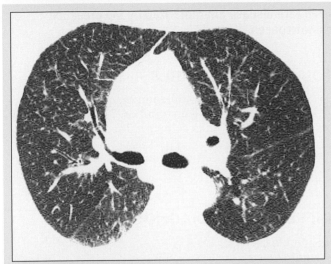

Figure 1. Niemann-Pick disease. High-resolution CT image at the level of bronchus intermedius in a 43-year-old man with Niemann-Pick disease shows thickening of the interlobular septa and patchy ground-glass opacities.

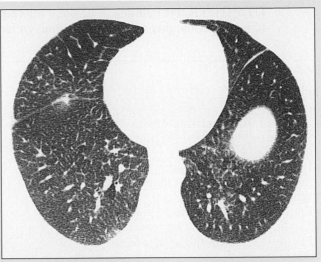

Figure 2. Niemann-Pick disease. High-resolution CT image at the level of lung bases in a 43-year-old man with Niemann-Pick disease shows thickening of the interlobular septa and patchy ground-glass opacities.

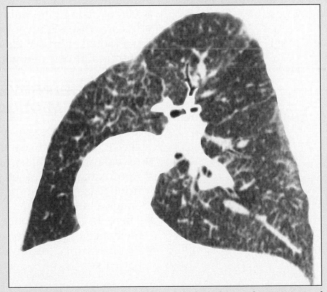

Figure 3. Niemann-Pick disease. Sagittal reformatted CT image of the right lung better demonstrates the overall distribution of the thickened interlobular septa and ground-glass opacities.

Pulmonary Alveolar Microlithiasis

DEFINITION: Pulmonary alveolar microlithiasis is a rare disease characterized by the presence of innumerable tiny calculi (microliths) within alveolar airspaces.

IMAGING

Radiography

Findings

- Fine sand-like micronodulation ("sandstorm lung") is diffuse but tends to be most severe in middle and lower lung zones.
- Deposits are usually identifiable as sharply defined nodules measuring less than 1 mm.
- Bullae occur in lung apices.
- Zone of increased lucency is between lung parenchyma and ribs ("black pleural line").
- Pleural calcification is evident.

Utility

- Characteristic appearance on the radiograph is often the first suggestion of the diagnosis.

CT

Findings

- Calcific nodules measuring less than 1mm in diameter that may be diffuse but tend to be distributed mainly in dorsal portions of lower lung zones
- Ground-glass opacities
- Interlobular septal thickening (often with apparent extensive calcification)
- Subpleural interstitial thickening
- Paraseptal emphysema

Utility

- Helpful particularly in patients with early or mild disease.

Nuclear Medicine

Findings

- ^{99m}Tc-MDP bone scintigraphy shows diffuse uptake of radiotracer in both lungs.

Utility

- Helpful particularly in patients with early or mild disease.

CLINICAL PRESENTATION

- Dyspnea on exertion
- Cough (occasionally)
- Respiratory insufficiency in association with cyanosis, clubbing of fingers, and evidence of pulmonary hypertension

DIAGNOSTIC PEARLS

- Sand-like nodules in a predominantly middle and lower lung zone distribution
- Calcified septal lines commonly seen on high-resolution CT
- Ground-glass opacities commonly seen on high-resolution CT

DIFFERENTIAL DIAGNOSIS

- Sarcoidosis
- Tuberculosis
- Talcosis (Talc embolism)

PATHOLOGY

- Pathogenesis of microlithiasis is unknown.
- Microliths consist of calcareous concentric lamellae placed around a central nucleus, mainly calcium phosphate.
- Microliths may fill pulmonary alveolar airspaces.
- In early disease, alveolar walls are normal; eventually, interstitial fibrosis develops, sometimes associated with multinucleated giant cell formation.

INCIDENCE/PREVALENCE AND EPIDEMIOLOGY

- Most reported cases have been in patients between the ages of 20 and 50 years.
- Alveolar microlithiasis is rare.
- Approximately 43% of cases came from Europe, 41% from Asia, with the remaining cases from the United States and elsewhere.
- There is no preference for a specific race, and the incidence is similar in both sexes.
- Family history for the disease is found in one third of patients.

Suggested Readings

Castellana G, Lamorgese V: Pulmonary alveolar microlithiasis: World cases and review of the literature. *Respiration* 70:549-555, 2003.

Lauta VM: Pulmonary alveolar microlithiasis: An overview of clinical and pathological features together with possible therapies. *Respir Med* 97:1081-1085, 2003.

Mariotta S, Ricci A, Papale M, et al: Pulmonary alveolar microlithiasis: Report on 576 cases published in the literature. *Sarcoidosis Vasc Diffuse Lung Dis* 21:173-181, 2004.

WHAT THE REFERRING PHYSICIAN NEEDS TO KNOW

- Chest radiograph often is highly suggestive of diagnosis.
- CT and scintigraphy can be helpful in confirming the diagnosis, particularly in patients with mild disease.

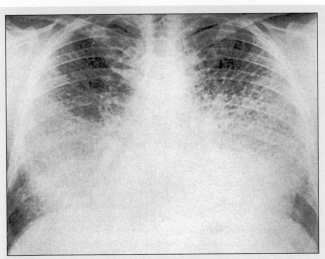

Figure 1. Alveolar microlithiasis. Posteroanterior radiograph of this 40-year-old asymptomatic man reveals a remarkably uniform opacification of both lungs. (*From Müller NL, Fraser RS, Colman NC, Paré PD: Radiologic Diagnosis of Diseases of the Chest. Philadelphia, WB Saunders, 2001.*)

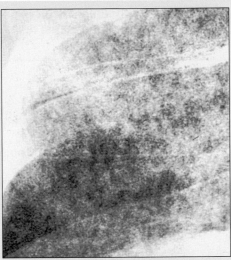

Figure 2. Alveolar microlithiasis. On close scrutiny, a multitude of tiny, discrete opacities of calcific density can be seen (same patient as in Fig. 1). Pulmonary function test results were normal except for a reduction in residual volume of 800 mL, representing the displacement of pulmonary volume by the microliths. (*From Müller NL, Fraser RS, Colman NC, Paré PD: Radiologic Diagnosis of Diseases of the Chest. Philadelphia, WB Saunders, 2001.*)

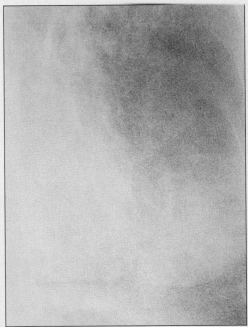

Figure 3. Alveolar microlithiasis. View of the left lung from a posteroanterior chest radiograph in a 60-year-old woman shows numerous small calcific opacities, resulting in a sandstorm appearance. (*Courtesy of Dr. Jim Barrie, University of Alberta Medical Centre. From Müller NL, Fraser RS, Colman NC, Paré PD: Radiologic Diagnosis of Diseases of the Chest. Philadelphia, WB Saunders, 2001.*)

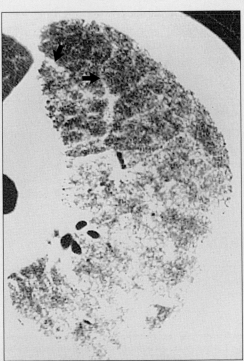

Figure 4. Alveolar microlithiasis. View of the left lung of the same patient as in Figure 3 from a high-resolution CT scan shows confluence of nodules in the dependent lung regions. A few thickened interlobular septa (*arrows*) can be seen anteriorly. (*Courtesy of Dr. Jim Barrie, University of Alberta Medical Centre. From Müller NL, Fraser RS, Colman NC, Paré PD: Radiologic Diagnosis of Diseases of the Chest. Philadelphia, WB Saunders, 2001.*)

Pulmonary Alveolar Proteinosis

DEFINITION: Pulmonary alveolar proteinosis is a rare disease characterized by the accumulation of protein- and lipid-rich material resembling surfactant within the parenchymal airspaces.

IMAGING

Radiography
Findings
- Bilateral patchy areas of consolidation with vaguely nodular appearance
- Consolidation often perihilar (bat wing or butterfly distribution)
- Consolidation may have peripheral or basal distribution
- Ground-glass opacities
- Linear interstitial pattern superimposed on areas of consolidation or ground-glass opacities

Utility
- Usually first imaging modality used in the assessment of these patients
- Limited value in the diagnosis

CT
Findings
- Bilateral ground-glass opacities
- Consolidation may be present particularly in dorsal lung regions
- "Crazy-paving" pattern
- Sharp demarcation between normal and abnormal parenchyma

Utility
- High-resolution CT is superior to conventional CT and chest radiography in assessment of pattern and distribution of abnormalities.

CLINICAL PRESENTATION

- Shortness of breath on exertion that is usually slowly progressive
- Cough (usually nonproductive)
- Low-grade fever
- Clubbing of fingers in about a third of patients

DIFFERENTIAL DIAGNOSIS

- Lipoid pneumonia
- Niemann-Pick disease

DIAGNOSTIC PEARLS

- "Crazy-paving" pattern on high-resolution CT
- Ground-glass opacities on high-resolution CT
- Consolidation is perihilar (bat wing or butterfly distribution) on the radiograph
- Chronic symptoms, dry cough and dyspnea

- Nonspecific interstitial pneumonia
- *Pneumocystis* pneumonia
- Pulmonary hemorrhage

PATHOLOGY

- Accumulation of protein- and lipid-rich material resembling surfactant occurs within parenchymal airspaces.
- Alveoli are filled with finely granular, lipoproteinaceous material that stains eosinophilic with hematoxylin and eosin and purple with periodic acid–Schiff.
- Alveolar architecture is usually preserved but septal thickening may occur due to edema or lymphocytic infiltration.
- Pulmonary function test results are normal or show restrictive ventilatory defect with reduction in vital capacity and total lung capacity.
- Extensive disease may result in hypoxemia and increased alveolar-arterial pressure gradient, which increases further with exercise.

INCIDENCE/PREVALENCE AND EPIDEMIOLOGY

- This disease is rare.
- Ninety percent of cases occur as an acquired disease of unknown etiology appearing related to antibody to granulocyte-macrophage colony-stimulating factor.
- It is associated with conditions resulting in functional impairment of alveolar macrophages.
- Incidence has been estimated to be approximately 4 per million persons.

WHAT THE REFERRING PHYSICIAN NEEDS TO KNOW

- When reviewing radiographic and CT images, it is important to also look for complications of pulmonary alveolar proteinosis.
- The main complication is infection, including community-acquired pneumonia and unusual organisms such as *Nocardia, Aspergillus,* and *Pneumocystis.*
- Rarely, patients with pulmonary alveolar proteinosis may develop interstitial fibrosis.
- Diagnosis can usually be confirmed by examination of bronchoalveolar lavage fluid.
- Treatment is with whole-lung lavage.

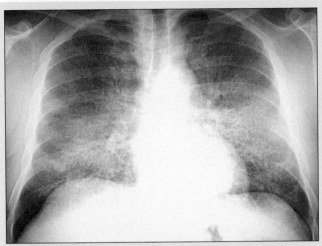

Figure 1. Pulmonary alveolar proteinosis: imaging findings. Posteroanterior chest radiograph shows airspace consolidation and ground-glass opacities mainly in the perihilar regions ("butterfly pattern") with sparing of the peripheral regions. Note vaguely nodular appearance.

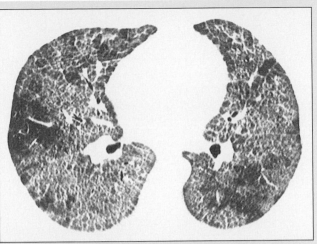

Figure 2. Pulmonary alveolar proteinosis: imaging findings. High-resolution CT demonstrates extensive bilateral areas of ground-glass opacities and a superimposed fine linear pattern forming polygonal arcades ("crazy-paving" pattern).

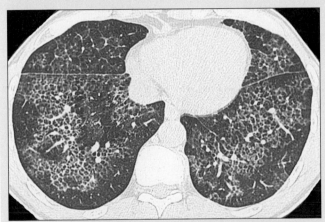

Figure 3. Pulmonary alveolar proteinosis: imaging findings. High-resolution CT shows bilateral ground-glass opacities and superimposed fine linear pattern forming polygonal arcades ("crazy-paving" pattern). Note the sharp demarcation between normal and abnormal parenchyma, a feature that usually reflects lobular boundaries. Also note presence of mild emphysema.

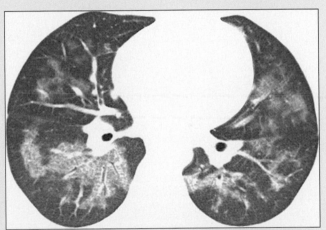

Figure 4. Pulmonary alveolar proteinosis in a patient with aplastic anemia. High-resolution CT shows bilateral ground-glass opacities with sparing of the peripheral lung. Mild superimposed linear opacities ("crazy-paving" pattern) are present in the lower lobes. The patient was an 11-year-old girl undergoing immunosuppressive therapy for aplastic anemia.

- Predominantly patients between 20 and 50 years of age are affected, and there is a male-to-female preponderance of about 2.5:1.
- Approximately 70% of patients are smokers.

Suggested Readings

Chung MJ, Lee KS, Franquet T, et al: Metabolic lung disease: Imaging and histopathologic findings. *Eur J Radiol* 54:233-245, 2005.

Seymour JF, Presneill JJ: Pulmonary alveolar proteinosis: Progress in the first 44 years. *Am J Respir Crit Care Med* 166:215-235, 2002.

Pulmonary Embolism, Hypertension, and Edema

Acute Pulmonary Embolism

DEFINITION: Acute blockage of one or more pulmonary arteries due to migration of clots that usually develop initially in the deep veins of the legs.

IMAGING

Radiography

Findings
- Chest radiograph may be normal.
- Radiographic findings are usually nonspecific.
- Infarction including a homogeneous wedge-shaped consolidation in periphery of lung with rounded, convex apex toward hilum (Hampton's hump) is uncommon.
- Peripheral oligemia (Westermark sign) is uncommon.
- Dilatation of major pulmonary artery (Fleischner sign) is uncommon.
- Pleural effusion(s) occur.

Utility
- Important in excluding other diagnoses that can mimic clinical picture of acute pulmonary embolism
- Insensitive and nonspecific test

CT

Findings
- Partial or complete filling defect within one or more pulmonary arteries on contrast-enhanced CT (CT angiography).
- Partial filing defect: intravascular central or marginal area of low attenuation surrounded by variable amount of contrast material.
- Complete filling defect: intraluminal area of low attenuation that occupies entire section.
- Enlargement of central pulmonary arteries.
- Signs of right ventricular strain or failure in severe acute pulmonary embolism, including enlargement of right ventricle and right atrium, bowing of interventricular septum to the left, and reflux of contrast into the inferior vena cava and hepatic veins.
- Peripheral areas of consolidation or ground-glass opacities due to pulmonary hemorrhage or infarction.
- Areas of decreased attenuation and vascularity possibly evident.
- Pleural effusion.

Utility
- CT is the imaging modality of choice for the diagnosis of acute pulmonary thromboembolism.
- CT usually allows confident diagnosis.
- It often allows suggestion of an alternate diagnosis in patients without pulmonary embolism.
- Cardiac functional information can be calculated from datasets required with electrocardiographic gating.
- Multidetector CT offers better diagnostic performance than single-detector row helical CT.
- Multidetector CT is an accurate and reliable noninvasive technique for evaluating right-sided heart failure.

MRI

Findings
- Filling defect(s) within one or more pulmonary arteries
- Segmental or subsegmental areas of decreased perfusion

Utility
- Allows direct and noninvasive demonstration of acute pulmonary embolism
- Advantage of not requiring radiation

WHAT THE REFERRING PHYSICIAN NEEDS TO KNOW
- Pulmonary embolism should prompt a search for venous thrombosis at level of lower extremities.
- Multidetector CT has replaced pulmonary angiography as the gold standard in diagnosis of acute pulmonary embolism.
- CT also provides important cardiac information, such as ejection fraction and signs of right ventricular strain.
- Ventilation-perfusion scintigraphy can be a useful diagnostic alternative to CT in patients with normal chest radiographs.
- Evaluation of clinical likelihood of acute pulmonary embolism is mandatory to optimize the use of diagnostic tests, especially in the emergency department.
- Potential consequences of acute pulmonary embolism are hemorrhage or infarction within lung parenchyma and acute pulmonary hypertension.
- Right ventricular dysfunction is responsible for ventricular failure due to impaired left ventricular preload and decreased ventricular coronary perfusion.

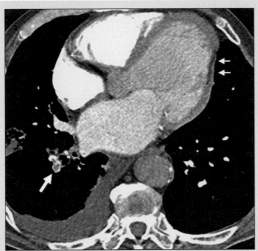

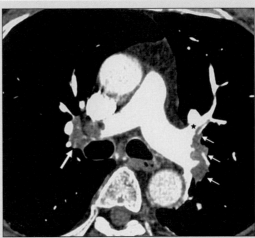

Figure 1. **Acute pulmonary embolism.** A 62-year-old patient with a previous history of ischemic heart disease presented with acute chest pain. Contrast-enhanced CT image obtained at the level of the lower lobes shows a partial filling defect within the posterobasal segmental artery of the right lower lobe (*large arrow*). Note the concurrent presence of an abnormal thinning of the myocardial wall with features of lipomatous metaplasia (*small arrows*), indicative of a previous history of myocardial infarction. (*Courtesy of Dr. Martine Remy-Jardin, Lille, France*)

Figure 2. **Acute pulmonary embolism.** Contrast-enhanced CT scan obtained at the level of the main bronchi shows endoluminal filling defects at the level of the right (*large arrow*) and left (*small arrows*) interlobar pulmonary arteries. The *large arrow* points to a complete filling defect. The *small arrows* point to partial filling defects extending into the anterior segmental artery of the left upper lobe (*star*). (*Courtesy of Dr. Martine Remy-Jardin, Lille, France*)

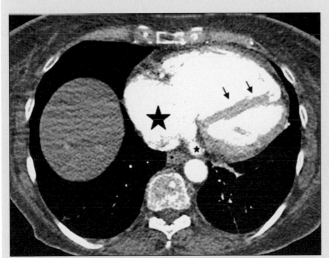

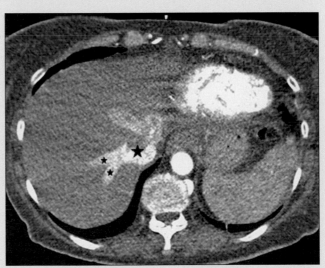

Figure 3. **Assessment of severity of pulmonary embolism: CT features of right-sided heart failure.** Contrast-enhanced CT image obtained at the level of the ventricular cavities shows a leftward shift of the interventricular septum (*arrows*) due to right ventricular dilatation. Note the enlarged right atrium (*large star*) and reflux of contrast medium within the coronary sinus (*small star*). (*Courtesy of Dr. Martine Remy-Jardin, Lille, France*)

Figure 4. **Assessment of severity of pulmonary embolism: CT features of right-sided heart failure.** CT image obtained at the level of the liver demonstrates reflux of contrast medium into the inferior vena cava (*large star*) and hepatic veins (*small stars*). (*Courtesy of Dr. Martine Remy-Jardin, Lille, France*)

- Accuracy high for MR angiography, MR pulmonary perfusion, real-time MRI, and combined protocols
- Seldom used in clinical practice except in patients with allergy to iodinated contrast

Nuclear Medicine
Findings
- Presence of ventilation in absence of perfusion distal to obstructing emboli.
Utility
- Ventilation-perfusion lung scans with ^{99m}Tc-MAA (radiolabeled albumin macroaggregates) are most helpful in patients with normal chest radiographs.

CLINICAL PRESENTATION

- Most common symptoms are dyspnea, tachypnea, and pleuritic chest pain.
- Sudden onset in absence of underlying respiratory disease is highly suggestive of acute pulmonary embolism.
- Clinical diagnosis of acute pulmonary embolism is difficult in a patient with chronic obstructive pulmonary disease and may mimic an exacerbation of this problem.

PATHOLOGY

- Embolic fragment in the pulmonary vasculature from migration of clots that usually develop in deep veins of the legs.

INCIDENCE/PREVALENCE AND EPIDEMIOLOGY

- Approximately 600,000 cases per year in United States.
- Third most common cause of death after myocardial ischemia and stroke.

Suggested Readings

Ghaye B, Ghuysen A, Bruyere PJ, et al: Can CT pulmonary angiography allow assessment of severity and prognosis in patients presenting with pulmonary embolism? What the radiologist needs to know. *RadioGraphics* 26:23-40, 2006.

Remy-Jardin M, Pistolesi M, Goodman LR, et al: Management of suspected acute pulmonary embolism in the era of CT angiography: A statement from the Fleischner Society. *Radiology* 245(2):315-329, 2007.

Wood KE: Major pulmonary embolism: Review of pathophysiologic approach to the golden hour of hemodynamically significant pulmonary embolism. *Chest* 121:877-905, 2002.

Chronic Pulmonary Embolism

DEFINITION: Chronic pulmonary thromboembolism results from incomplete resolution of thrombi, leading to complex restructuring processes within pulmonary arteries.

IMAGING

Radiography

Findings
- Enlargement of central pulmonary arteries and right ventricle in patients with pulmonary arterial hypertension
- Asymmetry in size of central pulmonary arteries
- Areas of relative hypoperfusion and hyperperfusion
- Parenchymal scars

Utility
- Usually first imaging modality performed in these patients
- Has main value in excluding other causes of shortness of breath
- Has limited value in diagnosis of acute or chronic pulmonary embolism

CT

Findings
- Eccentric filling defects contiguous with vessel wall; mean attenuation value of chronic clots higher than acute filling defects.
- Recanalization within area of arterial hypoattenuation.
- Arterial stenosis or web.
- Reduction of more than 50% of overall arterial diameter.
- Complete filling defect at level of stenosed pulmonary arteries.
- Lung windows frequently show areas of decreased attenuation and vascularity and areas of increased attenuation and vascularity (mosaic attenuation and perfusion pattern).
- Cylindric bronchial dilatation.
- Enlargement of central pulmonary arteries and dilatation of right ventricle in patients with pulmonary arterial hypertension.

Utility
- Contrast-enhanced CT is the imaging modality of choice.

MRI

Findings
- Eccentric filling defects contiguous with vessel wall on contrast-enhanced MR (MR angiography).
- Arterial stenosis or web.
- Segmental or subsegmental areas of hypoperfusion.

DIAGNOSTIC PEARLS

- Ventilation-perfusion scintigraphy is most sensitive imaging modality to detect chronic pulmonary embolism but has low specificity.
- Contrast-enhanced CT is the imaging modality of choice.
- Eccentric filling defects contiguous with vessel wall, arterial stenosis or web, complete filling defect at level of stenosed pulmonary arteries.
- Mosaic attenuation and perfusion pattern on lung windows.
- Enlarged central pulmonary arteries.

Utility
- Seldom used in clinical practice.
- Useful mainly in patients with allergy to iodinated contrast medium.

Nuclear Medicine

Findings
- Segmental or larger mismatched perfusion defects
- Areas of diminished isotopic activity.

Utility
- Most sensitive method to detect chronic pulmonary embolism; low specificity.

Pulmonary Angiography

Findings
- Irregularity of the lumen, eccentric filling defects, recanalization, arterial stenosis or web
- Segmental or subsegmental areas of hypoperfusion

Utility
- Main indication is in patients being considered for thromboendarterectomy for treatment of chronic thromboembolic pulmonary arterial hypertension.

CLINICAL PRESENTATION

- Pulmonary hypertension
- Progressive dyspnea and exercise intolerance

WHAT THE REFERRING PHYSICIAN NEEDS TO KNOW

- Diagnosis of chronic pulmonary thromboembolism should be considered in all patients who have dyspnea and no obvious other cause.
- Noninvasive diagnosis can be obtained with multidetector CT angiography.
- Scintigraphy has a high sensitivity but a low specificity.

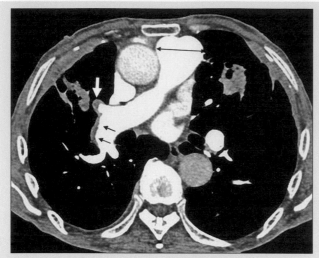

Figure 1. Chronic pulmonary thromboembolism. Transverse CT scan obtained at the level of bronchus intermedius showing a mural defect at the level of the outer wall of the right interlobar pulmonary artery (*small black arrows*). Note the additional presence of a complete defect within the right middle lobe pulmonary artery (*large white arrow*) and enlarged pulmonary arteries on both sides, suggestive of pulmonary hypertension. *Black double arrow* points to the enlarged pulmonary trunk. (*Courtesy of Dr. Martine Remy-Jardin, Lille, France*)

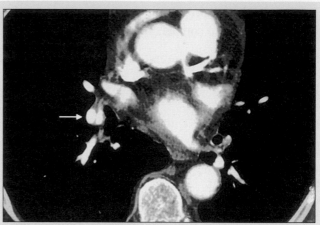

Figure 2. Chronic pulmonary thromboembolism. Transverse CT scan obtained at the level of the right interlobar pulmonary artery shows a thin web (*arrow*) within the arterial lumen, consistent with incomplete recanalization. (*Courtesy of Dr. Martine Remy-Jardin, Lille, France*)

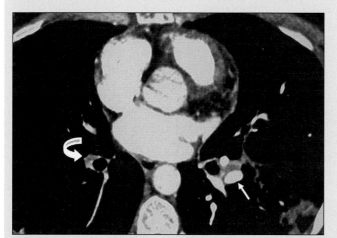

Figure 3. Chronic pulmonary thromboembolism. Transverse CT scan obtained at the level of the lower lobes shows complete obstruction and retraction of the right lower lobe pulmonary artery (*curved arrow*) in comparison with the normally perfused left lower lobe pulmonary artery (*straight arrow*). (*Courtesy of Dr. Martine Remy-Jardin, Lille, France*)

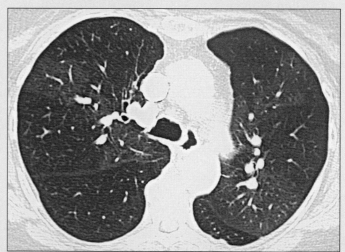

Figure 4. Chronic pulmonary thromboembolism. Transverse CT image obtained at the level of carina shows enlarged vessels within areas of increased attenuation while decreased vascularity and lower attenuation are found in the remaining portions of both lungs (mosaic attenuation and perfusion pattern). (*Courtesy of Dr. Martine Remy-Jardin, Lille, France*)

DIFFERENTIAL DIAGNOSIS

- Fibrosing mediastinitis
- Pulmonary sarcoma
- Takayasu arteritis
- Pulmonary stenosis

PATHOLOGY

- Fresh thrombus may fragment and disperse into smaller pulmonary arteries.
- Thrombotic emboli undergo organization and become firmly adherent to vessel wall.
- Thromboembolic material and breakdown products are incorporated into vessel wall and transformed into patches of intimal fibrosis.
- Long-standing increase in pulmonary artery pressure resulting from obstruction of pulmonary arterial bed leads to chronic thromboembolic pulmonary hypertension.

INCIDENCE/PREVALENCE AND EPIDEMIOLOGY

- Failure of thromboembolus resolution after single or recurrent thromboembolic events is a predisposing factor.
- Approximately 600,000 episodes of pulmonary embolism occur each year in the United States.
- Evolution toward chronic thromboembolic disease has been estimated to range between 2% and 18% of patients.
- Despite extensive investigation, the only identifiable thrombotic predisposition has been presence of lupus anticoagulant in approximately 10% of patients.
- Less than 1% of patients have had deficiencies of either antithrombin III, protein C, or protein S.
- With cor pulmonale and right-sided heart failure, there is poor prognosis, with 5-year survival rate of only 30%.

Suggested Readings

Coulden R: State-of-the-art imaging techniques in chronic thromboembolic pulmonary hypertension. *Proc Am Thorac Soc* 3(7): 577-583, 2006.

Doyle RL, McCrory D, Channick RN, et al: American College of Chest Physicians. Surgical treatments/interventions for pulmonary arterial hypertension: ACCP evidence-based clinical practice guidelines. *Chest* 126(1 Suppl):63S-71S, 2004.

Fedullo PF, Auger WR, Kerr KM, Rubin LJ: Chronic thromboembolic pulmonary hypertension. *N Engl J Med* 345:1465-1472, 2001.

Reddy GP, Gotway MB, Araoz PA: Imaging of chronic thromboembolic pulmonary hypertension. *Semin Roentgenol* 40(1):41-47, 2005.

Part 37

NONTHROMBOTIC PULMONARY EMBOLISM

Pulmonary Embolism: Fat

DEFINITION: Fat embolism refers to the presence of globules of free fat within the pulmonary vasculature.

IMAGING

Radiography

Findings

- Radiograph is often normal.
- Most common findings consist of bilateral hazy areas of increased opacity (ground-glass opacities) or patchy consolidation.
- Widespread consolidation may occur.

Utility

- First and frequently only modality used in the assessment of these patients.

CT

Findings

- Bilateral patchy or diffuse ground-glass opacities.
- Patchy or confluent areas of consolidation.
- Poorly defined centrilobular nodules.

Utility

- Superior to radiography in demonstrating presence and extent of parenchymal abnormalities.
- Contrast-enhanced CT helpful in excluding acute pulmonary thromboembolism.

CLINICAL PRESENTATION

- Dyspnea, neurologic symptoms, fever, and petechial rash develop 12 to 36 hours after injury.
- Cough, hemoptysis, and pleuritic chest pain occur occasionally.
- Acute cor pulmonale with cardiac failure, cyanosis, and circulatory shock may occur.

DIFFERENTIAL DIAGNOSIS

- Lung contusion
- Aspiration
- Pulmonary thromboembolism

PATHOLOGY

- Globules of free fat are present within the pulmonary vasculature.

DIAGNOSTIC PEARLS

- Dyspnea 12 to 36 hours after fractures of femur, tibia, or pelvis
- Bilateral ground-glass opacities
- Patchy or confluent areas of consolidation
- Poorly defined centrilobular nodules

- Mechanical vascular obstruction, predominantly by fat globules, is possibly enhanced by platelet or red blood cell aggregates.
- Conversion of neutral triglycerides into free fatty acids by endothelial lipases leads to endothelial damage and increased permeability pulmonary edema.
- Definitive histologic diagnosis requires use of fat-soluble dyes on unfixed (frozen) tissue or other special techniques.

INCIDENCE/PREVALENCE AND EPIDEMIOLOGY

- Fat embolism is very common among trauma patients, especially those with long bone or pelvic fractures.
- It is common after extensive injury to subcutaneous fat.
- Incidence of clinically significant disease in patients who have simple tibial or femoral fractures is 1% to 3%.
- Individuals who have severe trauma have an incidence of clinically evident embolism of 10% to 20%.
- May also occur after orthopedic surgery such as arthroplasty.

Suggested Readings

Han D, Lee KS, Franquet T, et al: Thrombotic and nonthrombotic pulmonary arterial embolism: Spectrum of imaging findings. *RadioGraphics* 23:1521-1539, 2003.

Husebye EE, Lyberg T, Roise O: Bone marrow fat in the circulation: Clinical entities and pathophysiological mechanisms. *Injury* 37(Suppl 4):S8-S18, 2006.

Talbot M, Schemitsch EH: Fat embolism syndrome: History, definition, epidemiology. *Injury* 37:S3-S7, 2006.

WHAT THE REFERRING PHYSICIAN NEEDS TO KNOW

- Dyspnea, neurologic symptoms, fever, and petechial rash typically develop 12 to 36 hours after injury.
- Resolution generally takes 7 to 10 days and occasionally as long as 4 weeks.
- Mainstay of treatment is supportive.

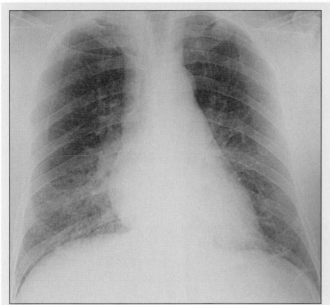

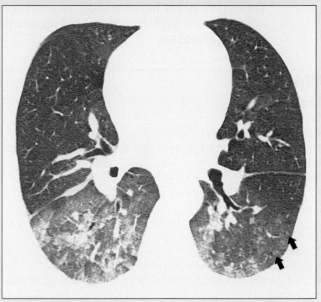

Figure 1. **Mild fat embolism: radiographic findings.**
Anteroposterior chest radiograph shows poorly defined areas of consolidation in the right lower lobe. The patient was a 53-year-old man with fat embolism syndrome after trauma sustained in a motor vehicle accident.

Figure 2. **Mild fat embolism: CT findings.** High-resolution CT image demonstrates patchy bilateral consolidation and ground-glass opacities in the lower lobes. Also noted are a few centrilobular nodules (*arrows*) in the left lower lobe. The patient was a 53-year-old man with fat embolism syndrome from trauma sustained in a motor vehicle accident.

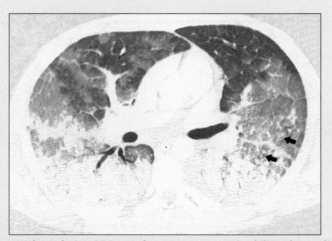

Figure 3. **Fat embolism: CT findings.** High-resolution CT image demonstrates extensive bilateral consolidation, ground-glass opacities, and a few poorly defined centrilobular nodules (*arrows*). The patient was a 17-year-old man with severe fat embolism syndrome after hip arthroplasty.

Pulmonary Embolism: Tumor

DEFINITION: Tumor emboli are made up of tumor fragments lodged within the pulmonary vessels where, once a sufficient amount of fragments have accumulated, they manifest as a pulmonary thromboembolism.

IMAGING

Radiography
Findings
- Small nodular opacities
- Occasionally enlargement of the central pulmonary arteries

Utility
- Intravascular tumor emboli are seldom recognized on chest radiographs.

CT
Findings
- Filling defects in central pulmonary arteries
- Nodular or beaded thickening of peripheral pulmonary arteries
- Nodular and branching centrilobular opacities ("tree-in-bud" pattern) representing enlarged centrilobular arteries

Utility
- CT is imaging modality of choice for assessment of pulmonary tumor embolism.

CLINICAL PRESENTATION

- Slowly progressive syndrome of dyspnea and pulmonary hypertension
- Occasionally acute cor pulmonale

DIFFERENTIAL DIAGNOSIS

- Pulmonary thromboembolism
- Sarcoidosis

DIAGNOSTIC PEARLS

- Intravascular filling defects
- Nodular or beaded thickening of the peripheral pulmonary arteries
- Nodular and branching centrilobular opacities ("tree-in-bud" pattern)

- Lymphangitic carcinomatosis
- Infectious bronchiolitis

PATHOLOGY

- Hematogenous pulmonary metastases derived from tumor fragments lodged within pulmonary vessels.

INCIDENCE/PREVALENCE AND EPIDEMIOLOGY

- Most commonly seen in metastatic renal cell carcinoma, hepatocellular carcinoma, and carcinoma of breast, stomach, and prostate.

Suggested Readings

Han D, Lee KS, Franquet T, et al: Thrombotic and nonthrombotic pulmonary arterial embolism: Spectrum of imaging findings. *RadioGraphics* 23:1521-1539, 2003.

Seo JB, Im JG, Goo JM, et al: Atypical pulmonary metastases: Spectrum of radiologic findings. *RadioGraphics* 21:403-417, 2001.

WHAT THE REFERRING PHYSICIAN NEEDS TO KNOW

- In vast majority of cases, tumor fragments are small and do not result in clinically or radiologically apparent vascular obstruction.
- Occasionally, extensive pulmonary tumor embolism may result in progressive shortness of breath or acute cor pulmonale.
- CT is imaging modality of choice for diagnosis of pulmonary tumor embolism.
- Tumor emboli are most commonly seen in metastatic renal cell carcinoma, hepatocellular carcinoma, and carcinoma of breast, stomach, and prostate.

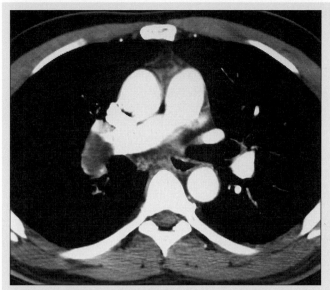

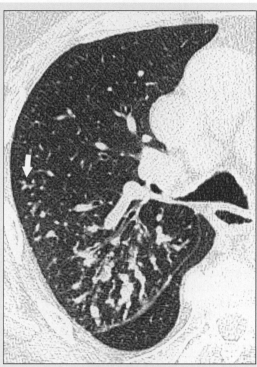

Figure 1. **Intravascular metastases.** Contrast-enhanced CT image at the level of the right interlobar pulmonary arteries demonstrates large intraluminal filling defects. The appearance is indistinguishable from that of pulmonary thromboembolism. The patient was a 63-year-old man with extensive intravascular metastases from renal cell carcinoma.

Figure 2. **Intravascular metastases.** View of the right lung at the level of the tracheal carina demonstrates nodular thickening of the pulmonary vessels and centrilobular nodular and branching opacities ("tree-in-bud" pattern) (*arrow*). The patient was a 78-year-old man with metastatic renal cell carcinoma.

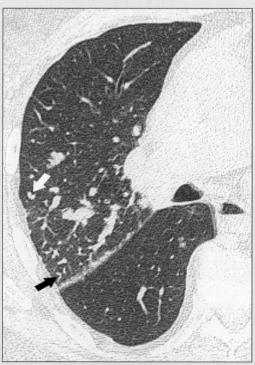

Figure 3. **Intravascular metastases.** View of the right lung at the level of the bronchus intermedius demonstrates nodular thickening of the pulmonary vessels and centrilobular nodular and branching opacities ("tree-in-bud" pattern) (*arrows*). The patient was a 78-year-old man with metastatic renal cell carcinoma.

Talcosis (Talc Embolism)

DEFINITION: Emboli of talc, starch, and cellulose are seen almost invariably in chronic intravenous drug users.

IMAGING

Radiography
Findings
- Diffuse fine nodular pattern
- Upper lobe conglomerate mass with associated superior retraction of hila
- Hyperlucency of lower lobes in panacinar emphysema

CT
Findings
- Diffuse ground-glass opacities
- Fine granular pattern
- Perihilar upper lobe conglomerate masses with foci of high attenuation
- Enlarged main pulmonary artery
- Fibrosis and honeycombing
- Bilateral, symmetric emphysema involving mainly lower lung zones (methylphenidate [Ritalin] abuse)

CLINICAL PRESENTATION
- Asymptomatic
- Symptoms develop only in very heavy intravenous drug users and consist of slowly progressive dyspnea and persistent cough
- Cor pulmonale

DIFFERENTIAL DIAGNOSIS
- Sarcoidosis
- Silicosis
- Coal worker's pneumoconiosis
- *Pneumocystis* pneumonia
- Alveolar microlithiasis

PATHOLOGY
- Insoluble fillers contained in tablets meant for oral use become trapped within pulmonary arterioles and capillaries and cause vascular occlusion.

DIAGNOSTIC PEARLS
- Upper lobe conglomerate masses with foci of high attenuation due to talc accumulation
- Widespread nodules ranging from barely visible to 1 mm in diameter
- Lower lobe panacinar emphysema in methylphenidate (Ritalin) users
- Enlarged central pulmonary arteries

- Foreign particles migrate through vessel wall, lie in adjacent perivascular/parenchymal interstitial tissue, and cause a foreign-body giant cell reaction and fibrosis.
- Talc is recognized as irregular, plate-like crystals that are strongly birefringent.

INCIDENCE/PREVALENCE AND EPIDEMIOLOGY
- Emboli of talc, starch, and cellulose are seen almost invariably in chronic intravenous drug users.
- Available estimates from 130 countries indicate the presence of 13.2 million intravenous drug users.

Suggested Readings

Aceijas C, Friedman SR, Cooper HL, et al: Estimates of injecting drug users at the national and local level in developing and transitional countries, and gender and age distribution. *Sex Transm Infect* 82(Suppl 3):iii10-iii17, 2006.

Aceijas C, Stimson G, Hickman M, et al: Global overview of injecting drug use and HIV infection among injecting drug users. *AIDS* 18:2295-2303, 2004.

Nguyen ET, Silva CI, Souza CA, Müller NL: Pulmonary complications of illicit drug use: Differential diagnosis based on CT findings. *J Thorac Imaging* 22:199-206, 2007.

Ward S, Heyneman LE, Reittner P, et al: Talcosis associated with IV abuse of oral medications: CT findings. *AJR Am J Roentgenol* 174:789-793, 2000.

WHAT THE REFERRING PHYSICIAN NEEDS TO KNOW
- Most patients are asymptomatic.
- Radiographic findings are nonspecific.
- Intravenous talcosis is seen almost exclusively in chronic intravenous drug users.
- Complication occurs with medications intended solely for oral use.

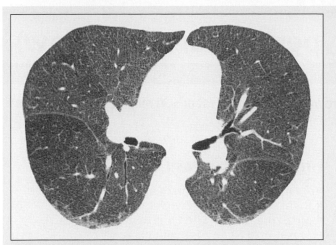

Figure 1. **Intravenous talcosis: diffuse pinpoint nodular pattern on CT.** High-resolution CT at the level of the bronchus intermedius demonstrates fine granular pattern throughout both lungs. The patient was a 42-year-old intravenous drug user.

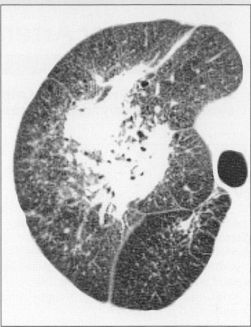

Figure 2. **Intravenous talcosis with conglomerate massive fibrosis.** High-resolution CT image of the right upper lobe shows numerous small nodules, diffuse ground-glass opacities, a conglomerate mass with associated distortion of the architecture, and anterior tenting of the interlobar fissure. The patient was a 30-year-old intravenous drug user.

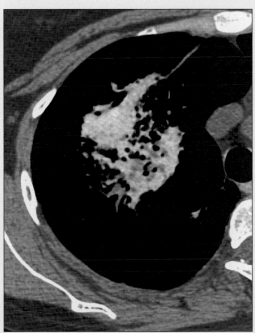

Figure 4. **Intravenous talcosis and panacinar emphysema.** High-resolution CT at the level of the lower lobe demonstrates extensive areas of decreased attenuation and focal areas of scarring. The patient was a 44-year-old woman who was a chronic intravenous user of methylphenidate (Ritalin) and developed severe panacinar emphysema.

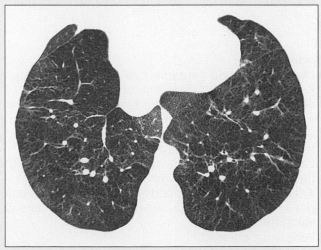

Figure 3. **Intravenous talcosis with conglomerate massive fibrosis.** High-resolution CT image using soft tissue windows demonstrates foci of high attenuation within the conglomerate mass consistent with talc deposition. The patient was a 30-year-old intravenous drug user.

Pulmonary Arterial Hypertension (Overview)

DEFINITION: Mean pulmonary arterial pressure of >25 mm Hg at rest or >30 mm Hg with exercise is considered pulmonary arterial hypertension.

IMAGING

Radiography

Findings

- Central pulmonary arterial dilatation to segmental level and attenuation of peripheral pulmonary vessels (peripheral pruning)
- Calcification within the pulmonary arteries
- Right ventricular enlargement causing reduction of retrosternal airspace on lateral radiograph
- Right atrial dilatation: widening of right-sided heart border on frontal projection

Utility

- Initial imaging study in patients with suspected pulmonary hypertension
- Useful to assess heart size, cardiac chamber dilatation, and proximal pulmonary arteries enlargement and to detect any underlying pulmonary parenchymal disorder
- Upper limit for transverse diameter of right interlobar artery measured from its lateral aspect to intermediate bronchus: normally <16 mm in men and <15 mm in women

CT

Findings

- Diameter of main pulmonary artery 30 mm or larger, exceeding thoracic aorta diameter.
- Segmental artery-to-bronchus ratio >1; abruptly tapering tortuous peripheral pulmonary vessels (pruning).
- Cardiac enlargement (right atrium >35 mm, right ventricle >45 mm); may have tricuspid regurgitation.
- Paradoxical bulging of the interventricular septum into the left ventricle during systole (septal bounce).
- Tricuspid regurgitation: early opacification of the inferior vena cava or hepatic veins on first-pass contrast-enhanced CT.
- Pericardial effusion.

DIAGNOSTIC PEARLS

- Dilated central pulmonary arteries
- Right cardiac chamber enlargement
- Mean pulmonary arterial pressure >25 mm Hg at rest or >30 mm Hg with exercise

- Ancillary findings: presence of ascites and features of hepatic congestion and cirrhosis.
- Septal thickening in pulmonary veno-occlusive disease.
- Poorly defined centrilobular nodules in pulmonary capillary hemangiomatosis, severe idiopathic pulmonary hypertension, and, occasionally, in veno-occlusive disease.
- Mosaic perfusion (attenuation) pattern.

Utility

- CT pulmonary angiography/high-resolution CT: comprehensive assessment of pulmonary vasculature/parenchyma, cardiac chamber dilatation, tricuspid regurgitation, limited right-sided heart function evaluation.
- Main pulmonary artery diameter of 30 mm or larger: 69%-87% sensitivity and 89%-100% specificity for pulmonary artery hypertension.
- Pulmonary artery/aorta diameter ratio: 92% specificity, 93% positive predictive value, 44% negative predictive value, and 70% sensitivity.

MRI

Findings

- Diameter of main pulmonary artery 30 mm or larger, exceeding thoracic aorta diameter
- Right ventricular hypertrophy and reversal of septal curvature
- Abnormal intravascular signal corresponding to slow pulmonary arterial blood flow
- Presence of left-to-right shunt

WHAT THE REFERRING PHYSICIAN NEEDS TO KNOW

- Not uncommonly, pulmonary hypertension can be misdiagnosed as asthma, hyperventilation syndrome, or lack of fitness.
- Echocardiography permits estimation of pulmonary artery pressure and is useful as screening tool and in follow-up.
- Diagnostic strategy should be tailored to suit individual institution, depending on local expertise, easy access, and cost.

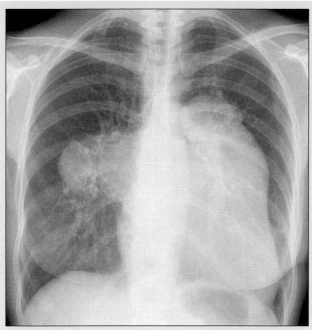

Figure 1. Posteroanterior chest radiograph demonstrates gross enlargement of the proximal pulmonary arteries with tapering of the peripheral vasculature (peripheral pruning) and cardiomegaly due to dilated right-sided heart chambers. (*Courtesy of Drs. Nicholas J. Screaton and Deepa Gopalan, Cambridge, UK*)

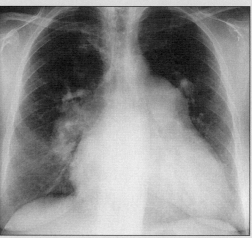

Figure 2. Pulmonary arterial hypertension caused by an atrial septal defect. Posteroanterior chest radiograph shows cardiomegaly and marked enlargement of the central pulmonary arteries. Although there is rapid tapering, increased vascularity still is present in the lung periphery, particularly evident on the right side. The patient was a 61-year-old woman. (*From Müller NL, Fraser RS, Colman NC, Paré PD: Radiologic Diagnosis of Diseases of the Chest. Philadelphia, WB Saunders, 2001.*)

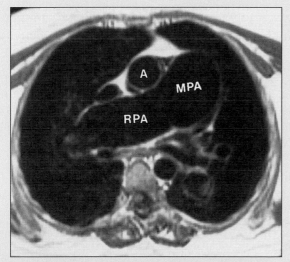

Figure 3. Pulmonary arterial hypertension caused by an atrial septal defect. Cardiac-gated spin-echo MR image shows enlargement of the main (MPA) and right (RPA) pulmonary arteries. The diameter of the MPA is considerably larger than that of the aorta (A). The patient was a 61-year-old woman. (*From Müller NL, Fraser RS, Colman NC, Paré PD: Radiologic Diagnosis of Diseases of the Chest. Philadelphia, WB Saunders, 2001.*)

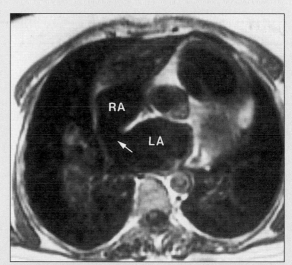

Figure 4. Pulmonary arterial hypertension caused by an atrial septal defect. MR image at the level of the right (RA) and left (LA) atrium shows an atrial septal defect (*arrow*). The patient was a 61-year-old woman. (*From Müller NL, Fraser RS, Colman NC, Paré PD: Radiologic Diagnosis of Diseases of the Chest. Philadelphia, WB Saunders, 2001.*)

Utility
- MRI enables noninvasive morphologic and functional assessment.
- MRI is the gold standard examination for evaluation of structural cardiac disease.

Nuclear Medicine
Findings
- Thromboembolic disease: segmental reduction in perfusion, maintenance of normal ventilation (ventilation-perfusion mismatch) in affected bronchopulmonary segment.
Utility
- Main role of ventilation-perfusion lung scintigraphy is to differentiate chronic thromboembolic disease from other pulmonary hypertension causes.
- Ventilation-perfusion scintigraphy has 90%-100% sensitivity and 94%-100% specificity for distinguishing between idiopathic pulmonary hypertension and chronic thromboembolic pulmonary hypertension.
- Mismatched segmental perfusion defects may be seen with other processes that result in obstruction of the central pulmonary arteries.

Pulmonary Angiography
Findings
- Signs of chronic pulmonary thromboembolism on angiography: pouch-like filling defects, webs or bands, intimal irregularities, abrupt vascular narrowing, and absent arterial segments.
Utility
- Measurement of oxygen saturations in vena cava, right-sided heart chambers, and pulmonary artery may identify previously unsuspected left-to-right shunting.
- This is the gold standard technique for defining pulmonary vascular anatomy, but CT and MRI are increasingly utilized as noninvasive alternatives.
- Most useful role is in chronic thromboembolic pulmonary hypertension and helping determine disease location and surgical accessibility in equivocal cases.

CLINICAL PRESENTATION
- Disease presents insidiously as nonspecific clinical findings.
- Exertional breathlessness, representing right-sided cardiac insufficiency, occurs in the presence of increased workload.
- As disease progresses, exercise tolerance steadily deteriorates and exertional syncope or chest pain may develop.

DIFFERENTIAL DIAGNOSIS
- Idiopathic dilatation of the pulmonary artery
- Pulmonary artery stenosis
- Pulmonary artery aneurysm
- Hilar lymphadenopathy

PATHOLOGY
- Intimal fibrosis of elastic and large muscular arteries and thickening of media of small muscular arteries; vessel diameter between 1 mm and 100 μm have walls replaced by smooth muscle.
- Cellular intimal proliferation and fibrosis, plexiform lesions, fibrinoid "necrosis," and vasculitis.
- Plexiform lesions: localized focus of vascular dilation associated with intraluminal plexus of slit-like vascular channels.
- Findings of pulmonary hypertension due to chronic thromboembolism: thrombi in various stages of organization in large/small pulmonary arteries.
- Veno-occlusive disease: stenosis or obliteration of lumens of small pulmonary veins and venules by intimal fibrous tissue.
- Pulmonary capillary hemangiomatosis: venular infiltration often accompanied by intimal fibrosis, which may lead to stenosis.

INCIDENCE/PREVALENCE AND EPIDEMIOLOGY
- The true prevalence of chronic thromboembolic pulmonary hypertension is unknown. It may complicate up to 3.8% of cases of acute pulmonary embolism.
- The incidence of idiopathic pulmonary hypertension is estimated at 1 to 2 cases per million population per year.
- The main pulmonary parenchymal causes of pulmonary hypertension are chronic obstructive pulmonary disease (COPD) and idiopathic pulmonary fibrosis.
- Pulmonary hypertension in collagen vascular disease may occur without or with parenchymal disease.

Suggested Readings

Coulden R: State-of-the-art imaging techniques in chronic thromboembolic pulmonary hypertension. *Proc Am Thorac Soc* 3(7): 577-583, 2006.

Landzberg MJ: Congenital heart disease associated pulmonary arterial hypertension. *Clin Chest Med* 28(1):243-253, 2007:x.

McGoon M, Gutterman D, Steen V, et al: Screening, early detection, and diagnosis of pulmonary arterial hypertension: ACCP evidence-based clinical practice guidelines. *Chest* 126(1 Suppl):14S-34S, 2004.

Nikolaou K, Schoenberg SO, Attenberger U, et al: Pulmonary arterial hypertension: Diagnosis with fast perfusion MR imaging and high-spatial-resolution MR angiography—preliminary experience. *Radiology* 236(2):694-703, 2005.

Sherrick AD, Swensen SJ, Hartman TE: Mosaic pattern of lung attenuation on CT scans: Frequency among patients with pulmonary artery hypertension of different causes. *AJR Am J Roentgenol* 169(1):79-82, 1997.

Simonneau G, Galie N, Rubin LJ, et al: Clinical classification of pulmonary hypertension. *J Am Coll Cardiol* 43(12 Suppl S): 5S-12S, 2004.

Trow TK, McArdle JR: Diagnosis of pulmonary arterial hypertension. *Clin Chest Med* 28(1):59-73, 2007:viii.

Chronic Thromboembolic Pulmonary Hypertension

DEFINITION: Thrombi from untreated or recurrent acute emboli organize and become incorporated into the walls of the pulmonary arteries.

IMAGING

Radiography

Findings

- Central pulmonary arteries are enlarged with peripheral pruning.
- Peripheral pulmonary vessels are disorganized with regional areas of hypoperfusion and hyperperfusion.
- Pleural thickening or effusions and peripheral scarring from previous infarction and atelectasis may be present.
- Enlargement of right ventricle is seen as reduction of retrosternal airspace on lateral radiograph.
- Right atrial dilatation is seen as widening of right-sided heart border on the frontal projection.

Utility

- Initial imaging study in patients with suspected pulmonary hypertension.
- Useful to assess heart size, cardiac chamber dilatation, proximal pulmonary artery enlargement, and underlying pulmonary parenchymal disorder.
- Transverse diameter of right interlobar artery measured from its lateral aspect to intermediate bronchus: normally <15 mm in women and <16 mm in men.
- Limited value in diagnosis of chronic pulmonary thromboembolism.

CT

Findings

- Enlarged main pulmonary artery (>30 mm), right ventricular dilatation (>45 mm transverse diameter).
- Eccentric flattened mural thrombi, which may be occlusive or have areas of recanalization.
- Segmental vessels absent or abruptly narrowed with distal pruning.
- Obstruction of vessels at point of origin, with fibrous pulmonary artery bands/webs that may traverse vascular lumen, resulting in stenosis.
- Mosaic attenuation and perfusion pattern.
- Areas of bronchial dilatation in segmental and subsegmental bronchi in poorly perfused lung regions.

DIAGNOSTIC PEARLS

- Usually bilateral central pulmonary artery obstruction
- Eccentric flattened mural thrombi, which may be occlusive or have areas of recanalization
- Segmental vessels completely absent or abruptly narrowed with distal pruning
- Pulmonary artery bands and webs, which may traverse the vascular lumen and result in stenosis
- Bronchial and nonbronchial systemic artery dilatation
- Mosaic attenuation and perfusion pattern

- Enlargement of bronchial (>1.5 mm) and nonbronchial systemic collateral arteries with resultant systemic to pulmonary venous shunting.

Utility

- Cross-sectional modality of choice for direct visualization of central and segmental vessel thromboembolism.
- More specific than scintigraphy.

MRI

Findings

- Enlarged main pulmonary artery (>30 mm), right ventricular dilatation (>45 mm transverse diameter).
- Paradoxical motion of interventricular septum.
- Eccentric flattened mural thrombi that may be occlusive or have areas of recanalization.
- Abrupt vessel cut-offs, intraluminal webs and bands, and abnormal proximal-to-distal tapering of the vessels.

Utility

- Low spatial resolution particularly for small pulmonary vessels and limited availability.
- Used mainly in patients with history of allergic reaction to iodinated contrast medium.

Nuclear Medicine

Findings

- One or more mismatched, segmental, or larger defects.

WHAT THE REFERRING PHYSICIAN NEEDS TO KNOW

- Ventilation-perfusion scintigraphy is a valuable screening test for chronic thromboembolic pulmonary hypertension.
- CT angiography is the imaging modality of choice for the diagnosis.
- Pulmonary endarterectomy has curative potential.
- Imaging plays a central role in patient selection, centering on identification of patients with predominantly proximal and surgically accessible disease.

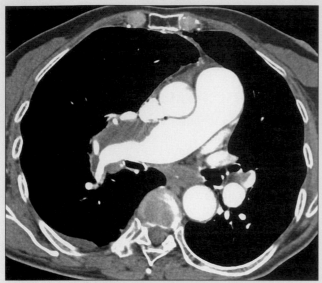

Figure 1. Contrast-enhanced CT image shows enlargement of the proximal pulmonary arteries with eccentric mural thickening involving the right pulmonary artery characteristic of chronic thromboembolic disease. (*Courtesy of Drs. Nicholas J. Screaton and Deepa Gopalan, Cambridge, UK*)

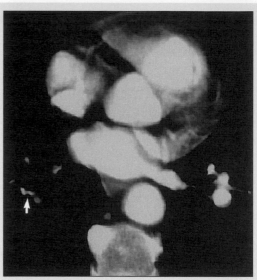

Figure 2. Chronic thromboembolism. Contrast-enhanced spiral CT scan image in a 71-year-old woman who had chronic pulmonary thromboembolism shows marked narrowing of the right lower lobe pulmonary arteries (*arrow*). Note normal tapering of the left lower lobe vessels. (*From Müller NL, Fraser RS, Colman NC, Paré PD: Radiologic Diagnosis of Diseases of the Chest. Philadelphia, WB Saunders, 2001.*)

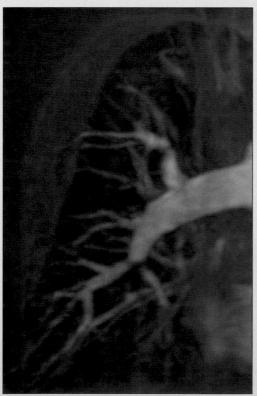

Figure 3. Chronic thromboembolic pulmonary hypertension. Contrast-enhanced MR pulmonary angiogram demonstrates multiple webs and segmental occlusions in the right upper and lower lobes in a patient with proximal chronic thromboembolic pulmonary hypertension. (*Courtesy of Drs. Nicholas J. Screaton and Deepa Gopalan, Cambridge, UK*)

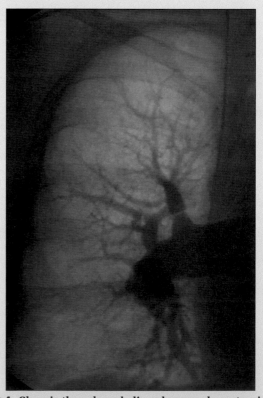

Figure 4. Chronic thromboembolic pulmonary hypertension. Pulmonary angiogram on a patient with proximal chronic thromboembolic pulmonary hypertension shows a proximal web in the right upper lobe artery with multiple segmental occlusions in the middle and lower lobes. (*Courtesy of Drs. Nicholas J. Screaton and Deepa Gopalan, Cambridge, UK*)

Utility

- High sensitivity but low specificity.
- Partial recanalization of organized thrombi may result in underestimate from perfusion scintigraphy of the magnitude of vascular compromise.

Pulmonary Angiography

Findings

- Characteristic findings on angiography include pouch-like filling defects, webs or bands, intimal irregularities, abrupt vascular narrowing, and complete vascular obstruction.
- Pouch defect is a partially or completely occlusive chronic thrombus that organizes in concave configuration toward the lumen.
- Pulmonary arterial webs or bands are seen as lines of decreased opacity that traverse the width of pulmonary artery, usually at the lobar or segmental level.

Utility

- Angiography is reference standard to confirm diagnosis, define extent of disease, and evaluate need for surgical endarterectomy.
- Improvement in noninvasive imaging is reducing its utilization.

CLINICAL PRESENTATION

- Exertional breathlessness
- Fatigue
- Chest pain

DIFFERENTIAL DIAGNOSIS

- Acute pulmonary embolism
- Pulmonary artery stenosis
- Fibrosing mediastinitis
- Mediastinal lymphadenopathy
- Idiopathic pulmonary hypertension
- Pulmonary hypertension in connective tissue disease

PATHOLOGY

- Thrombi from untreated or recurrent acute emboli organize and become incorporated into wall of pulmonary arteries.
- Thrombi in smaller vessels often recanalize, forming a trabecular mesh.
- Repeated cycles of thromboemboli organization leave endothelialized residua that obstruct or narrow pulmonary arteries, resulting in progressive pulmonary hypertension.

INCIDENCE/PREVALENCE AND EPIDEMIOLOGY

- True prevalence of chronic thromboembolic pulmonary hypertension is unknown because many cases may remain undiagnosed.
- It may complicate up to 3.8% of cases of acute pulmonary embolism.
- History of previous acute embolism is usual but not universal.

Suggested Readings

Bergin CJ, Sirlin CB, Hauschildt JP, et al: Chronic thromboembolism: Diagnosis with helical CT and MR imaging with angiographic and surgical correlation. *Radiology* 204(3):695-702, 1997.

Kreitner KF, Ley S, Kauczor HU, et al: Chronic thromboembolic pulmonary hypertension: Pre and postoperative assessment with breath-hold MR imaging techniques. *Radiology* 232:535-543, 2004.

McGoon M, Gutterman D, Steen V, et al: Screening, early detection, and diagnosis of pulmonary arterial hypertension: ACCP evidence-based clinical practice guidelines. *Chest* 126(1 Suppl):14S-34S, 2004.

Oikonomou A, Dennie CJ, Müller NL, et al: Chronic thromboembolic pulmonary arterial hypertension: Correlation of postoperative results of thromboendarterectomy with preoperative helical contrast-enhanced computed tomography. *J Thorac Imaging* 19(2):67-73, 2004.

Simonneau G, Galie N, Rubin LJ, et al: Clinical classification of pulmonary hypertension. *J Am Coll Cardiol* 43(12 Suppl S):5S-12S, 2004.

Idiopathic Pulmonary Hypertension

DEFINITION: Precapillary pulmonary hypertension without an identifiable cause is considered idiopathic.

IMAGING

Radiography

Findings

- Enlarged proximal pulmonary arteries with peripheral pruning, cardiomegaly with right-sided chamber enlargement, and pulmonary oligemia.
- Right interlobar artery diameter (lateral aspect to intermediate bronchus), posteroanterior view: >15 mm in women and >16 mm in men.
- Normal lungs.
- Left interlobar artery (left upper lobe bronchus circular lucency to posterior margin of vessel), lateral view: >18 mm.
- Reduction of retrosternal airspace on lateral radiograph from right ventricular enlargement.
- Right atrial dilatation: widening of right-sided heart border on frontal projection.

Utility

- Initial imaging study in patients with suspected pulmonary hypertension.
- Useful to assess heart size, pattern of cardiac chamber dilatation, and proximal pulmonary artery enlargement and to detect any underlying pulmonary parenchymal disorder.
- No correlation between extent of radiographic abnormalities and degree of pulmonary hypertension.
- Accuracy of chest radiograph in detecting pulmonary hypertension unknown.
- Abnormal radiograph at time of diagnosis in approximately 90% of patients.

CT

Findings

- Main pulmonary arteries 30 mm or larger, exceeding thoracic aorta diameter.
- Segmental artery-to-bronchus ratio >1; abruptly tapering tortuous peripheral pulmonary vessels (pruning).
- Cardiac enlargement (right atrium >35 mm, right ventricle >45 mm); may have tricuspid regurgitation.
- Severe disease: pericardial effusion.

DIAGNOSTIC PEARLS

- Main pulmonary arteries are dilated and abruptly tapering with tortuous peripheral pulmonary vessels.
- Right-sided cardiac chamber enlargement may or may not be associated with tricuspid regurgitation.
- Lungs are normal but may have mosaic pattern of lung attenuation.
- Perfusion scintiscan is either normal or shows patchy subsegmental areas of reduced perfusion or "mottling."

- Normal lungs; severe disease may show small, poorly defined, centrilobular nodules due to cholesterol granulomas or capillary congestion.
- Regional variations in parenchymal perfusion: mosaic attenuation/perfusion pattern.

Utility

- CT pulmonary angiography/high-resolution CT provides comprehensive assessment of pulmonary vasculature/parenchyma, cardiac chamber dilatation, tricuspid regurgitation, limited right-sided heart function evaluation.
- Main pulmonary artery diameter of 30 mm or larger has 69%-87% sensitivity, 89%-100% specificity for diagnosis of pulmonary artery hypertension.
- Pulmonary artery/aorta diameter ratio has 92% specificity, 93% positive predictive value, 44% negative predictive value, and 70% sensitivity for diagnosis of pulmonary artery hypertension.

MRI

Findings

- Right ventricular hypertrophy and dilatation
- Symmetrically enlarged central pulmonary arteries
- Diffuse pattern of abruptly tapering and pruned subsegmental vessels
- Reversal of septal curvature

WHAT THE REFERRING PHYSICIAN NEEDS TO KNOW

- Familial pulmonary arterial hypertension is clinically and radiologically indistinguishable from idiopathic pulmonary arterial hypertension.
- Plexiform lesion is not pathognomonic for idiopathic pulmonary arterial hypertension and can be seen in pulmonary hypertension secondary to shunts and chronic thromboembolic pulmonary hypertension.
- Distinguishing the idiopathic type from chronic thromboembolic pulmonary hypertension is critical because treatment options differ, being medical for the former and surgical for the latter.
- Lungs are normal in idiopathic pulmonary hypertension, enabling differentiation from pulmonary hypertension secondary to parenchymal lung disease.

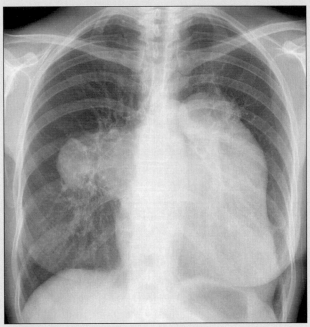

Figure 1. Idiopathic pulmonary arterial hypertension.
Posteroanterior chest radiograph demonstrates gross enlargement of the proximal pulmonary arteries with tapering of the peripheral vasculature (peripheral pruning) and cardiomegaly due to dilated right-sided heart chambers. (*Courtesy of Drs. Nicholas J. Screaton and Deepa Gopalan, Cambridge, UK*)

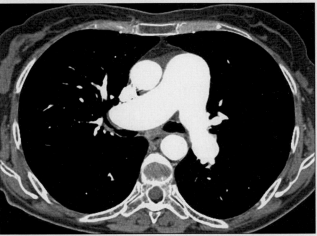

Figure 2. Idiopathic pulmonary arterial hypertension.
Contrast-enhanced CT image at the level of the right main pulmonary artery demonstrates dilatation of the main pulmonary artery, which is larger than the adjacent ascending aorta. (*Courtesy of Drs. Nicholas J. Screaton and Deepa Gopalan, Cambridge, UK*)

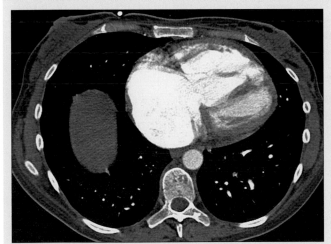

Figure 3. Idiopathic pulmonary arterial hypertension. CT image at the level of tricuspid valve shows enlargement of the right atrium and ventricle with bowing of the interventricular septum. (*Courtesy of Drs. Nicholas J. Screaton and Deepa Gopalan, Cambridge, UK*)

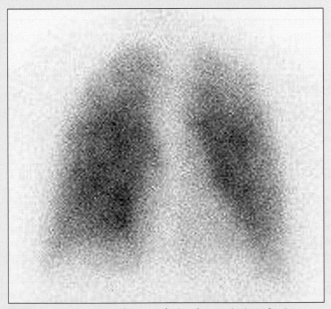

Figure 4. Anterior view from perfusion lung scintigraphy in a patient with idiopathic pulmonary arterial hypertension shows heterogeneous, mottled perfusion pattern. (*Courtesy of Drs. Nicholas J. Screaton and Deepa Gopalan, Cambridge, UK*)

- Abnormal intravascular signal corresponding to slow pulmonary arterial blood flow

Utility

- MRI enables noninvasive morphologic and functional assessment.

Pulmonary Angiography

Findings

- Symmetrically enlarged central pulmonary arteries on angiogram.
- Diffuse pattern of abruptly tapering and pruned subsegmental vessels.
- Filamentous or "corkscrew" peripheral arteries.

Utility

- Evaluation is possible of pulmonary hemodynamics, cardiac function, and assessment of dynamic response to pharmacologic stimuli.

Nuclear Medicine

Findings

- Normal.
- Patchy subsegmental areas of reduced perfusion or "mottling."
- Reversed mismatching in advanced cases: pulmonary perfusion of areas of lung showing little or no ventilation.

Utility

- Perfusion scintigraphy is key screening test in differentiating between idiopathic pulmonary arterial hypertension and chronic thromboembolic pulmonary hypertension.
- There is a potential fallibility of the perfusion lung scintiscan in making the differential diagnosis.

CLINICAL PRESENTATION

- Exertional breathlessness
- Chest pain
- Fatigue

DIFFERENTIAL DIAGNOSIS

- Chronic thromboembolic pulmonary hypertension
- Asthma
- Pulmonary hypertension in connective tissue disease
- Pulmonary hypertension in left-to-right shunts
- Pulmonary hypertension in parenchymal lung disease

PATHOLOGY

- Pathologic changes are largely confined to small (< 1 mm) muscular precapillary pulmonary arteries.
- Medial smooth muscle hypertrophy, intimal proliferation, and adventitial thickening are present in small pulmonary arteries.

- Plexiform lesion consists of localized focus of vascular dilation associated with an intraluminal plexus of slit-like vascular channels.
- Plexiform lesion tends to occur in arteries < 100 μm either at branching points or at origins of supernumerary arteries.
- Dilatation lesions and necrotizing arteritis with segmental destruction of arterial walls are seen.
- Cause is unknown.
- Acute and organizing thrombi due to intimal injury induced by long-standing pulmonary hypertension lead to development of in-situ thrombosis.

INCIDENCE/PREVALENCE AND EPIDEMIOLOGY

- Incidence is estimated at 1 to 2 cases per 1 million inhabitants per year.
- Mean age at onset is 36 years, with a 1.7:1 female-to-male preponderance and no racial predilection.
- About one tenth of patients are older than 60 years of age.
- Idiopathic cases outnumber familial cases of pulmonary hypertension by more than 10:1.
- National Institutes of Health data show median survival of 2.8 years and 1-year, 3-year, and 5-year survival rates of 68%, 48%, and 34%, respectively.
- Moderate pericardial thickening > 2 mm or effusion was seen in 53% of patients with severe pulmonary hypertension.
- Development of in-situ thrombosis is noted in over 50% of cases.

Suggested Readings

Bergin CJ, Hauschildt J, Rios G, et al: Accuracy of MR angiography compared with radionuclide scanning in identifying the cause of pulmonary arterial hypertension. *AJR Am J Roentgenol* 168(6):1549-1555, 1997.

Hansell DM: Small-vessel diseases of the lung: CT-pathologic correlates. *Radiology* 225(3):639-653, 2002.

McGoon M, Gutterman D, Steen V, et al: Screening, early detection, and diagnosis of pulmonary arterial hypertension: ACCP evidence-based clinical practice guidelines. *Chest* 126(1 Suppl):14S-34S, 2004.

Pietra GG, Capron F, Stewart S, et al: Pathologic assessment of vasculopathies in pulmonary hypertension. *J Am Coll Cardiol* 43(12 Suppl S):25S-32S, 2004.

Simonneau G, Galie N, Rubin LJ, et al: Clinical classification of pulmonary hypertension. *J Am Coll Cardiol* 43(12 Suppl S):5S-12S, 2004.

Pulmonary Hypertension in Left-to-Right Shunts

DEFINITION: Pulmonary hypertension can develop from a sustained congenital left-to-right shunt.

IMAGING

Radiography

Findings
- Enlarged central pulmonary arteries, rapidly tapering but prominent and tortuous peripheral vessels, vessels identifiable within 2 cm of pleural surface.
- Peripheral oligemia with rapid tapering of peripheral vessels and disparity between proximal and distal calibers (late manifestation).
- Atrial septal defects: characterized by cardiomegaly with enlargement of the right atrium and ventricle.
- Ventricular septal defects: characterized by right ventricular hypertrophy and dilatation of left ventricle and right atrium.
- Patent ductus arteriosus: enlargement of left atrium and rib notching, ascending aorta and arch, calcification of ductus diverticulum.

Utility
- Initial imaging study in patients with suspected pulmonary hypertension.
- Useful to assess heart size, pattern of cardiac chamber dilatation, and proximal pulmonary artery enlargement and to detect any underlying pulmonary parenchymal disorder.

CT

Findings
- Main pulmonary artery diameter 30 mm or larger, exceeding thoracic aorta diameter.
- Segmental artery-to-bronchus ratio >1; abruptly tapering tortuous peripheral pulmonary vessels (pruning).
- Linear calcification in the central pulmonary arteries.
- In-situ nonocclusive thrombus possible in central pulmonary arteries.
- Atrial septal defect: enlargement of the right atrium and ventricle; often evident on electrocardiographic gated contrast-enhanced CT angiography.
- Ventricular septal defect: right ventricular hypertrophy and dilatation of left ventricle and right atrium; often evident on electrocardiographic gated contrast-enhanced CT angiography.

DIAGNOSTIC PEARLS

- Atrioseptal defects are characterized by cardiomegaly with enlargement of the right atrium and ventricle.
- Ventriculoseptal defects are characterized by right ventricular hypertrophy and dilatation of the left ventricle and right atrium.
- Echocardiography and MRI are the imaging modalities of choice for detection of left-to-right shunts.
- Left-to-right shunts are increasingly found incidentally in patients undergoing contrast-enhanced CT for routine workup pulmonary hypertension.

- Patent ductus arteriosus: enlargement of left atrium and ascending aorta and arch; patent ductus evident on electrocardiographic gated contrast-enhanced CT angiography.

Utility
- Not the primary imaging modality in patients with known cardiac shunts.
- Frontline investigation in patients with suspected pulmonary hypertension.
- Limited use in functional evaluation of shunts.

MRI

Findings
- Main pulmonary artery diameter 30 mm or larger, or exceeding thoracic aorta diameter.
- Segmental artery-to-bronchus ratio >1; abruptly tapering tortuous peripheral pulmonary vessels (pruning).
- Shunt defects evident on electrocardiographic gated MR angiography.
- Atrial septal defect: enlargement of the right atrium and ventricle.
- Ventricular septal defect: right ventricular hypertrophy and dilatation of the left ventricle and right atrium.

WHAT THE REFERRING PHYSICIAN NEEDS TO KNOW

- Echocardiography permits estimation of pulmonary artery pressure and is useful as a screening tool and in follow-up.
- Echocardiography and MRI are the imaging modalities of choice for detection of cardiac abnormalities (e.g., shunts or raised left atrial pressure).
- Even after apparently effective corrective surgery patients may go on to develop significant pulmonary hypertension.

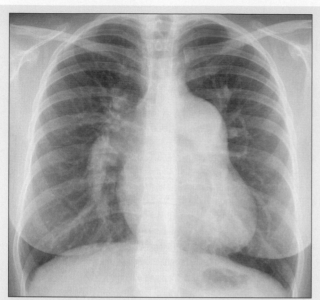

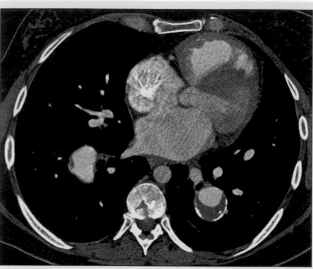

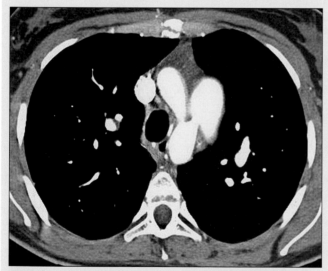

Figure 1. **Pulmonary hypertension due to left-to-right shunt.** Chest radiograph shows cardiomegaly and enlarged central pulmonary arteries in a patient with pulmonary hypertension secondary to an atrial septal defect. (*Courtesy of Drs. Nicholas J. Screaton and Deepa Gopalan, Cambridge, UK*)

Figure 2. **Pulmonary hypertension due to congenital shunt detected on routine workup for pulmonary hypertension.** CT angiogram depicts a large atrial septal defect with in-situ thrombus in the left lower lobe pulmonary artery. Peripheral calcification is seen around the thrombus. (*Courtesy of Drs. Nicholas J. Screaton and Deepa Gopalan, Cambridge, UK*)

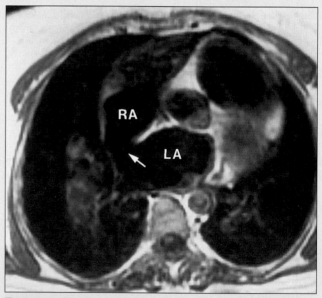

Figure 3. **Pulmonary hypertension due to congenital shunt detected on routine workup for pulmonary hypertension.** CT angiogram shows a communication between the left pulmonary artery and the aortic isthmus characteristic of a patent ductus arteriosus. (*Courtesy of Drs. Nicholas J. Screaton and Deepa Gopalan, Cambridge, UK*)

Figure 4. **Pulmonary arterial hypertension caused by atrial septal defect.** MR image at the level of the right (RA) and left (LA) atrium shows an atrial septal defect (*arrow*). The patient was a 61-year-old woman. (*From Müller NL, Fraser RS, Colman NC, Paré PD: Radiologic Diagnosis of Diseases of the Chest. Philadelphia, WB Saunders, 2001.*)

Utility

- Valuable tool for depicting cardiac anatomy, enabling not only the detection and localization of shunts but also their quantification.
- Useful for cardiac shunt evaluation in supracristal ventricular septal defect, atrioventricular septal defect, and partial anomalous pulmonary venous drainage.
- Shunt severity expressed quantitatively as the ratio of pulmonary flow to systemic flow.

Ultrasonography

Findings

- Echocardiography demonstrates presence of shunt and pulmonary arterial hypertension.

Utility

- Echocardiography and MRI are the imaging modalities of choice for detection of intracardiac shunts.

Nuclear Medicine

Findings

- Activity in kidney consistent with shunt

Utility

- In presence of right-to-left shunt, activity in thyroid or kidneys can be seen and used to calculate shunt fraction.

CLINICAL PRESENTATION

- Exertional breathlessness
- Chest pain
- Fatigue

DIFFERENTIAL DIAGNOSIS

- Idiopathic pulmonary hypertension
- Pulmonary hypertension in parenchymal lung disease
- Pulmonary hypertension in connective tissue disease
- Chronic thromboembolic pulmonary hypertension

PATHOLOGY

- Presence of shunt exposes pulmonary circulation to high flow, preventing it from adapting normally to extrauterine life.
- Ongoing high flow over extended periods results in progressive pulmonary vasculopathy with associated in-situ thrombosis.
- Rising pulmonary arterial pressures lead to bidirectional then reversed flow across shunt (Eisenmenger syndrome).
- Histologic features include plexiform lesions, aneurysmal muscular arteries, necrotizing arteritis, in-situ thrombi, medial hypertrophy with intimal proliferation, and laminar fibrosis.
- There is progressive vessel obliteration and irreversible smooth muscle proliferation of pulmonary arterioles.
- Position, size of cardiac defect, and magnitude of shunt govern time taken for pathologic changes to occur.

INCIDENCE/PREVALENCE AND EPIDEMIOLOGY

- Most common cause of left-to-right shunt in adults is atrial septal defect.

Suggested Readings

McGoon M, Gutterman D, Steen V, et al: Screening, early detection, and diagnosis of pulmonary arterial hypertension: ACCP evidence-based clinical practice guidelines. *Chest* 126(1 Suppl):14S-34S, 2004.

Rubin LJ: Pulmonary arterial hypertension. *Proc Am Thorac Soc* 3:111-115, 2006.

Simonneau G, Galie N, Rubin LJ, et al: Clinical classification of pulmonary hypertension. *J Am Coll Cardiol* 43(12 Suppl S):5S-12S, 2004.

Steiner RM, Reddy GP, Flicker S: Congenital cardiovascular disease in the adult patient: Imaging update. *J Thorac Imaging* 17:1-17, 2002.

Pulmonary Hypertension in Connective Tissue Disease

DEFINITION: Pulmonary hypertension occurs in a wide variety of collagen vascular diseases.

IMAGING

Radiography

Findings

- Enlarged proximal pulmonary arteries with peripheral pruning, cardiomegaly with right-sided chamber enlargement, and pulmonary oligemia
- Right interlobar artery diameter (lateral aspect to intermediate bronchus), posteroanterior view: >15 mm in women and >16 mm in men
- Left interlobar artery (left upper lobe bronchus circular lucency to posterior margin of vessel), lateral view: >18 mm
- Right ventricular enlargement resulting in reduction of retrosternal airspace on lateral radiograph
- Right atrial dilatation: widening of right-sided heart border on frontal projection
- May be sole manifestation of connective tissue disease or may occur in association with interstitial fibrosis

Utility

- Initial imaging study in patients with suspected pulmonary hypertension
- Useful to assess heart size, pattern of cardiac chamber dilatation, and proximal pulmonary artery enlargement and to detect any underlying pulmonary parenchymal disorder

CT

Findings

- Main pulmonary artery diameter of 30 mm or larger; greater than diameter of thoracic aorta at same level
- Segmental artery-to-bronchus ratio >1; abruptly tapering tortuous peripheral pulmonary vessels (pruning)
- May be sole manifestation of connective tissue disease or may occur in association with interstitial fibrosis
- Cardiac enlargement (right atrium >35 mm, right ventricle >45 mm); may have tricuspid regurgitation
- Severe disease: moderate pericardial thickening >2 mm or effusion

Utility

- CT pulmonary angiography/high-resolution CT: comprehensive assessment of pulmonary vasculature/

DIAGNOSTIC PEARLS

- Main pulmonary arteries are dilated and abruptly tapering with tortuous peripheral pulmonary vessels.
- Right-sided cardiac chamber enlargement may or may not be associated with tricuspid regurgitation.
- Interstitial fibrosis may be present.

parenchyma, cardiac chamber dilatation, tricuspid regurgitation, limited right-sided heart function evaluation.
- Main pulmonary artery diameter: measured at bifurcation level at right angle to long axis and just lateral to ascending aorta.
- Main pulmonary artery diameter of 30 mm or larger: 69%-87% sensitivity, 89%-100% specificity.
- Pulmonary artery/aorta diameter ratio: 92% specificity, 93% positive predictive value, 44% negative predictive value, and 70% sensitivity.

MRI

Findings

- Right ventricular hypertrophy and dilatation; reversal of septal curvature
- Symmetrically enlarged central pulmonary arteries
- Diffuse pattern of abruptly tapering and pruned subsegmental vessels
- Filamentous or "corkscrew" peripheral arteries
- Abnormal intravascular signal corresponding to slow pulmonary arterial blood flow

Utility

- Technique of choice when long-term follow-up is required.
- Permits monitoring of cardiac function in response to therapy without use of ionizing radiation.

Nuclear Medicine

Findings

- May be normal
- Patchy subsegmental areas of reduced perfusion or "mottling"

WHAT THE REFERRING PHYSICIAN NEEDS TO KNOW

- Pulmonary hypertension occurs in a wide variety of collagen vascular diseases and confers a worse prognosis.
- It may be the sole manifestation of connective tissue disease, or it may occur in association with interstitial fibrosis.
- Incidence varies among the diseases, being highest in scleroderma and occurring less frequently in systemic lupus erythematosus, rheumatoid arthritis, and polymyositis.
- Systemic lupus erythematosus can be complicated by a hypercoagulable state; therefore, chronic thromboembolic pulmonary hypertension should always be considered an alternative cause of pulmonary hypertension.

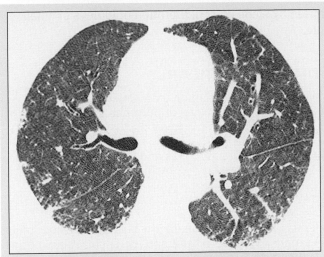

Figure 1. Pulmonary hypertension in systemic sclerosis and CREST syndrome. CT image at the level of the main bronchi shows mild peripheral reticulation in keeping with interstitial fibrosis in addition to subtle heterogeneity of lung attenuation consistent with a pulmonary vasculopathy. (*Courtesy of Drs. Nicholas J. Screaton and Deepa Gopalan, Cambridge, UK*)

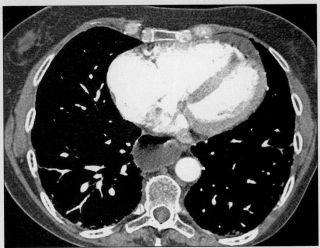

Figure 2. Pulmonary hypertension in systemic sclerosis and CREST syndrome. CT image at the level of tricuspid valve shows right-sided cardiac chamber enlargement, a small pericardial effusion, and a dilated fluid-filled esophagus in keeping with esophageal dysmotility. (*Courtesy of Drs. Nicholas J. Screaton and Deepa Gopalan, Cambridge, UK*)

- Reversed mismatching in advanced cases: pulmonary perfusion of areas of lung showing little or no ventilation

Utility
- Perfusion lung scan has potential fallibility in the differential diagnosis.

CLINICAL PRESENTATION

- Exertional breathlessness
- Fatigue
- Chest pain

DIFFERENTIAL DIAGNOSIS

- Chronic thromboembolic pulmonary hypertension
- Asthma
- Idiopathic pulmonary hypertension
- Pulmonary hypertension in parenchymal lung disease
- Pulmonary hypertension in left-to-right shunts

PATHOLOGY

- Pathologic changes are largely confined to small (<1 mm), muscular, precapillary pulmonary arteries.
- Medial smooth muscle hypertrophy, intimal proliferation, and adventitial thickening occur in the small pulmonary arteries.
- Pulmonary hypertension may be sole manifestation of connective tissue disease, or it may occur in association with interstitial fibrosis.

INCIDENCE/PREVALENCE AND EPIDEMIOLOGY

- Pulmonary hypertension occurs in a wide variety of collagen vascular diseases and confers a worse prognosis.
- Incidence varies among the diseases but is as high as 12% in patients with a limited form of scleroderma.
- It occurs less frequently in systemic lupus erythematosus, rheumatoid arthritis, and polymyositis.
- Pulmonary hypertension is the cause of up to 50% of disease-related deaths in patients with limited scleroderma.
- Isolated pulmonary hypertension is less common in diffuse scleroderma.
- Pulmonary hypertension is a common cause of death in patients with mixed connective tissue disease.

Suggested Readings

Hoeper MM: Pulmonary hypertension in collagen vascular disease. *Eur Respir J* 19:571-576, 2002.

McGoon M, Gutterman D, Steen V, et al: Screening, early detection, and diagnosis of pulmonary arterial hypertension: ACCP evidence-based clinical practice guidelines. *Chest* 126(1 Suppl):14S-34S, 2004.

Rubin LJ: Pulmonary arterial hypertension. *Proc Am Thorac Soc* 3:111-115, 2006.

Trad S, Amoura Z, Beigelman C, et al: Pulmonary arterial hypertension is a major mortality factor in diffuse systemic sclerosis, independent of interstitial lung disease. *Arthritis Rheum* 54(1):184-191, 2006.

Trow TK, McArdle JR: Diagnosis of pulmonary arterial hypertension. *Clin Chest Med* 28(1):59-73, 2007:viii.

Pulmonary Veno-Occlusive Disease

DEFINITION: Pulmonary hypertension that is caused by stenosis or obliteration of lumens of small pulmonary veins and venules by intimal fibrous tissue.

IMAGING

Radiography
Findings
- Enlarged proximal pulmonary arteries with peripheral pruning, cardiomegaly with right-sided chamber enlargement, and pulmonary oligemia.
- Right interlobar artery diameter (lateral aspect to intermediate bronchus), posteroanterior view: >15 mm in women and >16 mm in men.
- Right ventricular enlargement resulting in reduction of retrosternal airspace on lateral radiograph.
- Septal lines.

Utility
- Initial imaging study in patients with suspected pulmonary hypertension
- Useful to assess heart size, cardiac chamber dilatation pattern, and proximal pulmonary arteries enlargement and to detect any underlying pulmonary parenchymal disorder

CT
Findings
- Main pulmonary artery diameter 30 mm or larger, exceeding thoracic aorta diameter.
- Cardiac enlargement (right atrium >35 mm, right ventricle >45 mm); may have tricuspid regurgitation.
- Smooth interlobular septal thickening in pulmonary veno-occlusive disease; may have poorly defined centrilobular nodules.
- Central and gravity-dependent ground-glass opacity.

Utility
- CT pulmonary angiography/high-resolution CT: allows comprehensive assessment of pulmonary vasculature and lung parenchyma.

CLINICAL PRESENTATION

- Insidious onset of dyspnea
- Intermittent hemoptysis with reduced gas transfer and desaturation on exercise
- Symptoms usually progressive, ultimately resulting in death

DIAGNOSTIC PEARLS

- Triad of severe pulmonary arterial hypertension, radiographic evidence of pulmonary edema, and a normal pulmonary artery occlusion pressure is seen.
- Central pulmonary veins and the left atrium are not enlarged.

- Triad of severe pulmonary arterial hypertension, radiographic evidence of pulmonary edema, and normal pulmonary artery occlusion pressure

DIFFERENTIAL DIAGNOSIS

- Idiopathic pulmonary hypertension
- Chronic thromboembolic pulmonary hypertension
- Pulmonary hypertension in connective tissue disease
- Pulmonary hypertension in left-to-right shunts
- Chronic left heart failure

PATHOLOGY

- Unique histologic hallmarks of pulmonary veno-occlusive disease are webs, recanalized thrombosis (essential pathogenetic factor), and intimal fibrosis within pulmonary veins.
- Distribution of venous damage is characteristically localized and patchy.
- Pulmonary veins become occluded by fibrous tissue, ranging from loose edematous tissue to dense sclerotic tissue.
- Hydrostatic pressure rise causes focal areas of edema and hemorrhage as a result of capillary and lymphatic congestion.
- Cytotoxic drugs including bleomycin, herbal "bush" tea, bone marrow transplantation, and thoracic radiotherapy have all been implicated as causative.
- Majority of cases are currently considered idiopathic.

WHAT THE REFERRING PHYSICIAN NEEDS TO KNOW

- Symptoms are usually progressive, ultimately resulting in death within 3 years of diagnosis.
- Management is complicated by potential for poor outcome with targeted therapy.
- Some patients may respond to trial of targeted therapy, instituted cautiously and with close monitoring; if unsuccessful, transplantation may be needed.
- Diagnostic triad includes severe pulmonary arterial hypertension, pulmonary edema, and normal pulmonary artery occlusion pressure and can obviate need for tissue diagnosis.
- Indiscriminate vasodilator therapy can lead to fatal acute pulmonary edema.

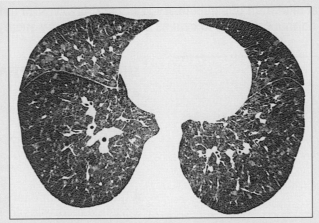

Figure 1. Pulmonary veno-occlusive disease. High-resolution CT image in patient with pulmonary hypertension secondary to pulmonary veno-occlusive disease shows widespread ground-glass opacities with centrilobular nodules and smooth interlobular septal thickening. (*Courtesy of Dr. Nicholas J. Screaton, Cambridge, UK*)

INCIDENCE/PREVALENCE AND EPIDEMIOLOGY

- Pulmonary veno-occlusive disease is rare, occurring 10 times less often than idiopathic pulmonary hypertension.
- Fewer than 200 cases of pulmonary veno-occlusive disease and pulmonary capillary hemangiomatosis have been reported in the literature.
- One third of cases occur in children, with equal sex distribution.
- There is a slight (2:1) male predominance in adult patients.
- The disease is usually fatal within 3 years of diagnosis.

Suggested Readings

Frazier AA, Franks TJ, Mohammed TL, et al: From the Archives of the AFIP: Pulmonary veno-occlusive disease and pulmonary capillary hemangiomatosis. *RadioGraphics* 27(3):867-882, 2007.

Holcomb BW Jr, Loyd JE, Ely EW, et al: Pulmonary veno-occlusive disease: A case series and new observations. *Chest* 118(6): 1671-1679, 2000.

Lantuéjoul S, Sheppard MN, Corrin B, et al: Pulmonary veno-occlusive disease and pulmonary capillary hemangiomatosis: A clinicopathologic study of 35 cases. *Am J Surg Pathol* 30(7): 850-857, 2006.

Mandel J, Mark EJ, Hales CA: Pulmonary veno-occlusive disease. *Am J Respir Crit Care Med* 162:1964 1973, 2000.

Resten A, Maitre S, Humbert M, et al: Pulmonary hypertension: CT of the chest in pulmonary veno-occlusive disease. *AJR Am J Roentgenol* 183(1):65-70, 2004.

Pulmonary Artery Aneurysm

DEFINITION: Focal dilatation of a pulmonary artery that involves all three layers of vessel wall, beyond its maximum normal caliber, is known as a pulmonary artery aneurysm.

IMAGING

Conventional Radiography
Findings
- Hilar enlargement or lung nodular opacity

Utility
- Usually first imaging modality used in assessment of patient
- Limited value in diagnosis

CT
Findings
- Focal dilatation of a pulmonary artery
- Mural calcification (results from atherosclerosis secondary to severe chronic pulmonary hypertension or calcified intramural thrombus)
- Pulmonary artery wall thickening, aneurysm, thrombus formation, hemorrhage in Behçet disease
- Ground-glass opacities in patients with associated pulmonary hemorrhage
- Scarring, bronchiectasis, and calcified granulomas in patients with pulmonary artery aneurysm related to previous tuberculosis (Rasmussen aneurysm)

Utility
- Diagnosis is usually confirmed with contrast-enhanced CT.

MRI
Findings
- Findings similar to those on CT

Utility
- Provides useful information regarding the size, number, location, and extent of aneurysms and pseudoaneurysms.

Pulmonary Angiography
Utility
- Pulmonary angiography is the gold standard technique for defining the pulmonary vascular anatomy.

CLINICAL PRESENTATION
- Hemoptysis

DIFFERENTIAL DIAGNOSIS
- Solitary lung nodule
- Hilar lymphadenopathy

DIAGNOSTIC PEARLS
- Focal dilatation of a pulmonary artery involves all three layers of vessel wall, beyond its maximum normal caliber.
- Pseudoaneurysm does not involve all layers of the arterial wall.
- Diagnosis usually readily made on contrast-enhanced CT.
- Causes of pulmonary artery aneurysms and pseudoaneurysms include Behçet disease, Hughes-Stovin syndrome, trauma, infection, and severe pulmonary arterial hypertension.

PATHOLOGY
- Vasculitis: pulmonary artery aneurysms typically involve right lower lobe arteries with frequent thrombosis and surrounding inflammation.
- Primary lung cancer and pulmonary metastasis may erode into pulmonary arteries and result in pseudoaneurysm formation.
- Iatrogenic: catheter tip eroding arterial wall causes weakening, dilatation, and vessel rupture; thrombus forms pseudoaneurysm.
- Rasmussen aneurysm: pseudoaneurysm results from weakening of pulmonary artery wall by adjacent cavitary tuberculosis.

INCIDENCE/PREVALENCE AND EPIDEMIOLOGY
- Pulmonary artery aneurysms and pseudoaneurysms are uncommon.
- Most common forms of vasculitis associated with pulmonary artery aneurysms are Behçet syndrome and Hughes-Stovin syndrome.
- Rasmussen aneurysms usually involve upper lobes and are associated with pulmonary hemorrhage and life-threatening hemoptysis.
- Pyogenic bacteria are an increasingly common cause of pulmonary artery pseudoaneurysm formation.

WHAT THE REFERRING PHYSICIAN NEEDS TO KNOW
- Pulmonary artery aneurysms associated with vasculitis may regress with immunosuppressive medication; embolization is often needed to prevent life-threatening hemoptysis.
- Contrast-enhanced CT is the imaging modality of choice for diagnosis.

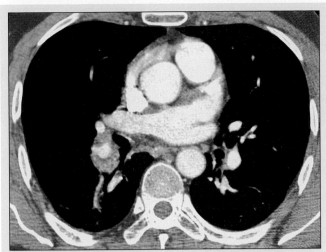

Figure 1. Behçet disease. Contrast-enhanced CT image shows partially thrombosed aneurysm of the right interlobar pulmonary artery. The patient was a 50-year-old man with Behçet disease, pulmonary artery aneurysm, and pulmonary hemorrhage.

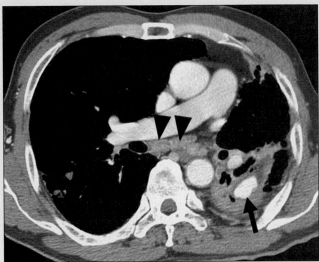

Figure 2. Rasmussen aneurysm in a 60-year-old man with chronic pulmonary tuberculosis. Contrast-enhanced CT image obtained at level of bronchus intermedius shows contrast filling aneurysm (*arrow*) within parenchymal consolidation in superior segment of left lower lobe. Also note enlarged subcarinal lymph nodes (*arrowheads*). (*Courtesy of Dr. Yeon Joo Jeong, Pusan National University Hospital, Pusan, Korea*)

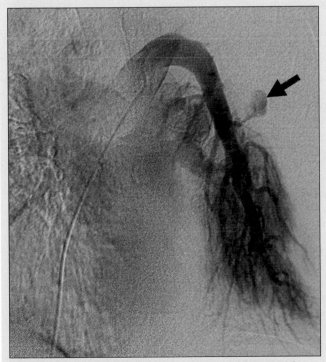

Figure 3. Rasmussen aneurysm in a 60-year-old man with chronic pulmonary tuberculosis. Nonselective left pulmonary angiogram shows contrast filling aneurysm (*arrow*) of left pulmonary artery branch. (*Courtesy of Dr. Yeon Joo Jeong, Pusan National University Hospital, Pusan, Korea.*)

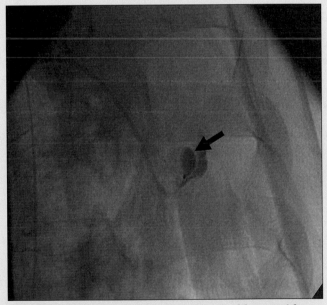

Figure 4. Rasmussen aneurysm in a 60-year-old man with chronic destructive pulmonary tuberculosis. Selective left pulmonary angiogram shows contrast filling aneurysm (*arrow*) of left pulmonary artery branch. (*Courtesy of Dr. Yeon Joo Jeong, Pusan National University Hospital, Pusan, Korea.*)

Suggested Readings

Bartter T, Irwin RS, Nash G: Aneurysms of the pulmonary arteries. *Chest* 94:1065-1075, 1988.

Castañer E, Gallardo X, Rimola J, et al: Congenital and acquired pulmonary artery anomalies in the adult: Radiologic overview. *RadioGraphics* 26(2):349-371, 2006.

Nguyen ET, Silva CI, Seely JM, et al: Pulmonary artery aneurysms and pseudoaneurysms in adults: Findings at CT and radiography. *AJR Am J Roentgenol* 188:W126-W134, 2007.

Part 39

PERMEABILITY PULMONARY EDEMA

Acute Respiratory Distress Syndrome

DEFINITION: Capillary endothelial injury and/or alveolar epithelial damage with resultant loss of fluid and protein into airspaces or interstitium is known as acute respiratory distress syndrome (ARDS).

IMAGING

Radiology
Findings
- Acute phase (first 12 hours): may be normal.
- Exudative phase: extensive bilateral, hazy, increased (ground-glass) opacities and consolidation with air bronchograms.
- Proliferative and fibrotic phases; coarse reticular pattern superimposed on ground-glass opacities and progressive volume loss.

Utility
- Has important role in diagnosis of ARDS, monitoring disease progression, and assessment of clinically suspected complications.

CT
Findings
- May be normal in acute phase.
- Exudative and early proliferative phase: extensive bilateral ground-glass opacities with or without associated consolidation.
- Exudative phase: consolidation more homogeneous and gravity dependent.
- "Crazy-paving" pattern (interlobular septal thickening and intralobular thickening superimposed on ground-glass opacities).
- Traction bronchiectasis and bronchiolectasis associated with lung volume loss (displacement or distortion of interlobular fissures, bronchi, or vessels).
- Fibrotic phase: coarse reticular opacities and small cystic spaces and patchy distribution with areas of relative sparing.
- Extrathoracic causes associated with extensive dependent consolidation; direct lung injury associated with more extensive nondependent consolidation.

DIAGNOSTIC PEARLS
- Acute onset of dyspnea and refractory hypoxemia
- Extensive bilateral ground-glass opacities and consolidation
- Septal lines superimposed on ground-glass opacities ("crazy-paving" pattern) on high-resolution CT
- Traction bronchiectasis and bronchiolectasis in the proliferative and fibrotic stages
- Superimposed coarse reticular pattern with progressive volume loss

Utility
- High-resolution CT findings have been shown to correlate well with pathologic phases of diffuse alveolar damage.
- Forty percent of cases of pneumothorax and 80% of cases of pneumomediastinum seen on CT may not be apparent on radiograph.
- CT is superior to radiography in the detection of complications.
- Several diffuse parenchymal lung diseases may present acutely and mimic ARDS.

CLINICAL PRESENTATION
- Acute onset of shortness of breath
- Refractory hypoxemia
- No evidence of left-sided heart failure
- Associated with other organ failure

DIFFERENTIAL DIAGNOSIS
- Bronchopneumonia
- Diffuse pulmonary hemorrhage
- Hydrostatic pulmonary edema

WHAT THE REFERRING PHYSICIAN NEEDS TO KNOW
- Chest radiography plays an important role in the diagnosis, monitoring disease progression, and detection of complications.
- CT is superior to chest radiography in the detection of complications.
- Radiographic findings are influenced by the stage of diffuse alveolar damage, positive end-expiratory pressure, inspiratory volume, and timing of x-ray exposure.
- Similar to radiography, high-resolution CT may be normal in early phase of ARDS but is usually abnormal within 12 hours.

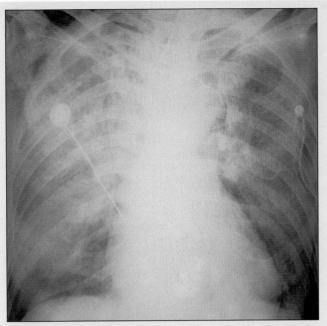

Figure 1. Acute exudative phase of diffuse alveolar damage in 54-year-old man with ARDS due to sepsis. Chest radiograph shows extensive bilateral, hazy, increased opacities (ground-glass opacities) and consolidation. (*Courtesy of Dr. Kazyua Ichikado, Kumamoto, Japan*)

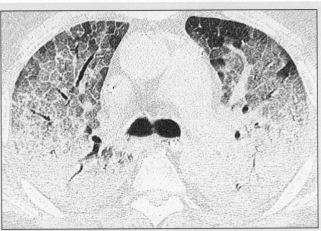

Figure 2. ARDS with "crazy-paving" pattern on CT. High-resolution CT image shows extensive ground-glass opacities with superimposed smooth septal thickening and intralobular lines. Also noted are bilateral areas of consolidation with air bronchograms in dependent lung regions. Patient was a 71-year-old man with ARDS.

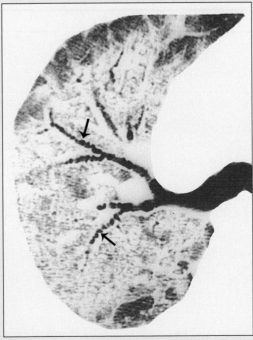

Figure 3. Subacute proliferative phase of diffuse alveolar damage in a 77-year-old man with ARDS due to viral pneumonia. High-resolution CT scan at level of right upper lobe bronchus shows extensive ground-glass opacities with associated reticulation and traction bronchiectasis (*arrows*). (*Courtesy of Dr. Kazyua Ichikado, Kumamoto, Japan*)

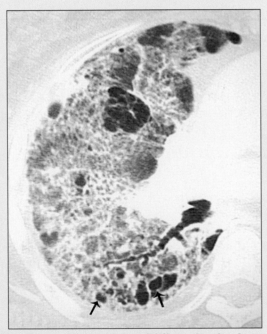

Figure 4. Chronic fibrotic phase of diffuse alveolar damage (2 weeks after onset of lung injury) in a 65-year-old woman with ARDS due to unknown etiology. High-resolution CT scan at level of right middle lobe shows extensive ground-glass opacities associated with reticulation ("crazy-paving" pattern), traction bronchiectasis, and cystic changes (*arrows*). (*Courtesy of Dr. Kazyua Ichikado, Kumamoto, Japan*)

PATHOLOGY

- Diffuse alveolar damage evolves from epithelial and endothelial necrosis to alveolar collapse, fibroblast proliferation, and fibrosis.
- Exudative phase is seen in first 7 days of injury and characterized by edema, intra-alveolar hemorrhage, and hyaline membrane formation.
- In the subacute proliferative phase, fibroblast proliferation and collagen deposition occur mainly within interstitium but also within airspaces.
- Chronic fibrotic phase develops approximately 2 weeks after injury.

INCIDENCE/PREVALENCE AND EPIDEMIOLOGY

- Incidence of ARDS is approximately 60 per 100,000 person-years.
- Risk for ARDS includes direct lung injury (pneumonia, gastric content aspiration) and indirect injury (sepsis, major trauma, multiple transfusions).

- Sepsis with multiorgan failure is the most common cause of death (30%-50%); respiratory failure results in smaller percentage of deaths (13%-19%).
- Complications include pneumothorax, pleural effusion, lung abscesses, pneumomediastinum, and subcutaneous emphysema.
- Mortality rate for patients with ARDS is 30%-40%.

Suggested Readings

Bernard GR: Acute respiratory distress syndrome: A historical perspective. *Am J Respir Crit Care Med* 172:798-806, 2005.

Desai SR: Acute respiratory distress syndrome: Imaging of the injured lung. *Clin Radiol* 57:8-17, 2002.

Fan E, Needham DM, Stewart TE: Ventilatory management of acute lung injury and acute respiratory distress syndrome. *JAMA* 294:2889-2896, 2005.

Gattinoni L, Caironi P, Pelosi P, Goodman LR: What has computed tomography taught us about the acute respiratory distress syndrome? *Am J Respir Crit Care Med* 164:1701-1711, 2001.

Rubenfeld GD, Caldwell E, Peabody E, et al: Incidence and outcomes of acute lung injury. *N Engl J Med* 353:1685-1693, 2005.

Part 40 HYDROSTATIC PULMONARY EDEMA

Hydrostatic Pulmonary Edema

DEFINITION: Increase in microvascular hydrostatic pressure or decrease in protein osmotic pressure in the microvascular lumen that results in transudation of fluid from microvessels into interstitial tissue.

IMAGING

Radiography
Findings
- Increase in caliber of upper zone vessels typically precedes evidence of overt edema.
- Artery becomes larger than accompanying bronchus.
- There is loss of definition of segmental and subsegmental pulmonary vessels and thickening of interlobular septa (Kerley A and B lines).
- Lamellar-shaped fluid collection conforms to shape of visceral pleura.
- Interstitial edema, haze that is predominantly lower zonal/perihilar in distribution, increase in bronchi wall thickness, and loss of sharp definition are noted.
- Airspace edema and symmetric patchy or confluent bilateral areas of consolidation involve perihilar regions and lower lung zones.
- Coalescence of areas of consolidation is seen with "bat wing" or "butterfly" edema.

Utility
- Redistribution of blood flow is assessed reliably only on radiographs performed at maximal inspiration in erect position.
- Radiography has an important role in initial evaluation and follow-up of patients.

CT
Findings
- Septal thickening and ground-glass opacities.
- Interlobular septal thickening that is smooth and uniform, except for focal nodular appearance due to prominent septal veins.
- Increased vascular caliber, perihilar peribronchovascular interstitium thickening, thickening of interlobar fissures, prominence of centrilobular structures due to interstitial edema, and pleural effusion.

DIAGNOSTIC PEARLS
- Dyspnea, tachypnea, and orthopnea
- Increased caliber of upper lobe vessels, loss of definition of subsegmental and segmental vessels, septal (Kerley) lines, thickening of interlobar fissures, and pleural effusion
- Presence of septal lines and pleural effusion, lack of air bronchograms, and predominantly central distribution of edema on radiograph
- Presence of septal lines and pleural effusion, lack of air bronchograms, and predominantly central or dependent distribution of ground-glass opacities on CT

- Ground-glass opacities and consolidation that tend to involve mainly perihilar and dependent lung regions.
- If with left-sided heart failure, may have enlarged mediastinal lymph nodes and hazy opacification of the mediastinal fat.

Utility
- Superior to the radiograph in the demonstration of the presence and extent of pulmonary edema but seldom required in the diagnosis.

CLINICAL PRESENTATION
- Dyspnea, tachypnea, and orthopnea
- Peripheral and central cyanosis, tachycardia, pallor, peripheral edema, elevated jugular venous pressure, and expectoration of frothy, blood-tinged fluid
- History of orthopnea and paroxysmal nocturnal dyspnea

WHAT THE REFERRING PHYSICIAN NEEDS TO KNOW
- Characteristic findings include pulmonary vascular redistribution, ill-defined pulmonary vascular markings, septal (Kerley B) lines, pleural effusions, and cardiomegaly.
- Cardiomegaly may not be present in patients with acute pulmonary edema.
- There may be a lag of 12 hours or more between development of edema and of radiologically visible abnormalities.
- Chest radiograph has limited accuracy in distinguishing between hydrostatic and permeability pulmonary edema.

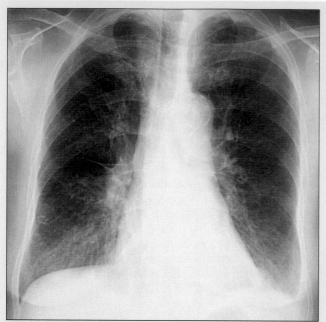

Figure 1. Septal pattern in interstitial pulmonary edema.
Posteroanterior chest radiograph shows numerous bilateral linear opacities. Also noted is a prominence of pulmonary vessels and small left pleural effusion. Patient was an 80-year-old woman with interstitial pulmonary edema due to left-sided heart failure.

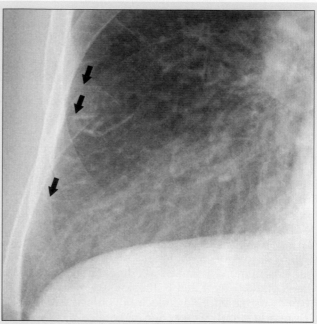

Figure 2. Septal pattern in interstitial pulmonary edema.
Magnified view of right lower lung zone shows linear opacities (*arrows*) measuring 1 to 2 cm in length and perpendicular to pleura. These represent septal (Kerley B) lines. Patient was an 80-year-old woman with interstitial pulmonary edema due to left-sided heart failure.

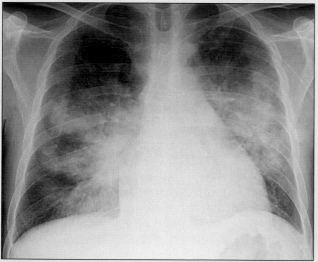

Figure 3. Bat wing pattern of pulmonary edema.
Posteroanterior radiograph shows consolidation of perihilar and medullary portion of both lungs creating a bat wing or butterfly appearance; cortex of both lungs is relatively unaffected. Also noted is a central venous line. Patient was a 38-year-old man with severe acute hydrostatic pulmonary edema.

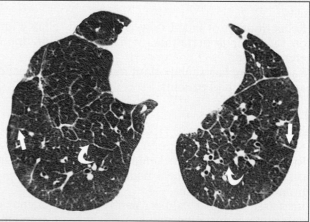

Figure 4. Interstitial pulmonary edema: CT findings. High-resolution CT image at level of lower lung zones shows smooth septal lines perpendicular to pleura (*straight arrows*) and more centrally as polygonal arcades (*curved arrows*). Patient was an 84-year-old woman with left-sided heart failure and interstitial pulmonary edema.

DIFFERENTIAL DIAGNOSIS

- Acute respiratory distress sundrome
- Bronchopneumonia
- Diffuse pulmonary hemorrhage

PATHOLOGY

- Rise in pulmonary venous pressure may be secondary to left-sided heart disease or pulmonary vein stenosis.
- Increase in microvascular hydrostatic pressure or decrease in protein osmotic pressure results in fluid transudation from microvessels into interstitial tissue.
- Edema develops in alveolar airspaces when storage capacity of interstitial space is exceeded.
- When pulmonary venous hypertension is moderate in degree (17-20 mm Hg or higher) fluid accumulates within perivascular interstitial tissue and interlobular septa.
- Airspace pulmonary edema tends to develop when transmural pressure becomes > 25 mm Hg.

INCIDENCE/PREVALENCE AND EPIDEMIOLOGY

- Most common cause is left-sided heart failure (cardiogenic pulmonary edema), acute and chronic renal disease, and fluid overload.
- Most common cause of asymmetric hydrostatic pulmonary edema is morphologic changes in lung parenchyma in chronic obstructive pulmonary disease.
- Asymmetric distribution occurs in 9% of adults with grade 3 or 4 mitral regurgitation.
- Acute mitral regurgitation due to papillary muscle dysfunction after myocardial infarction typically causes predominantly right upper lobe edema.

Suggested Readings

Gluecker T, Capasso P, Schnyder P, et al: Clinical and radiologic features of pulmonary edema. *RadioGraphics* 19:1507-1531, 1999.

Primack SL, Müller NL, Mayo JR, et al: Pulmonary parenchymal abnormalities of vascular origin: High-resolution CT findings. *RadioGraphics* 14:739-746, 1994.

Ware LB, Matthay MA: Clinical practice: Acute pulmonary edema. *N Engl J Med* 353:2788-2796, 2005.

Unilateral Pulmonary Edema

DEFINITION: Unilateral or markedly asymmetric pulmonary edema may occur in patients with parenchymal, airway, or pulmonary vascular disease; mitral regurgitation; and after drainage of large pneumothorax or pleural effusion.

IMAGING

Radiography
Findings
- Unilateral or markedly asymmetric pulmonary edema with hazy increased opacity or consolidation, poorly defined vascular markings, and septal lines.

Utility
- There may be a lag of 12 hours or more between development of edema and development of radiologically visible abnormalities.

CT
Findings
- Unilateral or markedly asymmetric pulmonary edema
- Ground-glass opacities, consolidation, and septal lines
- Extensive asymmetric parenchymal abnormalities, most commonly emphysema
- Extensive asymmetric pulmonary thromboembolism
- Unilateral venous obstruction

Utility
- May be helpful in determining cause for the unilateral or markedly asymmetric pulmonary edema

CLINICAL PRESENTATION

- Dyspnea, tachypnea, and orthopnea

DIFFERENTIAL DIAGNOSIS

- Pneumonia
- Aspiration pneumonia
- Pulmonary hemorrhage

PATHOLOGY

- Unilateral pulmonary edema occurs when a pathogenetic mechanism exists either on the same side (ipsilateral edema) or the opposite side (contralateral edema).
- In tuberculosis or sarcoidosis, edema occurs in regions less affected by these diseases, resulting in an asymmetric distribution.
- Edema associated with acute mitral regurgitation as may occur after myocardial infarctions typically

DIAGNOSTIC PEARLS

- Asymmetric patchy or confluent areas of consolidation
- Morphologic changes secondary to extensive emphysema, marked destruction, and fibrosis in tuberculosis or sarcoidosis
- Involves mainly right upper lobe in mitral regurgitation
- May occur after drainage of large pleural effusion or pneumothorax

involves mainly right upper lobe because the reflux stream is directed toward the right upper pulmonary vein.
- Pulmonary edema may result from ipsilateral pulmonary venous obstruction.
- Rapid re-expansion of the lung that occurs after chest tube drainage of a large pleural effusion or pneumothorax.
- Extensive pulmonary embolism involving predominantly one lung may result in pulmonary edema in the spared lung or lobe.

INCIDENCE/PREVALENCE AND EPIDEMIOLOGY

- Most common cause of asymmetric hydrostatic pulmonary edema is morphologic change in lung parenchyma in chronic obstructive pulmonary disease.
- Asymmetric distribution occurs in 9% of adults with grade 3 or 4 mitral regurgitation.

Suggested Readings

Agarwal R, Aggarwal AN, Gupta D: Other causes of unilateral pulmonary edema. *Am J Emerg Med* 25:129-131, 2007.

Gluecker T, Capasso P, Schnyder P, et al: Clinical and radiologic features of pulmonary edema. *RadioGraphics* 19:1507-1531, 1999.

Hassan W, El Shaer F, Fawzy ME, et al: Cardiac unilateral pulmonary edema: Is it really a rare presentation? *Congest Heart Fail* 11:220-223, 2005.

Schnyder PA, Sarraj AM, Duvoisin BE, et al: Pulmonary edema associated with mitral regurgitation: Prevalence of predominant involvement of the right upper lobe. *AJR Am J Roentgenol* 161:33-36, 1993.

WHAT THE REFERRING PHYSICIAN NEEDS TO KNOW

- Lag of 12 hours or more between the development of edema and radiologically visible abnormalities

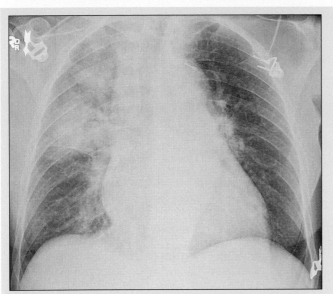

Figure 1. Right upper lobe pulmonary edema due to acute mitral regurgitation. Anteroposterior chest radiograph shows prominence and ill-defined pulmonary vascular markings and septal lines consistent with interstitial pulmonary edema. Also noted is extensive right upper lobe consolidation. Although upper lobe consolidation is most suggestive of pneumonia, it was proved to be due to airspace pulmonary edema secondary to acute mitral regurgitation after myocardial infarction. Patient was an 83-year-old woman.

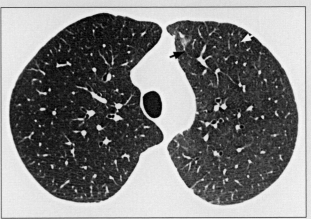

Figure 2. Unilateral pulmonary edema due to venous obstruction after radiofrequency ablation. High-resolution CT image at level of upper lobes demonstrates thickening of interlobular septa (*arrows*) and diffuse ground-glass opacities in left upper lobe. Patient was a 42-year-old man who had recently undergone radiofrequency ablation for treatment of atrial fibrillation.

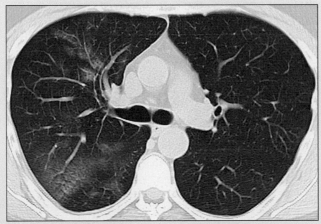

Figure 3. Re-expansion pulmonary edema. CT of the chest obtained 48 hours after drainage of large right pneumothorax demonstrates extensive ground-glass opacification in the right middle and lower lobes, in keeping with re-expansion pulmonary edema. The edema resolved within 24 hours.

Diseases of the Airways

Tracheal Stenosis

DEFINITION: Narrowing of the tracheal lumen that can result from a variety of inflammatory, infectious, neoplastic, or iatrogenic processes.

IMAGING

Radiography
Findings
- Airway narrowing

Utility
- Initial imaging test obtained for assessment of patients with central airway symptoms and suspected tracheal stenosis.
- Tracheal stenoses often overlooked on conventional radiographs because of their proximal location.

CT
Findings
- Eccentric or concentric soft tissue thickening with associated luminal narrowing.
- Hourglass-shaped focal stenosis postintubation.
- Focal or diffuse thickening of the tracheal wall.
- Thickening typically spares the posterior membrane in relapsing polychondritis and tracheobronchopathia osteochondroplastica.
- Thickening typically circumferential in amyloidosis and Wegener granulomatosis.

Utility
- CT is imaging modality of choice for detecting and characterizing tracheal stenosis.
- Multiplanar reformatted and 3D external rendering images help to detect focal stenoses and aid assessment of craniocaudal length.
- Dynamic expiratory CT sequence may be helpful to assess for coexisting tracheomalacia.

MRI
Findings
- Eccentric or concentric soft tissue thickening internal to tracheal cartilage

Utility
- MRI is alternative to CT in younger patients in whom radiation exposure may be a concern.
- Multiplanar images along the axis of trachea accurately depict the craniocaudal extent of stenosis.

DIAGNOSTIC PEARLS
- Focal tracheal stenosis with hourglass configuration in postintubation stenosis.
- Eccentric or concentric soft tissue thickening internal to the tracheal cartilage in postintubation stenosis.
- Thickening of tracheal wall typically spares the posterior membrane in relapsing polychondritis and tracheobronchopathia osteochondroplastica.
- Thickening typically circumferential in tracheobronchial amyloidosis and Wegener granulomatosis.

CLINICAL PRESENTATION
- Dyspnea on exertion, stridor, and wheezing are noted.
- Symptoms of upper airway obstruction are often delayed several weeks after extubation.
- Patients with mild stenoses may initially be asymptomatic.
- Patients may eventually develop symptoms when tracheal luminal narrowing is worsened by airway edema and secretions from coexistent respiratory infection.
- Lung function: flow-volume loops may show characteristic changes of airway obstruction.

PATHOLOGY
- Variety of iatrogenic, inflammatory, infectious, and neoplastic processes may result in focal or diffuse tracheal narrowing.
- Postintubation stenosis is characterized by eccentric or concentric tracheal wall thickening and associated luminal narrowing.
- Postintubation stenosis occurs secondary to tracheal injury from high pressure of endotracheal tube balloon against tracheal wall.

WHAT THE REFERRING PHYSICIAN NEEDS TO KNOW
- Chest CT with multiplanar reformatted images and 3D reconstructions is the study of choice for detection and characterization of tracheal stenosis.
- Additional dynamic expiratory CT sequences may be helpful to assess for coexisting tracheomalacia.

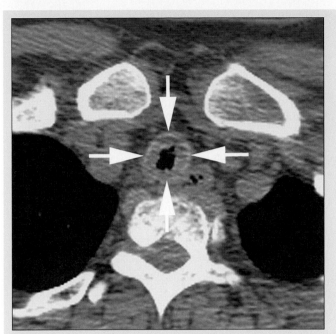

Figure 1. Postintubation stenosis. Axial image of proximal trachea demonstrates circumferential wall thickening (*arrows*) and luminal narrowing. (*Courtesy of Dr. Phillip M. Boiselle, Harvard Medical School, Boston*)

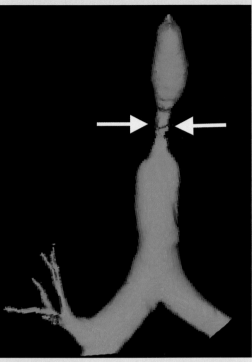

Figure 2. Postintubation stenosis. 3D external rendering of trachea demonstrates hourglass-shaped focal stenosis. Craniocaudal extent of stenosis (*arrows*) was more accurately assessed on 3D image than on contiguous axial CT images (see Fig. 1). (*Courtesy of Dr. Phillip M. Boiselle, Harvard Medical School, Boston*)

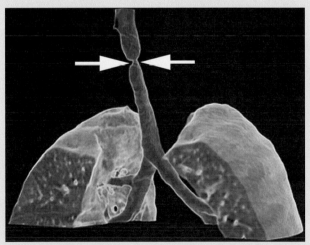

Figure 3. Postintubation stenosis. 3D external rendering of trachea demonstrates focal, high-grade subglottic stenosis (*arrows*). The stenosis was nearly overlooked on axial CT images (not shown). (*Courtesy of Dr. Phillip M. Boiselle, Harvard Medical School, Boston*)

- Sites include tracheostomy tube placement-stoma site and endotracheal intubation subglottic region at level of endotracheal balloon.
- Ischemic necrosis occurs due to compromise of blood supply to tracheal mucosa followed by superficial tracheitis with shallow ulcerations.
- Exposed cartilaginous rings subsequently soften and become fragmented, followed by fibrosis and granulation tissue formation.

INCIDENCE/PREVALENCE AND EPIDEMIOLOGY

- Postintubation stenosis is most common cause of acquired tracheal stenosis.

- Prevalence has decreased substantially to an estimated 1% after introduction of low-pressure cuff endotracheal tubes.
- Prevalence is estimated at approximately 30% after long-standing tracheostomy tube placement.
- Risk factors include difficult or prolonged intubation, infection, mechanical irritation, corticosteroid administration and use of positive-pressure ventilation.

Suggested Readings

Prince JS, Duhamel DR, Levin L, et al: Non-neoplastic lesions of the tracheobronchial wall: Radiographic findings with bronchoscopic correlation. *RadioGraphics* 22:S215-S230, 2002.

Webb EB, Elicker BM, Webb WR: Using CT to diagnose nonneoplastic tracheal abnormalities. *AJR Am J Roentgenol* 174:1315-1321, 2000.

Tracheal Neoplasms

DEFINITION: Tumors of the trachea can be benign or malignant.

IMAGING

Radiography

Findings

- Tracheal mass
- Extraluminal involvement not usually detectable unless it is sufficiently extensive to distort the normal mediastinal contours
- Severe, tracheal luminal narrowing

Utility

- First-line imaging test for patients presenting with central airway symptoms
- On radiography, careful scrutiny of airway needed because lesions often overlooked
- Difficult to distinguish intrinsic tracheal abnormality from extrinsic compression

CT

Findings

- Polypoid or sessile intraluminal mass of soft tissue density
- Necrosis and ulceration
- Hamartoma or lipoma: fat within a lesion
- Chondroid tumor: calcification within a lesion
- Regional lymph node metastases and complications (tracheoesophageal fistula)
- Circumferential tracheal wall thickening and luminal narrowing

Utility

- Multidetector CT is imaging modality of choice for detection and staging of tracheal neoplasms.
- CT has high sensitivity (>97%) for detecting tracheal neoplasms.
- CT has limited specificity in distinguishing between neoplastic cell types.
- Assessment of submucosal spread and local extratracheal invasion is possible.
- Multiplanar and 3D reconstructions complement axial images by improving assessment of craniocaudal extent of disease and degree of extratracheal involvement.
- CT does not reliably detect microscopic mediastinal invasion or neural invasion.

DIAGNOSTIC PEARLS

- Endoluminal tracheal nodule or mass
- Polypoid or sessile intraluminal mass of soft tissue density
- Adenoid cystic carcinoma may result in circumferential thickening of the tracheal wall
- CT has limited specificity in distinguishing benign from malignant tracheal tumors
- Findings which favor malignancy include large size (>2 cm diameter), irregular or lobulated margins, contiguous tracheal wall thickening, and mediastinal invasion.

MRI

Findings

- Intermediate signal intensity on T1-weighted images
- High signal intensity on T2-weighted images
- Tracheal wall thickening and luminal narrowing

Utility

- Second-line, problem-solving tool for assisting in tissue characterization and assessment of mediastinal invasion.

CLINICAL PRESENTATION

- Tumor is clinically silent until tracheal lumen is narrowed by approximately 75%.
- Symptoms include dyspnea, cough, hemoptysis, wheezing, and stridor.
- Squamous cell carcinoma: average age at presentation is between 50 and 60 years.
- Adenoid cystic carcinoma: average age at presentation is between 40 and 50 years.

DIFFERENTIAL DIAGNOSIS

- Wegener granulomatosis
- Tracheal stenosis

WHAT THE REFERRING PHYSICIAN NEEDS TO KNOW

- Tracheal neoplasm should be considered in patients with a history of "adult-onset asthma."
- Clinical symptoms of central airway obstruction overlap with other tracheal disorders, including tracheal stenosis and tracheomalacia.
- Biopsy is usually necessary to establish the diagnosis.
- Surgery is the treatment of choice.
- Majority of tracheal neoplasms are malignant in adults.
- CT is the imaging modality of choice for detection and staging.

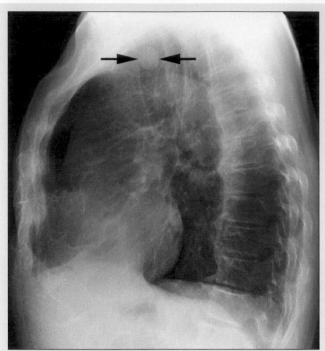

Figure 1. Tracheal neoplasm. Lateral chest radiograph demonstrates a smoothly marginated, round mass within the tracheal lumen. (*Courtesy of Dr. Phillip M. Boiselle, Harvard Medical School, Boston*)

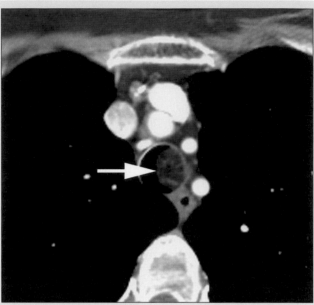

Figure 2. Tracheal hamartoma. CT image demonstrates a fat-attenuation tracheal mass (*arrow*) arising from the left lateral wall. Final diagnosis was lipomatous hamartoma. (*Courtesy of Dr. Phillip M. Boiselle, Harvard Medical School, Boston*)

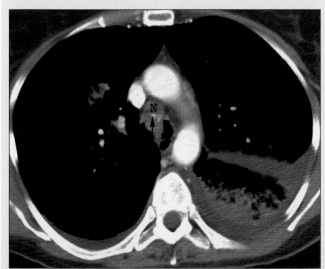

Figure 3. Malignant tracheal neoplasm. CT image at carina demonstrates a lobulated intraluminal mass with direct invasion through airway wall (anterior). Also note enlarged precarinal lymph node (N), left lower lobe consolidation, and bilateral pleural effusions. Final diagnosis was adenoid cystic carcinoma. (*Courtesy of Dr. Phillip M. Boiselle, Harvard Medical School, Boston*)

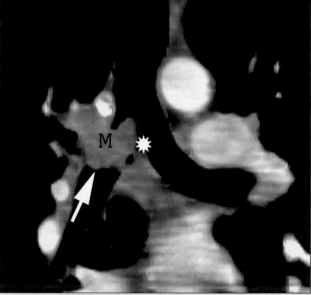

Figure 4. Coronal reformatted image demonstrates a mass (M) arising at level of carina (*asterisk*), with extension into right main bronchus (*arrow*) and paratracheal soft tissues. This image provided a better assessment of extent of disease than axial images and aided preoperative planning. Final diagnosis was adenoid cystic carcinoma. (*Courtesy of Dr. Phillip M. Boiselle, Harvard Medical School, Boston*)

- Tracheobronchial amyloidosis
- Tuberculosis
- Metastases

PATHOLOGY

- Approximately 80% of tracheal neoplasms are malignant and the great majority are adenoid cystic carcinomas and squamous cell carcinomas.
- Benign neoplasms include papillomas, hamartomas, schwannomas, hemangiomas, and chondromas.

INCIDENCE/PREVALENCE AND EPIDEMIOLOGY

- Primary tracheal neoplasms are rare.

- Primary tracheal tumor is roughly 180 times less common than a primary lung cancer.
- Squamous cell carcinoma and squamous cell papilloma have a male predominance and are associated with cigarette smoking.
- Adenoid cystic carcinoma has no sex predilection and is not related to smoking.

Suggested Readings

Kwak SH, Lee KS, Chung MJ, et al: Adenoid cystic carcinoma of the airways: Helical CT and histopathologic correlation. *AJR Am J Roentgnol* 183:277-281, 2004.

McCarthy MJ, Rosado-de-Christenson ML: Tumors of the trachea. *J Thorac Imaging* 10:180-198, 1995.

Parsons RB, Milestone BN, Adler LP: Radiographic assessment of airway tumors. *Chest Surg Clin North Am* 13:63-77, 2003.

Tracheomalacia

DEFINITION: Tracheomalacia is characterized by increased compliance and excessive collapsibility of the trachea due to weakness of the airway walls and/or supporting cartilage.

IMAGING

Radiography
Findings
- Inspiratory radiograph is usually normal

Utility
- May be detected on radiograph

CT
Findings
- Inspiratory CT may be normal.
- Smooth thickening of the tracheal wall with sparing of the posterior membrane in relapsing polychondritis.
- Inspiratory CT may show relative widening of coronal dimension resulting in a lunate shape of the trachea.
- Excessive expiratory collapse of the trachea, defined as >50% reduction in cross-sectional lumen of trachea during expiration.
- Crescentic, "frown-like" configuration of tracheal lumen with <6 mm distance between anterior and posterior walls on expiration.

Utility
- CT findings should be closely correlated with symptoms in patients at the low range of positive.
- Paired inspiratory–dynamic expiratory CT is imaging method of choice and provides simultaneous information about airway anatomy and compliance.
- Dynamic expiratory imaging during forced exhalation is more sensitive than end-expiratory imaging for detecting this condition.
- Cine-CT imaging during coughing maneuver is highly sensitive for detecting tracheomalacia; it requires multiple acquisitions to image the entire trachea.

MRI
Utility
- Dynamic MRI during breathing maneuvers or coughing may be used to diagnose tracheomalacia.
- MRI is an alternative imaging modality for younger patients and those undergoing serial follow-up examinations.

Fluoroscopy
Utility
- May be used to diagnose this condition
- Highly operator dependent
- Supplanted by cross-sectional imaging with CT or MRI

DIAGNOSTIC PEARLS
- Greater than 50% reduction in the cross-sectional lumen of the trachea during expiration
- Complete expiratory collapse
- Crescentic, "frown-like" configuration of tracheal lumen with <6 mm distance between anterior and posterior walls

CLINICAL PRESENTATION
- Congenital form typically presents in first weeks to months of life with symptoms of expiratory stridor, cough, difficulty feeding.
- Acquired form may present at any age.
- Intractable cough, dyspnea, and wheezing occur.
- Recurrent respiratory infections noted.
- Lung function tests show decreased FEV_1 and low peak flow rate with rapid decrease in flow.

DIFFERENTIAL DIAGNOSIS
- Emphysema
- Chronic bronchitis
- Asthma
- Relapsing polychondritis

PATHOLOGY
- Weakening of cartilage and/or posterior membranous wall, with degeneration and atrophy of longitudinal elastic fibers.
- Increased compliance and excessive collapsibility of trachea.
- May be congenital or acquired.
- Primary/congenital tracheomalacia: congenital airway wall weakness in setting of abnormal cartilaginous matrix, inadequate cartilage maturity, or congenital tracheoesophageal fistula.
- Secondary/acquired tracheomalacia: chronic obstructive pulmonary disease, prior intubation, prior surgery, radiation therapy, long-standing extrinsic compression, and chronic inflammation.

WHAT THE REFERRING PHYSICIAN NEEDS TO KNOW
- Tracheomalacia should be considered in patients with respiratory symptoms and risk factors for this disorder.
- Paired inspiratory–dynamic expiratory CT or dynamic CT during forced expiration is the imaging modality of choice.

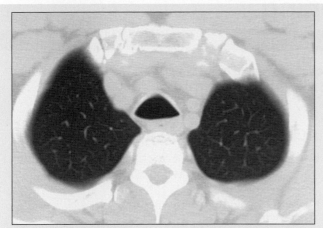

Figure 1. End-inspiratory CT. Axial CT image at end inspiration demonstrates patency of tracheal lumen. Note relative widening of coronal dimension with respect to the sagittal dimension ("lunate" shape). (*Courtesy of Dr. Phillip M. Boiselle, Harvard Medical School, Boston*)

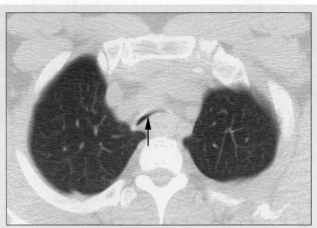

Figure 2. Dynamic expiratory CT. Axial CT image during dynamic expiration demonstrates near-complete collapse of tracheal lumen (*arrow*), consistent with tracheomalacia. (*Courtesy of Dr. Phillip M. Boiselle, Harvard Medical School, Boston*)

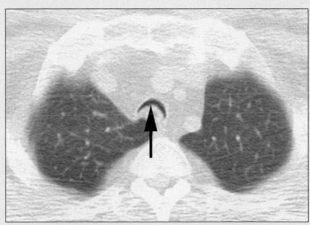

Figure 3. Frown sign. Dynamic expiratory CT image demonstrates "frown-like," crescentic configuration of tracheal lumen (*arrow*), highly suggestive of tracheomalacia. (*Courtesy of Dr. Phillip M. Boiselle, Harvard Medical School, Boston*)

- Acquired tracheomalacia: may also be idiopathic in some cases.

INCIDENCE/PREVALENCE AND EPIDEMIOLOGY

- True prevalence of tracheomalacia is unknown.
- Congenital form is most commonly observed in premature infants and often associated with cardiovascular abnormalities, bronchopulmonary dysplasia, and gastroesophageal reflux.
- Acquired form of tracheomalacia has been reported in 5%-23% of bronchoscopic studies performed in patients with respiratory symptoms.

Suggested Readings

Boiselle PM, Ernst A: Tracheal morphology in patients with tracheomalacia: Prevalence of inspiratory lunate and expiratory "frown" shapes. *J Thorac Imaging* 21:190-196, 2006.

Boiselle PM, Feller-Kopman D, Ashiku S, Ernst A: Tracheobronchomalacia: Evolving role of mutlislice helical CT. *Radiol Clin North Am* 41:627-636, 2003.

Carden K, Boiselle PM, Waltz D, Ernst A: Tracheomalacia and tracheobronchomalacia in children and adults: An in-depth review of a common disorder. *Chest* 127:984-1005, 2005.

Lee EY, Mason KP, Zurakowski D, et al: MDCT assessment of tracheomalacia in symptomatic infants with mediastinal aortic vascular anomalies: Preliminary technical experience. *Pediatr Radiol* 38:82-88, 2008.

Bronchial Wall Thickening

DEFINITION: Bronchi are considered thick walled if the wall is at least twice as thick as that of the normal airway or the internal diameter of the lumen is <80% of its external diameter.

IMAGING

Radiography
Findings
- Ring shadows or "tram tracks," particularly in patients with chronic bronchitis, bronchiectasis, and asthma.
- Increased lung markings due to superimposition of thickened bronchial walls and small airways disease in patients with chronic obstructive lung disease (COPD).
- Associated findings of pulmonary vascular redistribution, septal lines, cardiomegaly, and small pleural effusions in patients with hydrostatic pulmonary edema.

Utility
- Low sensitivity and specificity in the diagnosis of bronchial wall thickening.

CT
Findings
- Ring shadows or "tram tracks," particularly in patients with chronic bronchitis, bronchiectasis, and asthma.
- Emphysema common in patients with COPD related to cigarette smoking.
- Associated septal lines and, commonly, ground-glass opacities, thickening of interlobar fissures, cardiomegaly, and small pleural effusions in patients with hydrostatic pulmonary edema.

Utility
- CT is imaging modality of choice in the diagnosis of bronchiectasis.
- It has limited value in the diagnosis of chronic bronchitis and asthma.
- Apparent bronchial wall thickening may be mimicked by peribronchial ground-glass opacities or consolidation.
- The thickness of the bronchial wall on CT is influenced by technical parameters such as window width and level.

CLINICAL PRESENTATION

- Chronic bronchitis is characterized by productive cough occurring on most days for 3 or more months and for 2 or more successive years.

DIAGNOSTIC PEARLS

- Bronchi are considered thick-walled if the wall of the airway is at least twice as thick as that of the normal airway.
- Internal diameter of airway lumen is < 80% of its external diameter.
- Bronchial wall thickening is a common finding in patients with chronic bronchitis, bronchiectasis, and asthma.
- There is considerable interobserver variability in the diagnosis of bronchial wall thickening on the radiograph and CT.

PATHOLOGY

- Chronic inflammation and mucosal gland enlargement in chronic bronchitis and bronchiectasis.
- Edema and increase in airway smooth muscle and submucosal mucous glands in asthma.

INCIDENCE/PREVALENCE AND EPIDEMIOLOGY

- Bronchial wall thickening is a common finding in patients with chronic bronchitis, bronchiectasis, and asthma.
- Chronic bronchitis is usually due to cigarette smoking.

Suggested Readings

Gluecker T, Capasso P, Schnyder P, et al: Clinical and radiologic features of pulmonary edema. *RadioGraphics* 19:1507-1531, 1999.
McGuinness G, Naidich DP: CT of airways disease and bronchiectasis. *Radiol Clin North Am* 40:1-19, 2002.
Müller NL, Coxson H: Chronic obstructive pulmonary disease: 4. Imaging the lungs in patients with chronic obstructive pulmonary disease. *Thorax* 57:982-985, 2002.
Silva CI, Colby TV, Müller NL: Asthma and associated conditions: High-resolution CT and pathologic findings. *AJR Am J Roentgenol* 183:817-824, 2004.

WHAT THE REFERRING PHYSICIAN NEEDS TO KNOW

- High-resolution CT is the imaging modality of choice in the diagnosis of bronchiectasis and bronchial wall thickening.
- Chest radiography and CT have limited value in the diagnosis of chronic bronchitis and asthma.
- Radiographic and CT findings of bronchial wall thickening are nonspecific.
- There is considerable interobserver variability in the diagnosis of bronchial wall thickening on radiography and CT.

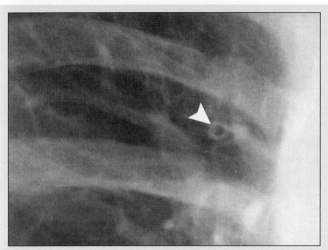

Figure 1. Asthma. View of the right lung from a frontal radiograph shows bronchial wall thickening (*arrowhead*).

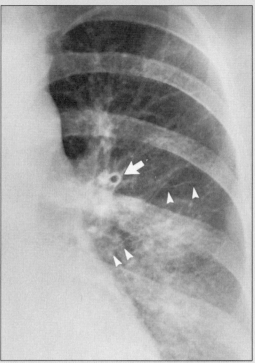

Figure 2. Peribronchial cuffing in pulmonary edema. Detail view of the upper half of the left lung from a posteroanterior chest radiograph shows distended upper lobe vessels, perihilar haze, septal A lines (*arrowheads*), and thickened bronchial wall viewed end on (*arrow*). The patient was a middle-aged woman with renal failure. (*From Müller NL, Fraser RS, Colman NC, Paré PD: Radiologic Diagnosis of Diseases of the Chest. Philadelphia, WB Saunders, 2001.*)

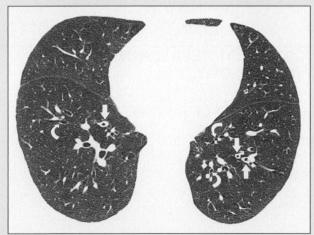

Figure 3. Bronchial wall thickening in chronic asthma. High-resolution CT image at the level of the lower lobes shows several bronchi with thickened walls (*straight arrows*). Also noted are several normal appearing bronchi (*curved arrows*). The patient was a 67-year-old man who was a nonsmoker with chronic asthma.

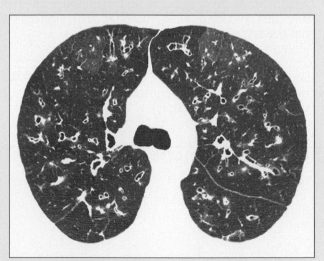

Figure 4. Cystic fibrosis. High-resolution CT scan in a 27-year-old man at the level of tracheal carina shows extensive bilateral bronchiectasis, bronchial wall thickening, and areas of decreased attenuation and vascularity.

Chronic Bronchitis

DEFINITION: Chronic bronchitis is a clinical diagnosis based on a history of chronic sputum expectoration (on most days) for 3 months of the year for 2 consecutive years.

IMAGING

Radiography

Findings

- Usually no demonstrable abnormality on plain radiography
- Bronchial wall thickening and general sense of increase in lung markings

Utility

- Imaging tests have a limited role in diagnosis of chronic bronchitis.
- Chest radiograph has greatest value in detection of infective consolidation and in exclusion of alternative diagnosis.

CT

Findings

- Bronchial wall thickening
- Signs of small airway involvement with focal areas of air trapping on expiratory CT

Utility

- Has limited role in the diagnosis and management of patients with chronic bronchitis

CLINICAL PRESENTATION

- History of chronic sputum expectoration (on most days) for 3 months of the year for 2 consecutive years is noted.
- Cough, productive sputum, and symptoms are typically first reported after subjects have smoked for some years.
- Acute exacerbations occur reasonably commonly and are usually ascribable to lower respiratory tract infections.
- On auscultation there may be inspiratory crackles, presumably related to presence of mucus in airways.

DIFFERENTIAL DIAGNOSIS

- Asthma
- Bronchiectasis
- Obliterative (constrictive) bronchiolitis
- Panbronchiolitis

DIAGNOSTIC PEARLS

- History of chronic sputum expectoration (on most days) for 3 months of the year for 2 consecutive years.
- Bronchial wall thickening.
- Imaging plays a limited role in the diagnosis and management of patients with chronic bronchitis.
- Main role of imaging is to assess for presence of superimposed complications such as pneumonia and carcinoma.

PATHOLOGY

- Dominant cause of chronic bronchitis is cigarette smoke with potential to regress on cessation of smoking.
- Respiratory bronchiolitis, shown as "pigmented" macrophage infiltration of the respiratory bronchioles, is almost invariably present in the lungs of smokers.
- There is a background of chronic inflammation with an increase in macrophages, T lymphocytes (predominantly CD8+), and neutrophils.
- These activated cells are known to release potent inflammatory mediators that cause lung damage and further sustain neutrophilic infiltration.
- Key pathologic finding is the presence of enlarged mucous glands and goblet cell hyperplasia.

INCIDENCE/PREVALENCE AND EPIDEMIOLOGY

- COPD taken as a whole has worldwide prevalence estimated as 9.3/1000 in males and 7.3/1000 in females.
- Chronic obstructive airways diseases represent a major global public health burden.

Suggested Reading

Müller NL, Coxson H: Chronic obstructive pulmonary disease: 4. Imaging the lungs in patients with chronic obstructive pulmonary disease. *Thorax* 57:982-985, 2002.

WHAT THE REFERRING PHYSICIAN NEEDS TO KNOW

- Clinical diagnosis is based on history of chronic sputum expectoration for 3 months of the year for 2 consecutive years.
- Imaging plays a limited role in evaluation of these patients except to exclude other findings, such as bronchiectasis.

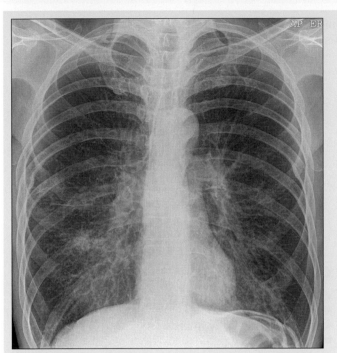

Figure 1. Chronic bronchitis. Chest radiograph in a patient with chronic bronchitis shows generalized increase in lung markings and bronchial wall thickening in the lower zones. An ill-defined opacity seen in the right lower zones was subsequently proven to be a bronchogenic carcinoma. (*Courtesy of Dr. Sujal R. Desai, London, UK*)

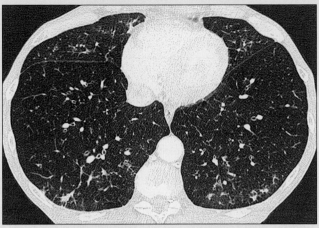

Figure 2. Chronic bronchitis. High-resolution CT image shows thick-walled (but nonbronchiectatic) subsegmental airways in both lower lobes. The patient was a 65-year-old smoker. (*Courtesy of Dr. Sujal R. Desai, London, UK*)

Bronchiectasis

DEFINITION: Abnormal, permanent dilatation of the airways with or without associated thickening of the walls of the airways is known as bronchiectasis.

IMAGING

Radiography

Findings
- Bronchial dilatation
- Poorly defined ring shadows (dilated bronchus with peribronchial inflammation when seen "end on") or "tram-track" opacities (denoting nontapering airway)
- With more severe disease, thin-walled cysts, with or without air-fluid levels, possibly apparent
- Tubular and branching opacities due to plugging of dilated airways with mucus, volume loss or hyperexpansion, and subsegmental atelectasis

Utility
- Generally the first imaging test requested by the physician when bronchiectasis is suspected
- Has limited value in the diagnosis

CT

Findings
- Bronchial dilatation
- Signet ring appearance
- Absence of normal tapering
- Bronchial wall thickening
- Airway plugging, mucous secretions within distal airways, and inflammatory thickening of bronchiolar walls seen as "tree-in-bud" pattern.

Utility
- High-resolution CT is as close to "gold standard" investigation as is currently available.
- Presence and extent of bronchiectasis are more accurately assessed using multidetector CT.

CLINICAL PRESENTATION

- Chronic cough
- Less commonly, mucopurulent sputum or intermittent hemoptysis
- Nonspecific findings on physical examination: early to mid inspiratory crackles and wheezing

DIAGNOSTIC PEARLS

- Bronchial dilatation
- Poorly defined ring shadows or "tram-track" opacities
- Ancillary CT features: bronchial wall thickening, mosaic attenuation pattern, airway plugging, volume loss, thickened interlobar septa

DIFFERENTIAL DIAGNOSIS

- Tracheobronchomegaly
- Decreased size of pulmonary vessels
- Lymphangioleiomyomatosis
- Pulmonary Langerhans cell histiocytosis

PATHOLOGY

- Initial damage to, or disruption of, process of normal mucociliary clearance occurs as a result of viral respiratory infection or genetic susceptibility.
- Organisms lead to further epithelial damage, reducing mucociliary clearance further and increasing susceptibility to microbial colonization.
- Inevitable inflammatory host response contributes to further airway damage and dilatation of the airways.
- Florid polymorphonuclear leukocytic infiltration into airway lumen and marked cytotoxic CD8+ T lymphocytes and macrophages increase in bronchial wall.
- Loss of the elastin layer in the bronchial wall and destruction of cartilage are noted.
- Patterns include *cylindrical,* uniform bronchial dilatation; *varicose,* focal narrowings along dilated airways; and *cystic,* grossly dilated airways with cystic appearance.

WHAT THE REFERRING PHYSICIAN NEEDS TO KNOW

- Patients may be asymptomatic or present with nonspecific symptoms such as cough, hemoptysis, or recurrent lower respiratory tract infections.
- Chest radiograph is of limited value in diagnosis.
- High-resolution CT performed at 10-mm intervals or volumetrically through the chest is the imaging modality of choice.
- Mainstay of therapy (no definite underlying cause) is effective clearance of airway secretions and vigorous treatment of infective exacerbations.

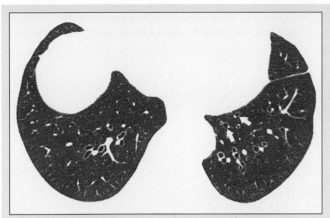

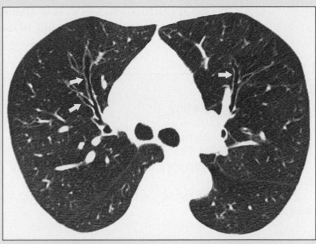

Figure 1. Bronchiectasis. High-resolution CT shows several bronchi with a luminal diameter greater than the diameter of the adjacent pulmonary artery. This appearance of a dilated airway and the normal size adjacent pulmonary artery in patients with bronchiectasis has been likened to a "signet ring" (*arrows*).

Figure 2. Bronchiectasis. High-resolution CT image shows bilateral upper lobe bronchiectasis (*arrows*) as denoted by the lack of tapering of the bronchi after they bifurcate.

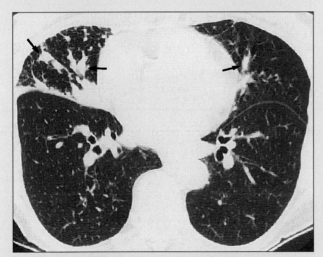

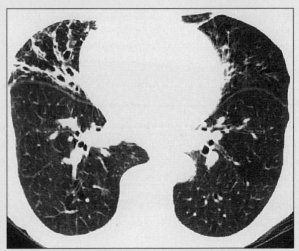

Figure 3. Mucus-filled bronchi. High-resolution CT image shows tubular and nodular (*arrows*) opacities in the right middle lobe and lingula. The patient was an 80-year-old woman who had bronchiectasis as a result of previous tuberculosis. (*From Müller NL, Fraser RS, Colman NC, Paré PD: Radiologic Diagnosis of Diseases of the Chest. Philadelphia, WB Saunders, 2001.*)

Figure 4. Mucus-filled bronchi. High-resolution CT performed after expectoration of the mucus shows that the opacities in Figure 3 represented ectatic bronchi filled with secretions. The patient was an 80-year-old woman who had bronchiectasis as a result of previous tuberculosis. (*From Müller NL, Fraser RS, Colman NC, Paré PD: Radiologic Diagnosis of Diseases of the Chest. Philadelphia, WB Saunders, 2001.*)

INCIDENCE/PREVALENCE AND EPIDEMIOLOGY

- Frequently related to previous infection, particularly childhood bronchopneumonia
- Prevalence of bronchiectasis high in select populations: indigenous Australians and native Alaskans
- Associated with a wide variety of causes
- Relatively common causes in the adult: previous infection, cystic fibrosis, asthma, allergic bronchopulmonary aspergillosis, and association with obliterative bronchiolitis

Suggested Readings

Bruzzi JF, Remy-Jardin M, Delhaye D, et al: Multi-detector row CT of hemoptysis. *RadioGraphics* 26:3-22, 2006.

McGuinness G, Naidich DP: CT of airways disease and bronchiectasis. *Radiol Clin North Am* 40:1-19, 2002.

Rosen MJ: Chronic cough due to bronchiectasis: ACCP evidence-based clinical practice guidelines. *Chest* 129(1 Suppl):122S-131S, 2006.

Bronchial Stenosis and Bronchomalacia

DEFINITION: Bronchial stenosis is abnormal narrowing of a bronchus. Bronchomalacia is increased compliance and excessive collapsibility of bronchi due to weakness of the airway walls and/or supporting cartilage.

IMAGING

Conventional Radiography
Findings
- Narrowing of bronchus
- Partial obstruction of main or lobar bronchus
- Air trapping on expiratory radiographs

Utility
- Limited value in diagnosis of bronchial narrowing and bronchomalacia

CT
Findings
- Decreased attenuation and vascularity (maximal inspiration)
- Air trapping on expiratory CT
- Narrowing of the bronchus
- Bronchial wall thickening
- Bronchomalacia: presence of excessive expiratory collapse, generally defined by > 50% reduction in cross-sectional lumen of bronchus during expiration

Utility
- Expiratory or dynamic CT required for diagnosis of bronchomalacia
- Multiplanar reconstructions obtained on multidetector scanners required for optimal assessment of presence and severity of airway stenosis.

CLINICAL PRESENTATION

- Cough, wheezing, shortness of breath

PATHOLOGY

- Bronchial stenosis due to focal or diffuse thickening of the wall or extrinsic compression
- Bronchomalacia: weakness of airway walls and/or supporting cartilage
- Intrinsic bronchial causes: inflammation (Wegener granulomatosis), infection (tuberculosis), tumor, trauma, and fibrosis

DIAGNOSTIC PEARLS

- Bronchial stenosis due to focal or diffuse thickening of the wall or extrinsic compression
- Hyperlucent lung
- Bronchomalacia: presence of excessive expiratory collapse, generally defined by > 50% reduction in cross-sectional lumen of bronchus during expiration

- Extrinsic causes: compression by tumor, enlarged lymph nodes, aortic aneurysm, mediastinal mass, or fibrosing mediastinitis
- Primary/congenital bronchomalacia: congenital weakness of airway wall due to abnormal cartilaginous matrix or inadequate cartilage maturity
- Secondary/acquired bronchomalacia: associated with chronic obstructive pulmonary disease, prior surgery, radiation therapy, long-standing extrinsic compression, and chronic inflammation (relapsing polychondritis)

INCIDENCE/PREVALENCE AND EPIDEMIOLOGY

- Bronchomalacia is particularly common in patients with chronic obstructive pulmonary disease.
- Narrowing of the bronchial lumen is common in central lung tumors.
- Bronchomalacia may occur in isolation or in association with tracheomalacia.

Suggested Readings

Grenier PA, Beigelman-Aubry C, Brillet PY: Nonneoplastic tracheal and bronchial stenoses. *Radiol Clin North Am.* 47:243-260, 2009.

Lee EY, Litmanovich D, Boiselle PM: Multidetector CT evaluation of tracheobronchomalacia. *Radiol Clin North Am.* 47:261-269, 2009.

WHAT THE REFERRING PHYSICIAN NEEDS TO KNOW

- Thin-section (≤1 mm) spiral CT with multiplanar reconstructions is required for optimal assessment of presence and severity of airway stenosis.
- Expiratory or dynamic CT is required for the diagnosis of bronchomalacia.

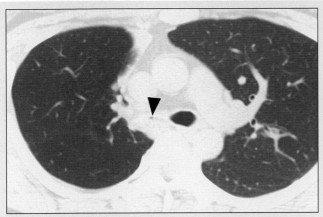

Figure 1. Bronchial tuberculosis in a 31-year-old woman. CT scan obtained at level of main bronchi demonstrates nearly completely obliterated right main bronchus lumen (*arrowhead*) with marked wall thickening. (*Courtesy of Dr. Kyung Soo Lee, Seoul, Korea*)

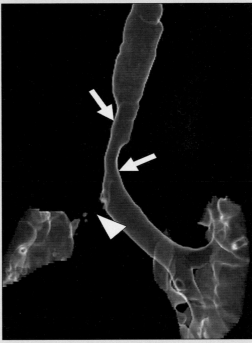

Figure 2. Bronchial tuberculosis in a 31-year-old woman. Volume-rendered image shows luminal narrowing of the lower trachea (*arrows*) and obliterated lumen of right main bronchus (*arrowhead*). (*Courtesy of Dr. Kyung Soo Lee, Seoul, Korea*)

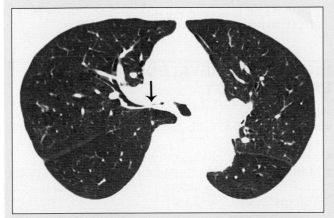

Figure 3. Tracheal and bronchial involvement in relapsing polychondritis. CT image shows marked narrowing of the right main and upper lobe bronchi (*arrow*) and mild narrowing of the left main bronchus.

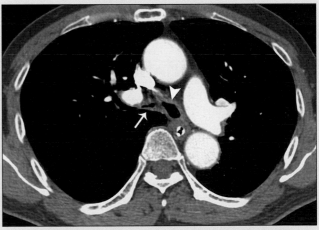

Figure 4. Tracheal and bronchial involvement in relapsing polychondritis. Soft tissue settings demonstrate thickening of the wall of the right (*arrow*) and left (*arrowhead*) main bronchus.

Broncholithiasis

DEFINITION: Broncholithiasis is a disorder characterized either by the presence of calcified or ossified material within the lumens of bronchi or the distortion of the tracheobronchial tree by calcified peribronchial nodes but without obvious erosion into the lumens.

IMAGING

Radiography
Findings
- Due to primary pathology: central/hilar or peripheral calcification
- Movement of previously noted focus of calcification in its relationship to an adjacent airway on serial radiographs
- Depending on severity and duration of obstruction: segmental atelectasis, lobar atelectasis, or recurrent infective consolidation
- "Middle lobe" syndrome in some patients

Utility
- Of limited value in diagnosis

CT
Findings
- Endobronchial broncholiths: calcified small nodular opacities within bronchus
- Peribronchial calcification
- Atelectasis

Utility
- CT is best noninvasive technique for the diagnosis of broncholithiasis.
- It is useful in identification of the effects of obstruction.
- Thinner CT section should be considered when diagnosis of broncholithiasis is suspected because anatomic relationships are optimized.
- Multidetector CT is recommended.

CLINICAL PRESENTATION

- Hemoptysis and nonproductive cough occur.
- Breathlessness, chest pain, and, because of obstructive effects, symptoms due to recurrent infections may occur.
- Lithoptysis (expectoration of calcific material) is a characteristic symptom but infrequently reported by patients.
- Rarely, broncholithiasis masquerades as asthma with wheeze as a dominant feature.

DIFFERENTIAL DIAGNOSIS

- Carcinoid tumor
- Hamartoma
- Foreign body

DIAGNOSTIC PEARLS

- Endobronchial broncholiths
- Segmental atelectasis, lobar atelectasis, or recurrent infective consolidation
- Calcified hilar and/or mediastinal lymph nodes

PATHOLOGY

- Broncholiths are seen due to extrusion of calcified material from adjacent lymph nodes and erosion into airways.
- Lymph node calcification is usually the consequence of chronic necrotizing granulomatous infection (usually tuberculosis or histoplasmosis).
- Luminal calcification occurs secondary to foreign-body calcification or calcific material migration from distant source through some putative fistulous communication.
- Basic pathogenetic mechanism is extrusion and subsequent erosion of dystrophic calcific material from lymph nodes into adjacent structures.
- Calcification typically affects the tracheobronchial tree, but erosions into lung parenchyma and mediastinum are known to occur.

INCIDENCE/PREVALENCE AND EPIDEMIOLOGY

- Uncommon
- Peak incidence in sixth decade, although broad overall age range
- No particular gender predilection
- Most commonly due to endobronchial erosion of calcified lymph nodes due to previous tuberculosis or histoplasmosis

Suggested Reading
Seo JB, Song KS, Lee JS, et al: Broncholithiasis: Review of the causes with radiologic-pathologic correlation. *RadioGraphics* 22(Spec No):S199-S213, 2002.

WHAT THE REFERRING PHYSICIAN NEEDS TO KNOW

- Broncholithiasis is the presence of calcified material within the lumens of bronchi.
- It is due to extrusion of calcified material from adjacent lymph nodes and erosion into airways from tuberculosis or histoplasmosis.
- CT, preferably with thin sections and performed on multidetector-row scanner, is the best noninvasive technique for the diagnosis.

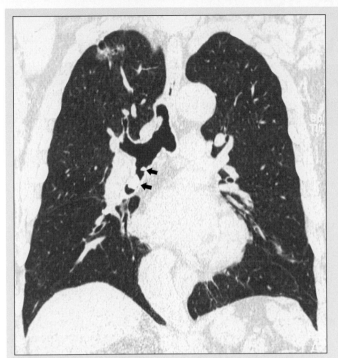

Figure 1. Broncholithiasis. Coronal reformatted image from a volumetric high-resolution CT of the chest demonstrates two nodular opacities (*arrows*) within the bronchus intermedius. Also noted is right upper lobe scarring related to previous tuberculosis.

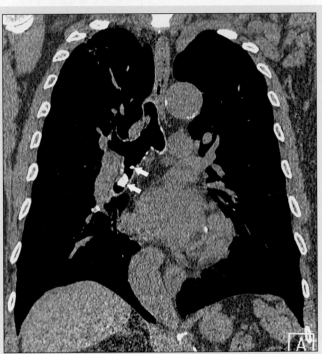

Figure 2. Broncholithiasis. Soft tissue windows demonstrate broncholiths (*arrows*). The patient was an 88-year-old man with previous tuberculosis.

Allergic Bronchopulmonary Aspergillosis

DEFINITION: Allergic bronchopulmonary aspergillosis is characterized by chronic airway inflammation and damage resulting from persistent colonization and sensitization by *Aspergillus fumigatus* and related species.

IMAGING

Radiography

Findings

- Homogeneous, branching opacities usually involve upper lobes and almost always are located in more central segmental bronchi rather than peripheral branches.
- Bifurcating opacities are described as having gloved-finger, inverted-Y or inverted-V, or cluster-of-grapes appearance.
- Transient parenchymal opacities due to eosinophilic lung disease may be evident.

Utility

- First and often only imaging modality performed in these patients.
- Radiographic findings relatively nonspecific.

CT

Findings

- Bronchiectasis and mucoid impaction involve mainly segmental and subsegmental bronchi of upper lobes.
- Centrilobular nodules and "tree-in-bud" pattern can be seen.
- Approximately 30% of patients with mucus plugs have high attenuation, presumably due to the presence of calcium salts.

Utility

- High-resolution CT is superior to radiography for assessment of this disease.

CLINICAL PRESENTATION

- Clinically, peripheral blood eosinophilia and pulmonary opacities are noted in patients who have asthma or cystic fibrosis.

DIAGNOSTIC PEARLS

- Central bronchiectasis, most commonly varicose
- Mucoid impaction
- Upper lobe predominance
- Occurs almost exclusively in patients with asthma or cystic fibrosis

---

- Patients are asymptomatic or present with worsening of asthma, increased cough, wheezing, and expectoration of a mucus plug.
- Physical examination is often normal except for underlying manifestations of asthma or cystic fibrosis.

DIFFERENTIAL DIAGNOSIS

- Asthma
- Cystic fibrosis
- Tuberculosis
- Infectious bronchiolitis
- Endobronchial tumor

PATHOLOGY

- Pathogenesis is unclear but it is believed that genetic factors and T-cell reactivity to *Aspergillus* play an important role.
- Eosinophils are numerous, cell debris consists of degenerate eosinophils with associated Charcot-Leyden crystals, and there are scattered, typically fragmented fungal hyphae.
- Patchy filling of alveolar airspaces by eosinophils (eosinophilic pneumonia) may be seen in adjacent lung parenchyma.

WHAT THE REFERRING PHYSICIAN NEEDS TO KNOW

- Asthmatics may have cylindrical bronchiectasis and filling of ectatic bronchi with secretions without having allergic bronchopulmonary aspergillosis.
- Patients often have more severe bronchiectasis (varicose rather than cylindrical) and more extensive bronchiectasis (several segments) than when having asthma alone.
- Diagnostic criteria include underlying asthma or cystic fibrosis, blood eosinophilia, reactivity to *Aspergillus fumigatus* antigen, anti-*A. fumigatus* antigen antibodies, elevated IgE levels, and imaging findings.
- Confidence in diagnosis depends on number and type of abnormalities, histologic findings on bronchoscopy specimens, and positive sputum culture for *Aspergillus* species.

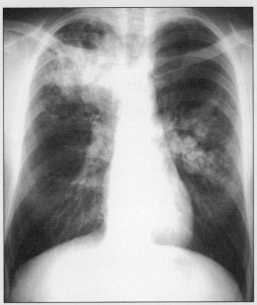

Figure 1. **Allergic bronchopulmonary aspergillosis.** Posteroanterior chest radiograph in a 31-year-old woman who had asthma and severe allergic bronchopulmonary aspergillosis shows tubular and nodular opacities in the upper lobes and foci of consolidation in the right upper lobe.

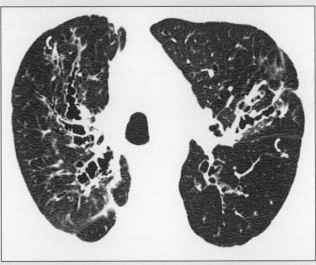

Figure 2. **Allergic bronchopulmonary aspergillosis in a 56-year-old man.** High-resolution CT image performed on multidetector CT through the upper lobes shows severe bilateral bronchiectasis and marked bronchial wall thickening. Also noted is mucoid impaction (*arrows*). (*From Silva CI, Colby TV, Müller NL: Asthma and associated conditions: High-resolution CT and pathologic findings. AJR Am J Roentgenol 183:817-824, 2004, with permission.*)

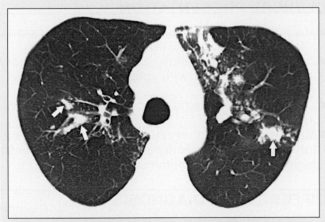

Figure 3. **Allergic bronchopulmonary aspergillosis.** CT image at the level of the aortopulmonary window in an asthmatic patient who had allergic bronchopulmonary aspergillosis shows tubular and branching opacities (*straight arrows*) due to mucoid impaction within bronchi and small centrilobular nodules and "tree-in-bud" pattern due to mucoid impaction within bronchioles. Also noted are localized areas of decreased attenuation and vascularity.

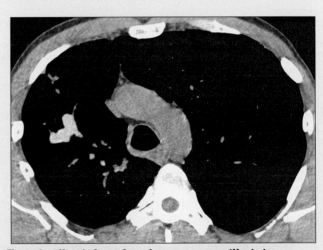

Figure 4. **Allergic bronchopulmonary aspergillosis in a 54-year-old asthmatic man.** CT image shows branching tubular opacity in right upper lobe and volume loss of the right lung with ipsilateral shift of the mediastinum. The tubular opacity has increased attenuation presumably due to deposition of calcium salts within the mucoid impaction.

INCIDENCE/PREVALENCE AND EPIDEMIOLOGY

- Occurs almost exclusively in patients with asthma or cystic fibrosis.
- Estimated prevalence: 2%-25% in patients with cystic fibrosis and 1%-8% in patients with asthma.

Suggested Readings

Franquet T, Müller NL, Gimenez A, et al: Spectrum of pulmonary aspergillosis: Histologic, clinical, and radiologic findings. *Radio-Graphics* 21:825-837, 2001.

Gibson PG: Allergic bronchopulmonary aspergillosis. *Semin Respir Crit Care Med* 27:185-191, 2006.

Virnig C, Bush RK: Allergic bronchopulmonary aspergillosis: A US perspective. *Curr Opin Pulm Med* 13:67-71, 2007.

Cystic Fibrosis

DEFINITION: Cystic fibrosis is an autosomal recessive hereditary disease. The fundamental abnormality consists of the production of abnormal secretions from exocrine glands, such as salivary and sweat glands, as well as pancreas, large bowel, and tracheobronchial tree.

IMAGING

Radiography

Findings

- Round or poorly defined linear opacities measuring 3-5 mm in diameter, located within 2-3 cm of pleura.
- Thickened bronchial walls (ring shadows) and hyperinflation.
- Increases in bronchial diameter, bronchial wall thickness, lung volume, and number and size of peripheral nodular opacities.
- Development of mucoid impaction and focal areas of consolidation.
- Recurrent foci of consolidation in most patients.

Utility

- Main imaging modality used in initial evaluation and follow-up.
- Of main value in assessment of complications such as pneumonia and pneumothorax.
- Of limited value in assessment of presence and extent of bronchiectasis.

CT

Findings

- Bronchiectasis: most severe in upper lobes, can be cylindrical, varicose, or cystic.
- Bronchial wall thickening, peribronchial interstitial thickening, and mucus plugging.
- Consolidation or atelectasis and cystic or bullous lung lesions.
- Branching or nodular centrilobular opacities ("tree-in-bud" pattern) frequently present and possible early sign of disease.
- Focal areas of decreased attenuation and vascularity on inspiratory CT and air trapping on expiratory CT common.

Utility

- High-resolution CT demonstrates abnormalities in patients who have early cystic fibrosis and normal chest radiographs.
- In young patients, radiation dose is minimized by using lowest dose possible (40-80 mA) and performing scanning only when clinically indicated.

DIAGNOSTIC PEARLS

- Bilateral symmetric distribution and upper lobe predominance
- Bronchiectasis: most severe in the upper lobes and cylindrical, varicose, or cystic
- Recurrent respiratory infections
- Pancreatic insufficiency
- Children and young adults

MRI

Findings

- Bronchiectasis
- Areas of consolidation
- Enlargement of central pulmonary arteries

Utility

- Used as alternative tool to assess parenchymal and functional abnormalities and monitoring treatment of cystic fibrosis.
- Has limited role in assessment of airway disease.

CLINICAL PRESENTATION

- Major clinical manifestations are recurrent respiratory infections and pancreatic insufficiency.
- Pulmonary manifestations are recurrent respiratory infections associated with productive cough, wheezing, and dyspnea.
- Common complications include hemoptysis and pneumothorax.
- Majority of patients eventually progress to respiratory insufficiency accompanied by pulmonary arterial hypertension and cor pulmonale.

DIFFERENTIAL DIAGNOSIS

- Allergic bronchopulmonary aspergillosis
- Ciliary dyskinesia
- Immunodeficiency
- Bronchiectasis due to previous infection

WHAT THE REFERRING PHYSICIAN NEEDS TO KNOW

- Diagnosis is made before age of 5 years in 80% of all individuals, in 10% during adolescence, and in 10% during adulthood.
- Radiographic findings are nonspecific, but diagnosis is suggested by family history, persistent respiratory disease, and pancreatic insufficiency.
- Confirmation of diagnosis requires positive sweat test or identification of two abnormal copies of the cystic fibrosis gene.
- High-resolution CT may demonstrate abnormalities in patients with normal radiographs.
- Main high-resolution CT manifestation is bronchiectasis.
- Use of routine CT scans should be avoided because of the risks of radiation.

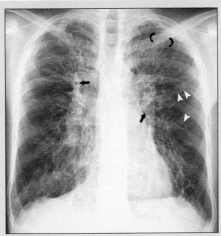

Figure 1. Cystic fibrosis. Posteroanterior chest radiograph in a 26-year-old man shows marked bronchial wall thickening (*straight arrows*) and extensive varicose (*arrowheads*) and cystic (*curved arrows*) bilateral bronchiectasis. Also noted are hyperinflation and enlarged central pulmonary arteries consistent with pulmonary arterial hypertension.

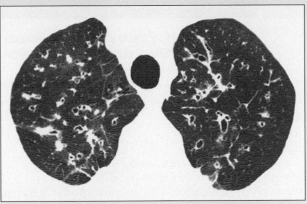

Figure 2. Cystic fibrosis. High-resolution CT scan in a 27-year-old man at the level of the lung apices shows extensive bilateral bronchiectasis and areas of decreased attenuation and vascularity.

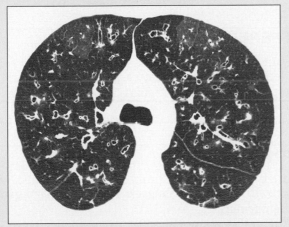

Figure 3. Cystic fibrosis. High-resolution CT in a 27-year-old man at the level of the tracheal carina shows extensive bilateral bronchiectasis, mucoid impaction, and areas of decreased attenuation and vascularity.

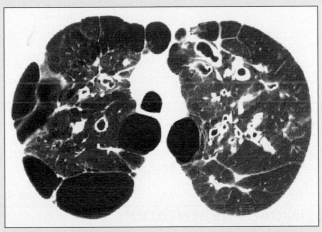

Figure 4. Cystic fibrosis. High-resolution CT scan in a 39-year-old woman at the level of the lung apices shows extensive bronchiectasis and bullous changes.

PATHOLOGY

- Histologic examination shows chronic inflammation/fibrosis of bronchial wall, partial/complete luminal occlusion by purulent material, focal epithelial ulceration, and cartilage destruction.
- Membranous bronchioles may have similar inflammatory changes or may show narrowing or obliteration due to fibrosis.
- Pancreatic Infufficiency
- Cystic fibrosis gene

INCIDENCE/PREVALENCE AND EPIDEMIOLOGY

- Most common lethal genetically transmitted disease in white persons, with estimated incidence being about 1 per 2000-3500 live births.
- It is uncommon in nonwhites.

- There is no sex predilection.
- Cystic fibrosis is most common cause of pulmonary insufficiency in first 3 decades of life.

Suggested Readings

Altes TA, Eichinger M, Puderbach M: Magnetic resonance imaging of the lung in cystic fibrosis. *Proc Am Thorac Soc* 4(4):321-327, 2007.

Aziz ZA, Davies JC, Alton EW, et al: Computed tomography and cystic fibrosis: Promises and problems. *Thorax* 62(2):181-186, 2007.

Cleveland RH, Zurakowski D, Slattery DM, Colin AA: Chest radiographs for outcome assessment in cystic fibrosis. *Proc Am Thorac Soc* 4(4):302-305, 2007.

de Jong PA, Tiddens HA: Cystic fibrosis specific computed tomography scoring. *Proc Am Thorac Soc* 4(4):338-342, 2007.

Long FR: High-resolution computed tomography of the lung in children with cystic fibrosis: Technical factors. *Proc Am Thorac Soc* 4(4):306-309, 2007.

Robinson TE: Computed tomography scanning techniques for the evaluation of cystic fibrosis lung disease. *Proc Am Thorac Soc* 4(4):310-315, 2007.

Nick JA, Rodman DM: Manifestations of cystic fibrosis diagnosed in adulthood. *Curr Opin Pulm Med* 11:513-518, 2005.

Primary Ciliary Dyskinesia (Dyskinetic Cilia Syndrome)

DEFINITION: Primary ciliary dyskinesia refers to a group of autosomal-recessive disorders associated with defective ciliary structure and function.

IMAGING

Radiography

Findings

- Bronchiectasis
- Nasal polyps or recurrent sinusitis
- Dextrocardia in approximately 50% of cases
- Areas of consolidation due to pneumonia frequently present

Utility

- Nonspecific features that resemble those of bronchiectasis from other causes.

CT

Findings

- Extensive central or diffuse bilateral bronchiectasis that involves predominantly or exclusively lower lobes.
- Centrilobular nodules and branching opacities ("tree-in-bud" pattern).
- Localized areas of decreased attenuation and vascularity due to obstructive bronchiolitis.
- Dextrocardia in approximately 50% of cases.
- Areas of consolidation due to pneumonia frequently present.

Utility

- Superior to chest radiography in determining presence and extent of bronchiectasis.

CLINICAL PRESENTATION

- Age at presentation ranges from 4 months to 51 years.
- Chronic rhinitis, sinusitis, and recurrent lower respiratory tract infections occur.
- Many patients develop mild to moderate air flow obstruction.
- Men have reduced fertility.
- Approximately 50% of patients with ciliary dyskinesia have triad of situs inversus totalis, bronchiectasis, and recurrent sinusitis (Kartagener syndrome).

DIAGNOSTIC PEARLS

- Radiographically, features progress from bronchial wall thickening to bronchiectasis, hyperinflation, segmental atelectasis, and consolidation.
- CT shows extensive central or diffuse bilateral bronchiectasis predominantly or exclusively in the lower lobes.
- Dextrocardia and situs inversus occur in half of cases.
- The combination of situs inversus totalis, bronchiectasis, and recurrent sinusitis is known as Kartagener syndrome.

DIFFERENTIAL DIAGNOSIS

- Cystic fibrosis
- Allergic bronchopulmonary aspergillosis
- Immunodeficiency
- Bronchiectasis due to childhood viral pneumonia

PATHOLOGY

- Variety of ultrastructural defects associated with clinical syndrome suggest considerable genetic heterogeneity.
- Structurally abnormal cilia move ineffectively and therefore predispose to sinusitis, recurrent pulmonary infections, and bronchiectasis.
- Reduced fertility is due to decreased motility of spermatozoa.
- Electron microscopic features include absent outer dynein arms, absent/short radial spokes, absent/defective inner dynein arms, absent/disoriented central microtubules, and peripheral microtubule transposition.

WHAT THE REFERRING PHYSICIAN NEEDS TO KNOW

- High-resolution CT is superior to chest radiography in determining presence and extent of bronchiectasis
- The radiologic findings, except for Kartagener syndrome, are nonspecific.
- Treatment consists mainly of antibiotics and physiotherapy.
- Prognosis is good; patients usually have normal life expectancy.
- Diagnosis is usually made by assessing ciliary motility in bronchial wall, nasal biopsy specimens, and semen samples; electron microscopy shows abnormal cilia morphology.

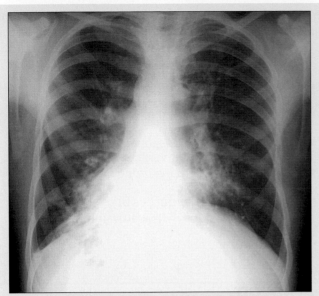

Figure 1. Kartagener syndrome: radiographic findings. Posteroanterior chest radiograph shows dextrocardia, situs inversus, bronchial wall thickening, and evidence of bronchiectasis.

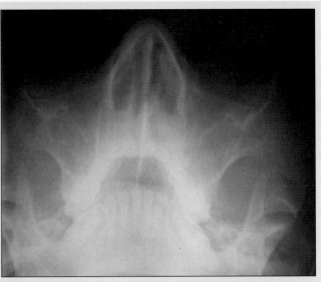

Figure 2. Kartagener syndrome: radiographic findings. View of the paranasal sinuses shows opacification of the maxillary sinuses consistent with chronic sinusitis. The triad of situs inversus totalis, bronchiectasis, and sinusitis is known as the Kartagener syndrome and occurs in approximately 50% of patients with primary ciliary dyskinesia.

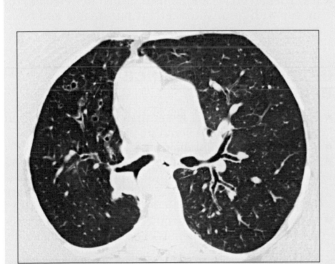

Figure 3. Kartagener syndrome. High-resolution CT in a 52-year-old woman at the level of the upper lobes shows dextrocardia and bilateral bronchiectasis.

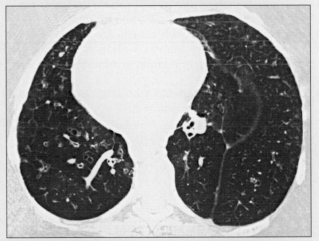

Figure 4. Kartagener syndrome. High-resolution CT in a 52-year-old woman at the level of the lung bases shows bilateral bronchiectasis and volume loss.

INCIDENCE/PREVALENCE AND EPIDEMIOLOGY

- Incidence in white persons is estimated to be between 1 in 12,500 and 1 in 40,000.
- Higher prevalence has been reported in Japan.
- Most common bacterial organism found in sputum is *Haemophilus influenzae.*
- Situs inversus totalis or heterotaxy is seen in approximately 50% of patients.
- Fifty percent of patients have Kartagener syndrome (situs inversus, sinusitis, and bronchiectasis).
- Pectus excavatum is seen in 9% of patients.

Suggested Readings

Jain K, Padley SP, Goldstraw EJ, et al: Primary ciliary dyskinesia in the paediatric population: Range and severity of radiological findings in a cohort of patients receiving tertiary care. *Clin Radiol* 62:986-993, 2007.

Kennedy MP, Noone PG, Leigh MW, et al: High-resolution CT of patients with primary ciliary dyskinesia. *AJR Am J Roentgenol* 188(5):1232-1238, 2007.

Morillas HN, Zariwala M, Knowles MR: Genetic causes of bronchiectasis: Primary ciliary dyskinesia. *Respiration* 74(3):252-263, 2007.

Rosen MJ: Chronic cough due to bronchiectasis: ACCP evidence-based clinical practice guidelines. *Chest* 129(1 Suppl):122S-131S, 2006.

Tracheomegaly and Tracheobronchomegaly

DEFINITION: Tracheomegaly and tracheobronchomegaly are rare conditions characterized by dilation of the tracheobronchial tree involving the trachea and main bronchi that may extend from the larynx to the lung periphery.

IMAGING

Radiography
Findings
- Calibers of trachea and major bronchi are increased.
- Air columns have an irregular corrugated appearance (tracheal diverticulosis).
- In women, transverse and sagittal diameters of trachea exceed 21 mm and 23 mm, respectively.
- In women, transverse diameters of right and left main bronchi exceed 19.8 mm and 17.4 mm, respectively.
- In men, transverse and sagittal diameters of the trachea exceed 25 mm and 27 mm, respectively.
- In men, transverse diameters of right and left main bronchi exceed 21.1 mm and 18.4 mm, respectively.

Utility
- Both tracheal dilation and tracheal diverticulosis are seen best in lateral projection.

CT
Findings
- Calibers of trachea and main bronchi are increased.
- Intrapulmonary bronchi are often dilated.
- Localized areas of bronchiectasis are seen.
- Dynamic CT and expiratory CT show ballooning of airways on inspiration and collapse of airways on expiration.
- Dilated bronchi of patients who have tracheobronchomegaly typically have thin walls.
- Recurrent infections may result in thick-walled bronchi and areas of consolidation.

Utility
- CT is superior to the radiograph in demonstrating dilatation of bronchi.

CLINICAL PRESENTATION

- May be asymptomatic or present as recurrent pneumonia.

PATHOLOGY

- Increased compliance of trachea results in abnormal flaccidity and easy collapsibility during forced expiration and coughing.
- Inefficient cough mechanism leads to retention of mucus with resultant recurrent pneumonia and bronchiectasis.

INCIDENCE/PREVALENCE AND EPIDEMIOLOGY

- This condition is rare; fewer than 100 cases had been reported in the world literature as of 2006.
- It is more common in males.
- Majority of cases are congenital; others are acquired as a complication of diffuse pulmonary fibrosis. Ankylosing spondylitis and rheumatoid arthritis are associated.
- Association occurs with other congenital abnormalities of the trachea, Ehlers-Danlos syndrome, and cutis laxa.
- Majority of patients are in their third and fourth decades of life (range: 18 months to 76 years).

WHAT THE REFERRING PHYSICIAN NEEDS TO KNOW
- Majority of cases are congenital; others are acquired as a complication of diffuse pulmonary fibrosis. Association with ankylosing spondylitis and rheumatoid arthritis may occur.
- Association occurs with other congenital abnormalities of the trachea, Ehlers-Danlos syndrome, and cutis laxa.
- Increased compliance of trachea results in abnormal flaccidity and easy collapsibility during forced expiration and coughing.
- Inefficient cough mechanism leads to retention of mucus with resultant recurrent pneumonia and bronchiectasis.
- Pulmonary function may be normal or show evidence of airflow obstruction due to associated small airway disease.

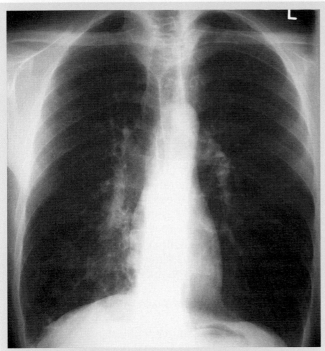

Figure 1. Tracheobronchomegaly (Mounier-Kuhn syndrome). Posteroanterior chest radiograph shows marked increase in caliber of the trachea and main bronchi.

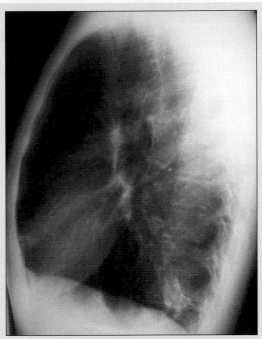

Figure 2. Tracheobronchomegaly (Mounier-Kuhn syndrome). Lateral chest radiograph shows marked increase in caliber of the trachea and main bronchi.

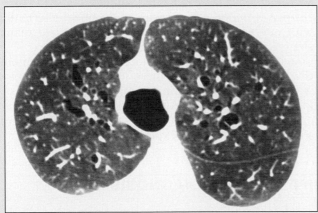

Figure 3. Tracheobronchomegaly (Mounier-Kuhn syndrome). High-resolution CT image at the level of the trachea shows tracheomegaly and increased caliber of the intraparenchymal bronchi. Note that the dilated intraparenchymal bronchi have thin walls, which is distinct from the bronchial wall thickening typically seen in patients who have bronchiectasis.

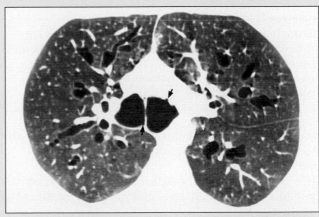

Figure 4. Tracheobronchomegaly (Mounier-Kuhn syndrome). High-resolution CT image at the level of the main bronchi shows increased caliber of the main bronchi and the intraparenchymal bronchi. Note that the dilated intraparenchymal bronchi have thin walls, which is distinct from the bronchial wall thickening typically seen in patients who have bronchiectasis. Minimal bilateral bronchial diverticulosis is also present (*arrows*).

Suggested Readings

Genta PR, Costa MV, Stelmach R, Cukier A: A 26-yr-old male with recurrent respiratory infections. *Eur Respir J* 22(3):564-567, 2003.

Ghanei M, Peyman M, Aslani J, Zamel N: Mounier-Kuhn syndrome: A rare cause of severe bronchial dilatation with normal pulmonary function test: A case report. *Respir Med* 101(8):1836-1839, 2007.

Hartman TE, Primack SL, Lee KS, et al: CT of bronchial and bronchiolar diseases. *RadioGraphics* 14:991-1003, 1994.

Kwong JS, Müller NL, Miller RR: Diseases of the trachea and mainstem bronchi: Correlation of CT with pathologic findings. *RadioGraphics* 12:645-657, 1992.

Marom EM, Goodman PC, McAdams HP: Diffuse abnormalities of the trachea and main bronchi. *AJR Am J Roentgenol* 176(3):713-717, 2001.

Asthma

DEFINITION: Asthma is an inflammatory disease characterized by increased airway reactivity and by air flow obstruction that is at least partially reversible and results in recurrent episodes of wheezing, breathlessness, and cough.

IMAGING

Radiography
Findings
- Often normal even during an acute attack
- Hyperinflation and bronchial wall thickening; ring shadows evident when viewed end on or "tram-track" opacities when viewed en face
- Prominence of hila, increased central lung markings, and peripheral oligemia
- Pulmonary hyperinflation, increase in depth of retrosternal space, increase in lung height, and flattening of diaphragm
- Complications: pneumonia, atelectasis, pneumomediastinum, and pneumothorax

Utility
- Of limited role in the diagnosis of asthma
- Important in excluding other conditions that cause wheezing and in identifying complications

CT
Findings
- Bronchial wall thickening and luminal narrowing.
- One or more bronchi dilated, typically cylindrical; bronchoarterial ratio usually < 1.5.
- Areas of decreased attenuation and vascularity.
- Air trapping on expiratory CT.
- Prominent centrilobular structures or small centrilobular opacities.
- Parenchymal abnormalities of hyperinflation, emphysema, and, occasionally, cystic spaces.

Utility
- Has limited role in diagnosis and management of patients with asthma and seldom indicated during an acute attack.
- Has value in diagnosis of endotracheal/endobronchial tumors that mimic asthma clinically and are difficult to visualize on radiography.
- Can distinguish asthma from tracheobronchomalacia.

DIAGNOSTIC PEARLS

- Chronic inflammatory disorder of the airways associated with exaggerated bronchoconstrictor response to a wide variety of stimuli, resulting in recurrent episodes of dyspnea and wheezing.
- Thickening of the airway walls by a combination of edema and increase in smooth muscle and in the size of the mucous glands.
- Hyperinflation and bronchial wall thickening on chest radiograph.
- Thickening and narrowing of the bronchi on high-resolution CT.
- Air trapping on expiratory high-resolution CT.

CLINICAL PRESENTATION

- High incidence of eczema and rhinitis.
- History of periodic paroxysms of dyspnea, alternating with intervals of complete or nearly complete remission.
- Cough prominent, and occasionally the only, symptom.
- Gradual increase in shortness of breath, cough, and wheezing and decrease in expiratory air flow.
- Physical findings: hyperventilation, inspiratory and expiratory rhonchi and wheezes, decreased breath sounds, and prolonged expiration.

DIFFERENTIAL DIAGNOSIS

- Tracheal neoplasms
- Tracheomalacia
- Aspiration of foreign bodies
- Bronchomalacia
- Endobronchial tumor

WHAT THE REFERRING PHYSICIAN NEEDS TO KNOW
- Chest radiograph has a limited role in the diagnosis of asthma. It is often normal, even during an acute attack; when it is abnormal, findings are nonspecific.
- Two main indications for imaging are to exclude other conditions that cause wheezing and to identify complications.
- CT is seldom indicated in diagnosis and management of patients with asthma.
- Main role of CT is assessment of tracheal and bronchial abnormalities that mimic asthma and assessment of complications of asthma, such as allergic bronchopulmonary aspergillosis.

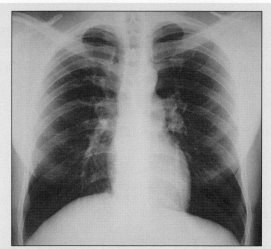

Figure 1. Acute asthma. Posteroanterior chest radiograph shows increased lung volumes and reduction of the peripheral vascular markings.

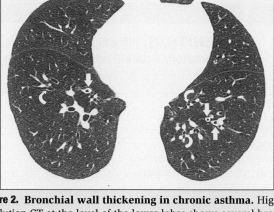

Figure 2. Bronchial wall thickening in chronic asthma. High-resolution CT at the level of the lower lobes shows several bronchi with thickened walls (*straight arrows*). Also noted are several normal appearing bronchi (*curved arrows*). The patient was a 67-year-old man who was a nonsmoker with chronic asthma.

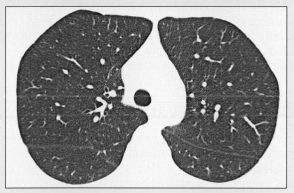

Figure 3. Air trapping in asthma. High-resolution CT performed at end inspiration shows subtle areas of decreased attenuation and vascularity. The patient was a 62-year-old man with wheezing and cough at the time of the CT.

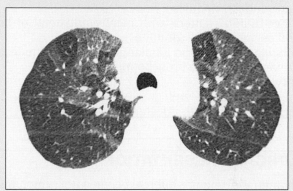

Figure 4. Air trapping in asthma. High-resolution CT performed after maximal expiration demonstrates extensive air trapping. The patient was a 62-year-old man with wheezing and cough at the time of the CT.

PATHOLOGY

- Pathophysiologic abnormality that determines the functional and symptomatic status of an asthmatic patient is airway narrowing.
- Chronic inflammation of the airways involves mainly the medium-sized and small bronchi.
- Air trapping reflects chronic inflammation, muscle hypertrophy of small airways, or development of obliterative bronchiolitis.
- This chronic inflammatory disorder of airways is associated with airway hyperresponsiveness and exaggerated bronchoconstrictor response to a wide variety of exogenous/endogenous stimuli.

INCIDENCE/PREVALENCE AND EPIDEMIOLOGY

- Affects 5%-25% of children and 2%-12% of adults.

- Highest prevalence found in United Kingdom, Australia, and New Zealand (approximately 12% each) and in Tristan da Cunha (56% of population).
- Prevalence before age of 10, incidence higher in boys than girls; after age of 10, incidence higher in females.
- United States: accounts for nearly 2 million emergency department visits, 500,000 hospitalizations, and 5,000 deaths each year.
- Australia, Canada, and Spain: acute asthma accounts for 1%-12% of all adult emergency department visits.
- France: 7% of adult patients with acute asthma in emergency department transferred to intensive care unit.

Suggested Readings

Global strategy for asthma management and prevention. Available at: http://www.ginasthma.com (2002). NIH publication 02–3659.

Rodrigo GJ, Rodrigo C, Hall JB: Acute asthma in adults: A review. *Chest* 125:1081-1102, 2004.

Silva CI, Colby TV, Müller NL: Asthma and associated conditions: High-resolution CT and pathologic findings. *AJR Am J Roentgenol* 183:817-824, 2004.

Infectious Bronchiolitis

DEFINITION: Infectious bronchiolitis is the presence of inflammatory cells in walls of airways and inflammatory exudate and mucus in airway lumens due to viral, bacterial, or fungal infection.

IMAGING

Radiography
Findings
- Bronchial wall thickening
- Hyperinflation due to partial small airway obstruction
- Bilateral nodular or reticulonodular pattern
- Patchy bilateral consolidation due to bronchopneumonia

Utility
- Radiograph often normal or shows nonspecific findings

CT
Findings
- Centrilobular nodules
- "Tree-in-bud" pattern with patchy unilateral or bilateral asymmetric distribution
- Airspace nodules and lobular ground-glass attenuation or consolidation in bronchopneumonia

Utility
- Superior to chest radiography in demonstrating findings consistent with infectious bronchiolitis

CLINICAL PRESENTATION

- Infants and young children begin with symptoms of upper respiratory tract infection and 2-3 days later have abrupt onset of dyspnea, tachypnea, and fever.
- Adults are probably infected with respiratory tract viruses as often as infants but not as severely.

DIFFERENTIAL DIAGNOSIS

- Tuberculosis
- Allergic bronchopulmonary aspergillosis
- Aspiration pneumonia
- Panbronchiolitis
- Bronchopneumonia
- Mucoid impaction in bronchiectasis
- *Mycobacterium avium-intracellulare* infection
- Proliferative bronchiolitis

DIAGNOSTIC PEARLS

- Centrilobular nodules and "tree-in-bud" pattern
- Bronchial wall thickening and peribronchial (central) areas of consolidation
- Centrilobular branching ("tree-in-bud" pattern) seen most commonly in infectious bronchiolitis, bronchopneumonia, tuberculosis, and mucoid impaction.

PATHOLOGY

- Presence of inflammatory cells in walls of airways and inflammatory exudate and mucus in airway lumens
- Inflammatory cells mainly neutrophils
- Necrosis of bronchiolar epithelium

INCIDENCE/PREVALENCE AND EPIDEMIOLOGY

- Disease is most common and severe in children.
- Incidence is as high as 10 per 100 children per year in first year of life in United States.
- Most common agents are viruses, particularly respiratory syncytial virus, adenoviruses, parainfluenzaviruses, influenzaviruses, and human metapneumovirus.
- Less common agents are *Mycoplasma*, *Chlamydia*, bacteria, and fungi (particularly *Aspergillus* in immunocompromised patients).

Suggested Readings

Colby TV: Bronchiolitis: Pathologic considerations. *Am J Clin Pathol* 109:101-109, 1998.
Pipavath SJ, Lynch DA, Cool C, et al: Radiologic and pathologic features of bronchiolitis. *AJR Am J Roentgenol* 185:354-363, 2005.
Pipavath SN, Stern EJ: Imaging of small airway disease (SAD). *Radiol Clin North Am* 47:307-316, 2009.
Ryu JH, Myers JL, Swensen SJ: Bronchiolar disorders. *Am J Respir Crit Care Med* 168:1277-1292, 2003.
Visscher DW, Myers JL: Bronchiolitis: The pathologist's perspective. *Proc Am Thorac Soc* 3:41-47, 2006.

WHAT THE REFERRING PHYSICIAN NEEDS TO KNOW

- Symptoms are often severe in infants.
- Disease is usually mild in adults.
- "Tree-in-bud" pattern is highly suggestive of small airway infection and seen commonly in infectious bronchiolitis, bronchopneumonia, and endobronchial spread of mycobacterial infection.

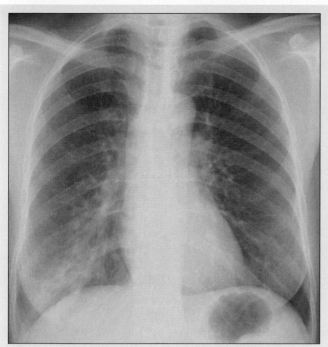

Figure 1. **Infectious bronchiolitis and bronchopneumonia.**
Posteroanterior chest radiograph shows poorly defined nodular
opacities and foci of consolidation in the right lower lobe. The
patient was a 48-year-old man with *Mycoplasma* bronchiolitis
and bronchopneumonia. (*Courtesy of Dr. Atsushi Nambu,
Department of Radiology, University of Yamanashi, Yamanashi,
Japan.*)

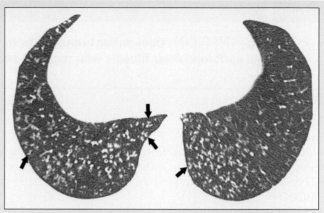

Figure 2. **"Tree-in-bud" pattern in infectious bronchiolitis.**
High-resolution CT image shows centrilobular branching nodular
and linear opacities resulting in a "tree-in-bud" appearance
(*arrows*). Patient was a 20-year-old woman with recurrent
respiratory tract infections.

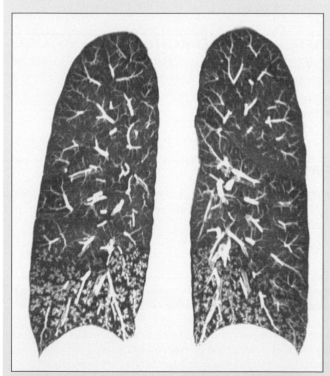

Figure 3. **"Tree-in-bud" pattern in infectious bronchiolitis.**
Coronal maximum intensity projection image demonstrates "tree-
in-bud" pattern in the lower lobes. Patient was a 20-year-old
woman with recurrent respiratory tract infections.

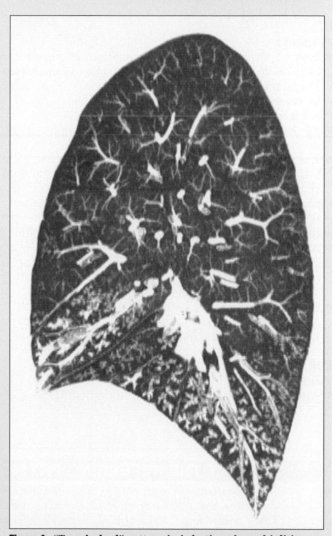

Figure 4. **"Tree-in-bud" pattern in infectious bronchiolitis.**
Sagittal maximum intensity projection image demonstrates "tree-
in-bud" pattern in right lower lobe and in the right middle lobe.
Patient was a 20-year-old woman with recurrent respiratory tract
infections.

Obliterative Bronchiolitis (Bronchiolitis Obliterans)

DEFINITION: Obliterative bronchiolitis (bronchiolitis obliterans) is characterized by submucosal and peribronchiolar fibrosis with resulting bronchiolar narrowing or obliteration of the bronchiolar lumen.

IMAGING

Radiography

Findings
- Often normal in patients with mild to moderate disease
- Peripheral attenuation of vascular markings
- Hyperinflation resulting in overall increase in lung volumes
- Flattening of diaphragm
- Increase in retrosternal airspace
- Ancillary findings: prominent bronchial markings, bronchiectasis, and nodular or reticulonodular opacities

Utility
- Of limited value in diagnosis

CT

Findings
- Mosaic perfusion pattern (mosaic attenuation pattern) (40%-80% of patients) is noted as areas of decreased attenuation and vascularity and as areas of normal/increased attenuation and vascularity.
- Air trapping seen on expiratory images.
- To be considered abnormal, air trapping needs to involve more than 25% of the lung.
- Ancillary findings (20%-90% of patients) include central and peripheral bronchial dilatation (bronchiectasis), bronchiolectasis, and bronchial wall thickening.

Utility
- CT is superior to chest radiography in the assessment of the presence and severity of obliterative bronchiolitis.
- Abnormalities may be subtle on inspiratory images.
- Expiratory CT images may demonstrate air trapping in patients with normal or subtle findings on inspiratory scans.
- Presence of air flow obstruction/air trapping is easier to detect on high-resolution CT performed at end expiration or during maximal expiration.

MRI

Findings
- Areas of decreased ventilation and perfusion

DIAGNOSTIC PEARLS

- Areas of decreased attenuation and vascularity and areas of increased attenuation and vascularity (mosaic attenuation/perfusion pattern) on inspiratory high-resolution CT
- Air trapping on expiratory CT can be seen normally in the dependent lung regions and tips of the middle lobe or lingula
- To be considered abnormal, air trapping has to involve more than 25% of the lung and/or areas of nondependent lung
- Bronchiectasis is commonly present

Utility
- Hyperpolarized ^{3}He-enhanced MRI allows earlier recognition of obstructive airway disease.
- Seldom used in clinical practice.

CLINICAL PRESENTATION

- Dry cough and progressive shortness of breath
- Chest pain, respiratory distress, and cyanosis
- Demonstration of air flow obstruction on pulmonary function tests

DIFFERENTIAL DIAGNOSIS

- Asthma
- Chronic bronchitis
- Emphysema
- Bronchomalacia
- Normal lungs

PATHOLOGY

- There is submucosal accumulation of mucopolysaccharide proteins and submucosal and peribronchiolar fibrosis.

WHAT THE REFERRING PHYSICIAN NEEDS TO KNOW

- Obliterative bronchiolitis is usually irreversible.
- The characteristic high-resolution CT manifestation of obliterative bronchiolitis consists of areas of decreased attenuation and vascularity on inspiratory CT and air trapping on expiratory CT
- Ancillary findings such as bronchiectasis, bronchiolectasis, and bronchial wall thickening are found in 20% to 90% of patients.
- Although CT findings can be highly suggestive of obliterative bronchiolitis, specific diagnosis requires correlation with clinical findings, pulmonary function tests, and, in some cases, lung biopsy.

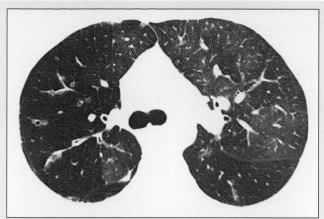

Figure 1. Obliterative bronchiolitis. High-resolution CT image shows extensive bilateral areas of decreased attenuation and vascularity (mosaic perfusion/attenuation pattern) mainly in right lung with blood flow redistribution to left upper lobe. Also note right upper lobe bronchiectasis. Patient was a 22-year-old man with obliterative bronchiolitis after stem cell transplantation for neuroblastoma in early childhood.

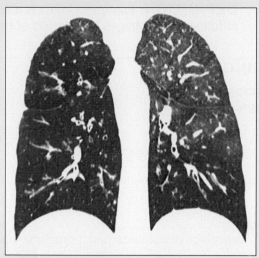

Figure 2. Obliterative bronchiolitis. Coronal reformatted high-resolution CT image demonstrates overall extent of abnormalities with severe disease in right lung and most of left lower lobe. Relative sparing of left upper lobe is associated with marked increase in vascularity (mosaic perfusion/attenuation pattern) due to blood flow redistribution. Patient was a 22-year-old man with obliterative bronchiolitis after stem cell transplantation for neuroblastoma in early childhood.

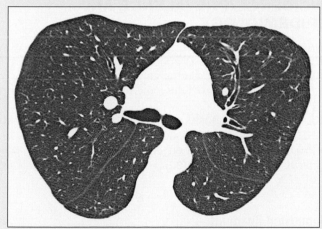

Figure 3. Obliterative bronchiolitis: value of expiratory high-resolution CT. Inspiratory high-resolution CT image shows subtle bilateral areas of decreased attenuation and vascularity. Patient had obliterative bronchiolitis after stem cell transplant for multiple myeloma.

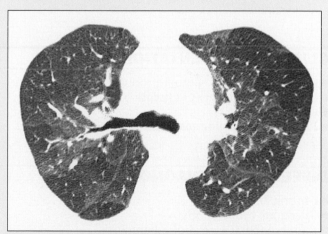

Figure 4. Obliterative bronchiolitis: value of expiratory high-resolution CT. Expiratory high-resolution CT image demonstrates extensive bilateral air trapping. Patient had obliterative bronchiolitis after stem cell transplant for multiple myeloma.

- Fibrosis surrounds rather than fills lumen and results in extrinsic compression and eventually complete obliteration of bronchiolar lumen.
- Areas of bronchiolar fibrosis are typically patchy.

INCIDENCE/PREVALENCE AND EPIDEMIOLOGY

- Obliterative bronchiolitis has been associated with a wide variety of causes and conditions.
- Relatively common causes in the adult include previous infection, connective tissue diseases, transplant, inhalational injuries, cigarette smoke, and drug reactions.

- It is commonly seen in association with large airway disease (e.g., bronchiectasis) and parenchymal disease (e.g., hypersensitivity pneumonitis).

Suggested Readings

Chan A, Allen R: Bronchiolitis obliterans: An update. *Curr Opin Pulm Med* 10:133-141, 2004.

Hansell DM, Rubens MB, Padley SP, Wells AU: Obliterative bronchiolitis: Individual CT signs of small airways disease and functional correlation. *Radiology* 203:721-726, 1997.

Lynch DA: Imaging of small airways disease and chronic obstructive pulmonary disease. *Clin Chest Med* 29:165-179, 2008.

Pipavath SN, Stern EJ: Imaging of small airway disease (SAD). *Radiol Clin North AM* 47:307-316, 2009.

Panbronchiolitis

DEFINITION: Panbronchiolitis is a disease of unknown etiology characterized by accumulation of foamy macrophages in the walls of respiratory bronchioles and alveolar ducts.

IMAGING

Radiography
Findings
- Diffuse nodules < 5 mm in diameter
- Reticulonodular pattern, bronchial wall thickening, and mild to moderate hyperinflation

Utility
- Of limited value in the diagnosis

CT
Findings
- Small centrilobular nodules and branching opacities ("tree-in-bud" pattern), bronchiolectasis, bronchiectasis, and mosaic perfusion pattern.
- Earliest manifestation is centrilobular nodular opacities, followed by branching opacities that connect to nodules, followed by bronchiolectasis, and, eventually, bronchiectasis.
- Cystic bronchiectasis in late stage.

Utility
- Superior to radiography in the detection of airway abnormalities.

CLINICAL PRESENTATION

- Cough, often with sputum production
- Progressive shortness of breath
- Chronic sinusitis
- Pulmonary function tests: air flow obstruction

DIFFERENTIAL DIAGNOSIS

- Chronic bronchitis
- Infectious bronchiolitis
- Endobronchial spread of tuberculosis
- *Mycobacterium avium-intracellulare* infection
- Bronchiectasis

PATHOLOGY

- Characterized histologically by accumulation of mononuclear inflammatory cells in walls of respiratory bronchioles, alveolar ducts, and adjacent alveoli.

DIAGNOSTIC PEARLS

- Occurs almost exclusively in Asia, particularly Japan.
- Chest radiograph shows diffuse small nodular pattern and hyperinflation.
- High-resolution CT shows small centrilobular nodules and branching opacities ("tree-in-bud" pattern), bronchiolectasis, bronchiectasis, and mosaic areas of decreased attenuation and vascularity.
- Chronic inflammation of paranasal sinuses is associated.

- Late stage of disease frequently complicated by colonization with *Pseudomonas aeruginosa*.

INCIDENCE/PREVALENCE AND EPIDEMIOLOGY

- Average age at onset is approximately 40 years.
- Male-to-female ratio is about 2:1.
- It occurs almost exclusively in Asia, particularly Japan, with few cases described in North America and Europe.
- A genetic predisposition located between HLA-A and HLA-B loci is highly associated.
- Prognosis is worse when infection with *Pseudomonas aeruginosa* is associated, with 10-year survival rate of 12%.

Suggested Readings

Azuma A, Kudoh S: Diffuse panbronchiolitis in East Asia. *Respirology* 11:249-261, 2006.

Iwata M, Colby TV, Kitaichi M: Diffuse panbronchiolitis: Diagnosis and distinction from various pulmonary diseases with centrilobular interstitial foam cell accumulations. *Hum Pathol* 25:357-363, 1994.

Lynch DA: Imaging of small airways disease and chronic obstructive pulmonary disease. *Clin Chest Med* 29:165-179, 2008.

Nishimura K, Kitaichi M, Izumi T, Itoh H: Diffuse panbronchiolitis: Correlation of high-resolution CT and pathologic findings. *Radiology* 184:779-785, 1992.

WHAT THE REFERRING PHYSICIAN NEEDS TO KNOW
- Disease occurs almost exclusively in Asia, particularly Japan.
- High-resolution CT typically shows bilateral centrilobular nodules, "tree-in-bud" pattern, and bronchiectasis.
- Majority of patients respond to low-dose macrolide therapy.
- Late stage of the disease is frequently complicated by colonization with *Pseudomonas aeruginosa*.

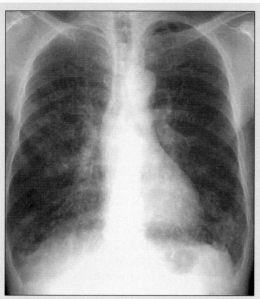

Figure 1. Diffuse panbronchiolitis: radiographic findings.
Chest radiograph in a patient with diffuse panbronchiolitis shows
bilateral reticulonodular pattern, bronchial wall thickening, and
increased lung volumes. (*Courtesy of Dr. Kyung Soo Lee, Samsung
Medical Center, Seoul, South Korea.*)

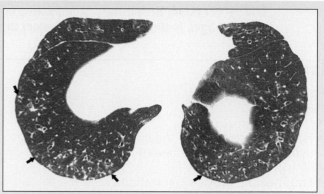

Figure 2. Diffuse panbronchiolitis. High-resolution CT at
presentation in a 47-year-old man with panbronchiolitis shows
centrilobular nodules and branching opacities resulting in a
"tree-in-bud" pattern (*straight arrows*), extensive bronchiectasis,
and localized areas of decreased attenuation and perfusion.

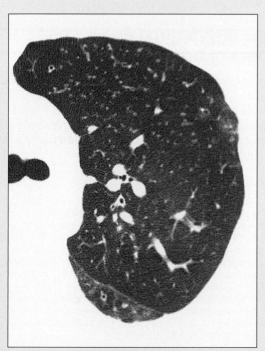

Figure 3. Diffuse panbronchiolitis. View of left upper lobe from
high-resolution CT scan in 44-year-old woman with severe long-
standing panbronchiolitis shows extensive areas of decreased
attenuation and vascularity, mild bronchiectasis, and a few
centrilobular nodules and branching opacities. (*Courtesy of Dr.
Noriyuki Tomiyama, Department of Radiology, Osaka University
Graduate School of Medicine, Osaka, Japan.*)

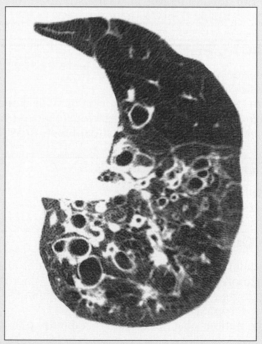

Figure 4. Diffuse panbronchiolitis. View of left lung at level
of inferior pulmonary vein from high-resolution CT scan in a
44-year-old woman with severe long-standing panbronchiolitis
shows cystic bronchiectasis in left lower lobe and lingula. Also
noted is diffuse decreased attenuation and vascularity in lingula.
(*Courtesy of Dr. Noriyuki Tomiyama, Department of Radiology,
Osaka University Graduate School of Medicine, Osaka, Japan.*)

Respiratory Bronchiolitis

DEFINITION: Respiratory bronchiolitis is characterized histologically by accumulation of pigmented macrophages in the lumens of respiratory bronchioles and adjacent alveoli.

IMAGING

Radiography

Findings
- Usually normal
- Poorly defined small nodular opacities or poorly defined areas of increased opacity (ground-glass opacities)
- Emphysema or bronchial wall thickening

Utility
- Rarely shows any demonstrable abnormality

CT

Findings
- Usually normal
- Centrilobular emphysema
- Poorly defined centrilobular nodules and/or patchy bilateral ground-glass opacities
- Ground-glass rather than soft tissue attenuation of nodules that measure 3-5 mm in diameter
- Can be diffuse but most commonly involves predominantly or exclusively upper lobes

Utility
- Superior to radiograph in demonstrating presence of parenchymal and airway abnormalities

CLINICAL PRESENTATION

- Not associated with symptoms
- Occasionally extensive
- When symptomatic or associated with functional evidence of lung disease, referred to as respiratory bronchiolitis–associated interstitial lung disease

DIFFERENTIAL DIAGNOSIS

- Chronic bronchitis
- Hypersensitivity pneumonitis

PATHOLOGY

- Characterized histologically by intraluminal and peribronchiolar airspace accumulation of macrophages containing a fine brown cytoplasmic pigment ("smoker's macrophages").
- Pigmentation most likely from metabolites of cigarette.

DIAGNOSTIC PEARLS

- Vast majority of cases occur in smokers.
- Characteristic findings in CT are poorly defined centrilobular nodules and/or patchy bilateral ground-glass opacities in the upper lobes.
- Upper lobe predominance of centrilobular nodules and association with emphysema favors the diagnosis of respiratory bronchiolitis, whereas diffuse parenchymal involvement associated with areas of lobular air trapping favors hypersensitivity pneumonitis.
- History of cigarette smoking is important because cigarette smokers have a lower prevalence of hypersensitivity pneumonitis than nonsmokers.

- Other findings: mild chronic inflammation and fibrosis of bronchiolar walls, mild peribronchiolar mononuclear inflammatory infiltrate, and mild peribronchiolar fibrosis.

INCIDENCE/PREVALENCE AND EPIDEMIOLOGY

- Vast majority of cases are associated with cigarette smoke.
- Occurrence is rare in nonsmokers.
- Intensity of macrophage pigmentation and of peribronchiolar fibrosis correlates with number of pack-years smoked.

Suggested Readings

Fraig M, Shreesha U, Savici D, Katzenstein AL: Respiratory bronchiolitis: A clinicopathologic study in current smokers, ex-smokers, and never-smokers. *Am J Surg Pathol* 26:647-653, 2002.

Heyneman LE, Ward S, Lynch DA, et al: Respiratory bronchiolitis, respiratory bronchiolitis-associated interstitial lung disease, and desquamative interstitial pneumonia: Different entities or part of the spectrum of the same disease process?. *AJR Am J Roentgenol* 173:1617-1622, 1999.

Kanne JP, Bilawich AM, Lee CH, et al: Smoking-related emphysema and interstitial lung diseases. *J Thorac Imaging* 22:286-291, 2007.

Visscher DW, Myers JL: Bronchiolitis: The pathologist's perspective. *Proc Am Thorac Soc* 3:41-47, 2006.

WHAT THE REFERRING PHYSICIAN NEEDS TO KNOW

- Condition is asymptomatic.
- Usually an incidental finding seen on high-resoultion CT or surgical biopsy specimens.
- When symptoms occur, condition is referred to as respiratory bronchiolitis–associated interstitial lung disease.
- Patients are almost always smokers; radiograph may demonstrate findings of emphysema.

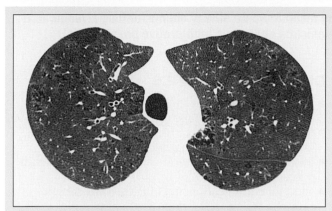

Figure 1. **Respiratory bronchiolitis.** High-resolution CT shows bilateral patchy ground-glass opacities, a few centrilobular nodules, and mild emphysema.

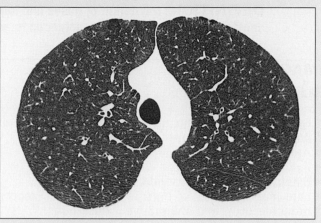

Figure 2. **Respiratory bronchiolitis.** High-resolution CT shows poorly defined bilateral centrilobular nodules and mild emphysema. (*Courtesy of Dr. Catherine Beigelman-Aubry, Pitié-Salpetriere Hospital, Paris.*)

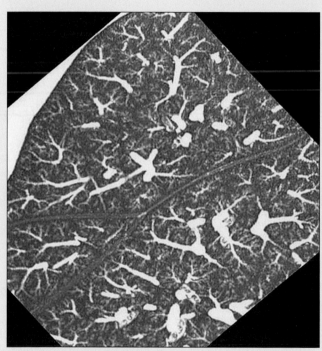

Figure 3. **Respiratory bronchiolitis.** Maximum intensity projection image better demonstrates the centrilobular nodules. (*Courtesy of Dr. Catherine Beigelman-Aubry, Pitié-Salpetriere Hospital, Paris.*)

Inhalation of Gases and Fumes

DEFINITION: Inhalation of gases and fumes may result in acute airway edema, diffuse alveolar damage, tracheal stenosis, bronchiectasis, and bronchiolitis obliterans (obliterative bronchiolitis).

IMAGING

Radiography
Findings
- Bronchial wall thickening, perivascular haziness, and poorly defined focal opacities
- Atelectasis and edema
- Patchy or diffuse bilateral consolidation
- Extensive bilateral consolidation
- Late manifestations of burn injury: tracheal stenosis, bronchiectasis, and obliterative bronchiolitis.

Utility
- Patients with abnormal radiograph within 48 hours after inhalation injury are more likely to require ventilatory support and have worse prognosis.
- Chest radiograph is much more likely to be abnormal 2-5 days after a burn.

CT
Findings
- Tracheal stenosis
- Bronchiectasis and areas of decreased attenuation and perfusion on inspiratory images and air trapping on expiratory CT are consistent with obliterative bronchiolitis

Utility
- Seldom performed after acute smoke inhalation
- Has main role in assessment of late complications

CLINICAL PRESENTATION

- Cough and shortness of breath are most common clinical manifestations.
- Severe exposure may result in respiratory failure and death.
- Abrupt onset of cough, dyspnea, weakness, and choking feeling are features of the earliest phase of silo filler's lung.
- Pulmonary edema can develop within 4 to 24 hours, clearing without residual lung damage if patient with silo filler's lung survives.
- At 2-5 weeks, symptoms abate during second phase.
- In third phase, progressive shortness of breath is due to obliterative bronchiolitis.

DIAGNOSTIC PEARLS

- Acute manifestations include airway edema and diffuse alveolar damage
- Bronchial wall thickening, perivascular haziness, and poorly defined focal opacities
- Patchy or diffuse bilateral consolidation in a small percentage of cases
- Chronic complications include tracheal stenosis, bronchiectasis, and evidence of obliterative bronchiolitis

DIFFERENTIAL DIAGNOSIS

- Bronchopneumonia
- Acute respiratory distress syndrome
- Hydrostatic pulmonary edema
- Bronchiolitis obliterans from other causes

PATHOLOGY

- Patients who inhale NO_2 will suffer bronchopulmonary irritation.
- Diffuse alveolar damage has also been documented in some patients.
- Airway abnormalities and pulmonary parenchymal disease are common and important complications of smoke inhalation.
- Direct trauma as a result of heat can cause severe tissue damage, particularly to airway mucosa.
- Smoke inhalation can also be associated with acute bronchiolitis; this often resolves but occasionally progresses to obliterative bronchiolitis.

INCIDENCE/PREVALENCE AND EPIDEMIOLOGY

- Pulmonary complications occur in 20%-30% of burn victims admitted to hospital.
- Bronchiolitis may be major manifestation or a minor component.

WHAT THE REFERRING PHYSICIAN NEEDS TO KNOW

- Chest radiograph is often initially normal.
- Pulmonary complications that typically become evident 2-5 days after a burn include atelectasis, edema, and pneumonia.
- Late manifestations of burn injury include tracheal stenosis, bronchiectasis, and obliterative bronchiolitis.

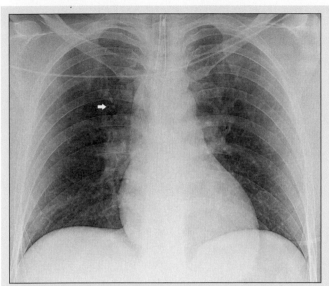

Figure 1. Acute smoke inhalation. Anteroposterior chest radiograph shows bronchial wall thickening (*arrow*), poorly defined small nodular opacities mainly in upper lobes, and prominence of pulmonary vessels. Patient was a 35-year-old man with acute smoke inhalation from a home fire.

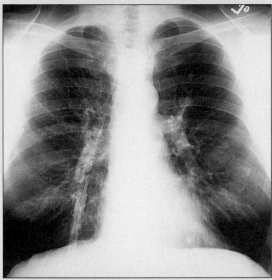

Figure 2. Obliterative bronchiolitis and bronchiectasis after smoke inhalation. Posteroanterior chest radiograph in a 33-year-old man shows increased lung volume, bronchiectasis, and decreased peripheral vascular markings. (*Courtesy of Dr. Christopher Griffin, Department of Radiology, Veterans Affairs Hospital, Portland, Oregon. From Müller NL, Fraser RS, Colman NC, Paré PD: Radiologic Diagnosis of Diseases of the Chest. Philadelphia, WB Saunders, 2001.*)

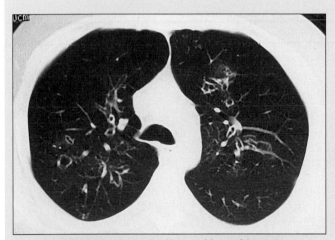

Figure 3. Obliterative bronchiolitis and bronchiectasis after smoke inhalation. High-resolution CT scan at the level of carina shows extensive central bronchiectasis and areas of decreased attenuation and vascularity as a result of obliterative bronchiolitis. The patient had experienced severe smoke inhalation several years earlier. (*Courtesy of Dr. Christopher Griffin, Department of Radiology, Veterans Affairs Hospital, Portland, Oregon. From Müller NL, Fraser RS, Colman NC, Paré PD: Radiologic Diagnosis of Diseases of the Chest. Philadelphia, WB Saunders, 2001.*)

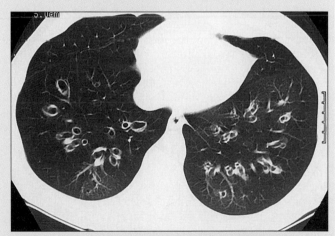

Figure 4. Obliterative bronchiolitis and bronchiectasis after smoke inhalation. High-resolution scan at the level of lung bases shows extensive bronchiectasis and areas of decreased attenuation and vascularity as a result of obliterative bronchiolitis. The patient had experienced severe smoke inhalation several years earlier. (*Courtesy of Dr. Christopher Griffin, Department of Radiology, Veterans Affairs Hospital, Portland, Oregon. From Müller NL, Fraser RS, Colman NC, Paré PD: Radiologic Diagnosis of Diseases of the Chest. Philadelphia, WB Saunders, 2001.*)

Suggested Readings

Lynch DA: Imaging of small airways disease and chronic obstructive pulmonary disease. *Clin Chest Med* 29:165-179, 2008.

Pipavath SJ, Lynch DA, Cool C, et al: Radiologic and pathologic features of bronchiolitis. *AJR Am J Roentgenol* 185:354-363, 2005.

Rabinowitz PM, Siegel MD: Acute inhalation injury. *Clin Chest Med* 23:707-715, 2002.

Ryu JH, Myers JL, Swensen SJ: Bronchiolar disorders. *Am J Respir Crit Care Med* 168:1277-1292, 2003.

Visscher DW, Myers JL: Bronchiolitis: The pathologist's perspective. *Proc Am Thorac Soc* 3:41-47, 2006.

Bronchiolitis Obliterans after Transplantation

DEFINITION: Obliterative bronchiolitis (bronchiolitis obliterans) is a common late complication following lung, heart-lung, and allogeneic hematopoietic stem cell transplantation.

IMAGING

Radiography
Findings
- Often normal in patients with mild to moderate disease
- Peripheral attenuation of the vascular markings and hyperinflation resulting in overall increase in lung volumes
- Flattening of the diaphragm
- Increase in the retrosternal airspace

Utility
- Chest radiography is of limited value in the diagnosis of patients with mild to moderate disease

CT
Findings
- Mosaic attenuation and perfusion pattern: areas of decreased attenuation and vascularity and areas of normal/increased attenuation and vascularity.
- Air trapping on expiratory CT.
- Ancillary findings: central and peripheral bronchial dilatation (bronchiectasis), bronchiolectasis and bronchial wall thickening, small centrilobular nodules, and "tree-in-bud" opacities.

Utility
- High-resolution CT is the imaging modality of choice in the diagnosis of obliterative bronchiolitis.
- Presence of air flow obstruction/air trapping is easier to detect on high-resolution CT performed at end expiration or during maximal expiration.
- Expiratory CT images may demonstrate air trapping in patients with normal or subtle findings on inspiratory scans.

MRI
Findings
- Hyperpolarized ³He-enhanced MRI demonstrates overall pulmonary ventilation and focal ventilation defects.

Utility
- Hyperpolarized ³He-enhanced MRI may allow earlier recognition of obstructive airway disease.
- MRI may be useful in early recognition and follow-up of obliterative bronchiolitis.
- Main advantages are functional imaging and lack of radiation.
- Not used in clinical practice.

DIAGNOSTIC PEARLS
- Presence of air trapping on expiratory CT scans
- Mosaic perfusion pattern
- Demonstration of air flow obstruction on pulmonary function tests

CLINICAL PRESENTATION
- Dry cough and progressive shortness of breath
- Chest pain, respiratory distress, and cyanosis
- Demonstration of air flow obstruction on pulmonary function tests

DIFFERENTIAL DIAGNOSIS
- Asthma
- Emphysema
- Chronic bronchitis
- Normal lung

PATHOLOGY
- Submucosal accumulation of mucopolysaccharide proteins and submucosal and peribronchiolar fibrosis

INCIDENCE/PREVALENCE AND EPIDEMIOLOGY
- Bronchiolitis is single leading cause of morbidity and mortality in patients with lung and heart-lung transplantation.
- Prevalence of obliterative bronchiolitis after lung transplantation is estimated at 20% at 1 year and greater than 50% at 3 to 5 years.
- It is the most common noninfectious late pulmonary complication of allogeneic hematopoietic stem cell transplantation.
- Bronchiolitis affects up to 20% of patients who receive allogeneic bone marrow transplants.

WHAT THE REFERRING PHYSICIAN NEEDS TO KNOW
- High-resolution CT plays a major role in diagnosis of bronchiolitis.
- Air trapping on expiratory CT scans is the most sensitive and accurate radiologic indicator of obliterative bronchiolitis after transplantation.

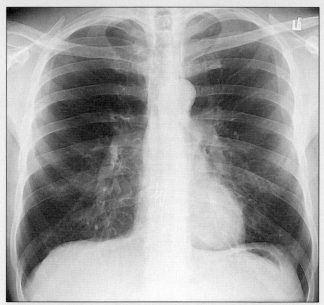

Figure 1. **Obliterative bronchiolitis.** Posteroanterior chest radiograph shows hyperinflation and marked attenuation of peripheral vascular markings. Patient was a 44-year-old man with obliterative bronchiolitis after bilateral lung transplantation for cystic fibrosis.

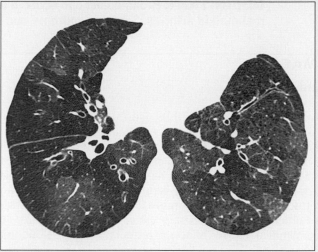

Figure 2. **Obliterative bronchiolitis.** High-resolution CT image shows extensive bilateral areas of decreased attenuation and vascularity and areas of normal or increased attenuation and vascularity (mosaic attenuation and perfusion pattern). Also note evidence of bronchiectasis. Patient was a 20-year-old woman with obliterative bronchiolitis after double-lung transplant for cystic fibrosis.

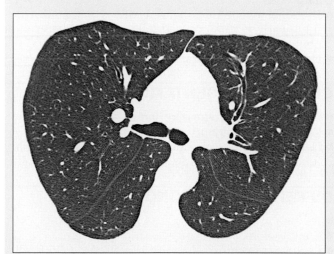

Figure 3. **Air trapping in obliterative bronchiolitis.** High-resolution CT image shows subtle areas of decreased attenuation and vascularity. The patient was a 54-year-old woman with obliterative bronchiolitis 4 months after stem cell transplantation for multiple myeloma.

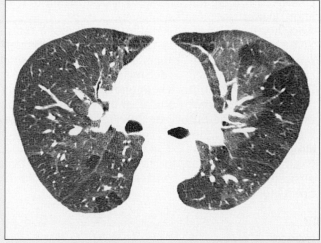

Figure 4. **Air trapping in obliterative bronchiolitis.** Expiratory CT demonstrates extensive bilateral air trapping. The patient was a 54-year-old woman with obliterative bronchiolitis 4 months after stem cell transplantation for multiple myeloma.

Suggested Readings

Boehler A, Estenne M: Post-transplant bronchiolitis obliterans. *Eur Respir J* 22:1007-1018, 2003.

Cooper JD, Billingham M, Egan T, et al: A working formulation for the standardization of nomenclature and for clinical staging of chronic dysfunction in lung allografts. International Society for Heart and Lung Transplantation. *J Heart Lung Transplant* 12:713-716, 1993.

Lynch DA. Imaging of small airways disease and chronic obstructive pulmonary disease. *Clin Chest Med* 29:165-179, 2008.

Ng YL, Paul N, Patsios D, et al: Imaging of lung transplantation: review. *AJR Am J Roentgenol* 192 (3 Suppl):S1-S13, Quiz S14-S19, 2009.

Soubani AO, Uberti JP: Bronchiolitis obliterans following haematopoietic stem cell transplantation. *Eur Respir J* 29:1007-1019, 2007.

Bronchiolitis in Connective Tissue Disease

DEFINITION: Bronchiolitis can occur in association with connective tissue disease such as rheumatoid arthritis, Sjögren syndrome, and systemic lupus erythematosus.

IMAGING

Radiography
Findings
- Obliterative bronchiolitis (bronchiolitis obliterans) commonly manifests as a normal finding.
- Severe obliterative bronchiolitis results in hyperinflation and attenuation of peripheral vascular markings.
- Mild to moderate bronchiectasis is difficult to detect on radiography; severe bronchiectasis results in tram-tracking and cystic changes.
- Follicular bronchiolitis: chest radiograph may be normal or show bilateral reticular or reticulonodular opacities.

Utility
- Limited value in diagnosis

CT
Findings
- Obliterative bronchiolitis: sharply defined areas of decreased lung attenuation associated with vessels of decreased caliber; blood flow redistribution to normal lung results in areas of increased attenuation and vascularity, a finding known as mosaic perfusion (attenuation) pattern.
- Ancillary findings of obliterative bronchiolitis: central and peripheral bronchial dilatation (bronchiectasis), bronchiolectasis and bronchial wall thickening, small centrilobular nodules, and "tree-in-bud" opacities.
- Follicular bronchiolitis (pulmonary lymphoid hyperplasia): bilateral centrilobular and peribronchial nodules that may be diffuse or involve mainly the lower lung zones.

Utility
- Expiratory CT is superior to inspiratory CT in demonstrating findings consistent with obliterative bronchiolitis.

MRI
Findings
- Obliterative bronchiolitis: areas of decreased ventilation and perfusion.

DIAGNOSTIC PEARLS

- Clinical history of dry cough and progressive shortness of breath; demonstration of air flow obstruction on pulmonary function tests.
- Obliterative bronchiolitis: sharply defined areas of decreased lung attenuation associated with vessels of decreased caliber; air trapping on expiratory CT.
- Occurs most commonly in rheumatoid arthritis.
- Air trapping can be seen in normal lungs in the most dependent lung regions and the tips of the middle lobe and lingula.
- Ancillary findings of obliterative bronchiolitis: central and peripheral bronchial dilatation (bronchiectasis), bronchiolectasis, and bronchial wall thickening.
- Follicular bronchiolitis (pulmonary lymphoid hyperplasia): bilateral centrilobular and peribronchial nodules.

Utility
- Hyperpolarized ^{3}He-enhanced MRI is potentially useful in early recognition and follow-up of patients with obliterative bronchiolitis.
- Not used in clinical practice.

CLINICAL PRESENTATION

- Dry cough and progressive shortness of breath
- Chest pain, respiratory distress, and cyanosis
- Demonstration of air flow obstruction on pulmonary function tests of patients with obliterative bronchiolitis

DIFFERENTIAL DIAGNOSIS

- Asthma
- Emphysema
- Chronic bronchitis
- Drug reaction
- Normal lung

WHAT THE REFERRING PHYSICIAN NEEDS TO KNOW

- Obliterative bronchiolitis in connective tissue disease is heterogeneous in severity and progression.
- Expiratory high-resolution CT is the imaging modality of choice for the demonstration of findings consistent with bronchiolitis obliterans.
- Penicillamine therapy and gold therapy are potential contributive causative agents of obliterative bronchiolitis in some patients with rheumatoid arthritis.
- Specific diagnosis requires correlation with clinical findings and, frequently, laboratory and bronchoalveolar lavage findings.
- Symptomatic pulmonary lymphoid hyperplasia occurs most commonly in patients with rheumatoid arthritis; the radiologic findings are nonspecific.

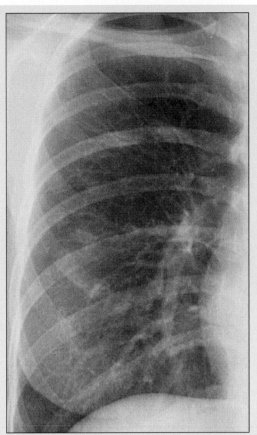

Figure 1. Pulmonary lymphoid hyperplasia in rheumatoid arthritis. View of the right lung from posteroanterior chest radiograph shows ill-defined nodular opacities. A similar pattern was present in the left lung. The patient was a 24-year-old woman who had rheumatoid disease and biopsy-proven pulmonary lymphoid hyperplasia (follicular bronchiolitis). (*From Müller NL, Fraser RS, Colman NC, Paré PD: Radiologic Diagnosis of Diseases of the Chest, WB Saunders, Philadelphia, 2001.*)

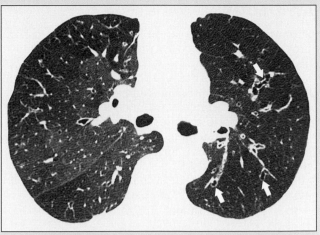

Figure 2. Obliterative bronchiolitis in rheumatoid arthritis. High-resolution CT shows "mosaic attenuation" pattern, with areas of decreased attenuation and vascularity, bronchiectasis (*arrows*), and bronchial wall thickening.

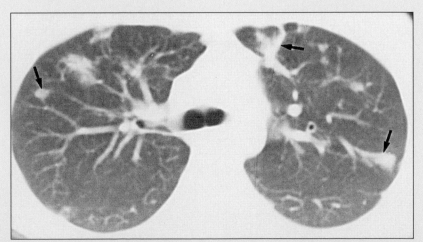

Figure 3. Pulmonary lymphoid hyperplasia in rheumatoid arthritis. Conventional 10-mm collimation CT scan shows focal nodular areas of consolidation in both lungs, located in a predominantly peribronchovascular distribution (*arrows*). The patient was a 24-year-old woman who had rheumatoid disease and biopsy-proven pulmonary lymphoid hyperplasia (follicular bronchiolitis). (*From Müller NL, Fraser RS, Colman NC, Paré PD: Radiologic Diagnosis of Diseases of the Chest, WB Saunders, Philadelphia, 2001.*)

PATHOLOGY

- Submucosal accumulation of mucopolysaccharide proteins and submucosal and peribronchiolar fibrosis occur.
- Fibrosis surrounds rather than fills lumen and results in extrinsic compression and eventually complete obliteration of bronchiolar lumen.
- Areas of bronchiolar fibrosis are typically patchy.
- Obstructive bronchiolitis in the setting of connective tissue disease is seen most commonly in patients with rheumatoid arthritis.
- Follicular bronchiolitis is characterized by lymphoid hyperplasia of bronchus-associated lymphoid tissue with follicles distributed along bronchioles.

INCIDENCE/PREVALENCE AND EPIDEMIOLOGY

- Obliterative bronchiolitis as sole presenting feature of rheumatoid arthritis is rare.
- Bronchiolitis is less commonly associated with Sjögren syndrome, systemic lupus erythematosus, and scleroderma.

- Patients with rheumatoid arthritis who develop bronchiolitis obliterans most commonly are women in their fifth to sixth decades of life with long-standing disease.

Suggested Readings

Hakala M, Paakko P, Sutinen S, et al: Association of bronchiolitis with connective tissue disorders. *Ann Rheum Dis* 45:656-662, 1986.

Howling SJ, Hansell DM, Wells AU, et al: Follicular bronchiolitis: thin-section CT and histologic findings. *Radiology* 212 637-642, 1999.

Lynch DA: Imaging of small airways disease and chronic obstructive pulmonary disease. *Clin Chest Med* 29:165-179, 2008.

Tanaka N, Kim JS, Newell JD, et al: Rheumatoid arthritis-related lung diseases: CT findings. *Radiology* 232:81-91, 2004.

White ES, Tazelaar HD, Lynch JP 3rd: Bronchiolar complications of connective tissue diseases. *Semin Respair Crit Care Med* 24: 543-566, 2003.

Woodhead F, Wells AU, Desai SR: Pulmonary complications of connective tissue diseases. *Clin Chest Med* 29:149-164, 2008.

Emphysema

DEFINITION: Emphysema is characterized by abnormal, permanent enlargement of airspaces distal to the terminal bronchiole, accompanied by destruction of their walls.

IMAGING

Radiography

Findings

- Direct sign: presence of bullae, which are focal areas of increased lucency.
- Indirect signs: focal absence of pulmonary vessels and reduction of vessel caliber with tapering toward lung periphery.
- Flattening of diaphragm and increased retrosternal space on lateral view.

Utility

- Limitations: low specificity, low sensitivity in mild disease, interobserver variability in interpretation of findings, inability to quantify severity.

CT

Findings

- Areas of low attenuation contrast to surrounding lung parenchyma with normal attenuation.
- Mild to moderate centrilobular emphysema is characterized by multiple rounded, small unwalled areas of low attenuation, with diameters of several millimeters.
- Lesions have no walls and are grouped around the center of secondary pulmonary lobules.
- Panlobular emphysema has a widespread and relatively homogeneous pattern of low attenuation involving the entire lung or mainly the lower lobes.
- Paraseptal emphysema involves single or multiple bullae adjacent to pleura or along the interlobular septa that is isolated or with centrilobular and/or panlobular emphysema.

Utility

- High-resolution CT (approximately 1-mm section thickness) volumetrically on multidetector scanners is imaging modality of choice for assessment of presence, distribution, and severity of emphysema.
- High-resolution CT reflects the macroscopic pathologic findings.
- Very mild emphysema can be missed on CT.

DIAGNOSTIC PEARLS

- Centrilobular emphysema: multiple rounded, small unwalled areas of low attenuation, with diameters of several millimeters with upper lobe predominance.
- Panlobular emphysema: widespread and relatively homogenous patterns of low attenuation involving entire lung or lower lobe predominance.
- Paraseptal emphysema: single or multiple bullae adjacent to pleura or along interlobular septa.

- Minimum intensity projection technique is more sensitive than conventional high-resolution CT in detection of subtle emphysema.

CLINICAL PRESENTATION

- During early stages, no symptoms may manifest and the disease may be detected only as an incidental finding on CT.
- Breathlessness can occur either with exertion or at rest.

DIFFERENTIAL DIAGNOSIS

- Pulmonary Langerhans histiocytosis
- Obliterative bronchiolitis
- Lymphangiomyomatosis

PATHOLOGY

- Centrilobular emphysema results from dilatation or destruction of respiratory bronchioles, associated with cigarette smoking.
- Panlobular emphysema is associated with α_1-antitrypsin deficiency, resulting in even dilatation and destruction of entire acinus.

WHAT THE REFERRING PHYSICIAN NEEDS TO KNOW

- Up to 30% of lung parenchyma must be destroyed before pulmonary function test results become abnormal.
- Chest radiography has low sensitivity to detect mild and moderate disease.
- High-resolution CT has high sensitivity in detecting mild and/or clinically silent disease.
- CT protocols can be tailored such that radiation exposure for the patient is minimal.
- No intravenous contrast material is required.

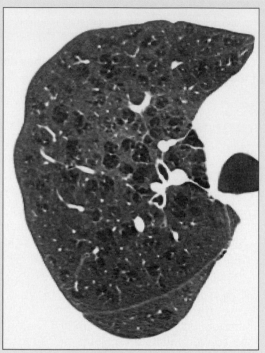

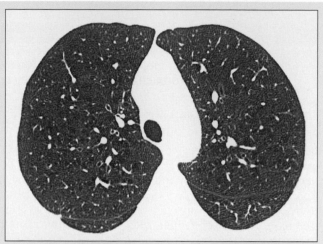

Figure 2. High-resolution CT image shows mild centrilobular emphysema in the upper lobes.

Figure 1. Centrilobular emphysema: classic CT findings. CT image targeted to the right lung shows well-defined "holes" in the centrilobular portions of the secondary pulmonary lobule surrounding small vessels. Note the lack of visible walls. The findings are typical of centrilobular emphysema.

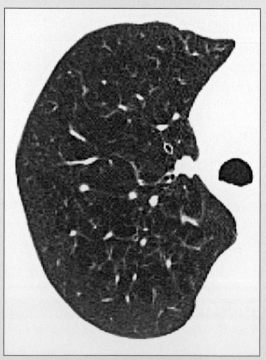

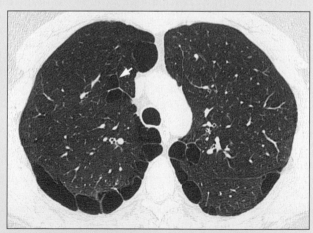

Figure 4. Paraseptal emphysema: typical CT findings. CT image at the level of aortic arch shows multiple bullae adjacent to the pleura and along interlobular septa (*arrow*).

Figure 3. Panlobular emphysema. High-resolution CT section through the right upper lobe shows extensive emphysematous destruction. The lack of lung structures gives the resulting areas of hypoattenuation a relatively homogeneous appearance. (*Courtesy of Alexander Bankier, Harvard Medical School, Boston*)

- In panlobular emphysema loss of contrast between alveolar sac and duct occurs with uniform destruction of secondary pulmonary lobule.

INCIDENCE/PREVALENCE AND EPIDEMIOLOGY

- Only 40% of heavy smokers develop substantial lung destruction due to emphysema.
- Occasionally emphysema is found in individuals with normal lung function and who have never smoked.
- Prevalence of emphysema strongly depends on regional factors such as smoking habits, social standards, and environmental air pollution.
- In late 1990s, up to 15% of the U.S. population suffered from COPD, accounting for 9% of hospitalization and 30 deaths/100,000 population.

Suggested Readings

Coxson HO, Rogers RM: Quantitative computed tomography of chronic obstructive pulmonary disease. *Acad Radiol* 12:1457-1463, 2005.

Goldin JG: Imaging the lungs in patients with pulmonary emphysema. *J Thorac Imaging* 24:163-170, 2009.

Litmanovich D, Boiselle PM, Bankier AA: CT of pulmonary emphysema—current status, challenges, and future directions. *Eur Radiol* 19:537-551, 2009.

Madani A, De Maertelaer V, Zanen J, Gevenois PA: Pulmonary emphysema: Radiation dose and section thickness at multidetector CT quantification–comparison with macroscopic and microscopic morphometry. *Radiology* 243:250-257, 2007.

Mannino DM: COPD: Epidemiology, prevalence, morbidity and mortality, and disease heterogeneity. *Chest* 121:121S-126S, 2002.

Thurlbeck WM, Müller NL: Emphysema: Definition, imaging, and quantification. *AJR Am J Roentgenol* 163:1017-1025, 1994.

Hemoptysis

DEFINITION: Hemoptysis may be secondary to focal or diffuse pulmonary hemorrhage.

IMAGING

Radiography

Findings

- Focal hazy area of increased opacity or consolidation
- Multifocal or diffuse airspace consolidation that tends to involve mainly middle and lower lung zones.

Utility

- Initial modality used in the evaluation of patients with hemoptysis
- May be normal in patients with diffuse pulmonary hemorrhage or focal abnormalities such as bronchiectasis and small endobronchial tumors

CT

Findings

- Focal ground-glass opacities or consolidation
- Bilateral patchy or confluent consolidations and/or ground-glass opacities.
- Interlobular septal thickening and poorly defined centrilobular nodular opacities (as hemorrhage resolves)
- May show underlying abnormality in patients with hemoptysis due to bronchiectasis or carcinoma

Utility

- Useful diagnostic tool for differential diagnosis and detection of underlying disease and complications.

CLINICAL PRESENTATION

- Hemoptysis may range from mild to copious and life-threatening.

DIFFERENTIAL DIAGNOSIS

- Bronchiectasis
- Chronic bronchitis
- Pulmonary carcinoma
- Endobronchial carcinoid tumor
- Goodpasture syndrome
- Wegener granulomatosis
- Microscopic polyangiitis
- Systemic lupus erythematosus

DIAGNOSTIC PEARLS

- Focal ground-glass or consolidation: most commonly due to airway abnormality or neoplasm
- Diffuse ground-glass or consolidation: most commonly due to vasculitis

PATHOLOGY

- Pulmonary hemorrhage should be considered particularly in patients with hemoptysis and in cases with blunt trauma.
- Causes of focal pulmonary hemorrhage and hemoptysis include carcinoma, bronchiectasis, and pulmonary embolism.
- Causes of multifocal/diffuse hemorrhage include Wegener granulomatosis, Goodpasture syndrome, microscopic polyangiitis, and systemic lupus erythematosus.

INCIDENCE/PREVALENCE AND EPIDEMIOLOGY

- Hemoptysis is a common manifestation of endobronchial carcinoids and pulmonary carcinoma.
- Wegener granulomatosis: hemoptysis occurs in 30%-40% of patients, and diffuse alveolar hemorrhage occurs in 10%.
- Goodpasture syndrome: hemoptysis is the most common presenting symptom, occurring in 80%-90% of patients.

Suggested Readings

Bruzzi JF, Rémy-Jardin M, Delhaye D, et al: Multi-detector row CT of hemoptysis. *RadioGraphics* 26(1):3-22, 2006.

Khalil A, Fartoukh M, Tassart M, et al: Role of MDCT in indentification of the bleeding site and the vessels causing hemoptysis. *AJR Am J Roentgenol* 188:W117-W125, 2007.

Primack SL, Miller RR, Müller NL: Diffuse pulmonary hemorrhage: Clinical, pathologic, and imaging features. *AJR Am J Roentgenol* 164:295-300, 1995.

WHAT THE REFERRING PHYSICIAN NEEDS TO KNOW

- In the majority of patients clinical and plain radiographic appearances are sufficient for diagnosis.
- CT is a useful diagnostic tool for differential diagnosis and detection of underlying disease and complications.
- CT is particularly helpful in excluding bronchiectasis or pulmonary carcinoma as a cause of hemoptysis.
- CT is of limited value in patients with diffuse pulmonary hemorrhage and pulmonary renal syndrome.

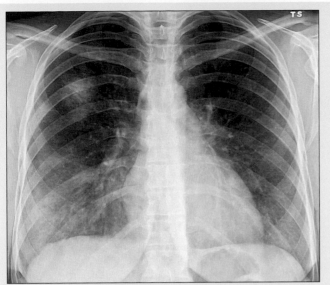

Figure 1. Multifocal consolidation in diffuse pulmonary hemorrhage. Posteroanterior chest radiograph shows dense consolidation in the right upper lobe and poorly defined areas of consolidation and ground-glass opacities in the lower lung zones. The patient was a 35-year-old man with Wegener granulomatosis and diffuse pulmonary hemorrhage.

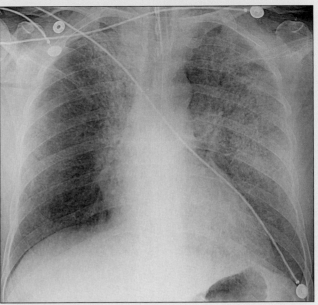

Figure 2. Diffuse pulmonary hemorrhage. Anteroposterior chest radiograph shows extensive bilateral areas of consolidation. Endotracheal and nasogastric tubes are in place. The patient was a 51-year-old man with Wegener granulomatosis and diffuse pulmonary hemorrhage.

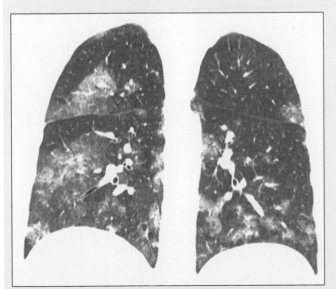

Figure 3. Multifocal consolidation in diffuse pulmonary hemorrhage. Coronal reformatted image from a multidetector helical CT scan demonstrates multifocal areas of consolidation and ground-glass opacities. The patient was a 35-year-old man with Wegener granulomatosis and diffuse pulmonary hemorrhage.

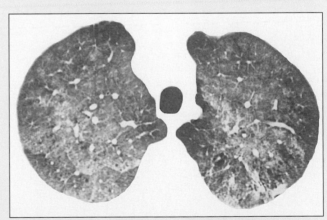

Figure 4. Diffuse pulmonary hemorrhage. High-resolution CT image shows extensive bilateral ground-glass opacities, small areas of consolidation, and poorly defined small nodular opacities. The patient was a 43-year-old man with Wegener granulomatosis and diffuse pulmonary hemorrhage.

Inhalational Diseases and Aspiration

Part 48

SILICOSIS AND COAL WORKER'S PNEUMOCONIOSIS

Silicosis

DEFINITION: Silicosis is an occupational lung disease caused by exposure to excessive amounts of respirable crystalline silica.

IMAGING

Radiography

Findings
- Small well-defined nodules that may have calcification
- Diffuse or predominantly upper lung distribution
- Hilar lymphadenopathy
- Focal, diffuse, or eggshell calcification of lymph nodes
- Silicoproteinosis: extensive bilateral ground-glass opacities

Utility
- Chest radiograph initial and usually only imaging modality required in the diagnosis and follow-up of patients
- Relatively insensitive to early disease and nonspecific
- Describes findings using International Labour Organization (ILO) 2000 terminology
- Radiographically indistinguishable from coal worker's pneumoconiosis
- Accelerated silicosis findings similar to classic silicosis

CT

Findings
- Well-defined 2- to 5-mm centrilobular and subpleural nodules that may have calcification.
- Diffuse distribution with posterior and upper lung predominance.
- Hilar and mediastinal lymphadenopathy.
- Focal, diffuse, or eggshell calcification of lymph nodes.
- Silicoproteinosis: diffuse ground-glass opacities, "crazy-paving" pattern, poorly defined nodules, dorsal lower lung consolidation.

Utility
- May demonstrate findings in patients with normal radiographs.

DIAGNOSTIC PEARLS
- Small, well-defined centrilobular and subpleural nodules
- Diffuse distribution with posterior and upper lobe predominance
- Hilar lymphadenopathy with eggshell calcification
- History of exposure to silica dust mainly in mining, quarrying, and sandblasting.

- CT findings similar to those of coal worker's pneumoconiosis.

Positron Emission Tomography

Findings
- Increased uptake may be seen in complicated lesions and enlarged lymph nodes.

Utility
- PET/CT used for silicosis complicated by progressive massive fibrosis.
- Conflicting data; potentially useful in differentiating progressive massive fibrosis from lung carcinoma and staging of coexistent disease.

CLINICAL PRESENTATION

- Classic silicosis: patient remains asymptomatic until after 10-20 years of continuous exposure; dyspnea on exertion, then at rest.
- Acute silicosis/silicoproteinosis: few months/years of exposure; rapidly progressive dyspnea, cough, weight loss, development of cyanosis and respiratory failure; may develop superimposed mycobacterial infection.

WHAT THE REFERRING PHYSICIAN NEEDS TO KNOW

- ILO 2000 International Classification of Radiographs of Pneumoconiosis is the most widely accepted classification of extent of disease.
- Chest radiograph is first and foremost imaging modality in initial evaluation and follow-up of suspected or proven cases.
- CT is helpful in case assessment and suspected pulmonary complications (carcinoma, pulmonary hypertension, right-sided heart failure, tuberculosis)
- PET/CT may be helpful in evaluating complications of silicosis but may be falsely positive in progressive massive fibrosis.
- Lung function impairment is related to the degree of nodulation, progressive massive fibrosis, and emphysema.

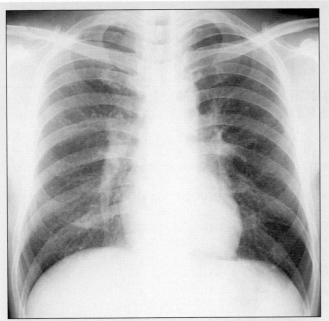

Figure 1. Silicosis in a 68-year-old construction site worker. Posteroanterior chest radiograph shows multiple small diffuse nodules with some lower zone sparing. (*Courtesy of Dr. Clara Ooi, Hong Kong*)

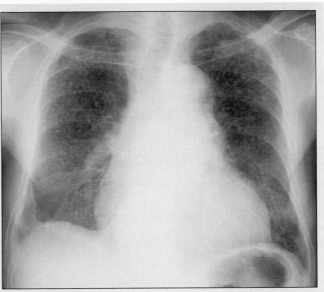

Figure 2. Silicosis. Posteroanterior chest radiograph shows multiple nodules in both lungs. Note upper lobe predominance. (*Courtesy of Dr. Clara Ooi, Hong Kong*)

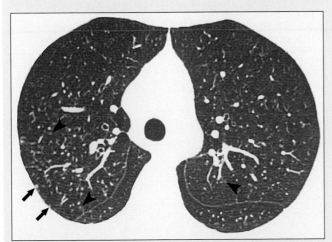

Figure 3. Silicosis. High-resolution CT image shows small, well-defined nodules mainly in the dorsal half of the upper lobes. Some of the nodules can be seen to be in a subpleural (*arrows*) and centrilobular (*arrowheads*) distribution. (*Case courtesy of Dr. Ericson Bagatin, Area of Occupational Health, State University of Campinas [UNICAMP], Campinas, São Paulo, Brazil.*)

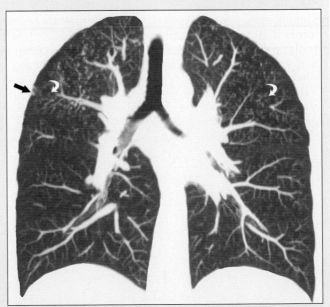

Figure 4. Silicosis. Coronal maximum intensity projection image better demonstrates the nodules and their predominantly centrilobular (*curved arrows*) distribution. Also noted are a few subpleural nodules (*straight arrow*). (*Case courtesy of Dr. Ericson Bagatin, Area of Occupational Health, State University of Campinas (UNICAMP), Campinas, São Paulo, Brazil.*)

- Death from respiratory failure within short period of time despite intensive treatment.
- Accelerated silicosis: 5-10 years' exposure, breathlessness after <1 year of exposure, progression to respiratory failure in 5 years.
- Breathlessness as early as 1 year after exposure with patient's condition rapidly deteriorating to hypoxic respiratory failure and death.

DIFFERENTIAL DIAGNOSIS

- Coal worker's pneumoconiosis
- Sarcoidosis
- Pulmonary alveolar proteinosis
- Tuberculosis
- Welder's pneumoconiosis (welder's lung)

PATHOLOGY

- Silica inhalation causes inflammatory lung fibrosis and parenchymal destruction.
- Lamellated whorled inflammatory and fibrotic nodules are formed by collagen deposition and hyalinization.
- Pulmonary changes continue even after exposure has ceased, eventually leading to progressive massive fibrosis.
- Silicoproteinosis is characterized by pulmonary edema, interstitial inflammation, surfactant-filled alveoli, eosinophilic exudate with fine granular appearance, and sparse and poorly demarcated/absent nodules.

- Accelerated disease includes exudative alveolar lipoproteinosis with chronic inflammation and association with fibrotic granulomas containing collagen, reticulin, and a large number of silica particles.

INCIDENCE/PREVALENCE AND EPIDEMIOLOGY

- Risk increases with increased amount and duration of silica exposure.
- Approximately 1500 cases are diagnosed annually in the United States.
- Workers in India (quarrying shale sedimentary rocks) have a 55% prevalence rate.
- Fifty percent of Latin American miners older than age 55 years develop silicosis.

Suggested Readings

Antao VC, Pinheiro GA, Terra-Filho M, et al: High-resolution CT in silicosis: Correlation with radiographic findings and functional impairment. *J Comput Assist Tomogr* 29(3):350-356, 2005.

Chong S, Lee KS, Chung MJ, et al: Pneumoconiosis: Comparison of imaging and pathologic findings. *RadioGraphics* 26:59-77, 2006.

International Labour Office Guidelines for the use of ILO International Classification of Radiographs of Pneumoconiosis: *Occupational Safety and Health Series No 22.* Geneva, 2000, International Labor Office.

Kim JS, Lynch DA: Imaging of nonmalignant occupational lung disease. *J Thorac Imaging* 17:238-260, 2002.

Marchiori E, Souza CA, Barbassa TG, et al: Silicoproteinosis: High-resolution CT findings in 13 patients. *AJR Am J Roentgenol* 189(6):1402-1406, 2007.

Progressive Massive Fibrosis

DEFINITION: Progressive pneumoconiotic lung disease with coalescence of nodules to form focal opacities greater than 1 cm in diameter is known as progressive massive fibrosis.

IMAGING

Radiography
Findings
- Coalescent upper lobe nodules forming opacities > 1 cm in diameter (large opacities).
- May have smooth or irregular borders (angel's wing appearance).
- Upper lobe volume loss with paracicatricial emphysema between lesion and pleura.
- Hilar lesions with sharply defined lateral margin.
- Punctate or diffuse calcification.
- Parenchymal nodules with hilar or mediastinal lymphadenopathy.
- Lymph nodes with focal, eggshell, or diffuse calcification.

Utility
- Usually only imaging modality required in diagnosis and follow-up

CT
Findings
- Mass-like consolidation greater than 1 cm in diameter on background of small nodules.
- Located in apical and posterior segments of upper and lower lobes.
- Distortion of parenchyma due to fibrosis.
- Small centrilobular nodules.
- Adjacent paracicatricial emphysema with smooth sharply defined flattened border of lesion.
- Punctate, curvilinear, or massive calcification.
- Parenchymal destruction, cavitation.
- Hilar and mediastinal lymphadenopathy.
- Lymph nodes with focal, eggshell, or diffuse calcification.

Utility
- Conglomeration of nodules is apparent earlier on CT than with radiography.
- CT may be helpful in distinguishing conglomerate masses of progressive massive fibrosis from pulmonary carcinoma.

DIAGNOSTIC PEARLS
- Coalescence of nodules to form focal opacity > 1 cm in diameter
- Distortion of parenchyma due to fibrosis
- Adjacent emphysema with abrupt sharp lateral lesion border
- Nonenhancement or slow enhancement on MRI with gadolinium

MRI
Findings
- Hyperintense to isointense to muscle on T1-weighted images depending on mineral dust content
- Hypointense to isointense on T2-weighted images
- Internal focal hyperintense area suggestive of necrosis
- Generally nonenhancing; may have rim enhancement
- Coexistent lung carcinoma: focal high signal separate from progressive massive fibrosis

Utility
- MRI with gadolinium enhancement is potentially useful in identifying lung cancer.

Positron Emission Tomography
Findings
- Increased uptake may be present in lesions and enlarged lymph nodes.

Utility
- Conflicting data; potentially useful in differentiating progressive massive fibrosis from lung carcinoma and staging of coexistent disease.

CLINICAL PRESENTATION
- Prior diagnosis of, or symptoms referable to, silicosis or coal worker's pneumoconiosis
- Patient may be asymptomatic or have mild cough and dyspnea on exertion.
- Progress to pulmonary hypertension with right ventricular and respiratory failure

---

WHAT THE REFERRING PHYSICIAN NEEDS TO KNOW
- Chest radiograph is first and foremost imaging modality in initial evaluation and follow-up of suspected or proven cases.
- CT is helpful in case assessment and when pulmonary complications (carcinoma, pulmonary hypertension, right-sided heart failure, tuberculosis) are suspected.
- PET/CT may be helpful in evaluating complicated disease but may be falsely positive.
- Lung function impairment is related to the degree of nodulation, progressive massive fibrosis, and emphysema.

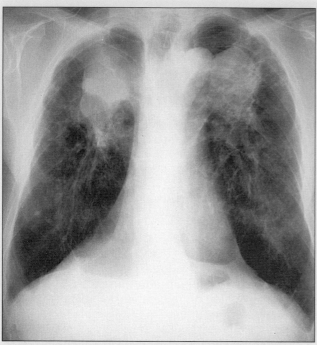

Figure 1. Silicosis with conglomeration. Posteroanterior chest radiograph shows large opacities in the upper lung zones associated with marked retraction of the hila superiorly. Several nodular opacities can be seen, mainly in the mid-lung zones. The patient was a 70-year-old man with long-standing silicosis related to mining of hard rock. (*From Müller NL, Fraser RS, Colman NC, Paré PD: Radiologic Diagnosis of Diseases of the Chest. Philadelphia, WB Saunders, 2001.*)

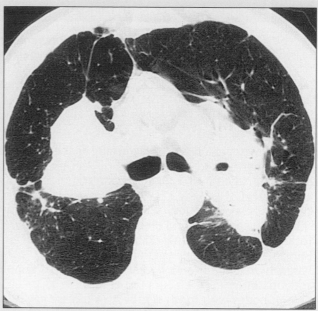

Figure 2. Silicosis with conglomeration. High-resolution CT scan shows conglomerate masses and extensive emphysema. The patient was a 70-year-old man with long-standing silicosis related to mining of hard rock. (*From Müller NL, Fraser RS, Colman NC, Paré PD: Radiologic Diagnosis of Diseases of the Chest. Philadelphia, WB Saunders, 2001.*)

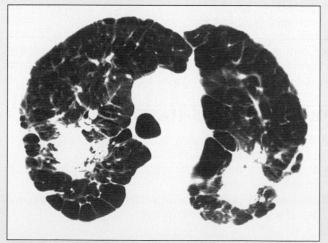

Figure 3. Progressive massive fibrosis. High-resolution CT scan showing masses in the upper lobes with paracicatricial emphysema and well-defined small centrilobular nodules. (*Courtesy of Dr. Clara Ooi, Hong Kong*)

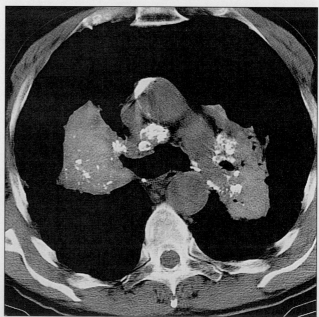

Figure 4. Silicosis with conglomeration. Soft tissue windows show calcification within the lung parenchyma and within mediastinal and hilar lymph nodes. The patient was a 70-year-old man with long-standing silicosis related to mining of hard rock. (*From Müller NL, Fraser RS, Colman NC, Paré PD: Radiologic Diagnosis of Diseases of the Chest. Philadelphia, WB Saunders, 2001.*)

DIFFERENTIAL DIAGNOSIS

- Sarcoidosis
- Talcosis
- Lung cancer
- Tuberculosis

PATHOLOGY

- Profusion, enlargement, and coalescence of pneumoconiotic nodules occurs.
- Silicotic nodules are composed of dense lamellar collagen that may become hyalinized or calcified.
- Individual nodules or conglomerates of lesions > 1 cm in diameter are defined as large opacities or progressive massive fibrosis.
- Large opacities may undergo necrosis and cavitation.
- Progressive massive fibrosis lesions migrate to hila leaving emphysematous lung adjacent to pleura.
- Destruction of lung parenchyma, bronchioles, and blood vessels occurs.
- Cavitation is secondary to infection by anaerobic organisms, tuberculosis, or ischemia.

INCIDENCE/PREVALENCE AND EPIDEMIOLOGY

- Progressive massive fibrosis is seen most commonly in patients with silicosis.
- Occupations associated with silicosis include rock mining, quarrying, stone cutting, engraving, and sandblasting.
- Progressive massive fibrosis may also occur in coal worker's pneumoconiosis.

Suggested Readings

Chong S, Lee KS, Chung MJ, et al: Pneumoconiosis: Comparison of imaging and pathologic findings. *RadioGraphics* 26:59-77, 2006.

International Labour Office Guidelines for the use of ILO International Classification of Radiographs of Pneumoconiosis: *Occupational Safety and Health Series No 22*. Geneva, 2000, International Labor Office.

Marchiori E, Ferreira A, Saez F, et al: Conglomerated masses of silicosis in sandblasters: High-resolution CT findings. *Eur J Radiol* 59:56-59, 2006.

Matsumoto S, Mori H, Miyake H, et al: MRI signal characteristics of progressive massive fibrosis in silicosis. *Clin Radiol* 53:510-514, 1998.

O'Connell M, Mennedy M: Progressive massive fibrosis secondary to pulmonary silicosis appearance on F-18 fluorodeoxyglucose PET/CT. *Clin Nucl Med* 29:754-755, 2004.

Coal Worker's Pneumoconiosis

DEFINITION: Diffuse nodular or reticulonodular lung disease caused by exposure to respirable carbonaceous material (coal dust) is referred to as coal worker's pneumoconiosis.

IMAGING

Radiography

Findings
- Simple type: diffuse bilateral small round nodules
- Complicated type: lesions > 1 cm (large opacities)
- Atypical: lower lung reticulation, decreased lung volumes, traction bronchiectasis, and honeycombing
- Hilar and mediastinal lymphadenopathy
- Calcification of nodules possible

Utility
- Chest radiograph usually only imaging modality required in diagnosis and follow-up
- Relatively insensitive to early disease
- Describes findings using International Labour Organization (ILO) 2000 terminology
- Disease radiographically indistinguishable from silicosis, although nodules may be less well defined and granular

CT

Findings
- Simple type: small nodules with upper lobe predominance that may occasionally calcify
- Small branching linear or ill-defined punctate attenuation
- Subpleural nodules adjacent to visceral pleura (pseudoplaques)
- Complicated type: lesions > 1 cm (large opacities)
- Mediastinal or hilar lymphadenopathy

Utility
- CT, particularly volumetric CT, superior to chest radiography in demonstrating presence of nodules
- Similar findings to silicosis

CLINICAL PRESENTATION

- Usually asymptomatic
- Chronic cough that persists even after patient leaves the workplace
- Coal dust exposure > 20 years

DIAGNOSTIC PEARLS

- Small nodular opacities mainly in upper lobes
- Subpleural nodules adjacent to visceral pleura (pseudoplaques)
- Coal miner

DIFFERENTIAL DIAGNOSIS

- Silicosis
- Sarcoidosis
- Tuberculosis
- Welder's pneumoconiosis (welder's lung)

PATHOLOGY

- Histologic landmark: black coal dust macule represents focal deposition of coal dust and pigment-laden macrophages around respiratory bronchioles.
- Macules enlarge and coalesce, forming a discrete network of interstitial fibrosis, resulting in respiratory bronchiole dilatation and emphysema.
- Increased exposure to coal mine dust causes development of nodular lesions at bifurcations of respiratory bronchiole against background of macules.
- Nodules are composed of heavily coal dust–laden macrophages interlaced with collagen fibers oriented in a haphazard manner microscopically.
- With chronic dust exposure, simple nodules coalesce to produce black, rubbery parenchymal fibrous masses resulting in complicated disease and progressive massive fibrosis.

INCIDENCE/PREVALENCE AND EPIDEMIOLOGY

- Prevalence of 2%-12% in American coal miners
- Predicted prevalence of 9% in British coal miners

WHAT THE REFERRING PHYSICIAN NEEDS TO KNOW

- ILO 2000 International Classification of Radiographs of Pneumoconiosis is the most widely accepted classification of extent of disease.
- Chest radiograph is the first and foremost imaging modality in initial evaluation and follow-up of suspected or proven cases.
- CT is helpful in case assessment and suspected pulmonary complications (carcinoma, pulmonary hypertension, right-sided heart failure, tuberculosis).
- PET/CT may be helpful in evaluating complicated disease but may be falsely positive in progressive massive fibrosis.
- Lung function impairment is related to the degree of nodulation, progressive massive fibrosis, and emphysema.

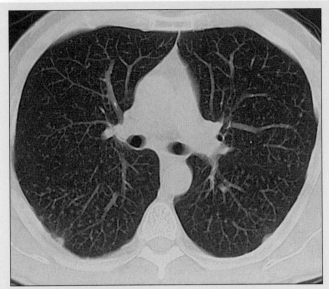

Figure 1. Coal worker's pneumoconiosis. Ten-millimeter collimation CT scan shows small nodules in both lungs. Subpleural nodules mimicking pleural plaques are evident posteriorly. (*Courtesy of Dr. Martine Remy-Jardin, Centre Hospitalier Regional et Universitaire de Lille, Lille, France; from Müller NL, Fraser RS, Colman NC, Paré PD: Radiologic Diagnosis of Diseases of the Chest. Philadelphia, WB Saunders, 2001.*)

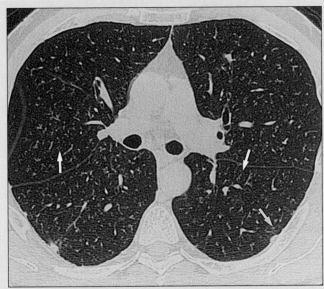

Figure 2. Coal worker's pneumoconiosis. On high-resolution CT the nodules are more difficult to distinguish from vessels. The nodular and branching opacities have a centrilobular distribution (*arrows*). The subpleural pseudoplaques are defined better with high-resolution CT. (*Courtesy of Dr. Martine Remy-Jardin, Centre Hospitalier Regional et Universitaire de Lille, Lille, France; from Müller NL, Fraser RS, Colman NC, Paré PD: Radiologic Diagnosis of Diseases of the Chest. Philadelphia, WB Saunders, 2001.*)

- Atypical type seen in 10%-20%, with higher risk of carcinoma
- Increased risk of developing active tuberculosis and nontuberculous mycobacterial infections

Suggested Readings

Chong S, Lee KS, Chung MJ, ct al: Pneumoconiosis: Comparison of imaging and pathologic findings. *RadioGraphics* 26:59-77, 2006.

Gevenois PA, Pichot E, Dargent F, et al: Low grade coal worker's pneumoconiosis: Comparison of CT and chest radiography. *Acta Radiol* 35:351-356, 1994.

International Labour Office Guidelines for the use of ILO International Classification of Radiographs of Pneumoconiosis: *Occupational Safety and Health Series No 22.* Geneva, 2000, International Labor Office.

Remy-Jardin M, Remy J, Farre I, Marquette CH: Computed tomographic evaluation of silicosis and coal workers' pneumoconiosis. *Radiol Clin North Am* 30:1155-1176, 1992.

Vallyathan V, Brower PS, Green FHY, Attfield MD: Radiographic and pathologic correlation of coal workers' pneumoconiosis. *Am J Respir Crit Care Meal* 154:741-748, 1996.

Asbestos-Related Pleural Plaques

DEFINITION: Pleural plaques are dense, almost acellular collagen with a basketweave pattern; they are usually bilateral and may be asymmetric.

IMAGING

Radiography
Findings
- Focal, pleural-based opacities with irregular margins
- Smooth-surfaced plaques or of fine or coarse nodularity that can be round, elliptical, or irregularly shaped
- Calcification: punctate, linear, or coalescent

Utility
- Only allows detection of plaques in 50%-80% of cases
- Limited specificity in cases of mild pleural disease, which may be difficult to distinguish from extrapleural fat

CT
Findings
- Circumscribed areas of pleural thickening separated from underlying ribs and extrapleural soft tissues by thin layer of fat
- Calcification

Utility
- High-resolution CT has greater sensitivity than conventional CT or chest radiography for detection of pleural plaques.
- Diaphragmatic pleural plaques are more readily detected on coronal or sagittal reformatted images of volumetric high-resolution performed on multidetector scanner.

CLINICAL PRESENTATION

- Usually first seen 20-30 years after exposure
- Pleural plaques do not cause any symptoms

DIFFERENTIAL DIAGNOSIS

- Previous tuberculosis
- Previous trauma
- Previous hemothorax

DIAGNOSTIC PEARLS

- Focal, pleural-based opacities with irregular margins
- Typical distribution: posterolateral chest wall, lateral chest wall, dome of diaphragm, and paravertebral pleura
- Usually bilateral; may be asymmetric
- Latency time for development of pleural plaques is 20-30 years
- Calcification is seldom evident until > 30 years after exposure.

PATHOLOGY

- Pleural plaques are dense, almost acellular collagen with basketweave pattern; they are usually bilateral and may be asymmetric.
- Major determinant of thickness of pleural plaques is duration from first exposure.
- Pleural plaques are usually limited to the parietal pleura.
- Asbestos fibers transported to pleural surface along lymphatic channels and/or by direct penetration result in pleural inflammation and fibrosis.

INCIDENCE/PREVALENCE AND EPIDEMIOLOGY

- Pleural plaques are the most common manifestation of asbestos exposure and invariably are bilateral.
- Prevalence of patients with asbestos-related pulmonary and pleural complications has been increasing.
- Symptoms are usually first seen 20-30 years after exposure.
- Ten percent to 15% of pleural plaques calcify; calcification is seldom evident until > 30 years after exposure.

WHAT THE REFERRING PHYSICIAN NEEDS TO KNOW

- Latency time for development of pleural plaques is usually 20-30 years.
- Most patients who have asbestos-related pleuropulmonary disease are asymptomatic; main symptom is shortness of breath.
- Chest radiograph has an important role in detection of asbestos-related pleural and parenchymal abnormalities and assessment of progression of disease.
- Radiograph is falsely negative in 20%-50% of patients with pleural plaques.
- High-resolution CT is superior to radiography in detection of pleural plaques.
- Asbestos-related pleural disease can be seen in 95%-100% of patients who have evidence of asbestosis on high-resolution CT.
- Isolated plaques and diffuse pleural thickening are also seen in tuberculosis, trauma, and hemothorax.

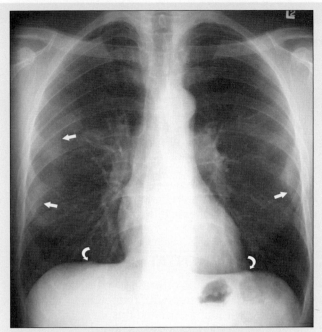

Figure 1. Pleural plaques. Posteroanterior chest radiograph shows multiple focal pleural-based opacities along the chest wall (*straight arrows*) and diaphragm (*curved arrows*) characteristic of pleural plaques. The patient was a 51-year-old shipyard worker.

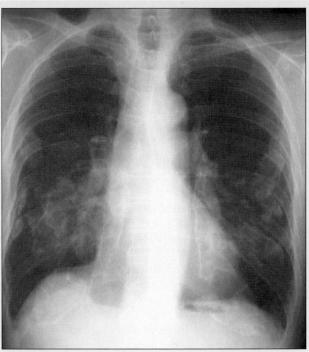

Figure 2. Calcified pleural plaques. Posteroanterior chest radiograph shows numerous bilateral calcified pleural plaques. The patient was an 82-year-old man who had worked for many years in a shipyard.

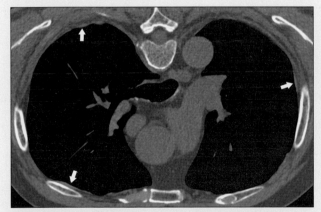

Figure 3. Pleural plaques. High-resolution CT image shows characteristic appearance of pleural plaques as sharply circumscribed focal areas of pleural thickening (*arrows*) separated from the underlying ribs and extrapleural soft tissues by a thin layer of fat.

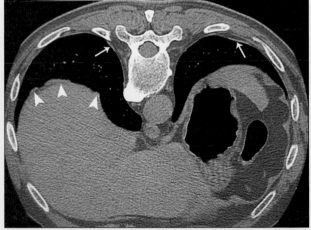

Figure 4. Diaphragmatic and costal pleural plaques. High-resolution CT image shows parietal pleural plaques along the intercostal spaces and paravertebral region (*arrows*) and along the right hemidiaphragm (*arrowheads*). (*Courtesy of Dr. Jorge Kavakama, São Paulo, Brazil.*)

Suggested Readings

Chapman SJ, Cookson WO, Musk AW, Lee YC: Benign asbestos pleural diseases. *Curr Opin Pulm Med* 9:266-271, 2003.

Cugell DW, Kamp DW: Asbestos and the pleura: A review. *Chest* 125:1103-1117, 2004.

Roach HD, Davies GJ, Attanoos R, et al: Asbestos: When the dust settles: An imaging review of asbestos-related disease. *RadioGraphics* 22(Spec No):S167-S184, 2002.

Asbestos-Related Diffuse Pleural Thickening

DEFINITION: Asbestos-related pleural disease results from pleural inflammation and fibrosis extending into the visceral pleura.

IMAGING

Radiography

Findings

- Smooth, uninterrupted pleural density extends over at least a fourth of the chest wall on radiography.
- There is a generalized, more or less uniform increase in pleural width.
- Pleural thickening is diffuse only in presence of, and in continuity with, an obliterated costophrenic angle.
- Fibrous strands ("crow's feet") extending into parenchyma are associated.
- Both circumscribed and diffuse pleural thickening may be present in same hemithorax.

Utility

- Used with pulmonary function tests for monitoring every 3-5 years to identify onset of asbestos-related disease.
- Limited accuracy in distinguishing pleural thickening from extrapleural fat.

CT

Findings

- Sheet of thickened pleura at least 5 cm in lateral dimension and 8 cm in craniocaudal dimension.
- Considered diffuse only in presence of, and in continuity with, an obliterated costophrenic angle.
- May calcify; usually focal but occasionally extensive.
- Margin between area of diffuse pleural thickening and adjacent lung frequently irregular as a result of parenchymal fibrosis.
- Rarely involves mediastinal pleura; frequently affects parietal pleura, abutting paravertebral gutters.

Utility

- High-resolution CT is more sensitive than plain chest radiography or conventional CT.
- High-resolution CT allows distinction of pleural thickening from extrapleural fat.

CLINICAL PRESENTATION

- Patients asymptomatic or present with dyspnea
- Restrictive lung function with reduction in vital capacity, with or without associated dyspnea
- Latency period of 10-40 years or more

DIFFERENTIAL DIAGNOSIS

- Malignant mesothelioma
- Pleural effusion
- Sequela of tuberculosis
- Sequela of previous trauma
- Sequela of previous surgery

PATHOLOGY

- Asbestos-related pleural disease resulting from pleural inflammation and fibrosis extending into the visceral pleura.
- Diffuse pleural thickening: may calcify: usually focal but occasionally extensive.
- Frequently develops after benign asbestos-related pleural effusion.
- Less commonly caused by extension of interstitial fibrosis to visceral pleura, consistent with pleural migration of asbestos fibers.

WHAT THE REFERRING PHYSICIAN NEEDS TO KNOW

- Diffuse pleural thickening is manifested radiologically as generalized, more or less uniform increase in pleural width.
- Circumscribed and diffuse pleural thickening may be present in the same hemithorax.
- Frequency of diffuse pleural thickening increases with time from first exposure and is believed to be dose related.
- Thickening frequently develops after benign asbestos-related pleural effusion.
- Presence of pleural effusion or circumferential pleural thickening should raise the possibility of mesothelioma.
- Isolated plaques and diffuse pleural thickening are also seen in tuberculosis, trauma, and hemothorax.

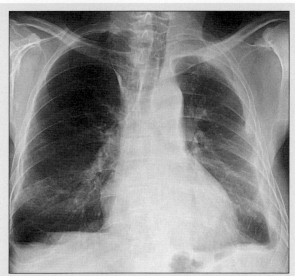

Figure 1. Diffuse pleural thickening. Chest radiograph shows diffuse left pleural thickening. The pleural thickening along the lateral chest wall is seen in profile as a broad band of homogenous increased opacity, whereas the thickening along the posterior chest wall is seen en face as a hazy increased opacity over the left lower hemithorax.

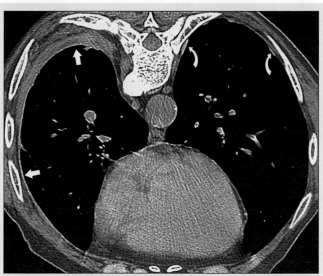

Figure 2. Diffuse pleural thickening. CT image in a patient with previous asbestos exposure shows diffuse pleural thickening (*straight arrows*) on the right and pleural plaques (*curved arrows*) on the left. (*Courtesy of Dr. Jorge Kavakama, São Paulo, Brazil.*)

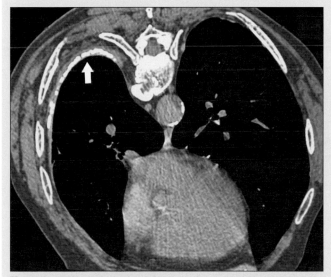

Figure 3. Diffuse pleural thickening. CT image obtained 6 years later in same patient as in Figure 2 shows extensive calcification (*arrow*) of the diffuse pleural thickening. (*Courtesy of Dr. Jorge Kavakama, São Paulo, Brazil.*)

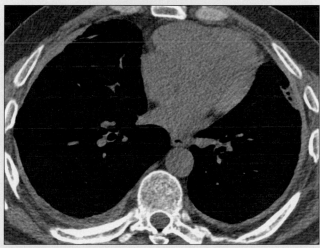

Figure 4. Diffuse pleural thickening. CT image in a patient with previous asbestos exposure shows diffuse bilateral pleural thickening involving the paravertebral pleura and costal pleura but sparing of the mediastinal pleura. Sparing of the mediastinal pleura is helpful in distinguishing benign from malignant pleural thickening.

INCIDENCE/PREVALENCE AND EPIDEMIOLOGY

- In United States, 8-9 million people have had occupational exposure to asbestos.
- Diffuse pleural thickening occurs in 9%-22% of asbestos-exposed workers with pleural disease.
- Frequency increases with time from first exposure and is believed to be dose related.

Suggested Readings

American Thoracic Society: Diagnosis and initial management of non-malignant diseases related to asbestos. *Am J Respir Crit Care Med* 170:691-715, 2004.

International Labour Office (ILO): Guidelines for the Use of the ILO International Classification of Radiographs of Pneumoconioses. Revised Edition 2000 (2002) International Labour Office: Geneva. (Occupational Safety and Health Series, No. 22).

Roach HD, Davies GJ, Attanoos R, et al: Asbestos: When the dust settles: An imaging review of asbestos-related disease. *RadioGraphics* 22(Spec No):S167-S184, 2002.

Asbestos-Related Parenchymal Disease

DEFINITION: Pulmonary abnormalities related to asbestos exposure include asbestosis, rounded ateletasis, and lung cancer.

IMAGING

Radiography

Findings
- Asbestosis is evident as reticular, small irregular opacities; shaggy heart sign may be seen.
- Rounded atelectasis is characterized by rounded pleural-based opacity, loss of volume, and comet tail sign and commonly occurs in middle and lower lung.
- Opacity of rounded atelectasis typically abuts area of pleural thickening or pleural effusion.
- Rounded atelectasis is static or grows very slowly and is distinguished from carcinoma by convergence of bronchovascular markings around edges.

Utility
- Radiography is performed routinely in the evaluation of patients with suspected asbestosis.
- Finding of asbestosis along with a compatible history of exposure is adequate for diagnosis.
- Sensitivity and specificity are limited in cases of mild fibrosis.
- Chest radiograph is falsely negative in 15%-20% of patients with asbestosis.

CT

Findings
- Asbestosis: intralobular linear opacities, irregular interlobular septa thickening, subpleural small rounded or branching opacities, subpleural curvilinear opacities, and parenchymal bands, pleural plaques or diffuse pleural thickening in vast majority of patients; tends to progress over time even after cessation of exposure.
- Round atelectasis: peripheral round or oval opacity with comet tail sign; acute/obtuse angles; volume loss proportional to size of opacity; abuts pleural thickening; can be unilateral or bilateral; enhances markedly with intravenous administration of a contrast agent.
- Lung cancer: similar manifestations to other non–asbestos-related carcinoma.

Utility
- High-resolution CT allows detection of parenchymal abnormalities not evident on chest radiography.

DIAGNOSTIC PEARLS

- Asbestosis: intralobular linear opacities, irregular interlobular septal thickening, ground-glass opacities; small round subpleural opacities; subpleural curvilinear opacities; parenchymal bands; pleural plaques or diffuse pleural thickening.
- Round atelectasis: peripheral round opacity, abuts pleural thickening; vessels and bronchi curving toward pleura and parenchymal opacity; volume loss proportional to size of opacity.
- Asbestos-related pleural disease is seen in 95%-100% of patients who have evidence of asbestosis on high-resolution CT.

- Patient is placed prone during imaging to distinguish dependent opacity due to atelectasis from mild fibrosis in dorsal basal lung regions.
- Findings of early asbestosis are neither sensitive nor specific.
- Condition is diagnosed with confidence only if parenchymal abnormalities are bilateral, present at multiple levels, and associated with pleural plaques.

CLINICAL PRESENTATION

- Most patients are asymptomatic.
- Progressive shortness of breath may occur.
- Nonproductive cough may be present.
- Weight loss, anorexia, malaise, cough, and hemoptysis occur in lung cancer.

DIFFERENTIAL DIAGNOSIS

- Idiopathic pulmonary fibrosis
- Nonspecific interstitial pneumonia

WHAT THE REFERRING PHYSICIAN NEEDS TO KNOW

- Latency time for development of asbestosis is 20-40 years, with that of lung cancer 10-60 years.
- Chest radiograph has important role in detection of asbestosis and assessment of disease progression; findings appear normal in up to 20% of patients with asbestosis.
- High-resolution CT findings of early asbestosis are neither sensitive nor specific.
- Asbestosis is diagnosed with reasonable confidence when it is bilateral, present at multiple levels, and associated with pleural plaques and diffuse pleural thickening.
- Asbestos-related pleural disease is seen in 95%-100% of patients who have evidence of asbestosis on high-resolution CT.
- Lung cancer is most common in patients with radiologic evidence of asbestosis.

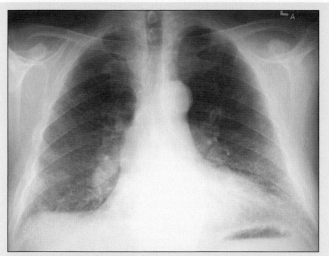

Figure 1. Asbestosis. Chest radiograph shows extensive bilateral reticulation and hazy increased opacity (ground-glass opacities) mainly in the lower lobes. Also note enlargement of the hilar pulmonary arteries consistent with pulmonary arterial hypertension. The patient was a 59-year-old man with end-stage asbestosis confirmed at lung transplantation.

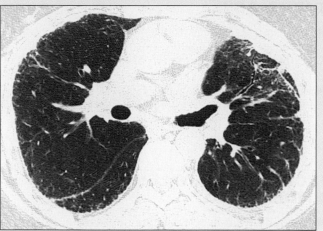

Figure 2. Asbestosis. High-resolution CT image performed with the patient supine shows bilateral predominantly subpleural intralobular lines and irregular thickening of interlobular septa. Also noted are nondependent ground-glass opacities and architectural distortion in the anterolateral aspect of the left upper lobe. The patient was a 76-year-old man with many years of asbestos exposure as a shipyard worker.

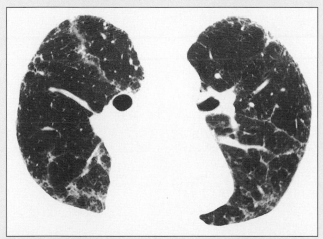

Figure 3. Asbestosis. High-resolution CT image performed with the patient prone shows bilateral predominantly subpleural intralobular lines and irregular thickening of interlobular septa with associated architectural distortion and mild subpleural honeycombing. Also noted are nondependent ground-glass opacities. The high-resolution CT findings resemble those of idiopathic pulmonary fibrosis. The patient was a 60-year-old man with proven asbestosis.

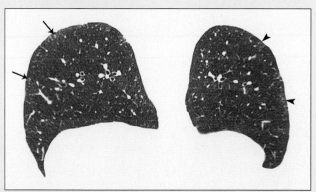

Figure 4. Subpleural nodules in early asbestos-related lung disease. High-resolution CT image with the patient prone shows small, round (dot-like) subpleural opacities (*arrows*) and localized traction bronchiectasis (*arrowheads*). They reflect the earliest pulmonary abnormality seen in association with asbestos exposure, that is, fibrosis in the walls of respiratory bronchioles. (*Courtesy of Dr. Jorge Kavakama, São Paulo, Brazil.*)

PATHOLOGY

- Appearance varies from slight interstitial collagen increase to complete normal lung architecture obliteration, with formation of thick fibrous bands and honeycombing.
- Microscopic diagnosis of asbestosis determined by evidence of diffuse interstitial fibrosis and asbestos bodies (fibers of asbestos to which lung has added iron-protein coating).

INCIDENCE/PREVALENCE AND EPIDEMIOLOGY

- Mortality from asbestosis has increased steadily, with it being now the most frequently recorded pneumoconiosis on death certificates.
- In United States, 8-9 million people have had occupational exposure to asbestos, resulting in 300,000 deaths.
- Asbestosis is seen mainly in asbestos miners and millers, asbestos textile workers, and asbestos insulators.
- Mean latency period for development of carcinoma is 45.8 ± 9.4 years, and mean patient age is 67.6 ± 8.4 years.

- Asbestos-related lung cancer likely accounts for 2%-3% of all lung cancer deaths among males in Great Britain.

Suggested Readings

Akira M, Yokoyama K, Yamamoto S, et al: Early asbestosis: Evaluation with high-resolution CT. *Radiology* 178:409-416, 1991.

American Thoracic Society: Diagnosis and initial management of nonmalignant diseases related to asbestos. *Am J Respir Crit Care Med* 170:691-715, 2004.

Friedman AC, Fiel SB, Fisher MS, et al: Asbestos-related pleural disease and asbestosis: A comparison of CT and chest radiography. *AJR Am J Roentgenol* 150:268-275, 1988.

Gamsu G, Salmon CJ, Warnock ML, Blanc PD: CT quantification of interstitial fibrosis in patients with asbestosis: A comparison of two methods. *AJR Am J Roentgenol* 164:63-68, 1995.

McHugh K, Blaquiere RM: CT features of rounded atelectasis. *AJR Am J Roentgenol* 153:257-260, 1989.

Ohar J, Sterling DA, Bleecker E, Donohue J: Changing patterns in asbestos-induced lung disease. *Chest* 125:744-753, 2004.

Roach HD, Davies GJ, Attanoos R, et al: Asbestos: When the dust settles: An imaging review of asbestos-related disease. *RadioGraphics* 22(Spec No):S167-S184, 2002.

Asbestos-Related Neoplastic Complications

DEFINITION: Asbestos-related neoplastic complications include lung cancer and mesothelioma.

IMAGING

Radiography
Findings
- Lung nodule or mass
- Hilar and mediastinal lymphadenopathy
- Pleural effusion
- Unilateral sheet-like or lobulated pleural thickening

Utility
- Plays important role in detection of asbestos-related pleural and parenchymal abnormalities and in assessment of disease progression.
- Limited accuracy in distinguishing benign from malignant pleural disease.

CT
Findings
- Lung nodule or mass
- Hilar and mediastinal lymphadenopathy
- Occasionally may simulate rounded atelectasis: irregular shape, increased opacity out of proportion for volume loss; no curving of adjacent vessels
- Pleural effusion
- Circumferential pleural thickening
- Nodular pleural thickening
- Mediastinal pleural thickening
- Marked enhancement with intravenous contrast
- Pleural plaques may or may not be seen

Utility
- CT findings suggestive of mesothelioma include unilateral pleural effusion, nodular pleural thickening, mediastinal pleural thickening, circumferential rind-like pleural thickening, and interlobar fissure thickening.

MRI
Findings
- Lung nodule or mass
- Hilar and mediastinal lymphadenopathy
- Pleural effusion
- Diffuse pleural thickening
- Mesothelioma: isointense or slightly hyperintense relative to adjacent chest wall muscle on T1-weighted

DIAGNOSTIC PEARLS
- Findings suggestive of mesothelioma include nodular pleural thickening, mediastinal pleural thickening, circumferential pleural thickening, and interlobar fissure thickening
- Mesothelioma should be suspected in patients with history of asbestos exposure and unilateral pleural effusion

images and moderately hyperintense on proton density- and T2-weighted images
- Marked enhancement of mesothelioma with gadolinium-based contrast agent on T1-weighted images

Utility
- MRI has limited value in the assessment of lung cancer.
- In patients with mesothelioma, MRI is usually only performed in cases in which contrast-enhanced CT is contraindicated or when extrapleural infiltration has not been clearly demonstrated on CT.

Positron Emission Tomography
Findings
- Positive uptake on FDG-PET in lung cancer and in mesothelioma
- False-positive findings in inflammatory lesions and infection

Utility
- Main value is detection of extrathoracic metastases.

CLINICAL PRESENTATION
- Pleuritic chest pain may accompany development of benign asbestos effusion or mesothelioma.
- Latency time for lung cancer is 10 to > 60 years (mean, 46 years).
- Latency time for development of mesothelioma is 25-60 years.
- Symptoms of lung cancer include cough, dyspnea, hemoptysis, weight loss, and chest pain.

WHAT THE REFERRING PHYSICIAN NEEDS TO KNOW
- Asbestos-related cancers can occur anywhere in the lungs and be of any cell type, but there is a greater likelihood in the lower lungs.
- Risk of mesothelioma is much greater after exposure to amphiboles, particularly crocidolite (blue asbestos) than after exposure to chrysotile (white asbestos).
- Chrysotile itself can cause malignant mesothelioma, although the risk is much lower than for amphiboles.
- Mesothelioma should be suspected in patients with asbestos exposure and unilateral pleural effusion and/or nodular, mediastinal, or circumferential pleural thickening.

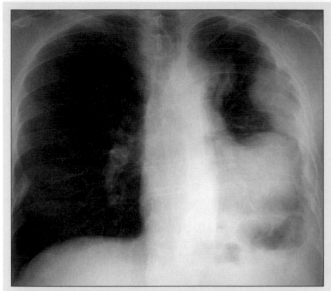

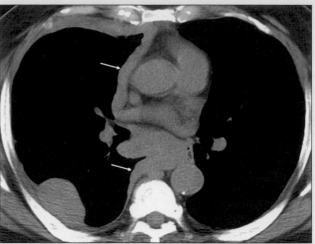

Figure 2. **Mesothelioma.** Non–contrast-enhanced CT shows nodular, circumferential, and mediastinal (*arrows*) pleural thickening of right hemithorax, in keeping with biopsy-proven mesothelioma. (*Courtesy of Dr. Jean M. Seely, University of Ottawa, Canada*)

Figure 1. **Mesothelioma.** Chest radiograph demonstrates left nodular and circumferential pleural thickening, with associated volume loss of the left hemithorax, ipsilateral mediastinal shift, and elevation of the hemidiaphragm. (*Courtesy of Dr. Jean M. Seely, University of Ottawa, Canada*)

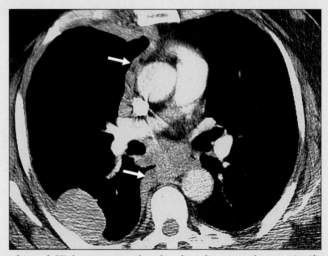

Figure 3. **Mesothelioma.** A contrast-enhanced CT demonstrates that the pleural tumor enhances significantly (same patient as in Fig. 2). Mediastinal pleural thickening is seen clearly (*arrows*). No pleural fluid was present. (*Courtesy of Dr. Jean M. Seely, University of Ottawa, Canada*)

- Symptoms of mesothelioma are chest pain, cough, dyspnea, and weight loss.

DIFFERENTIAL DIAGNOSIS

- Asbestos-related diffuse pleural thickening
- Round atelectasis
- Benign pleural effusion
- Pleural metastases

PATHOLOGY

- Amphiboles, particularly crocidolite, are more potent than chrysotile in inducing lung cancer.
- Mechanism of carcinogenesis is unclear.
- Asbestos-related cancers can occur anywhere in lungs and be of any cell type.
- It is controversial whether asbestos-related lung cancer arises only in the presence of pulmonary fibrosis.
- Pathogenesis of mesothelioma remains unclear.

INCIDENCE/PREVALENCE AND EPIDEMIOLOGY

- Asbestos exposure is associated with increased risk of small cell and non–small cell lung carcinoma and mesothelioma.

- The risk of lung cancer is magnified severalfold in cigarette smokers.
- Asbestos-related lung cancer likely accounts for 2%-3% of all lung cancer deaths among men in Great Britain.
- Number of asbestos-related lung cancers is between two-thirds and one death for every mesothelioma death.

Suggested Readings

British Thoracic Society Standards of Care Committee: BTS statement on malignant mesothelioma in the UK, 2007. Thorax 62 (Suppl 2): ii1–ii19, 2007.

Hodgson JT, Darnton A: The quantitative risks of mesothelioma and lung cancer in relation to asbestos exposure. *Ann Occup Hyg* 44:565-601, 2000.

Robinson BW, Lake RA: Advances in malignant mesothelioma. *N Engl J Med* 353:1591-1603, 2005.

Robinson BW, Musk AW, Lake RA: Malignant mesothelioma. *Lancet* 366:397-408, 2005.

Roggli VL, Sharma A, Butnor KJ, et al: Malignant mesothelioma and occupational exposure to asbestos: A clinicopathological correlation of 1445 cases. *Ultrastruct Pathol* 26:55-65, 2002.

Aluminum Pneumoconiosis

DEFINITION: Inhalation of aluminum dust can result in interstitial fibrosis and patchy granulomatous pneumonitis.

IMAGING

Radiography
Findings
- Bilateral hazy opacities or small nodular opacities more pronounced in upper or middle zones
- Reticulation and honeycombing (sometimes diffuse)
Utility
- Radiography is main imaging modality used in initial assessment and follow-up of patients.
- Chest findings become apparent after few months or several years of exposure.

CT
Findings
- Well-defined nodules of 2-5 mm in diameter or ill-defined centrilobular nodules diffusely throughout both lungs
- Small ill-defined, rounded, centrilobular opacities mainly in upper lobes in early stages
- Fibrosis, resulting in reticular pattern and honeycombing
- Ground-glass opacities with or without traction bronchiectasis
- Increased attenuation of mediastinal lymph nodes
Utility
- Higher sensitivity and specificity
- May show abnormalities in patients with normal radiograph

CLINICAL PRESENTATION

- Cough and dyspnea on exertion
- Spontaneous pneumothorax
- Pulmonary function test results consistent with reduced lung volumes and decreased transfer factor (DLCO)

DIFFERENTIAL DIAGNOSIS

- Nonspecific interstitial pneumonia
- Idiopathic pulmonary fibrosis
- Sarcoidosis

DIAGNOSTIC PEARLS

- Diffuse interstitial fibrosis
- Most severe in upper lung zones, although it may be diffuse
- Centrilobular nodules, bilateral reticulation, and ground-glass opacities
- Exposure to aluminum dust and pot room fumes

- Hypersensitivity pneumonitis
- Drug-induced lung disease

PATHOLOGY

- Stearin-coated, mineral oil–coated, and bare aluminum metal may be all equally effective in producing fibrosis.
- Subpleural and interstitial fibrosis occurs with scar emphysema and spotted granulomatous pneumonitis with giant cells.
- Histologic examination shows interstitial fibrosis, typically most severe in upper lobes, and patchy granulomatous pneumonitis with giant cells.
- High interstitial concentrations of aluminum are found.
- Desquamative interstitial pneumonia, granulomatous lung reaction, and pulmonary alveolar proteinosis have been described after exposure to fumes from aluminum welding.

INCIDENCE/PREVALENCE AND EPIDEMIOLOGY

- Aluminum pneumoconiosis is rare, although exposure to aluminum is very common.
- Small irregular opacities were observed in 7%-8% of 788 male employees of one aluminum production company.
- Prevalence is < 10% in individuals exposed at the workplace.
- Work in aluminum smelters is associated with asthma and chronic air flow obstruction.

WHAT THE REFERRING PHYSICIAN NEEDS TO KNOW

- Clinical symptoms consist of cough and dyspnea on exertion.
- Histologic examination shows interstitial fibrosis that is most severe in upper lobes and patchy granulomatous pneumonitis with giant cells.
- Most common radiologic manifestations consist of centrilobular nodules, bilateral reticulation, and ground-glass opacities that are diffuse or involve mainly upper lobes.

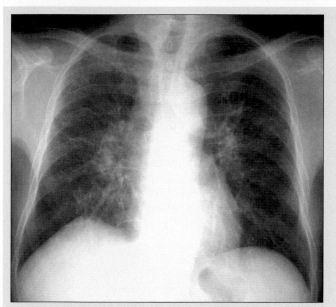

Figure 1. Aluminum pneumoconiosis. Chest radiograph shows ground-glass opacities mainly in the upper and middle lung zones. Also noted is mild cephalad displacement of the hila. (*Courtesy of Dr. Masanori Akira, Osaka, Japan*)

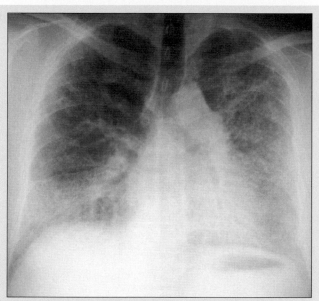

Figure 2. Aluminum pneumoconiosis. Chest radiograph shows extensive bilateral reticulonodular pattern. (*Courtesy of Dr. Masanori Akira, Osaka, Japan*)

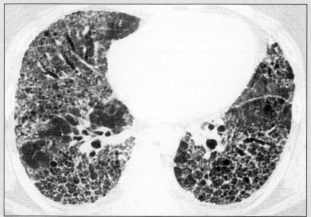

Figure 3. Aluminum pneumoconiosis. High-resolution CT scan reveals extensive reticulation, traction bronchiectasis, traction bronchiolectasis, and honeycombing. (*Courtesy of Dr. Masanori Akira, Osaka, Japan*)

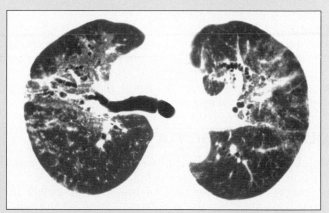

Figure 4. Aluminum pneumoconiosis. High-resolution CT scan demonstrates ground-glass opacities mainly in the central lung regions, a few small nodular and irregular linear opacities, and traction bronchiectasis. (*Courtesy of Dr. Masanori Akira, Osaka, Japan*)

Suggested Readings

Akira M: High-resolution CT in the evaluation of occupational and environmental disease. *Radiol Clin North Am* 40:43-59, 2002.

Akira M: Uncommon pneumoconioses: CT and pathologic findings. *Radiology* 197:403-409, 1995.

Chong S, Lee KS, Chung MJ, et al: Pneumoconiosis: Comparison of imaging and pathologic findings. *RadioGraphics* 26:59-77, 2006.

Hull MJ, Abraham JL: Aluminum welding fume-induced pneumoconiosis. *Hum Pathol* 33 (8):819-825, 2002.

Hard Metal Lung Disease

DEFINITION: Occupational exposure to hard metal (tungsten carbide in cobalt matrix) typically results in giant cell interstitial pneumonia.

IMAGING

Radiography
Findings
- Small irregular opacities, predominantly in middle and lower lung zones.
- Small nodular opacities and diffuse reticulonodular or ground-glass opacities

Utility
- Main imaging modality used in initial assessment and follow-up of patients with hard metal lung disease
- May appear normal despite presence of symptoms and functional impairment

CT
Findings
- Ground-glass opacities, reticulation
- Upper lobe nodular peribronchovascular thickening, subpleural lines, peripheral cystic spaces (paraseptal emphysema)
- Bilateral ground-glass and irregular linear opacities mainly in lower lung zones
- Ground-glass opacities to dense consolidation
- May result in honeycombing

Utility
- Appearance is variable; disease may mimic nonspecific interstitial pneumonia, usual interstitial pneumonia, or sarcoidosis.
- High-resolution CT may be useful in detecting the early parenchymal changes.

CLINICAL PRESENTATION

- Cough, wheeze, dyspnea, chest tightness, and rhinitis occur after 4-6 hours at workplace.
- Cough, gradual shortness of breath, and weight loss occur, with cyanosis and finger clubbing present in more advanced stages.

DIFFERENTIAL DIAGNOSIS

- Hypersensitivity pneumonitis
- Nonspecific interstitial pneumonia
- Drug-induced interstitial pneumonia
- Sarcoidosis
- Idiopathic pulmonary fibrosis

DIAGNOSTIC PEARLS

- Small nodular opacities and diffuse reticulonodular or ground-glass opacities are found in mid and lower lung zones.
- Upper lobe nodular peribronchovascular thickening, subpleural lines, and peripheral cystic spaces are consistent with paraseptal emphysema.
- Appearance may mimic nonspecific interstitial pneumonia, usual interstitial pneumonia, or sarcoidosis.

PATHOLOGY

- Exposure to cobalt is generally considered main cause of hard metal lung disease.
- Biologic reactivity to mixture of cobalt and tungsten carbide is much greater than that to cobalt alone.
- Disease is more likely to occur in poorly regulated workplaces.
- Infiltration of interstitium with lymphocytes and plasma cells, hyperplasia of alveolar epithelium, and cellular accumulation within alveolar lumen are evident.
- Most characteristic finding in hard metal lung disease is multinucleated giant cells in interstitium and alveoli/giant cell interstitial pneumonia.

INCIDENCE/PREVALENCE AND EPIDEMIOLOGY

- Hard metal lung disease occurs in workers engaged in manufacture, utilization, or maintenance of tools composed of hard metal.
- It is more likely to occur in poorly regulated workplaces.
- There is a low prevalence in exposed workers; lack of correlation with intensity and duration of exposure suggests possible genetic susceptibility.
- In one study, 10.9% had work-related wheeze and 0.7% had radiographic interstitial lung disease.
- In another study, 11 of 69 (14%) workers had pulmonary fibrosis.

WHAT THE REFERRING PHYSICIAN NEEDS TO KNOW

- Main respiratory complications are asthma, hypersensitivity pneumonitis, and pulmonary fibrosis.
- Bronchoalveolar lavage may show characteristic multinucleated "cannibalistic" giant cells.
- Most common radiographic abnormality of hard metal pneumoconiosis is small irregular opacities in middle and lower lung zones.
- Most common presentation on CT is that of bilateral ground-glass opacities and reticulation mimicking nonspecific interstitial pneumonia.

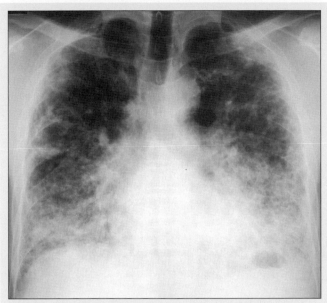

Figure 1. **Hard metal interstitial lung disease.** Posteroanterior chest radiograph reveals coarse reticular pattern and patchy ground-glass opacities involving predominantly the peripheral lung regions and the lower lung zones.(*Courtesy of Dr. Masanori Akira, Osaka, Japan*)

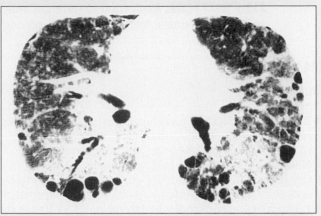

Figure 2. **Hard metal interstitial lung disease.** High-resolution CT scan demonstrates extensive bilateral ground-glass opacities, foci of consolidation, centrilobular nodular opacities, mild reticulation, traction bronchiectasis, and several bullae.(*Courtesy of Dr. Masanori Akira, Osaka, Japan*)

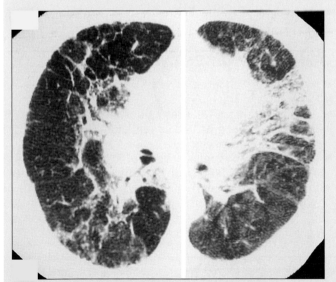

Figure 3. **Hard metal interstitial lung disease.** High-resolution CT shows multilobular ground-glass opacities, areas of consolidation, mild reticulation, and traction bronchiectasis. (*Courtesy of Dr. Masanori Akira, Osaka, Japan*)

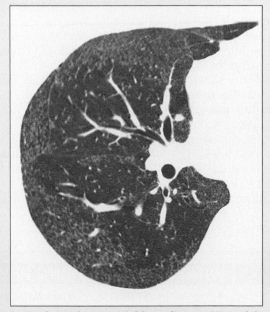

Figure 4. **Hard metal interstitial lung disease.** View of the right lung from a high-resolution CT scan reveals fine nodular opacities in the peripheral lung regions.(*Courtesy of Dr. Masanori Akira, Osaka, Japan*)

Suggested Readings

Akira M: High-resolution CT in the evaluation of occupational and environmental disease. *Radiol Clin North Am* 40:43-59, 2002.

Chong S, Lee KS, Chung MJ, et al: Pneumoconiosis: Comparison of imaging and pathologic findings. *RadioGraphics* 26:59-77, 2006.

Dunlop P, Müller NL, Wilson J, et al: Hard metal lung disease: High resolution CT and histologic correlation of the initial findings and demonstration of interval improvement. *J Thorac Imaging* 20(4):301-304, 2005.

Nemery B, Verbeken EK, Demedts M: Giant cell interstitial pneumonia (hard metal lung disease, cobalt lung). *Semin Respir Crit Care Med* 22:435-448, 2001.

Talc Pneumoconiosis

DEFINITION: Aspiration of pure talc may result in acute or chronic bronchitis, centrilobular nodules, interstitial fibrosis, and, occasionally, pleural plaques.

IMAGING

Radiography
Findings
- Inhalational talcosis: nodular pattern consists of opacities of 3.0-5.0 mm in diameter; may be diffuse or involve mainly middle or upper lung zones
- Nodular, linear, conglomerate fibrosis
- Conglomeration of nodules that may result in large opacities that may show evidence of cavity formation
- Bilateral pleural plaques in lateral parts of lower thorax and diaphragmatic plaques with calcification
- Pure talcosis: mixture of rounded and irregular opacities, which appear in middle zones and are often perihilar
- Intravenous talcosis: small nodular opacities that may progress to large masses or mass-like areas of consolidation

Utility
- Chest radiography is the main imaging modality in initial assessment and follow-up of talc pneumoconiosis.
- Nodular conglomeration resembles silicosis and progressive massive fibrosis.

CT
Findings
- Inhalational talcosis: small centrilobular and subpleural nodules and conglomerated masses containing focal areas of high attenuation
- Septal lines, subpleural lines, ground-glass opacity, and lobular areas of low attenuation
- Lymph node enlargement containing focal areas of high attenuation
- Chronic intravenous talcosis: diffuse small nodules (micronodules), ground-glass opacities, perihilar conglomerate masses with areas of high attenuation, and lower lobe panacinar emphysema
- Talc pleurodesis: high-density areas of pleural thickening

DIAGNOSTIC PEARLS
- Centrilobular nodules and high density areas due to talc accumulation.
- Conglomerated masses containing focal areas of high attenuation.
- Lower lobe panacinar emphysema in intravenous talcosis.
- Lymph node enlargement, pleural plaques.

Utility
- CT is more sensitive in detecting pleural plaques and lymph node enlargement with areas of high attenuation.
- High attenuation within perihilar massive areas of fibrosis in intravenous drug users is virtually diagnostic of talcosis.

Positron Emission Tomography
Findings
- Talc pleurodesis: increased FDG uptake on PET
Utility
- Limited value in the diagnosis

CLINICAL PRESENTATION
- Dyspnea and cough
- Cyanosis and finger clubbing
- Initially symptom free; resembles mild asbestosis as it progresses; accompanied by reduction in lung volumes and diffusing capacity
- Progressive dyspnea, weight loss from labored breathing, hypoxia, and cor pulmonale with eventual right-sided heart failure even after cessation of exposure

---

WHAT THE REFERRING PHYSICIAN NEEDS TO KNOW
- Aspiration of pure talc may result in acute or chronic bronchitis, centrilobular nodules, interstitial fibrosis, and, occasionally, pleural plaques.
- Talc may be contaminated with other substances, particularly silica and asbestos.
- Talc may be detected in bronchoalveolar lavage fluid.
- The most common radiologic findings consist of centrilobular nodules and high-density areas due to talc accumulation.
- Differential diagnosis of talcoasbestosis includes all other types of interstitial pneumonias.
- Intravenous talcosis occurs in intravenous drug users who inject medications intended for oral use; the most commonly used fillers in pills are talc, cornstarch, and microcrystalline cellulose.
- Intravenous talcosis may result in diffuse micronodules, perihilar conglomerate masses of fibrosis with characteristic areas of high attenuation on CT, and, particularly in patients with talcosis secondary to methylphenidate abuse, panacinar emphysema.

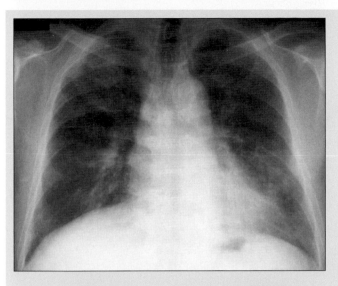

Figure 1. **Talc pneumoconiosis.** Chest radiograph shows poorly defined small nodular opacities diffusely distributed throughout both lungs. Also noted are confluent opacities. (*Courtesy of Dr. Masanori Akira, Osaka, Japan*)

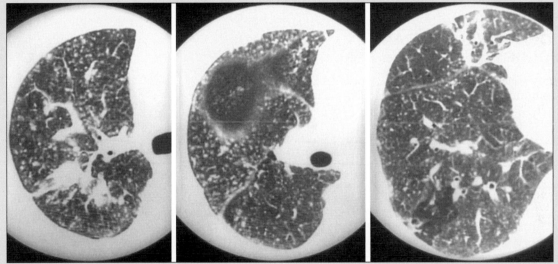

Figure 2. **Talc pneumoconiosis.** Views of the right lung from high-resolution CT scans at three different levels show small centrilobular nodules in all lung zones. Also noted is a focal large opacity in the right upper lobe. Incidental note is made of mild right middle and lower lobe consolidation. (*Courtesy of Dr. Masanori Akira, Osaka, Japan*)

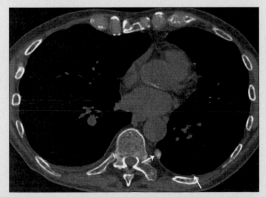

Figure 3. **Talc pleurodesis in a 77-year-old man with chronic obstructive airway disease and emphysema.** CT image photographed at soft tissue windows demonstrates left pleural thickening containing focal areas of high attenuation due to talc accumulation (*arrows*). Also noted is a small right pleural effusion. The patient underwent left talc pleurodesis for recurrent pneumothorax 7 years before the CT.

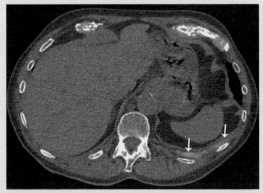

Figure 4. **Talc pleurodesis in a 77-year-old man with chronic obstructive airway disease and emphysema.** CT image photographed at soft tissue windows demonstrates left pleural thickening containing focal areas of high attenuation due to talc accumulation (*arrows*). The patient underwent left talc pleurodesis for recurrent pneumothorax 7 years before the CT.

DIFFERENTIAL DIAGNOSIS

- Drug-induced interstitial pneumonia
- Sarcoidosis
- Silicosis
- Nonspecific interstitial pneumonia
- Hypersensitivity pneumonitis

PATHOLOGY

- Inhalation of talc (inhalational talcosis): acute or chronic bronchitis, interstitial fibrosis.
- Intravenously administered talc: interstitial and perivascular granulomatous reaction, interstitial fibrosis, vascular thrombotic lesions, and pulmonary hypertension.
- Birefringent particulate material (talc) in the interstitium.

INCIDENCE/PREVALENCE AND EPIDEMIOLOGY

- In one study of 176 individuals who worked exclusively in talc industry, 46 (27%) developed pneumoconiosis.

- In another study of workers exposed to talc (free of asbestos, silica), 10% had diffuse small rounded or irregular opacities on radiography.
- Intravenous talcosis occurs in intravenous drug users who inject medications intended for oral use; the most commonly used fillers in pills are talc, cornstarch, and microcrystalline cellulose.
- Lower lobe panacinar emphysema is more common in intravenous talcosis in methylphenidate abusers.

Suggested Readings

Akira M: High-resolution CT in the evaluation of occupational and environmental disease. *Radiol Clin North Am* 40:43-59, 2002.

Chong S, Lee KS, Chung MJ, et al: Pneumoconiosis: Comparison of imaging and pathologic findings. *RadioGraphics* 26:59-77, 2006.

Marchiori E, Souza AS Jr, Müller NL: Inhalational pulmonary talcosis: High-resolution CT findings in 3 patients. *J Thorac Imaging* 19(1):41-44, 2004.

Ward S, Heyneman LE, Reittner P, et al: Talcosis associated with IV abuse of oral medications: CT findings. *AJR Am J Roentgenol* 174(3):789-793, 2000.

Welder's Pneumoconiosis (Welder's Lung)

DEFINITION: Exposure to welding fumes is a risk factor for developing pneumoconiosis, chronic bronchitis, and lung cancer.

IMAGING

Radiography
Findings
- Very fine nodules most prominent in middle third of lungs, perihilar regions, or lower lung zones
- Resolves after removal of patients from occupational exposure
- Pulmonary fibrosis

Utility
- Initial imaging modality

CT
Findings
- Ill-defined micronodules and fine branching lines are diffusely distributed in lung.
- Most micronodules have centrilobular distribution.
- Coalescence of micronodules and fine branching lines result in fine reticular pattern.
- Honeycomb pattern and ground-glass opacities are seen.
- Conglomerated masses with areas of high attenuation indicating organizing pneumonia have been reported.

Utility
- CT may show parenchymal abnormalities in patients with normal radiographs.

CLINICAL PRESENTATION

- Seldom results in symptoms
- Irreversible restrictive effect on pulmonary function studies
- Dyspnea on effort and cough

DIFFERENTIAL DIAGNOSIS

- Hypersensitivity pneumonitis
- Respiratory bronchiolitis
- Respiratory bronchiolitis/interstitial lung disease
- Pneumonia: *Mycoplasma*

DIAGNOSTIC PEARLS

- Ill-defined micronodules and fine branching lines diffusely distributed in lung
- Honeycomb pattern, ground-glass opacities, emphysema
- Elevation of ferritin levels in serum and bronchoalveolar lavage fluid possible

PATHOLOGY

- Iron dust and dust-laden macrophages associated with minimal fibrosis.
- Collections of dust along the interlobular septa and pleural lymphatics.
- Rounded ferruginous bodies with round or polygonal black cores.
- Micronodules evident as radiopaque accumulations of iron particles that lie within macrophages, aggregated along perivascular and peribronchial lymphatic vessels.

INCIDENCE/PREVALENCE AND EPIDEMIOLOGY

- Survey of chest radiographic abnormalities in 661 employed British electric arc welders found 7% prevalence of small rounded opacities.
- Small centrilobular nodules were seen on high-resolution CT in 81.8% of cases.
- Emphysematous changes were found in 27.3%.
- Fibrosis was found in 27.3% of cases.

Suggested Readings

Akira M: High-resolution CT in the evaluation of occupational and environmental disease. *Radiol Clin North Am* 40:43-59, 2002.

Chong S, Lee KS, Chung MJ, et al: Pneumoconiosis: Comparison of imaging and pathologic findings. *RadioGraphics* 26:59-77, 2006.

Sferlazza SJ, Beckett WS: The respiratory health of welders: State of the art. *Am Rev Respir Dis* 143:1134-1148, 1991.

Yoshii C, Matsuyama T, Takazawa A, et al: Welder's pneumoconiosis: Diagnostic usefulness of high-resolution computed tomography and ferritin determinations in bronchoalveolar lavage fluid. *Intern Med* 41(12):1111-1117, 2002.

WHAT THE REFERRING PHYSICIAN NEEDS TO KNOW

- Principal component of welding fumes is iron oxide.
- Ferritin levels may be elevated in serum and in bronchoalveolar lavage fluid.
- Main radiologic finding is the presence of small rounded opacities.
- Most common high-resolution CT findings consist of bilateral ill-defined centrilobular nodules and fine branching linear opacities.
- Appearance in high-resolution CT may mimic hypersensitivity pneumonitis.

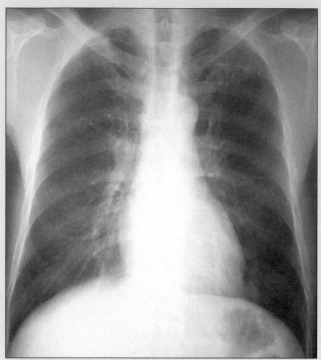

Figure 1. Welder's pneumoconiosis. Posteroanterior chest radiograph reveals fine nodular opacities that are most prominent in the middle third of the lungs. (*Courtesy of Dr. Masanori Akira, Osaka, Japan*)

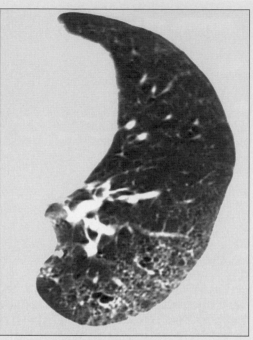

Figure 2. Welder's pneumoconiosis. View of the left lung from a CT scan shows ground-glass opacities, reticulation, traction bronchiectasis, and mild emphysema. (*Courtesy of Dr. Masanori Akira, Osaka, Japan*)

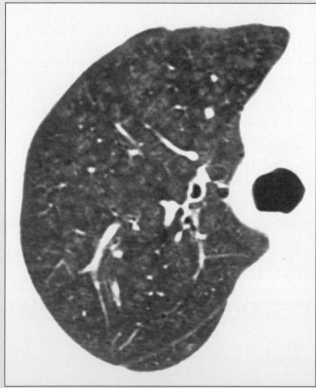

Figure 3. Welder's pneumoconiosis. View of the right upper lobe from a high-resolution CT scan shows ill-defined centrilobular nodules. (*Courtesy of Dr. Masanori Akira, Osaka, Japan*)

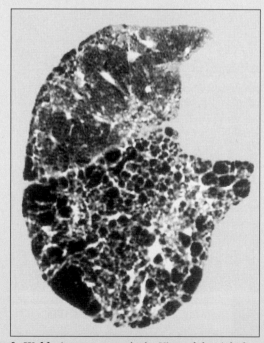

Figure 4. Welder's pneumoconiosis. View of the right lung from a CT scan shows ground-glass opacities, extensive reticulation, and honeycombing. Also noted is centrilobular and paraseptal emphysema. (*Courtesy of Dr. Masanori Akira, Osaka, Japan*)

Aspiration Bronchiolitis

DEFINITION: Aspiration bronchiolitis is a chronic inflammatory reaction to recurrent aspirated foreign particles in the bronchioles.

IMAGING

Radiography
Findings
- Poorly defined small nodular opacities mainly in dependent lung regions

Utility
- Radiographic findings are nonspecific.

CT
Findings
- Unilateral or bilateral centrilobular nodular and branching opacities ("tree-in-bud" pattern) and 5-10 mm diameter, poorly defined airspace nodules
- Abnormalities mainly in dependent lung regions
- Fluid within bronchi
- Presence of fluid-filled esophagus or hiatal hernia helpful in diagnosis

Utility
- Diagnosis often first suggested on CT

CLINICAL PRESENTATION

- Cough and dysphagia

DIFFERENTIAL DIAGNOSIS

- Panbronchiolitis
- Infectious bronchiolitis
- Bronchopneumonia

PATHOLOGY

- Chronic inflammatory reaction to recurrent aspirated foreign particles in the bronchioles

INCIDENCE/PREVALENCE AND EPIDEMIOLOGY

- Patients with neurologic disorders and esophageal conditions such as achalasia, Zenker diverticulum, or esophageal carcinoma are at risk for aspiration bronchiolitis.

DIAGNOSTIC PEARLS

- Unilateral or bilateral centrilobular nodular and branching opacities ("tree-in-bud" pattern)
- Involves mainly dependent regions but can be diffuse
- Presence of predisposing neurologic disorders and esophageal conditions such as achalasia, Zenker diverticulum, or esophageal carcinoma

Suggested Readings

Barnes TW, Vassallo R, Tazelaar HD, et al: Diffuse bronchiolar disease due to chronic occult aspiration. *Mayo Clin Proc* 81:172-176, 2006.

Marom EM, McAdams HP, Sporn TA, Goodman PC: Lentil aspiration pneumonia: Radiographic and CT findings. *J Comput Assist Tomogr* 22:598-600, 1998.

Matsuse T, Oka T, Kida K, Fukuchi Y: Importance of diffuse aspiration bronchiolitis caused by chronic occult aspiration in the elderly. *Chest* 110:1289-1293, 1996.

Mukhopadhyay S, Katzenstein AL: Pulmonary disease due to aspiration of food and other particulate matter: A clinicopathologic study of 59 cases diagnosed on biopsy or resection specimens. *Am J Surg Pathol* 31:752-759, 2007.

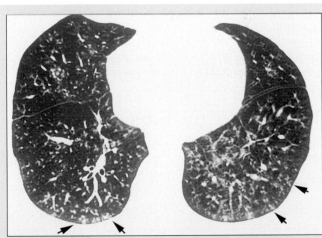

Figure 1. Aspirative cellular bronchiolitis in a 32-year-old woman with recurrent aspirations. High-resolution CT obtained at the level of the lung bases shows centrilobular nodules and branching opacities, resulting in a "tree-in-bud" appearance (*arrows*).

WHAT THE REFERRING PHYSICIAN NEEDS TO KNOW

- Pulmonary complications due to aspiration typically involve mainly dependent lung regions, most commonly the posterior segment of upper lobes and/or superior segment of lower lobes.

Aspiration of Foreign Bodies

DEFINITION: A foreign body in the airway can result in obstruction, air trapping, and inflammation.

IMAGING

Radiography
Findings
- Endotracheal or endobronchial soft tissue or high density
- Obstructive lobar or segmental overinflation or atelectasis
- Chronic loss of volume in the affected lobe; recurrent pneumonias
- Development of bronchiectasis

Utility
- Usually first and only imaging modality used in the assessment of these patients

CT
Findings
- Endotracheal or endobronchial soft tissue density
- Decreased attenuation and vascularity and air trapping in partial obstruction
- Atelectasis in complete bronchial obstruction

Utility
- More sensitive than chest radiography at demonstrating radiolucent foreign bodies

CLINICAL PRESENTATION

- Clinically, most patients are children with varying degrees of cough and recent history of foreign-body aspiration.
- Once the foreign body is within the lung parenchyma, prolonged irritation with intermittent infections may result in hemoptysis.

DIFFERENTIAL DIAGNOSIS

- Squamous cell carcinoma
- Carcinoid tumor
- Asthma

DIAGNOSTIC PEARLS

- Acute cough and shortness of breath
- Most commonly child or adult with impaired consciousness
- Obstructive lobar or segmental overinflation or atelectasis
- Chronic loss of volume in the affected lobe; recurrent pneumonias
- Centrally located mass with lobar or segmental atelectasis

- Pneumonia
- Bronchiectasis
- Bronchiolithiasis

PATHOLOGY

- In adults, most inhaled foreign bodies are food and broken fragments of teeth that frequently lodge in the main or lobar bronchus.
- Occasionally, the development of chronic inflammatory reaction around the inhaled material may lead to intrabronchial mass formation.

INCIDENCE/PREVALENCE AND EPIDEMIOLOGY

- Foreign-body aspiration is the most common cause of intraluminal airway abnormality in childhood.
- Foreign-body aspiration is unusual in adults.

Suggested Readings

Franquet T, Gimenez A, Roson N, et al: Aspiration diseases: Findings, pitfalls, and differential diagnosis. *RadioGraphics* 20:673-685, 2000.
Marik PE: Aspiration pneumonitis and aspiration pneumonia. *N Engl J Med* 344:665-671, 2001.
Zissin R, Shapiro-Feinberg M, Rozenman J, et al: CT findings of the chest in adults with aspirated foreign bodies. *Eur Radiol* 11:606-611, 2001.

WHAT THE REFERRING PHYSICIAN NEEDS TO KNOW

- Diagnosis requires careful integration of clinical data and radiographic findings.
- Definitive diagnosis is usually made by chest radiography and bronchoscopy.
- Diagnosis is sometimes difficult because the patient may not be aware of having aspirated.
- Foreign-body aspiration is unusual in adults and is often overlooked as a cause of airway obstruction.

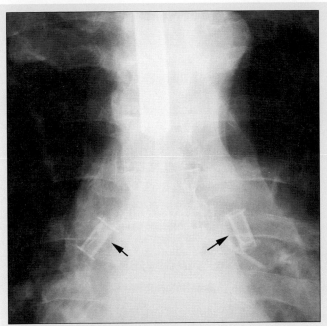

Figure 1. Aspiration of esophageal speech devices. A close-up view of the chest radiograph shows two esophageal speech devices in the bronchus intermedius and left lower bronchus (*arrows*). (*Courtesy of Dr. Tomás Franquet, Barcelona, Spain*)

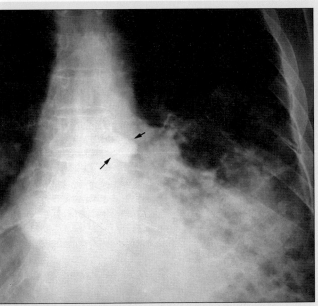

Figure 2. Aspiration of a tooth. This 75-year-old man developed recurrent episodes of infection in the left lower lobe after inadvertent aspiration of a tooth. Close-up view of a posterior chest radiograph shows an endobronchial tooth (*arrows*) and multiple rounded lucencies in the left lower lung representing postobstructive bronchiectasis. (*Courtesy of Dr. Tomás Franquet, Barcelona, Spain*)

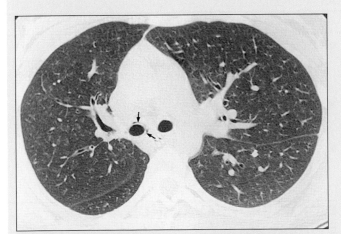

Figure 3. Foreign body aspiration. A 23-year-old drug addict presented with a 3-month history of cough productive of increasing amounts of green sputum. High-resolution CT scan shows tubing within the lumen of the right main bronchus (*arrows*). A small amount of secretions within the bronchial lumen and decreased attenuation, vascularity, and volume of the right lung are evident. The plastic tube was removed bronchoscopically. (*From Müller NL, Fraser RS, Colman NC, Paré PD: Radiologic Diagnosis of Diseases of the Chest. Philadelphia, WB Saunders, 2001.*)

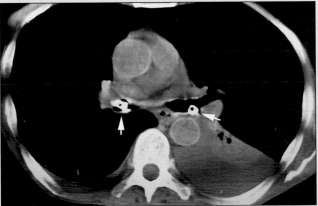

Figure 4. Aspiration of esophageal speech devices. Nonenhanced CT nicely depicts the intrabronchial devices (*arrows*). A left lower lobe atelectasis and bilateral pleural effusions are also present. The patient was a 56-year-old mentally retarded man treated with radical laryngectomy. (*Courtesy of Dr. Tomás Franquet, Barcelona, Spain*)

Aspiration Pneumonia

DEFINITION: Aspiration pneumonia is a pulmonary infection caused by aspiration of colonized oropharyngeal secretions.

IMAGING

Radiography
Findings
- Unilateral or bilateral patchy or confluent airspace consolidation involving mainly the dependent lung regions
- Recumbent patients: diffuse perihilar consolidation reflecting involvement of posterior segments of upper lobes or superior segments of lower lobes
- Upright patients: consolidation seen mainly in basal segments of the lower lobes
- Lung abscess formation of single or multiple masses usually measuring 2.0-6.0 cm in diameter that frequently cavitate

Utility
- Helpful in suggesting diagnosis in the appropriate clinical setting

CT
Findings
- Unilateral or bilateral patchy or confluent consolidation and ground-glass opacities involving mainly the dependent lung regions
- Poorly defined centrilobular nodules, presence of bronchiolitis and peribronchiolar inflammation, and presence of fluid or debris within dependent airways
- Abscess formation; single or multiple masses that frequently cavitate
- Fluid within bronchi

Utility
- Greater sensitivity and specificity than radiography in making the diagnosis

CLINICAL PRESENTATION

- Acute aspiration results in cough, wheezing, cyanosis, dyspnea, and tachypnea.
- Fever, cough, and purulent sputum are noted.
- Signs and symptoms of pneumonia may be milder or even absent in the elderly.
- Silent aspiration occurs during anesthesia or while a patient is intubated in the intensive care unit.

DIAGNOSTIC PEARLS

- Unilateral or bilateral patchy areas of consolidation
- Dependent distribution
- Abscess formation
- Aspiration of foreign material into the lungs may result in infection (pneumonia), chemical pneumonitis, or lipoid pneumonia
- Chemical pneumonitis due to aspiration of large quantities of sterile gastric fluid is also known as Mendelson syndrome

DIFFERENTIAL DIAGNOSIS

- Aspiration pneumonitis due to aspiration of sterile gastric fluid
- Bronchopneumonia
- Pulmonary hemorrhage
- Pulmonary edema

PATHOLOGY

- Pneumonia results from aspiration of secretions containing a variety of bacteria that are normally present in the oropharynx.
- Failure of mechanical defenses, defects in phagocytosis/ciliary function, neutropenia, and hypogammaglobulinemia result in increased frequency or severity of pneumonia.
- Patients with poor dental hygiene or advanced periodontal disease are at particular risk for development of aspiration pneumonia.
- Histologic findings include bronchopneumonia and foreign body granulomas.

INCIDENCE/PREVALENCE AND EPIDEMIOLOGY

- Ninety percent of aspiration pneumonias are caused by polymicrobial flora that include aerobic and anaerobic organisms.

WHAT THE REFERRING PHYSICIAN NEEDS TO KNOW

- Complications associated with aspiration pneumonia include abscess formation, necrotizing pneumonia, pleural effusion, and empyema.
- Prolonged clinical course or large aspirations may result in severe necrotizing bronchopneumonia or lung abscess formation.
- Imaging examinations are interpreted with awareness of clinical findings, including duration of symptoms and presence of fever, cough, dyspnea, and leukocytosis.

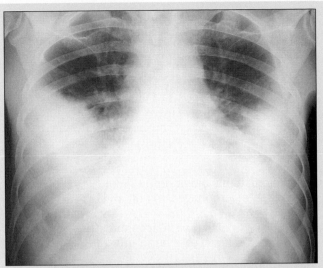

Figure 1. Acute aspiration pneumonia in 65-year-old alcoholic man. Anteroposterior chest radiograph shows extensive bilateral consolidation. (*Courtesy of Dr. Tomás Franquet, Barcelona, Spain*)

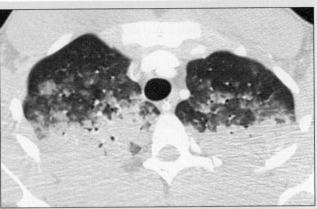

Figure 2. Acute aspiration pneumonia in 45-year-old man after a motor vehicle accident. A CT image shows extensive bilateral consolidation and poorly defined centrilobular nodules involving the dependent lung regions. (*Courtesy of Dr. Tomás Franquet, Barcelona, Spain*)

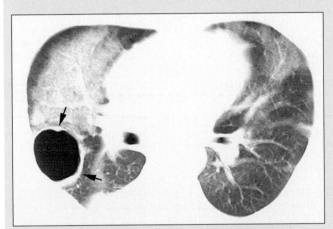

Figure 3. Acute aspiration pneumonia in 52-year-old man. A CT image obtained 3 days after aspiration shows extensive bilateral ground-glass opacities in upper lobes. A thin-walled abscess is present in the right lung (*arrows*). Also noted is a right pleural effusion. (*Courtesy of Dr. Tomás Franquet, Barcelona, Spain*)

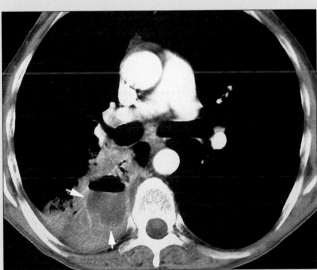

Figure 4. Acute aspiration pneumonia with abscess formation in a 56-year-old alcoholic man. A contrast-enhanced CT image shows airspace consolidation in the superior segment of the right lower lobe. An abscess with an air-fluid level is present within the parenchymal consolidation (*arrows*). (*Courtesy of Dr. Tomás Franquet, Barcelona, Spain*)

■ During sleep, 50% of normal individuals aspirate small volumes of oropharyngeal secretions.
■ The most common cause of lung abscess is aspiration.
■ Aspiration is estimated to account for 5% to 15% of community acquired pneumonias.
■ Aspiration occurs mainly in patients with reduced consciousness (general anesthesia, seizures, head trauma, alcoholism), neurologic disorders (multiple sclerosis, dementia) and esophageal disorders (dysphagia, gastroesophageal reflux).

Suggested Readings

Franquet T, Gimenez A, Roson N, et al: Aspiration diseases: Findings, pitfalls, and differential diagnosis. *RadioGraphics* 20:673-685, 2000.
Marik PE: Aspiration pneumonitis and aspiration pneumonia. *N Engl J Med* 344:665-671, 2001.

Lipoid Pneumonia

DEFINITION: Lipoid pneumonia results from repetitive aspiration or inhalation of mineral oil or a related material into the distal lung.

IMAGING

Radiography
Findings
- Single or multiple areas of consolidation
- May have mass-like appearance

Utility
- Helpful in demonstrating presence of parenchymal abnormality
- Nonspecific findings

CT
Findings
- Single or multiple areas of consolidation
- Focal areas of fat density
- "Crazy-paving" pattern may be seen

Utility
- Method of choice in establishing diagnosis

CLINICAL PRESENTATION

- Often asymptomatic
- Cough and low-grade fever

DIFFERENTIAL DIAGNOSIS

- Bronchopneumonia
- Lung abscess
- Pulmonary carcinoma
- Lymphoma
- Organizing pneumonia

PATHOLOGY

- Chronic exogenous lipoid pneumonia results from repetitive aspiration or inhalation of mineral oil or related material into distal lung.

DIAGNOSTIC PEARLS

- Single or multiple areas of consolidation
- Focal areas of fat density
- "Crazy-paving" pattern on high-resolution CT

- Characteristic histologic finding consists of numerous lipid-laden macrophages that fill and distend the alveolar walls and interstitium.
- Disease is associated with accumulation of lipid material, inflammatory cellular infiltration, and variable amount of fibrosis.
- Lipoid pneumonia in children is usually caused by aspiration of cod liver oil or milk.

INCIDENCE/PREVALENCE AND EPIDEMIOLOGY

- Most common cause: mineral oil for treatment of constipation and frequent use of oily nose drops for chronic rhinitis
- Occurs most often in young children and in the elderly

Suggested Readings

Franquet T, Gimenez A, Roson N, et al: Aspiration diseases: Findings, pitfalls, and differential diagnosis. *RadioGraphics* 20:673-685, 2000.
Gaerte SC, Meyer CA, Winer-Muram HT, et al: Fat-containing lesions of the chest. *RadioGraphics* 22(Spec No):S61-S78, 2002.
Lee KS, Müller NL, Hale V, et al: Lipoid pneumonia: CT findings. *J Comput Assist Tomogr* 19:48-51, 1995.

WHAT THE REFERRING PHYSICIAN NEEDS TO KNOW

- Lipoid pneumonia results from chronic aspiration of mineral, animal, or vegetable oils into the lungs.
- CT, particularly high-resolution CT, is imaging modality of choice for the diagnosis.
- Characteristic areas of fat density are evident within the consolidation in up to 80% of cases.

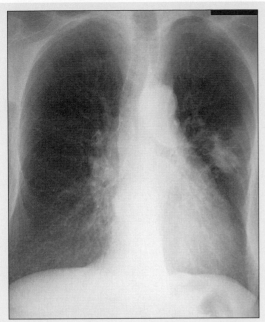

Figure 1. Lipoid pneumonia: mass lesion. Chest radiograph in an 80-year-old woman shows consolidation in the left upper lobe. (*From Müller NL, Fraser RS, Colman NC, Paré PD:* Radiologic Diagnosis of Diseases of the Chest. *Philadelphia, WB Saunders, 2001.*)

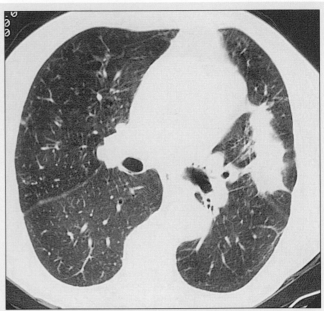

Figure 2. Lipoid pneumonia: mass lesion. High-resolution CT scan in an 80-year-old woman shows focal area of consolidation with surrounding linear opacities and architectural distortion consistent with fibrosis. (*From Müller NL, Fraser RS, Colman NC, Paré PD:* Radiologic Diagnosis of Diseases of the Chest. *Philadelphia, WB Saunders, 2001.*)

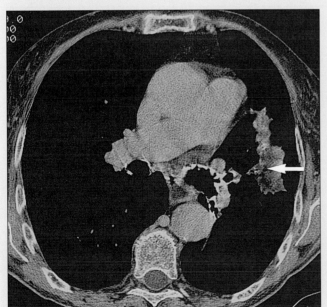

Figure 3. Lipoid pneumonia: mass lesion. High-resolution CT scan in an 80-year-old woman shows focal area of consolidation with surrounding linear opacities and architectural distortion consistent with fibrosis. Localized areas of fat attenuation are present within the consolidation (*arrow*), permitting the diagnosis of lipoid pneumonia. The diagnosis was confirmed by fine-needle aspiration biopsy. The patient had a history of intake of mineral oil for constipation. (*From Müller NL, Fraser RS, Colman NC, Paré PD:* Radiologic Diagnosis of Diseases of the Chest. *Philadelphia, WB Saunders, 2001.*)

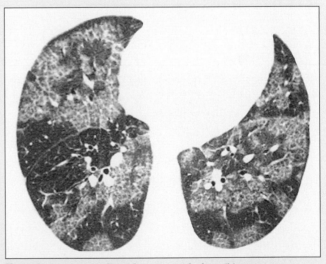

Figure 4. Exogenous lipoid pneumonia in a 54-year-old woman with mild dyspnea. High-resolution CT scan through lung bases shows patchy ground-glass opacities and superimposed fine reticulation resulting in a "crazy-paving" pattern. (*Courtesy of Dr. Tomás Franquet, Barcelona, Spain*)

SECTION XV

Iatrogenic Lung Disease and Trauma

Drug-Induced Nonspecific Interstitial Pneumonia

DEFINITION: Nonspecific interstitial pneumonia is a common reaction pattern to drugs.

IMAGING

Radiography
Findings
- Bilateral ground-glass opacities frequently with associated reticulation and volume loss

Utility
- Usually first imaging modality used in diagnosis

CT
Findings
- Extensive bilateral ground-glass opacities
- Disease progression with superimposed reticulation, traction bronchiectasis, and bronchiolectasis
- May have upper or lower lung predominance

Utility
- More precise assessment of presence and characterization of pattern and distribution of parenchymal and airway abnormalities than chest radiography
- May demonstrate abnormalities in patients with normal radiographs
- Best noninvasive method to assess presence of drug-induced lung disease and to predict underlying histologic pattern

CLINICAL PRESENTATION

- Cough
- Dyspnea
- Fatigue
- Fever
- Chest pain
- Weight loss

DIFFERENTIAL DIAGNOSIS

- Radiation-induced lung disease
- Hypersensitivity pneumonitis
- Collagen vascular disease
- Pneumonia
- Diffuse pulmonary hemorrhage

DIAGNOSTIC PEARLS

- Characterized histologically by varying proportions of interstitial inflammation and fibrosis that are temporally uniform
- Radiographic appearance of bilateral ground-glass opacities frequently with associated reticulation and volume loss
- May be diffuse or involve mainly lower lung zones, with traction bronchiectasis and bronchiolectasis commonly seen on CT
- Nonspecific interstitial pneumonia is a common pulmonary reaction pattern to drugs.

PATHOLOGY

- Adverse reactions to drugs include drug side effect, drug interaction, drug overdose, drug intolerance, drug idiosyncrasy, and drug allergy.
- Nonspecific interstitial pneumonia and other interstitial pneumonias are relatively common manifestations of drug-induced lung disease.
- Drugs most commonly associated with a nonspecific interstitial pneumonia–like pattern include amiodarone, methotrexate, nitrofurantoin, bleomycin, hydrochlorothiazide, and carmustine.

INCIDENCE/PREVALENCE AND EPIDEMIOLOGY

- Individuals aged 65 years or older twice as more likely to develop adverse drug events than younger persons.
- Common drug reaction pattern.

Suggested Readings

Flieder DB, Travis WD: Pathologic characteristics of drug-induced lung disease. *Clin Chest Med* 25:37-45, 2004.
Silva CI, Müller NL: Drug-induced lung diseases: Most common reaction patterns and corresponding high-resolution CT manifestations. *Semin Ultrasound CT MR* 27:111-116, 2006.

WHAT THE REFERRING PHYSICIAN NEEDS TO KNOW

- Common causes of nonspecific interstitial pneumonia include amiodarone, methotrexate, nitrofurantoin, bleomycin, hydrochlorothiazide, and carmustine.
- Clinical, radiologic, and histologic manifestations of pulmonary drug reactions are nonspecific and mimic various acute and chronic lung diseases.

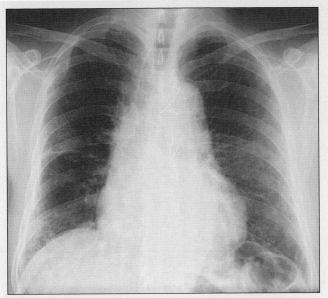

Figure 1. **Nonspecific interstitial pneumonia due to amiodarone.** Chest radiograph shows bilateral poorly defined ground-glass opacities and mild reticulation.

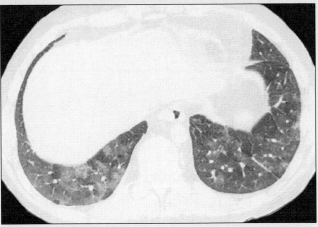

Figure 2. **Nonspecific interstitial pneumonia due to busulfan.** High-resolution CT image at level of lung bases demonstrates diffuse bilateral ground-glass opacities.

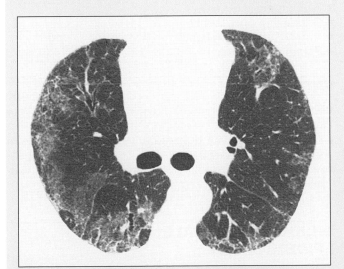

Figure 3. **Nonspecific interstitial pneumonia due to nitrofurantoin.** High-resolution CT image at level of main bronchi shows bilateral ground-glass opacities and reticulation mainly in peripheral lung regions.

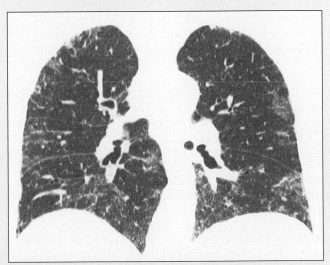

Figure 4. **Nonspecific interstitial pneumonia due to nitrofurantoin.** Coronal reformatted image demonstrates involvement of all lung zones and predominantly peripheral and basal distribution of ground-glass opacities and mild reticulation.

Drug-Induced Diffuse Alveolar Damage

DEFINITION: Drug-induced diffuse alveolar damage is a drug reaction that manifests as diffuse alveolar damage, which is a histopathologic finding corresponding to the clinical entity of acute respiratory distress syndrome.

IMAGING

Radiography

Findings

- Initially consists of bilateral homogeneous or heterogeneous opacities, often in mid and lower lung distribution.
- Commonly progresses to diffuse bilateral opacification.

Utility

- Radiographic manifestations of drug reaction are protean and mimic those of other interstitial and airspace lung diseases.
- Radiographic findings are similar to those from other causes of acute respiratory distress syndrome.

CT

Findings

- Bilateral ground-glass opacities and areas of consolidation typically involve mainly dependent lung regions.
- Predominant finding in early exudative phase is ground-glass opacities, initially patchy, that have a geographic appearance with adjacent areas of lobular sparing.
- Ground-glass opacities rapidly become confluent, with focal lobular sparing, and are associated with smooth linear opacities ("crazy-paving" pattern) and areas of consolidation.
- Further progression of disease is seen predominantly as consolidation.
- Organizing phase involves architectural distortion and traction bronchiectasis.
- Chronic fibrotic phase involves extensive reticulation; honeycombing may be seen.

Utility

- High-resolution CT findings of drug-induced diffuse alveolar damage are similar to those of other causes of ARDS.
- High-resolution CT allows for more precise assessment of presence and characterization of pattern and distribution of parenchymal/airway abnormalities than chest radiography.

DIAGNOSTIC PEARLS

- Initially, bilateral homogeneous or heterogeneous opacities, often in mid and lower lung distribution
- "Crazy-paving" pattern
- Focal lobular sparing commonly seen on CT
- Diagnostic criteria: drug exposure history, consistent radiologic findings, histologic evidence of diffuse alveolar damage, exclusion of other causes of injury

CLINICAL PRESENTATION

- Most common clinical manifestations: cough and rapidly progressive dyspnea
- Clinical entity of ARDS

DIFFERENTIAL DIAGNOSIS

- Pneumonia
- Organizing pneumonia
- Diffuse pulmonary hemorrhage
- Pulmonary edema

PATHOLOGY

- Edema and hyaline membrane formation in acute exudative phase
- Proliferation of type II pneumocytes and fibroblasts in chronic reparative phase
- Marked cytologic atypia in patients with diffuse alveolar damage secondary to busulfan

INCIDENCE/PREVALENCE AND EPIDEMIOLOGY

- Diffuse alveolar damage is one of the most common histologic manifestations of pulmonary drug toxicity.

WHAT THE REFERRING PHYSICIAN NEEDS TO KNOW

- Diagnostic criteria include drug exposure history, consistent radiologic findings, histologic evidence of lung damage, and exclusion of other causes of injury.
- It is most commonly due to chemotherapeutic drugs used in treatment of malignant neoplasms, particularly busulfan, cyclophosphamide, carmustine, and bleomycin.
- Histologic features seldom allow distinction of drug reaction from other common causes of diffuse alveolar damage.
- A complete list of drugs that may result in pulmonary toxicity and the types of reaction associated with various drugs can be found at http://www.pneumotox.com.
- Differential diagnosis includes opportunistic infection, radiation pneumonitis, pulmonary thromboembolism, and pulmonary edema from other causes.

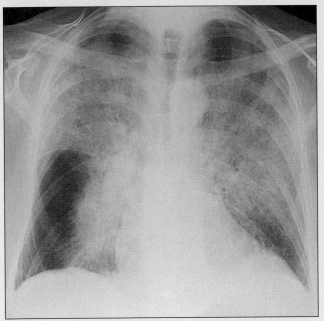

Figure 1. Diffuse alveolar damage due to amiodarone. Chest radiograph reveals extensive bilateral areas of consolidation with relative sparing of right lower and middle lobes. Patient presented with progressive shortness of breath and developed respiratory failure.

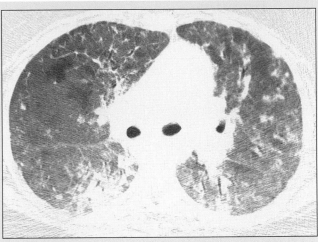

Figure 2. Diffuse alveolar damage caused by cocaine abuse. High-resolution CT image demonstrates extensive ground-glass opacities and dependent consolidation consistent with diffuse alveolar damage.

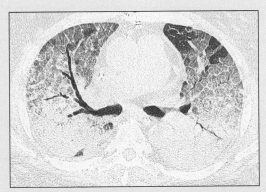

Figure 3. Diffuse alveolar damage due to amiodarone. High-resolution CT image demonstrates extensive bilateral ground-glass opacities and dependent areas of consolidation. Note focal lobular areas of sparing and smooth lines superimposed on ground-glass opacities resulting in "crazy-paving" pattern. Patient presented with progressive shortness of breath and developed respiratory failure.

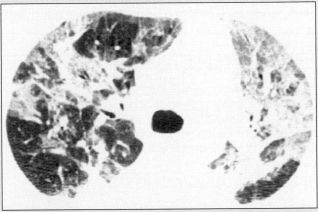

Figure 4. Diffuse alveolar damage due to bleomycin. High-resolution CT image shows extensive bilateral areas of consolidation and ground-glass opacities.

■ It is observed most commonly as a reaction to chemotherapeutic drugs used in the treatment of malignant neoplasms, particularly busulfan, cyclophosphamide, carmustine, bleomycin, paclitaxel, and docetaxel.

Suggested Readings

Foucher P, Camus P: The drug-induced lung diseases. Available at: http://www.pneumotox.com. Accessed May 8, 2009.

Gotway MB, Marder SR, Hanks DK, et al: Thoracic complications of illicit drug use: An organ system approach. *RadioGraphics* 22 (Spec No):S119-S135, 2002.

Myers JL, Limper AH, Swensen SJ: Drug-induced lung disease: A pragmatic classification incorporating HRCT appearances. *Semin Respir Crit Care Med* 24:445-453, 2003.

Nguyen ET, Silva CI, Souza CA, Müller NL: Pulmonary complications of illicit drug use: Differential diagnosis based on CT findings. *J Thorac Imaging* 22(2):199-206, 2007.

Silva CI, Müller NL: Drug-induced lung diseases: Most common reaction patterns and corresponding high-resolution CT manifestations. *Semin Ultrasound CT MR* 27:111-116, 2006.

Drug-Induced Eosinophilic Pneumonia

DEFINITION: A pulmonary drug reaction may occur that is characterized by areas of pulmonary consolidation consisting of eosinophilic infiltrates.

IMAGING

Radiography
Findings
- Migratory ground-glass opacities and consolidation
- Persistent bilateral upper lobe peripheral consolidation

Utility
- Radiographic findings similar to those of eosinophilic pneumonia of other causes

CT
Findings
- Airspace consolidation and ground-glass opacities often in predominantly peripheral distribution
- Focal areas of ground-glass attenuation surrounded by crescent or ring of consolidation ("reverse halo sign")
- Less common findings: small nodules, septal thickening, and reticulation

Utility
- High-resolution CT allows more precise assessment of presence/characterization of pattern and distribution of parenchymal and airway abnormalities than chest radiography.
- High-resolution CT findings are similar to those of eosinophilic pneumonias of other causes and overlap with those described in bronchiolitis obliterans organizing pneumonia.

CLINICAL PRESENTATION
- Cough, dyspnea, fatigue, fever, chest pain, and weight loss are the most common clinical presentations of pulmonary drug reaction.
- Onset may be acute or course may be insidious with progression over several months.

DIFFERENTIAL DIAGNOSIS
- Pneumonia
- Organizing pneumonia
- Pulmonary hemorrhage
- Radiation-induced lung disease

DIAGNOSTIC PEARLS
- Migratory areas of consolidation
- Usually symmetric, predominantly in upper and mid lung zone and in a peripheral distribution
- Eosinophilia in peripheral blood, lung biopsy, or bronchoalveolar lavage

PATHOLOGY
- Presence of eosinophils in alveolar airspaces and/or pulmonary interstitium.
- Common causes: amiodarone, bleomycin, nitrofurantoin, phenytoin, β-blockers, nonsteroidal anti-inflammatory drugs, antidepressants, hydrochlorothiazide, minocycline, sulfonamides, sulfasalazine, and mesalamine.

INCIDENCE/PREVALENCE AND EPIDEMIOLOGY
- Peripheral eosinophilia is described in 40% to 86% of patients.
- Drug reaction is one of the most common causes of eosinophilic pneumonia.

Suggested Readings

Foucher P, Camus P: The drug-induced lung diseases. Available at: http://www.pneumotox.com. Accessed June 1, 2007.

Jeong YJ, Kim KI, Seo IJ, et al: Eosinophilic lung diseases: A clinical, radiologic, and pathologic overview. *RadioGraphics* 27:617-637, 2007; discussion 637-639.

Myers JL, Limper AH, Swensen SJ: Drug-induced lung disease: A pragmatic classification incorporating HRCT appearances. *Semin Respir Crit Care Med* 24:445-453, 2003.

Silva CI, Müller NL: Drug-induced lung diseases: Most common reaction patterns and corresponding high-resolution CT manifestations. *Semin Ultrasound CT MR* 27:111-116, 2006.

Souza CA, Müller NL, Johkoh T, Akira M: Drug-induced eosinophilic pneumonia: High-resolution CT findings in 14 patients. *AJR Am J Roentgenol* 186:368-373, 2006.

WHAT THE REFERRING PHYSICIAN NEEDS TO KNOW
- Drug reaction is one of the most common causes of eosinophilic pneumonia.
- Radiologic findings are similar to those of eosinophilic pneumonias of other causes.
- A complete list of drugs that may result in pulmonary toxicity and the types of reaction associated with various drugs can be found at http://www.pneumotox.com.
- Diagnosis is shown by pulmonary infiltrates on chest radiographs, eosinophilia in peripheral blood, lung biopsy, or bronchoalveolar lavage, and association with drug administration.
- It is essential to rule out other causes of pulmonary infiltrates and eosinophilia, such as parasitic infestation, fungal infection, and immunologic or systemic diseases.

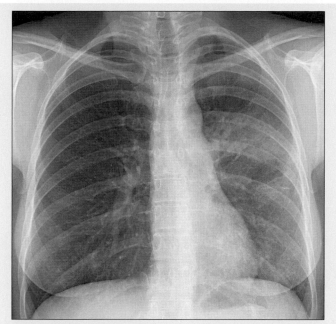

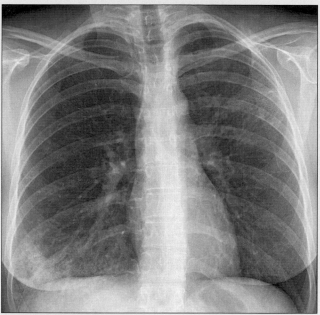

Figure 1. Eosinophilic lung disease due to mesalamine used for treatment of ulcerative colitis. Chest radiograph shows patchy consolidation in the left upper and lower lobes. The patient also had peripheral eosinophilia.

Figure 2. Eosinophilic lung disease due to mesalamine used for treatment of ulcerative colitis. Chest radiograph 22 days later shows resolution of the previous areas of consolidation but development of new areas of consolidation in the left upper and right lower lobes. Fleeting, migratory areas of consolidation are characteristic of eosinophilic lung disease. The patient also had peripheral eosinophilia.

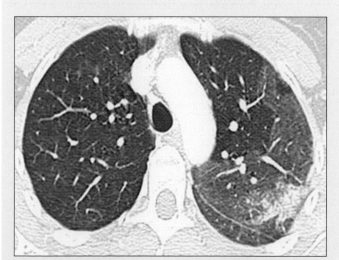

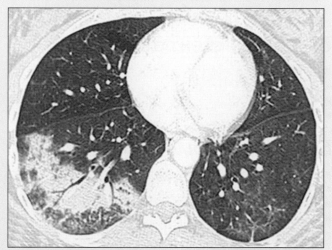

Figure 3. Eosinophilic lung disease due to mesalamine used for treatment of ulcerative colitis. High-resolution CT image at level of upper lobes shows ground-glass opacities and focal consolidation in peripheral regions of left upper lobe.

Figure 4. Eosinophilic lung disease due to mesalamine used for treatment of ulcerative colitis. High-resolution CT image at level of lower lobes shows peripheral consolidation and ground-glass opacities in right lower lobe. Mild ground-glass opacities and linear opacities are seen in left lower lobe. Patient also had peripheral eosinophilia.

Drug-Induced Hypersensitivity Pneumonitis

DEFINITION: Hypersensitivity pneumonitis is an uncommon manifestation of drug-induced lung disease characterized by the presence of noncaseating granulomas and bronchiolocentric cellular interstitial pneumonia.

IMAGING

Radiography
Findings
- Bilateral ground-glass opacities with or without associated poorly defined small nodular opacities

Utility
- Less sensitive modality than CT

CT
Findings
- Diffuse bilateral ground-glass opacities and/or small poorly defined centrilobular nodules
- Lobular areas of decreased attenuation and vascularity that show air trapping on CT images obtained at end of maximal expiration

Utility
- CT provides a more precise assessment of presence and characterization of pattern and distribution of parenchymal and airway abnormalities than chest radiography.
- CT may demonstrate abnormalities in patients with normal radiographs.
- High-resolution CT has value in identifying findings suggestive of alternative diagnosis and monitoring response to treatment.

CLINICAL PRESENTATION

- Cough
- Dyspnea
- Fatigue
- Fever

DIFFERENTIAL DIAGNOSIS

- Radiation-induced lung disease
- Pneumonia
- Nonspecific interstitial pneumonia
- Respiratory bronchiolitis

DIAGNOSTIC PEARLS

- Bilateral ground-glass opacities
- Poorly defined small nodular opacities on CT
- Lobular areas of decreased attenuation and vascularity on CT

PATHOLOGY

- Drugs associated with hypersensitivity pneumonitis include methotrexate, cyclophosphamide, mesalamine, fluoxetine, amitriptyline, and paclitaxel.
- Histologically, there are noncaseating granulomas and cellular interstitial pneumonia composed predominantly of lymphocytes.

INCIDENCE/PREVALENCE AND EPIDEMIOLOGY

- Hypersensitivity pneumonitis is a relatively uncommon manifestation of drug-induced lung disease.
- It is described most commonly with methotrexate, cyclophosphamide, mesalamine, fluoxetine, amitriptyline, and paclitaxel.

Suggested Readings

Ellis SJ, Cleverley JR, Müller NL: Drug-induced lung disease: High-resolution CT findings. *AJR Am J Roentgenol* 175:1019-1024, 2000.

Myers JL, Limper AH, Swensen SJ: Drug-induced lung disease: A pragmatic classification incorporating HRCT appearances. *Semin Respir Crit Care Med* 24:445-454, 2003.

Silva CI, Müller NL: Drug-induced lung diseases: Most common reaction patterns and corresponding high-resolution CT manifestations. *Semin Ultrasound CT MR* 27:111-116, 2006.

Silva CI, Churg A, Müller NL: Hypersensitivity pneumonitis: Spectrum of high-resolution CT and pathologic findings. *AJR Am J Roentgenol* 188:334-344, 2007.

Wong P, Leung AN, Berry GJ, et al: Paclitaxel-induced hypersensitivity pneumonitis: Radiographic and CT findings. *AJR Am J Roentgenol* 176:718-720, 2001.

WHAT THE REFERRING PHYSICIAN NEEDS TO KNOW

- Histopathologic/radiologic features are similar to those seen in hypersensitivity pneumonitis secondary to an immunologic reaction to inhaled organic antigens.
- A complete list of drugs that may result in pulmonary toxicity and the types of reaction associated with various drugs can be found at http://www.pneumotox.com.
- Clinical, radiologic, and histologic manifestations of pulmonary drug reactions are nonspecific and mimic those of various acute/chronic lung disease.
- Differential diagnosis includes opportunistic infection, radiation pneumonitis, nonspecific interstitial pneumonia and respiratory bronchiolitis.
- Treatment involves discontinuance of the drug and corticosteroid therapy.

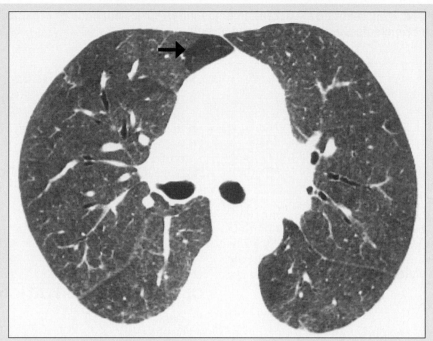

Figure 1.　Hypersensitivity pneumonitis due to cyclophosphamide. High-resolution CT image shows extensive bilateral ground-glass opacities and a few poorly defined small centrilobular nodules. Also noted is a lobular area of decreased attenuation and vascularity (*arrow*). (*From Silva CI, Müller NL: Drug-induced lung diseases: Most common reaction patterns and corresponding high-resolution CT manifestations.* Semin Ultrasound CT MR *27:111-116, 2006.*)

Drug-Induced Organizing Pneumonia

DEFINITION: Drug reaction may result in lung injury/repair with buds of organizing granulation tissue in respiratory bronchioles, alveolar ducts, and alveoli.

IMAGING

Radiography
Findings
- Bilateral scattered heterogeneous and homogeneous opacities consist mainly of areas of consolidation.
- Areas of consolidation can be patchy or confluent and may involve any lung zone but tend to have a peripheral or peribronchial distribution.

Utility
- Features resemble those seen in patients with idiopathic bronchiolitis obliterans organizing pneumonia (cryptogenic organizing pneumonia).
- First and often only imaging modality used in the assessment of these patients.

CT
Findings
- Airspace consolidation in subpleural and/or peribronchial distribution, with symmetric or asymmetric bilateral distribution and no zonal predominance
- Perilobular opacities
- Ground-glass opacities: bilateral asymmetric and random distribution
- Amiodarone toxicity: areas of high lung attenuation, often accompanied by high attenuation in liver and/or spleen
- May manifest as solitary nodule and/or multiple focal opacities; may mimic infection or neoplastic process
- Centrilobular nodules uncommon

Utility
- High-resolution CT: more precise assessment of presence and characterization of pattern and distribution of parenchymal/airway abnormalities than chest radiography
- May demonstrate abnormalities in patients with normal radiographs
- Best noninvasive method to assess presence of drug-induced lung disease and to predict underlying histologic pattern

DIAGNOSTIC PEARLS
- Airspace consolidation in subpleural and/or peribronchial distribution
- Perilobular opacities
- Areas of consolidation possibly of high attenuation on CT, often accompanied by high attenuation in liver and/or spleen in amiodarone toxicity
- Reversible after drug cessation or corticosteroid therapy
- Organizing pneumonia is an increasingly recognized manifestation of drug reaction

CLINICAL PRESENTATION
- Cough
- Dyspnea
- Fatigue
- Fever
- Chest pain
- Weight loss

DIFFERENTIAL DIAGNOSIS
- Eosinophilic pneumonia
- Cryptogenic organizing pneumonia (idiopathic bronchiolitis obliterans organizing pneumonia)
- Radiation-induced lung disease
- Bacterial, fungal, and viral pneumonia

PATHOLOGY
- Presence of buds of organizing granulation tissue in respiratory bronchioles, alveolar ducts, and adjacent alveoli.

WHAT THE REFERRING PHYSICIAN NEEDS TO KNOW
- Clinical, radiologic, and histologic manifestations of pulmonary drug reactions are nonspecific and mimic those of various acute and chronic lung diseases.
- A complete list of drugs that may result in pulmonary toxicity and the types of reaction associated with various drugs can be found at http://www.pneumotox.com.
- Only drug reaction that results in characteristic appearance on CT is amiodarone lung.
- Amiodarone lung is characterized by areas of high attenuation (82-175 Hounsfield units) in approximately 70% of patients who have symptoms of pulmonary toxicity.
- Drug-induced organizing pneumonia resembles cryptogenic organizing pneumonia, and features can overlap with those of eosinophilic pneumonia.
- Differential diagnosis also includes opportunistic infection, radiation pneumonitis, pulmonary thromboembolism, and progression of the primary illness.
- Biopsy is seldom performed, and the diagnosis is based primarily on clinical and radiologic findings.
- Treatment is with drug discontinuance and administration of corticosteroids.

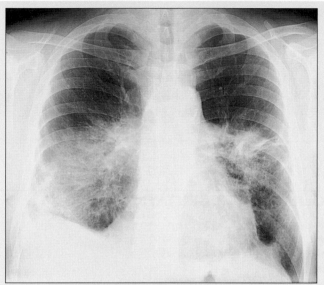

Figure 1. Organizing pneumonia due to sirolimus drug reaction in renal transplant patient. Chest radiograph shows asymmetric bilateral areas of consolidation and right pleural effusion.

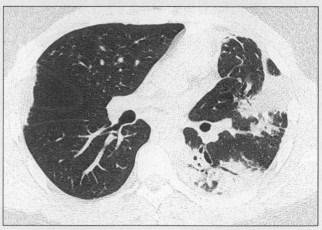

Figure 2. Organizing pneumonia (bronchiolitis obliterans organizing pneumonia–like reaction) due to mesalamine used for treatment of ulcerative colitis. High-resolution CT shows subpleural consolidation in right lung and peribronchial and peripheral consolidation in left lung.

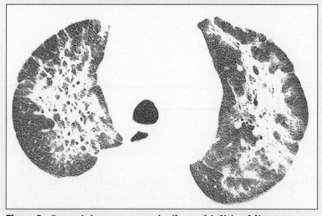

Figure 3. Organizing pneumonia (bronchiolitis obliterans organizing pneumonia–like reaction) due to amiodarone. Cross-sectional image of high-resolution CT performed on multidetector CT scanner demonstrates extensive bilateral areas of consolidation in peribronchial distribution. (*From Silva CI, Müller NL: Drug-induced lung diseases: Most common reaction patterns and corresponding high-resolution CT manifestations. Semin Ultrasound CT MR 27:111-116, 2006, with permission.*)

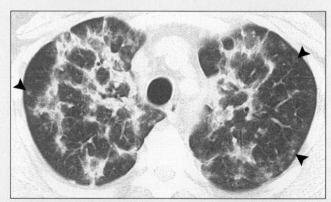

Figure 4. Organizing pneumonia (bronchiolitis obliterans organizing pneumonia–like reaction) due to mesalamine used for treatment of ulcerative colitis. CT image at level of upper lobes shows perilobular distribution of bilateral areas of consolidation, a characteristic feature of organizing pneumonia. Few poorly defined centrilobular nodules (*arrows*) are also evident.

- Most commonly associated with amiodarone, acebutolol, minocycline, nitrofurantoin, bleomycin, gold salts, cyclophosphamide, methotrexate, penicillamine, phenytoin, carbamazepine, mesalamine, hydralazine, and interferon.

INCIDENCE/PREVALENCE AND EPIDEMIOLOGY

- Increasingly recognized manifestation of drug reaction.
- Most commonly associated with amiodarone, acebutolol, minocycline, nitrofurantoin, bleomycin, gold salts, cyclophosphamide, methotrexate, penicillamine, phenytoin, carbamazepine, mesalamine, hydralazine, and interferon.

Suggested Readings

American Thoracic Society/European Respiratory Society: International Multidisciplinary Consensus Classification of the Idiopathic Interstitial Pneumonias. *Am J Respir Crit Care Med* 165:277-304, 2002.

Budnitz DS, Pollock DA, Weidenbach KN, et al: National surveillance of emergency department visits for outpatient adverse drug events. *JAMA* 296:1858-1866, 2006.

Dodd JD, Lee KS, Johkoh T, Müller NL: Drug-associated organizing pneumonia: High-resolution CT findings in 9 patients. *J Thorac Imaging* 21:22-26, 2006.

Epler GR: Drug-induced bronchiolitis obliterans organizing pneumonia. *Clin Chest Med* 25:89-94, 2004.

Lynch DA, Travis WD, Müller NL, et al: Idiopathic interstitial pneumonias: CT features. *Radiology* 236:10-21, 2005.

Silva CI, Müller NL: Drug-induced lung diseases: Most common reaction patterns and corresponding high-resolution CT manifestations. *Semin Ultrasound CT MR* 27:111-116, 2006.

Drug-Induced Pulmonary Hemorrhage

DEFINITION: Alveolar hemorrhage may be caused by drug toxicity.

IMAGING

Radiography
Findings
- Patchy or confluent hazy areas of increased opacity (ground-glass opacities) and bilateral areas of consolidation.
- Opacities usually widespread but may be more prominent in perihilar areas and in mid and lower lung zones.
- Lung apices and region of costophrenic angles usually spared.

Utility
- Main role is in the confirmation of the presence of pulmonary intrathoracic complications.

CT
Findings
- Extensive bilateral ground-glass opacities with patchy or diffuse distribution.
- With or without associated areas of consolidation.
- Decrease in ground-glass opacities and consolidation 2-3 days after acute episode.
- Presence of small poorly defined centrilobular nodules and, less commonly, interlobular septal thickening.
- Crack lung: transient ground-glass opacities or consolidation clearing rapidly after cessation of crack use.

Utility
- More precise assessment of presence and characterization of pattern and distribution of parenchymal and airway abnormalities than chest radiography.
- May demonstrate abnormalities in patients with normal radiographs.
- Has value in identifying findings suggestive of alternative diagnosis and monitoring response to treatment.
- Best noninvasive method to assess presence of drug-induced lung disease and to predict underlying histologic pattern.

DIAGNOSTIC PEARLS

- Patchy or confluent ground-glass opacities
- Bilateral areas of consolidation
- Transient opacities that improve after a few days
- Uncommon manifestation of drug reaction

CLINICAL PRESENTATION

- Cough, dyspnea
- Chest pain
- Fatigue, fever, weight loss
- Hemoptysis
- May present as an acute, subacute, or chronic process

DIFFERENTIAL DIAGNOSIS

- Pneumonia
- Radiation-induced lung disease
- Acute pulmonary embolism
- Pulmonary edema

PATHOLOGY

- Histologic findings of pulmonary drug reactions are often nonspecific and mimic those of various acute and chronic lung diseases.
- Drugs associated with alveolar hemorrhage include anticoagulants, amphotericin B, amiodarone, cyclophosphamide, carbamazepine, methotrexate, mitomycin, nitrofurantoin, penicillamine, phenytoin, and propylthiouracil.

WHAT THE REFERRING PHYSICIAN NEEDS TO KNOW

- Clinical, radiologic, and histologic manifestations of pulmonary drug reactions are nonspecific and mimic those of various acute/chronic lung diseases.
- A complete list of drugs that may result in pulmonary toxicity and the types of reaction associated with various drugs can be found at http://www.pneumotox.com.
- Pulmonary hemorrhage is an uncommon manifestation of drug toxicity.
- Most common drugs associated with alveolar hemorrhage are anticoagulants, amphotericin B, amiodarone, cyclophosphamide, carbamazepine, methotrexate, mitomycin, nitrofurantoin, penicillamine, phenytoin, and propylthiouracil.
- Differential diagnosis includes pneumonia, radiation pneumonitis, and pulmonary thromboembolism.
- Treatment is with drug discontinuance and corticosteroid therapy.

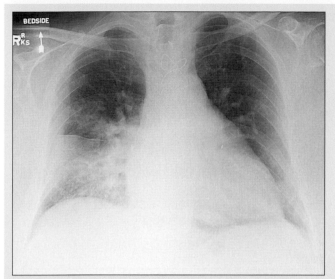

Figure 1. Pulmonary hemorrhage due to warfarin toxicity. Chest radiograph shows extensive consolidation mainly in right upper and lower lobes. Patient presented with hemoptysis.

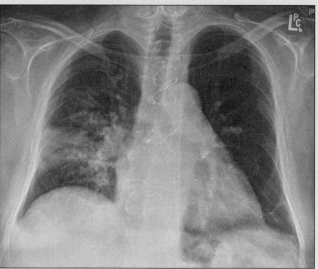

Figure 2. Pulmonary hemorrhage due to warfarin toxicity. Same patient as in Figure 1. Chest radiograph 24 hours later shows considerable improvement.

INCIDENCE/PREVALENCE AND EPIDEMIOLOGY

- Pulmonary hemorrhage is an uncommon manifestation of drug toxicity.
- Most common drugs associated with alveolar hemorrhage are anticoagulants, amphotericin B, amiodarone, cyclophosphamide, carbamazepine, methotrexate, mitomycin, nitrofurantoin, penicillamine, phenytoin, and propylthiouracil.

Suggested Readings

Foucher P, Camus P: The drug-induced lung diseases. Available at: http://www.pneumotox.com. Accessed June 1, 2007.

Gotway MB, Marder SR, Hanks DK, et al: Thoracic complications of illicit drug use: An organ system approach. *RadioGraphics* 22 (Spec No):S119-S135, 2002.

Myers JL, Limper AH, Swensen SJ: Drug-induced lung disease: A pragmatic classification incorporating HRCT appearances. *Semin Respir Crit Care Med* 24:445-453, 2003.

Nguyen ET, Silva CI, Souza CA, Müller NL: Pulmonary complications of illicit drug use: Differential diagnosis based on CT findings. *J Thorac Imaging* 22:199-206, 2007.

Silva CI, Müller NL: Drug-induced lung diseases: Most common reaction patterns and corresponding high-resolution CT manifestations. *Semin Ultrasound CT MR* 27:111-116, 2006.

Amiodarone Lung

DEFINITION: Pulmonary toxicity in patients treated with amiodarone is known as amiodarone lung. Common reaction patterns include diffuse alveolar damage, nonspecific interstitial pneumonia, and organizing pneumonia.

IMAGING

Radiography

Findings
- Bilateral reticular pattern or bilateral areas of consolidation are evident.
- Consolidation may be peripheral in distribution and involve upper lobes predominantly.
- Less common manifestations include focal consolidation and nodular opacities.

Utility
- Helpful in detecting parenchymal abnormalities and useful in monitoring progression and resolution of disease.

CT

Findings
- Parenchymal abnormalities may consist of bilateral symmetric or asymmetric areas of consolidation, ground-glass opacities, reticular pattern, linear atelectasis, or focal round areas of consolidation.
- High-attenuation (82-175 Hounsfield units) pulmonary abnormalities are seen in 70% of patients with symptoms of pulmonary toxicity.
- Pleural effusions are seen in 50% of cases.
- Characteristic high attenuation of liver is due to accumulation of amiodarone in reticuloendothelial cells.

Utility
- High-resolution CT allows more precise assessment of presence and characterization of pattern of distribution of pulmonary abnormalities than chest radiography.

CLINICAL PRESENTATION

- Most patients have received ≥400 mg/day of amiodarone before pulmonary disease occurs.
- Problems have occurred with maintenance doses of <400 mg/day in some patients.
- Lung damage generally has onset months after initiation of therapy.

DIFFERENTIAL DIAGNOSIS

- Bronchopneumonia
- Cryptogenic organizing pneumonia
- Hypersensitivity pneumonitis
- Pulmonary edema

PATHOLOGY

- Hyperplasia of type II pneumocytes and increase in macrophages in alveolar airspaces
- Macrophages and pneumocytes with coarsely vacuolated cytoplasm containing lysosomal inclusions composed of osmiophilic lamellae surrounded by amorphous electron-dense material
- Common pulmonary complications: diffuse alveolar damage, nonspecific interstitial pneumonia, and organizing pneumonia (BOOP [bronchiolitis obliterans organizing pneumonia]-like reaction)

INCIDENCE/PREVALENCE AND EPIDEMIOLOGY

- Pulmonary toxicity occurs in approximately 5% of patients.

WHAT THE REFERRING PHYSICIAN NEEDS TO KNOW

- Amiodarone is used in treatment of cardiac arrhythmias.
- Pulmonary toxicity is estimated to occur in about 5% of treated patients.
- Most patients have received ≥400 mg/day or more of amiodarone before appearance of pulmonary disease.
- However, problems have occurred with maintenance doses of <400 mg/day in some patients.
- Diagnostic criteria include history of drug exposure, consistent radiologic findings, histologic evidence of lung damage, and exclusion of another cause.
- In clinical practice, biopsy is seldom performed and diagnosis is based primarily on clinical and radiologic findings.
- Preferential concentration of drug in the lung and its very long half-life result in slow resolution of toxicity after discontinuation.

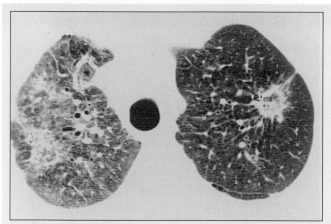

Figure 1. Amiodarone toxicity. High-resolution CT scan shows extensive ground-glass attenuation in the right upper lobe, a focal area of ground-glass attenuation in the left upper lobe, and bilateral irregular linear opacities. The patient was a 61-year-old man who had clinical findings consistent with amiodarone pulmonary toxicity.

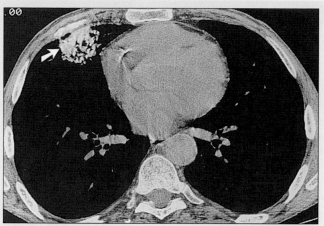

Figure 3. Amiodarone toxicity. High-resolution CT scan at the level of the inferior pulmonary veins and photographed using soft tissue windows shows that the consolidation in the right middle lobe (*arrow*) has an attenuation greater than that of chest wall and cardiac muscle. The patient was a 61-year-old man who had clinical findings consistent with amiodarone pulmonary toxicity.

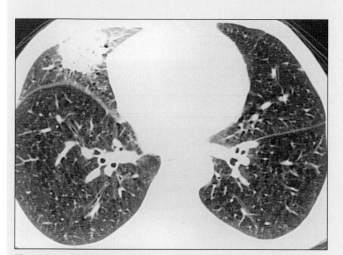

Figure 2. Amiodarone toxicity. High-resolution CT scan at the level of the inferior pulmonary veins shows a focal area of consolidation in the right middle lobe. The patient was a 61-year-old man who had clinical findings consistent with amiodarone pulmonary toxicity.

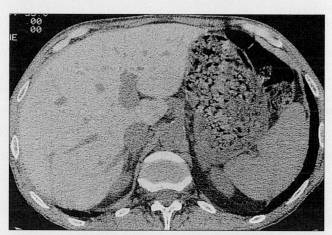

Figure 4. Amiodarone toxicity. High-resolution CT scan through the upper abdomen shows high attenuation of the liver. The patient was a 61-year-old man who had clinical findings consistent with amiodarone pulmonary toxicity.

Suggested Readings

Foucher P, Camus P: The drug-induced lung diseases. Available at: http://www.pneumotox.com.

Myers JL, Limper AH, Swensen SJ: Drug-induced lung disease: A pragmatic classification incorporating HRCT appearances. *Semin Respir Crit Care Med* 24:445-453, 2003.

Silva CI, Müller NL: Drug-induced lung diseases: Most common reaction patterns and corresponding high-resolution CT manifestations. *Semin Ultrasound CT MR* 27:111-116, 2006.

Drug-Induced Lung Diseases: Cocaine and Crack

DEFINITION: Cocaine and crack can result in pulmonary edema, hemorrhage, eosinophilic lung disease, organizing pneumonia, and barotrauma.

IMAGING

Radiography
Findings
- Bilateral ground-glass opacities or consolidation, predominantly perihilar in distribution, but not associated with septal lines, pleural effusion, or cardiomegaly.
- Pulmonary hemorrhage, resulting in transient focal or diffuse bilateral ground-glass opacities or consolidation.
- Pneumomediastinum, pneumothorax, and, occasionally, pneumopericardium.
Utility
- Usually the first and only imaging modality used to assess these patients.

CT
Findings
- High-resolution CT typically shows multifocal or confluent bilateral ground-glass opacities.
- Often, there are superimposed smooth septal lines and intralobular lines resulting in a "crazy-paving" pattern.
Utility
- High-resolution CT is of value in identifying findings suggestive of an alternative diagnosis and in monitoring presence of complications.
- High-resolution CT is seldom required in the assessment of these patients.

CLINICAL PRESENTATION

- Drug-induced lung disease may present as acute, subacute, or chronic process.
- Respiratory failure appearing shortly after using crack is also known as "crack lung."
- Abnormalities generally resolve within 24-72 hours, regardless of treatment.
- Most common clinical manifestations of pulmonary drug reaction are chest pain, cough, dyspnea, fatigue, fever, and weight loss.

DIAGNOSTIC PEARLS

- Pulmonary edema resulting in bilateral ground-glass opacities or consolidation, predominantly perihilar in distribution, but not associated with septal lines, pleural effusion, or cardiomegaly
- Pulmonary hemorrhage, resulting in transient focal or diffuse bilateral ground glass opacities or consolidation
- Pneumomediastinum and pneumothorax

DIFFERENTIAL DIAGNOSIS

- Pneumonia
- Aspiration
- Vasculitis
- Cryptogenic organizing pneumonia

PATHOLOGY

- Cocaine can result in pulmonary hemorrhage, increased pulmonary capillary permeability, and cardiogenic pulmonary edema.
- Organizing pneumonia (bronchiolitis obliterans–like reaction) and eosinophilic lung disease may be seen.
- Cardiovascular complications include myocardial infarction, cardiomyopathy, congestive heart failure, pulmonary arterial hypertension, and aortic dissection.
- Barotrauma from crack cocaine smoking may result in pneumothorax, pneumomediastinum, and pneumopericardium.

INCIDENCE/PREVALENCE AND EPIDEMIOLOGY

- Crack cocaine is the most frequently abused controlled substance in United States.
- The illicit use of crack cocaine is a major health problem in urban and suburban settings.

WHAT THE REFERRING PHYSICIAN NEEDS TO KNOW
- Main role of imaging is in the confirmation of the presence of pulmonary intrathoracic complications.
- Best noninvasive method to assess presence of drug-induced lung disease and predict underlying histologic pattern is high-resolution CT.
- Criteria for diagnosis include drug exposure, consistent radiologic findings, histologic evidence of lung damage, and exclusion of another cause.
- In clinical practice, however, biopsy is seldom performed and diagnosis is based primarily on clinical and radiologic findings.

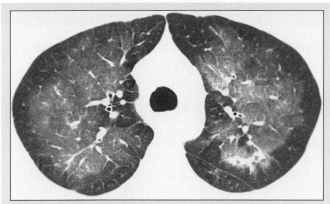

Figure 1. Crack lung. High-resolution CT image shows bilateral ground-glass opacities and small area of consolidation. The patient was a 34-year-old man who presented with marked shortness of breath after a "crack binge."

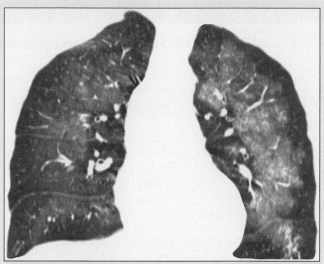

Figure 2. Crack lung. Same patient as Figure 1. Coronal reformatted image better demonstrates the overall distribution of the abnormalities. The patient was a 34-year-old man who presented with marked shortness of breath after a "crack binge."

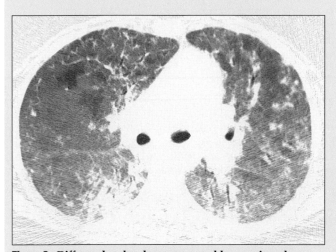

Figure 3. Diffuse alveolar damage caused by cocaine abuse. High-resolution CT image demonstrates extensive ground-glass opacities and dependent consolidation consistent with diffuse alveolar damage.

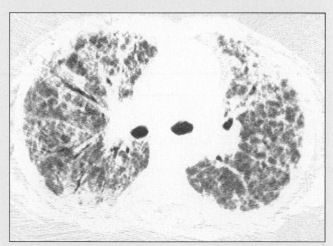

Figure 4. Diffuse alveolar damage caused by cocaine abuse. Follow-up high-resolution CT performed at the same level as in Figure 3 demonstrates extensive ground-glass opacities, foci of consolidation, and reticulation consistent with the fibrotic phase of diffuse alveolar damage.

Suggested Readings

Hagan IG, Burney K: Radiology of recreational drug abuse. *Radio-Graphics* 27:919-940, 2007.

Nguyen ET, Silva CI, Souza CA, Müller NL: Pulmonary complications of illicit drug use: Differential diagnosis based on CT findings. *J Thorac Imaging* 22:199-206, 2007.

Restrepo CS, Carrillo JA, Martinez S, et al: Pulmonary complications from cocaine and cocaine-based substances: Imaging manifestations. *RadioGraphics* 27:941-956, 2007.

Drug-Induced Lung Diseases: Opiates (Narcotics)

DEFINITION: Pulmonary disease can result from opiate use or overdose and use of contaminated needles.

IMAGING

Radiography

Findings

- Permeability edema evident as bilateral ground-glass opacities or consolidation often in a predominantly perihilar distribution but may be unilateral or markedly asymmetric.
- Aspiration pneumonia results in areas of consolidation in the dependent lung regions.
- Septic embolism is evident as bilateral nodules, frequently cavitated, and peripheral wedge-shaped opacities measuring 1-3 cm in diameter.
- Bronchiectasis is identified in some individuals, presumably related to recurrent infection and aspiration.
- Pneumothorax, hemothorax, hemopneumothorax, and pyopneumothorax are reported as complications of attempted intravenous injections in the supraclavicular fossa.

Utility

- Helpful in demonstrating presence of parenchymal abnormalities and in monitoring response to treatment.

CT

Findings

- Septic embolism evident as bilateral nodules, frequently cavitated, and peripheral wedge-shaped opacities measuring 1-3 cm in diameter.
- Nodules tend to be most numerous in peripheral lung regions and lower lobes.
- Pneumothorax, hemothorax, hemopneumothorax, and pyopneumothorax are reported as complications of attempted intravenous injections in the supraclavicular fossa.

Utility

- High-resolution CT allows more precise assessment of presence and characterization of pattern of distribution of pulmonary abnormalities than chest radiography.

DIAGNOSTIC PEARLS

- Bilateral ground-glass opacities or consolidation is often in a predominantly perihilar distribution.
- Aspiration pneumonia results in areas of consolidation that affect dependent lung regions.
- Septic emboli manifest as multiple nodules and wedge-shaped peripheral opacities.

CLINICAL PRESENTATION

- Altered mental status, decreased respiratory drive, pinpoint pupils, circumstantial evidence of drug use.

DIFFERENTIAL DIAGNOSIS

- Acute pulmonary embolism
- Septic embolism
- Aspiration pneumonia
- Bronchopneumonia

PATHOLOGY

- Common thoracic complications: noncardiogenic pulmonary edema, aspiration pneumonia, septic embolism, pneumothorax, hemothorax, vertebral body osteomyelitis, costochondritis, and septic arthritis.

INCIDENCE/PREVALENCE AND EPIDEMIOLOGY

- Use of heroin has increased considerably in past 2 decades.
- In some western cities, death toll from heroin overdoses has become largest category of preventable deaths.

WHAT THE REFERRING PHYSICIAN NEEDS TO KNOW

- Illicit use is common, particularly in urban centers.
- Opiate overdose diagnosis is made clinically with presence of altered mental status, decreased respiratory drive, pinpoint pupils, and evidence of drug use.
- Criteria for diagnosis include history of drug exposure, consistent radiologic findings, histologic evidence of lung damage, and exclusion of another cause.
- In clinical practice, however, biopsy is seldom performed and diagnosis is based primarily on clinical and radiologic findings.
- Other causes of pulmonary injury include opportunistic infection, radiation pneumonitis, and pulmonary thromboembolism.

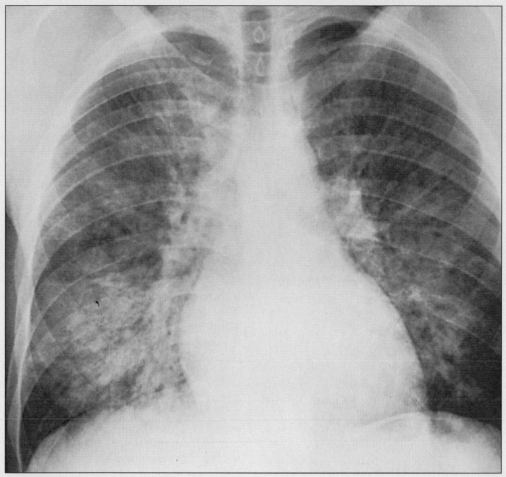

Figure 1. Acute pulmonary edema due to opiates. Posteroanterior chest radiograph shows airspace consolidation typical of acute pulmonary edema. Several hours previously, this 19-year-old man had injected a high dose of meperidine and methadone intravenously. He had an uneventful recovery.

- Vast majority of patients with fatal overdose have noncardiogenic pulmonary edema.

Suggested Readings

Gotway MB, Marder SR, Hanks DK, et al: Thoracic complications of illicit drug use: An organ system approach. *RadioGraphics* 22(Spec No):S119-S135, 2002.

Hagan IG, Burney K: Radiology of recreational drug abuse. *RadioGraphics* 27:919-940, 2007.

Nguyen ET, Silva CI, Souza CA, Müller NL: Pulmonary complications of illicit drug use: Differential diagnosis based on CT findings. *J Thorac Imaging* 22:199-206, 2007.

Lung Toxicity: Bleomycin

DEFINITION: Symptomatic lung toxicity occurs in approximately 3% - 5% of patients being treated with the chemotherapeutic drug bleomycin.

IMAGING

Radiography

Findings
- Patchy or confluent consolidation.
- With more severe disease, abnormalities may extend into middle and upper lung zones.
- Bibasilar reticular, reticulonodular, or fine nodular opacities often show striking peripheral distribution.
- Secondary organizing pneumonia may result in multiple nodules 5 mm to 3 cm in diameter that are usually subpleural.
- Nodules can be sharply or poorly marginated and can simulate metastatic disease radiologically.

Utility
- Abnormalities usually appear 6 weeks to 3 months after start of therapy.
- They may be seen before, synchronous with, or after the appearance of clinical symptoms.

CT

Findings
- Most common manifestations: extensive bilateral ground-glass opacities or consolidation due to diffuse alveolar damage.
- Bilateral ground-glass opacities with or without associated reticulation related to nonspecific interstitial pneumonia.
- Focal areas of consolidation in predominantly subpleural distribution due to organizing pneumonia.

Utility
- High-resolution CT is of value in monitoring appearance, progression, and resolution of disease.
- High-resolution CT allows more precise assessment of presence and characterization of pattern of distribution of pulmonary abnormalities than chest radiographs.

CLINICAL PRESENTATION

- Progressive shortness of breath and cough occur.
- Diffuse alveolar disease corresponds to clinical entity of acute respiratory distress syndrome.

DIAGNOSTIC PEARLS

- Bibasilar consolidation, reticular or reticulonodular opacities, on radiographs, often show a striking peripheral distribution.
- Extensive bilateral ground-glass opacities or consolidation are most common finding on CT.
- Secondary organizing pneumonia may result in multiple nodules 5 mm to 3 cm in diameter that are usually subpleural.

DIFFERENTIAL DIAGNOSIS

- Pneumonia
- Radiation-induced lung disease
- Pulmonary embolism
- Pulmonary edema

PATHOLOGY

- Most common pulmonary manifestation of bleomycin toxicity is diffuse alveolar damage.
- Less common complications include nonspecific interstitial pneumonia, organizing pneumonia, and, occasionally, eosinophilic pneumonia.

INCIDENCE/PREVALENCE AND EPIDEMIOLOGY

- Symptomatic pulmonary complications probably occur in 3%-5% of patients.
- Risk of pulmonary drug reaction is increased in patients receiving combined cytotoxic drug therapy (particularly with cyclophosphamide).
- Risk is also increased with high concentration of inspired oxygen or radiation therapy.

WHAT THE REFERRING PHYSICIAN NEEDS TO KNOW

- Symptomatic pulmonary complications occur in 3%-5% of patients.
- Manifestations include diffuse alveolar damage, nonspecific interstitial pneumonia, and organizing pneumonia.
- Criteria for diagnosis include drug exposure, consistent radiologic findings, histologic evidence of lung damage, and exclusion of another cause.
- In clinical practice, however, biopsy is seldom performed and diagnosis is based primarily on clinical and radiologic findings.
- Other causes of pulmonary injury include opportunistic infection, radiation pneumonitis, pulmonary thromboembolism, and progression of primary illness.

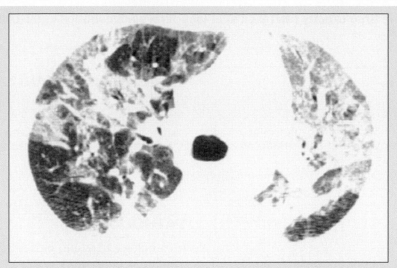

Figure 1. **Diffuse alveolar damage due to bleomycin.** High-resolution CT image shows extensive bilateral areas of consolidation and ground-glass opacities.

Suggested Readings

Foucher P, Camus P: The drug-induced lung diseases. Available at http://www.pneumotox.com

Myers JL, Limper AH, Swensen SJ: Drug-induced lung disease: A pragmatic classification incorporating HRCT appearances. *Semin Respir Crit Care Med* 24:445-453, 2003.

Silva CI, Müller NL: Drug-induced lung diseases: Most common reaction patterns and corresponding high-resolution CT manifestations. *Semin Ultrasound CT MR* 27:111-116, 2006.

Lung Toxicity: Busulfan

DEFINITION: Drug toxicity can result after long-term administration of the chemotherapeutic drug busulfan.

IMAGING

Radiography
Findings
- Bilateral reticular or reticulonodular pattern, which may be diffuse or have lower lung zone predominance

Utility
- Of value in monitoring appearance, progression, and resolution of disease

CT
Findings
- Most common manifestation on high-resolution CT consists of extensive bilateral ground-glass opacities with or without associated reticulation.

Utility
- High-resolution CT allows more precise assessment of presence and characterization of pattern of distribution of pulmonary abnormalities than chest radiography.

CLINICAL PRESENTATION

- Clinically apparent pulmonary toxicity that typically occurs with long-term use, from 8 months to 10 years (average, 3-4 years)
- Dyspnea

DIFFERENTIAL DIAGNOSIS

- Pneumonia
- Radiation-induced lung disease
- Pulmonary edema

DIAGNOSTIC PEARLS

- Bilateral reticular or reticulonodular pattern on radiograph
- Ground-glass opacities with or without reticulation on CT
- Lower lung zone distribution or diffuse

PATHOLOGY

- Pathologic finding most characteristic of busulfan-induced pulmonary disease is presence of large, cytologically atypical type II pneumocytes.
- There is marked extent and severity of atypia with busulfan, compared with pulmonary pathology caused by other drugs.

INCIDENCE/PREVALENCE AND EPIDEMIOLOGY

- Clinically recognized pulmonary toxicity occurs in 5% of patients.
- Previous use of other cytotoxic drugs or radiation therapy increases risk.

Suggested Readings

Foucher P, Camus P: The drug-induced lung diseases. Available at: http://www.pneumotox.com.

Myers JL, Limper AH, Swensen SJ: Drug-induced lung disease: A pragmatic classification incorporating HRCT appearances. *Semin Respir Crit Care Med* 24:445-453, 2003.

Silva CI, Müller NL: Drug-induced lung diseases: Most common reaction patterns and corresponding high-resolution CT manifestations. *Semin Ultrasound CT MR* 27:111-116, 2006.

WHAT THE REFERRING PHYSICIAN NEEDS TO KNOW

- Clinically recognized pulmonary toxicity occurs in approximately 5% of patients.
- Common complication is interstitial fibrosis, particularly nonspecific interstitial pneumonia.
- Criteria for diagnosis include history of drug exposure, consistent radiologic findings, histologic evidence of lung damage, and exclusion of another cause.
- In clinical practice, however, biopsy is seldom performed and diagnosis is based primarily on clinical and radiologic findings.
- Other causes of pulmonary injury include opportunistic infection, radiation pneumonitis, pulmonary thromboembolism, and progression of primary illness.

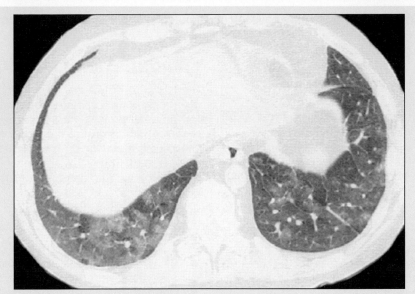

Figure 1. Nonspecific interstitial pneumonia due to busulfan. High-resolution CT image at the level of the lung bases demonstrates diffuse bilateral ground-glass opacities.

Lung Toxicity: Methotrexate

DEFINITION: Methotrexate may cause acute, subacute, or chronic drug reaction involving the lung.

IMAGING

Radiography
Findings
- Basal or diffuse reticular or ground-glass pattern, with rapid progression to patchy consolidation.

Utility
- Radiographic manifestations of drug reaction are protean and mimic those of other interstitial and airspace lung diseases.

CT
Findings
- Bilateral ground-glass opacities with or without associated intralobular linear opacities are seen.
- Less frequent findings include centrilobular nodular opacities or areas of consolidation.

Utility
- High-resolution CT allows more precise assessment for presence, pattern, and distribution of parenchymal and airway abnormalities than radiography.
- High-resolution CT can also be of value in identifying findings suggestive of alternative diagnosis and monitoring response to treatment.

CLINICAL PRESENTATION

- Most common clinical manifestations of pulmonary drug reaction are cough, dyspnea, fatigue, fever, chest pain, and weight loss.
- Drug-induced lung disease may present as acute, subacute, or chronic process.
- The condition clears after discontinuation of the drug.

DIFFERENTIAL DIAGNOSIS

- Pneumonia
- Pulmonary edema
- Eosinophilic pneumonia
- Hypersensitivity pneumonitis

DIAGNOSTIC PEARLS

- Basal or diffuse ground-glass pattern, with rapid progression to patchy consolidation
- Bilateral ground-glass opacities with or without associated intralobular linear opacities
- Centrilobular nodular opacities or areas of consolidation
- Radiologic findings are nonspecific

PATHOLOGY

- This reversible pulmonary disease is probably a result of a hypersensitivity reaction to methotrexate.
- Common complications of methotrexate are nonspecific interstitial pneumonia and hypersensitivity pneumonitis.
- Histologic findings of pulmonary drug reactions are often nonspecific and mimic those of various acute and chronic lung diseases.

INCIDENCE/PREVALENCE AND EPIDEMIOLOGY

- Incidence of disease in patients receiving low-dose methotrexate for rheumatoid arthritis is 2%-5%.
- Transient symptoms developed in 20% of patients treated with methotrexate for trophoblastic tumors.

Suggested Readings

Arakawa H, Yamasaki M, Kurihara Y, et al: Methotrexate-induced pulmonary injury: Serial CT findings. *J Thorac Imaging* 18:231-236, 2003.

Lateef O, Shakoor N, Balk RA: Methotrexate pulmonary toxicity. *Expert Opin Drug Saf* 4:723-730, 2005.

Silva CI, Müller NL: Drug-induced lung diseases: Most common reaction patterns and corresponding high-resolution CT manifestations. *Semin Ultrasound CT MR* 27:111-116, 2006.

WHAT THE REFERRING PHYSICIAN NEEDS TO KNOW

- Main role of imaging is in confirmation of presence of pulmonary intrathoracic complications.
- Best noninvasive method to assess presence of drug-induced lung disease and predict underlying histologic pattern is high-resolution CT.
- Criteria for diagnosis include drug exposure, consistent radiologic findings, histologic evidence of lung damage, and exclusion of another cause.
- In clinical practice, however, biopsy is seldom performed and diagnosis is based primarily on clinical and radiologic findings.
- Other causes of pulmonary injury include opportunistic infection, radiation pneumonitis, pulmonary thromboembolism, and progression of primary illness.

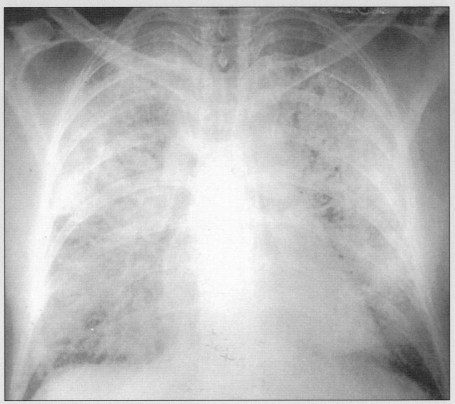

Figure 1. Methotrexate toxicity. Posteroanterior radiograph shows massive bilateral airspace consolidation containing a well-defined air bronchogram. The heart size is within normal limits. This appearance is highly suggestive of permeability pulmonary edema.

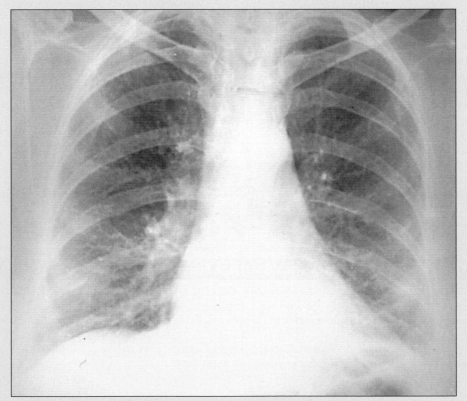

Figure 2. Methotrexate toxicity. Same patient as in Figure 1. Almost 2 weeks later, after cessation of methotrexate therapy for rheumatoid arthritis, the consolidation had cleared almost completely.

Part 53

RADIATION-INDUCED LUNG DISEASE

Radiation-Induced Lung Disease

DEFINITION: Irradiation of normal lung adjacent to an intrathoracic malignancy may result in radiation pneumonitis, radiation fibrosis, and, less commonly, organizing pneumonia and eosinophilic pneumonia.

IMAGING

Radiography

Findings

- Radiation pneumonitis: ground-glass opacities and or consolidation in the treatment field.
- Ipsilateral pleural effusions.
- Radiation fibrosis, with well-defined area of volume loss, linear scarring, consolidation, and traction bronchiectasis.
- Consolidation that usually coalesces and typically has a relatively sharp margin that conforms to the treatment field rather than to anatomic boundaries.
- Ipsilateral displacement of mediastinum and adjacent pleural thickening or effusion.

Utility

- Useful in initial assessment and follow-up.

CT

Findings

- Radiation pneumonitis: ground-glass opacities and loss of volume in the treatment field a few weeks after completion of radiation therapy.
- Radiation pneumonitis: may result in irregular, poorly defined nodular opacities.
- Radiation fibrosis: well-defined area of volume loss, linear scarring, consolidation, and traction bronchiectasis that conforms to treatment field.
- Ipsilateral displacement of mediastinum and adjacent pleural thickening or effusion.
- Less extensive consolidation, volume loss and bronchiectasis, scar-like and mass-like patterns in non–small cell lung cancer treated with 3D-conformal radiation therapy (3D-CRT).

DIAGNOSTIC PEARLS

- Radiation pneumonitis and fibrosis are typically limited to the irradiated field.
- Radiologic evidence of radiation pneumonitis usually becomes evident 4-8 weeks after completion of radiotherapy.
- Radiation fibrosis becomes evident after 3-4 months and becomes stable 9-12 months after completion of radiotherapy.

- Parenchymal opacities confined to the anterolateral subpleural region of the lung in breast cancer irradiated with tangential radiation fields.
- Radiation pneumonitis and fibrosis in the paramediastinal areas and apices after radiation therapy for mediastinal lymphoma.
- Paramedial opacities in the lower lobes in esophageal cancer.
- Organizing pneumonia (bronchiolitis obliterans–like reaction) related to radiation therapy: migratory areas of consolidation, and ground-glass opacities typically outside the radiation treatment field.

Utility

- More sensitive than chest radiographs in detecting radiation-induced lung disease.
- Radiation pneumonitis evident on CT before being evident on radiograph.
- Optimal modality for assessment of evolution and chronic manifestations of lung injury and for detection of locoregional recurrence of malignancy.

WHAT THE REFERRING PHYSICIAN NEEDS TO KNOW

- Radiation-induced lung disease rarely occurs with fractionated total doses <20 Gy but is commonly present with doses >60 Gy.
- Radiation induced lung disease is affected by the volume of lung irradiated and the fractions into which the total dose is divided.
- Results are affected by age, low performance status, cigarette smoking, preexisting lung disease, prior radiation therapy, and prior or concomitant chemotherapy.
- Intensity-modulated radiotherapy (IMRT), 3D conformal radiotherapy (3D-CRT), and altered fractionation can modify development and extent of lung injury.
- Decreases occur in vital capacity, inspiratory capacity, total lung capacity, residual volume, FEV_1, and DL_{CO}.
- Organizing pneumonia and chronic eosinophilic pneumonia may also be associated with thoracic radiotherapy.

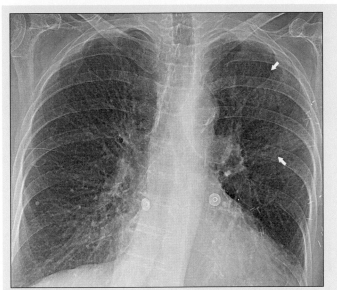

Figure 1. Radiation pneumonitis in an 86-year-old woman with non–small cell lung cancer in the left lung. Chest radiograph obtained 1 month after completion of radiation therapy shows radiation pneumonitis manifesting as diffuse increased hazy opacities (ground-glass opacities) in left lung (*arrows*) within the radiation field. (*Courtesy of Dr. Jeremy Erasmus, University of Texas M.D. Anderson Cancer Center, Texas*)

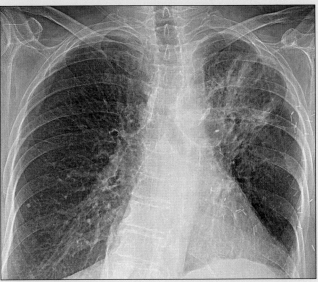

Figure 2. Radiation pneumonitis in an 86-year-old woman with non–small cell lung cancer in the left lung. Chest radiograph obtained 2 months after completion of radiation therapy shows evolution of radiation fibrosis manifesting as volume loss and consolidation. (*Courtesy of Dr. Jeremy Erasmus, University of Texas M.D. Anderson Cancer Center, Texas*)

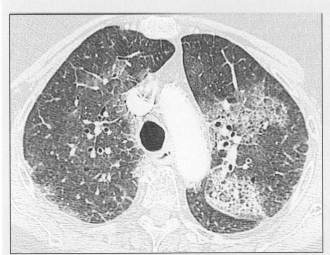

Figure 3. Radiation pneumonitis in an 86-year-old woman with non–small cell lung cancer after intensity-modulated radiation therapy (**IMRT**). CT image obtained 3 weeks after completion of IMRT shows radiation pneumonitis manifesting as diffuse ground-glass opacities and thickening of interlobular septa and intralobular lines ("crazy-paving" pattern). (*Courtesy of Dr. Jeremy Erasmus, University of Texas M.D. Anderson Cancer Center, Texas*)

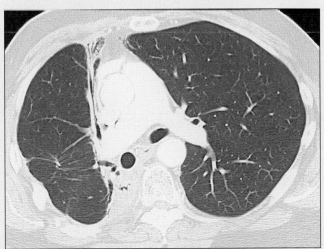

Figure 4. Radiation fibrosis in a 61-year-old man after resection of right lower lobe non–small cell lung cancer and conventional radiation therapy. CT image obtained 10 months after completion of radiation therapy shows radiation fibrosis. Note bronchiectasis, volume loss, and sharp demarcation between normal lung and fibrosis. (*Courtesy of Dr. Jeremy Erasmus, University of Texas M.D. Anderson Cancer Center, Texas*)

Positron Emission Tomography
Findings
- Acute radiation pneumonitis results in increased FDG activity.
- In patients with radiation fibrosis, increased FDG uptake in the radiated lung is suggestive of malignancy.

Utility
- FDG-PET imaging and PET/CT are more accurate than conventional imaging in evaluation of recurrent malignancy after radiation therapy.
- CT/PET is useful in localization of increased FDG uptake, facilitates directed biopsy, and improves accuracy in diagnosing recurrent or persistent malignancy.
- FDG-PET can give false-positive results within first 6 months after completion of radiation therapy.

CLINICAL PRESENTATION

- Generally, clinical symptomatology is proportional to extent of radiation-induced lung injury and pretreatment pulmonary function of the patient.
- Typically, patient presents with cough and mild to moderate dyspnea, although severe respiratory compromise can occur.
- Occasionally, patient presents with chest pain and fever associated with nonproductive cough or cough productive of small amounts of blood-tinged sputum.
- Chronic respiratory failure and cor pulmonale secondary to fibrosis of large volume of lung occasionally occur as late manifestations.

DIFFERENTIAL DIAGNOSIS

- Pneumonia
- Drug reaction
- Previous infection

PATHOLOGY

- Factors that increase lung injury after radiation therapy include age, cigarette smoking, and preexisting lung disease before irradiation.
- Radiation therapy initiates a sequence of molecular and genetic changes resulting in lung injury.
- Endothelial cell damage, proteinaceous material exudation into alveoli, and inflammatory cell infiltration result.
- Progression to fibrosis occurs typically limited to the radiation field.
- Organizing pneumonia and eosinophilic pneumonia may occur outside of the radiation field.

INCIDENCE/PREVALENCE AND EPIDEMIOLOGY

- Radiation-induced lung injury is common in patients with lung, breast, and thymic malignancies and with malignant pleural mesothelioma and lymphoma.
- Moderate to severe radiation-induced pneumonitis is estimated to occur in 10,000-20,000 of patients with lung cancer in United States per year.
- It is uncommon in patients receiving < 20 Gy of radiation and common in patients who receive > 60 Gy.

Suggested Readings

Abid SH, Malhotra V, Perry MC: Radiation-induced and chemotherapy-induced pulmonary injury. *Curr Opin Oncol* 13:242-248, 2001.

Loyer E, Fuller L, Libshitz HI, Palmer JL: Radiographic appearance of the chest following therapy for Hodgkin disease. *Eur J Radiol* 35:136-148, 2000.

Mehta V: Radiation pneumonitis and pulmonary fibrosis in non-small cell lung cancer: Pulmonary function, prediction, and prevention.. *Int J Radiat Oncol Biol Phys* 63:5-24, 2005.

Mesurolle B, Qanadli SD, Merad M, et al: Unusual radiologic findings in the thorax after radiation therapy. *RadioGraphics* 20:67-81, 2000.

Park KJ, Chung JY, Chun MS, Suh JH: Radiation-induced lung disease and the impact of radiation methods on imaging features. *RadioGraphics* 20:83-98, 2000.

Lung Contusion and Laceration

DEFINITION: Pulmonary laceration is a tear in lung parenchyma whereas pulmonary contusion represents pulmonary hemorrhage and edema from disruption of the alveolar capillary membrane.

IMAGING

Radiography

Findings

- Focal, patchy, or diffuse ground-glass opacities or parenchymal consolidation at site of impact and adjacent to rib fractures.
- Absent air bronchograms
- Nonsegmental distribution
- Pulmonary lacerations often initially obscured by pulmonary contusion
- As contusion resolves, lacerations visible as thin-walled cystic spaces (traumatic pneumatocele) or soft tissue masses (hematomas).
- Pneumothorax common particularly in pulmonary laceration

Utility

- Frontal chest radiograph is often initial screening test in thoracic trauma in emergency department.
- Contused lung is usually present within 6 hours after the inciting injury.
- Conspicuity of pulmonary opacities peaks at 24-72 hours and gradually diminishes over 1 week.
- Severe contusions may be radiographically evident for up to 2 weeks.
- Radiographic resolution of traumatic lung cysts occurs over weeks to months.

CT

Findings

- Dense consolidative opacity.
- Type 1 lacerations: most common type; pneumatoceles or partially fluid-filled cysts formed after sudden compressive force resulting in alveolar rupture.
- Type 2 lacerations: shear injury of lower lung near spine as compressive force causes lung to shift across vertebral column.

DIAGNOSTIC PEARLS

- Focal, patchy, or diffuse ground-glass opacities or parenchymal consolidation at the site of impaction and adjacent to rib fractures
- Pulmonary laceration presenting as traumatic pneumatocele or hematoma
- Pulmonary lacerations often initially obscured by pulmonay confusion

- Type 3 lacerations: lung cysts near chest wall adjacent to rib fracture fragment that has directly punctured pulmonary parenchyma.
- Type 4 lacerations: occur when previously formed pleuropulmonary adhesions tear lung after sudden movement or fracture of attached chest wall.

Utility

- Allows for evaluation of airways, pulmonary parenchyma, aorta, great vessels, pericardium, pleura, chest wall, diaphragm, and osseous structures
- Is superior to chest radiography in detection of pulmonary contusion and laceration
- May demonstrate pulmonary laceration and pneumothorax not evident on the radiograph

CLINICAL PRESENTATION

- Hypoxia
- Mild fever
- Hemoptysis
- Dyspnea
- Possibility of acute respiratory failure, requiring intubation and mechanical ventilation

---

WHAT THE REFERRING PHYSICIAN NEEDS TO KNOW

- Supportive therapy is the mainstay in management of pulmonary contusion and laceration.
- Intubation and respiratory support with mechanical ventilation are indicated in cases of impending respiratory failure.
- Long-term sequelae of pulmonary contusion include decreased functional residual capacity and pulmonary fibrosis.
- Pneumothorax is the most common complication associated with pulmonary laceration.

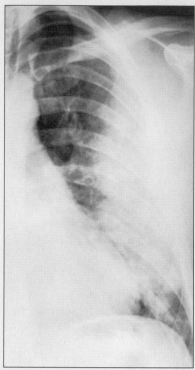

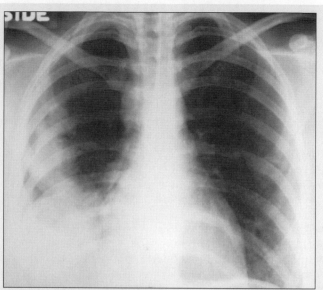

Figure 2. Multiple unilateral pulmonary hematomas. This 17-year-old girl was involved in a two-car collision in which she sustained fractures of the right scapula and humerus. The day after admission, an anteroposterior radiograph showed extensive parenchymal consolidation in the lower two thirds of the right lung in a nonsegmental distribution; the left lung was clear. There was some widening of the superior mediastinum from venous hemorrhage. (*From Müller NL, Fraser RS, Colman NC, Paré PD:* Radiologic Diagnosis of Diseases of the Chest. *Philadelphia, WB Saunders, 2001.*)

Figure 1. Pulmonary contusion. Six hours before radiographic examination, this 33-year-old man was involved in an automobile accident in which he suffered severe trauma to the posterior portion of his left chest. View of the left hemithorax from the anteroposterior radiograph shows homogeneous consolidation of the posterolateral portion of the left lung in a nonsegmental distribution. The margins of the consolidation are defined indistinctly, and there is no air bronchogram. No ribs were fractured. (*From Müller NL, Fraser RS, Colman NC, Paré PD:* Radiologic Diagnosis of Diseases of the Chest. *Philadelphia, WB Saunders, 2001.*)

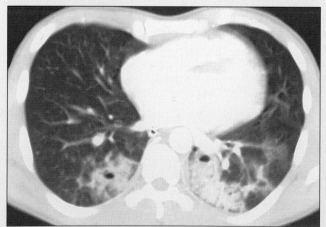

Figure 3. Pulmonary contusion and traumatic lungs cysts. CT image at the level of inferior pulmonary veins demonstrates lower lobe contusions, both of which contain pneumatoceles. (*Courtesy of Dr. Steven L. Primack, Oregon Health and Science University, Portland, Oregon*)

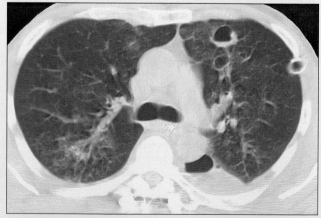

Figure 4. Traumatic lungs cysts. CT image of trauma patient shows type 1 (anterior left mid lung) and type 2 (paraspinal) pneumatoceles in the left lung. (*Courtesy of Dr. Steven L. Primack, Oregon Health and Science University, Portland, Oregon*)

DIFFERENTIAL DIAGNOSIS

- Aspiration pneumonia
- Atelectasis
- Pulmonary edema

PATHOLOGY

- Pulmonary contusion is a direct blow to the chest wall with injury of adjacent lung; rib fracture fragments may lacerate the lung.
- Contrecoup injuries are common, parenchymal contusions seen when lungs have been compressed against denser heart, liver, chest wall, and spine.
- Disruption of alveolar capillary membrane occurs via spallation (spalling effect) and implosion.
- Spallation is a bursting phenomenon that occurs when pressure waves deposit energy at liquid-gas interfaces, such as blood-air interface of alveolus.
- Implosion occurs after transmission of pressure wave through alveolus, when there is overexpansion of alveolar gas.
- Deceleration injuries occur when the alveolar capillary membrane is disrupted as lower-density alveoli shear from higher-density bronchovascular bundles.
- Shear forces, spallation, and implosion can all cause pulmonary laceration.

INCIDENCE/PREVALENCE AND EPIDEMIOLOGY

- Pulmonary contusion is seen in 30%-70% of patients with blunt thoracic injury.
- Pulmonary contusion is most common cause of pulmonary parenchymal opacification on chest radiography in blunt thoracic trauma.

Suggested Readings

Cohn SM: Pulmonary contusion: Review of the clinical entity. *J Trauma* 42:973-979, 1997.

Costantino M, Gosselin MV, Primack SL: The ABC's of thoracic trauma imaging. *Semin Roentgenol* 41:209-225, 2006.

Kishikawa M, Yoshioka T, Shimazu T, et al: Pulmonary contusion causes long-term respiratory dysfunction with decreased functional residual capacity. *J Trauma* 31:1203-1208, 1991.

Miller PR, Croce MA, Bee TK, et al: ARDS after pulmonary contusion: Accurate measurement of contusion volume identifies high-risk patients. *J Trauma* 51:223-230, 2001.

Rivas LA, Fishman JE, Múnera F, Bajayo DE: Multislice CT in thoracic trauma. *Radiol Clin North Am* 41:599-616, 2003.

Van Hise ML, Primack SL, Israel RS, Müller N: CT in blunt chest trauma: Indications and limitations. *RadioGraphics* 18:1071-1084, 1998.

Wanek S, Mayberry JC: Blunt thoracic trauma: Flail chest, pulmonary contusion, and blast injury. *Crit Care Clin* 20:71-81, 2004.

Aortic Injury

DEFINITION: Traumatic aortic injury is a common complication of blunt chest trauma.

IMAGING

Radiography
Findings
- Mediastinal hematoma or widening
- Loss of aortic arch definition, increased aortic arch opacity, increased width and density of descending aorta
- Rightward deviation of trachea
- Rightward deviation of enteric tube
- Thickening of right paratracheal stripe
- Downward displacement of left main-stem bronchus
- Left apical cap

Utility
- Frontal chest radiograph is often initial screening test in thoracic trauma obtained in emergency department.
- Radiography is used to evaluate for mediastinal hematoma and for exclusion of aortic injury.
- Negative predictive value of properly obtained chest radiograph is 98%.
- Positive predictive value, however, is low at 15%.
- Supine imaging, magnification factors, and rotational factors can all lead to radiographic mimics of mediastinal hematoma.

CT
Findings
- Irregularity of wall of aorta, abrupt caliber change of aorta
- Presence of pseudoaneurysm.
- Intimal flap
- Extravasation of contrast material
- Periaortic hematoma
- Diffuse circumferential perimural hematoma that extends down to abdominal aorta
- Polypoid intraluminal clot or low-density filling defect

Utility
- CT allows for evaluation of airways, pulmonary parenchyma, aorta, great vessels, pericardium, pleura, chest wall, diaphragm, and osseous structures.
- Multidetector helical CT is very sensitive diagnostic tool for exclusion of aortic injury.

DIAGNOSTIC PEARLS

- Mediastinal widening on radiograph
- Rightward deviation of trachea and enteric tube on radiograph
- Irregularity of wall of aorta on CT
- Intimal flap
- Pseudoaneurysm
- Intraluminal filling defect

- Morphologically normal aorta with no mediastinal hematoma has virtually 100% negative predictive value for exclusion of aortic injury.
- Positive predictive value is unclear at this time with equivocal studies (hematoma only) requiring aortography or close clinical follow-up.

Ultrasonography
Findings
- Aortic transection
- Irregularity of wall of aorta

Utility
- Transesophageal echocardiography is a valid option for exclusion of aortic injury if there are no contraindications.
- Disadvantages are the time required to logistically perform the study and user dependence.

CLINICAL PRESENTATION

- Clinical signs of traumatic aortic injury are seldom present; the diagnosis is based on mechanism of injury (major blunt trauma) and the results of imaging studies.

DIFFERENTIAL DIAGNOSIS

- Primary aortic intramural hematoma
- Aortic aneurysm
- Venous bleeding

WHAT THE REFERRING PHYSICIAN NEEDS TO KNOW

- Surviving trauma patients require prompt and accurate diagnosis to allow for timely repair of injury.
- Majority of blunt aortic injuries occur at the level of the aortic isthmus just distal to origin of the subclavian artery.
- Morphologically normal aorta with no mediastinal hematoma on CT has virtually 100% negative predictive value for exclusion of aortic injury.
- Positive predictive value for CT is unclear with equivocal studies (hematoma only) requiring aortography or close clinical follow-up.
- Treatment of traumatic aortic injury is increasingly being performed with endovascular stents.
- Alternative options of treatment include direct repair with surgical closure versus open surgical graft interposition.

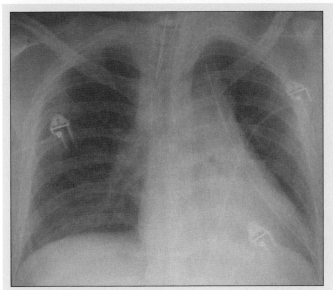

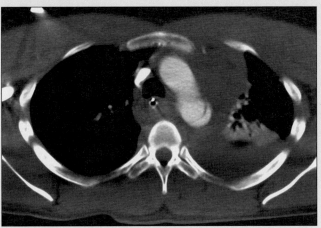

Figure 1. Thoracic aortic injury. Frontal chest radiograph in a 25-year-old man involved in a motor vehicle accident shows indistinct aortic arch, dense superior mediastinum, and deviation of both the enteric tube and the trachea to the right and bilateral apical caps. (*Courtesy of Dr. Steven L. Primack, Oregon Health and Science University, Portland, Oregon*)

Figure 2. Thoracic aortic injury. Contrast-enhanced CT scan shows posterior aortic wall contour abnormality with luminal flap and pseudoaneurysm with large surrounding periaortic hematoma in the region of the aortic isthmus. (*Courtesy of Dr. Steven L. Primack, Oregon Health and Science University, Portland, Oregon*)

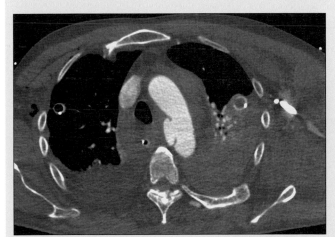

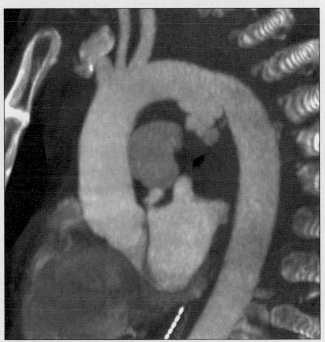

Figure 3. Thoracic aortic injury. Contrast-enhanced CT shows medial aortic wall transection with pseudoaneurysm. Note the large mediastinal and periaortic hematoma. (*Courtesy of Dr. Steven L. Primack, Oregon Health and Science University, Portland, Oregon*)

Figure 4. Thoracic aortic injury. Sagittal CT reconstruction shows a large irregular aortic wall pseudoaneurysm distal to the origin of the left subclavian artery. (*Courtesy of Dr. Steven L. Primack, Oregon Health and Science University, Portland, Oregon*)

PATHOLOGY

- Portion of aorta has been compromised, which can be either partial or complete rupture due to blunt trauma.
- Mechanism of injury includes high-speed motor vehicle collisions >30 mph, falls from heights >10 feet, and pedestrians struck by vehicles.
- Osseous pinch mechanism suggests that isthmus becomes compressed between spine and sternum.
- Shearing stress is caused by sudden deceleration with force vectors pointing in opposite directions centered at aortic isthmus.
- Water hammer effect is the sudden increase in intra-aortic pressure at the time of trauma.
- Viscous response theory is that velocity of compression is the most important determinant in internal chest trauma.
- A spectrum of vessel damage results ranging from microscopic intimal hemorrhage to gross transection of all three vessel layers.

INCIDENCE/PREVALENCE AND EPIDEMIOLOGY

- Thoracic aortic injury is a common cause of prehospital mortality, accounting for 15%-20% of prehospital traumatic deaths.
- Seventy percent of those with aortic injury die at the trauma scene.
- Ascending aorta is injured in less than 5% of patients with blunt aortic injury who survive transport for further treatment.
- Approximately 60% of tears involve intima and media with an intact adventitia.

Suggested Readings

Alkhadi H, Wildermuth S, Desbiolles L, et al: Vascular emergencies of the thorax after blunt and iatrogenic trauma: Multi-detector row CT and three-dimensional imaging. *RadioGraphics* 24:1239-1255, 2004.

Creasy J, Chiles C, Routh WD, Dyer RB: Overview of traumatic injury of the thoracic aorta. *RadioGraphics* 17:27-45, 1997.

Mayberry J: Imaging in thoracic trauma: The trauma surgeon's perspective. *J Thorac Imaging* 15:76-85, 2000.

Mirvis SE: Thoracic vascular injury. *Radiol Clin North Am* 44:181-197, 2006:vii.

Patel N, Stephens KE Jr, Mirvis SE, et al: Imaging of acute thoracic aortic injury due to blunt trauma: A review. *Radiology* 208:335-348, 1998.

Sammer M, Wang E, Blackmore CC, et al: Indeterminate CT angiography in blunt thoracic trauma: Is CT angiography enough?. *AJR Am J Roentgenol* 189:603-608, 2007.

Van Hise ML, Primack SL, Israel RS, Müller N: CT in blunt chest trauma: Indications and limitations. *RadioGraphics* 18:1071-1084, 1998.

Cardiac and Pericardial Injury

DEFINITION: Blunt trauma may result in cardiac injury and pericardial rupture.

IMAGING

Radiography

Findings

- Hemopericardium: may or may not be evident at presentation
- Unusual position/configuration of heart if cardiac herniation is present

Utility

- Initial screening test in thoracic trauma is frontal chest radiograph obtained in emergency department.

CT

Findings

- Hemopericardium: hyperdense fluid collection in pericardial space.
- Focal pericardial defect with "collar sign" of herniating cardiac tissue.
- Pneumopericardium: conforms more tightly to cardiac contour; if significant may result in diminutive cardiac size secondary to compression.

Utility

- Allows for evaluation of airways, pulmonary parenchyma, aorta, great vessels, pericardium, pleura, chest wall, diaphragm, and osseous structures.
- Imaging modality of choice for assessment of pericardial injury.
- Limited role in the assessment of cardiac injury.

DIFFERENTIAL DIAGNOSIS

- Pneumomediastinum
- Pericardial effusion
- Congenital absence of left pericardium

PATHOLOGY

- Injuries can affect pericardium, myocardium, coronary vessels, chordae, papillary muscles, and valves.
- Pericardial rupture can occur along its pulmonary or diaphragmatic borders (or both).

DIAGNOSTIC PEARLS

- Hemopericardium
- Hyperdense fluid collection in the pericardial space on CT
- "Collar sign" of herniating cardiac tissue
- Pneumopericardium

- Pericardial rupture becomes significant when heart herniates through tear, resulting in cardiac filling impedance and coronary vessel occlusion.
- Cardiac herniation through pericardial defect may not be present initially but may occur after administration or discontinuance of positive-pressure ventilation.

INCIDENCE/PREVALENCE AND EPIDEMIOLOGY

- Significant cardiac injuries are uncommon in patients with blunt trauma who are seen in the emergency department.
- Cardiac contusion is the most innocuous and most common of these injuries.
- Pericardial rupture more commonly occurs on the left side.
- Most commonly ruptured cardiac chamber discovered at autopsy is the right ventricle.
- Atria are the most commonly ruptured chambers in those who survive to hospitalization.
- Pneumopericardium is rarely seen in the trauma setting.

Suggested Readings

Pretre R: Blunt trauma to the heart and great vessels. *N Engl J Med* 336:626-632, 1997.

Restrepo CS, Lemos DF, Lemos JA, et al: Imaging findings in cardiac tamponade with emphasis on CT. *RadioGraphics* 27:1595-1610, 2007.

Rivas LA, Fishman JE, Múnera F, Bajayo DE: Multislice CT in thoracic trauma. *Radiol Clin North Am* 41:599-616, 2003.

WHAT THE REFERRING PHYSICIAN NEEDS TO KNOW

- Cardiac contusion is a clinical diagnosis with little imaging evidence to support the diagnosis.
- Hemopericardium will usually be managed via pericardial decompression/drainage.
- It is difficult to diagnose pericardial rupture with cardiac herniation even with CT.
- Not all pericardial tears are associated with cardiac herniation; therefore, chest radiography and CT may be unrevealing.
- Presence of adjacent pneumothorax and/or pneumomediastinum may complicate diagnosis because pericardium may be mistaken for pleura.
- Pericardial rupture may be diagnosed at a time remote from traumatic injury given the paucity of clinical and imaging findings.

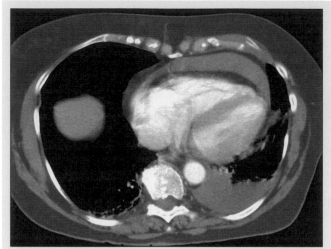

Figure 1. Hemopericardium. Contrast-enhanced CT image in a patient involved in a head-on motor vehicle collision shows hyperdense pericardial fluid compatible with hemopericardium. Note adjacent left anterior displaced rib fracture. (*Courtesy of Dr. Steven L. Primack, Oregon Health and Science University, Portland, Oregon*)

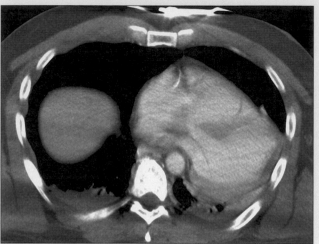

Figure 2. Pericardial rupture and cardiac herniation. Contrast-enhanced CT image in a 55-year-old man involved in a high-speed motor vehicle collision reveals abnormal cardiac configuration with "collar sign" best appreciated just adjacent to the aorta, indicating cardiac herniation through a pericardial tear. The patient had hemodynamic instability with the echocardiogram showing left atrium compression. A large left pericardial tear was repaired surgically. Notably the chest radiograph was unrevealing in this case, as is often the case with pericardial tears. (*Courtesy of Dr. Steven L. Primack, Oregon Health and Science University, Portland, Oregon*)

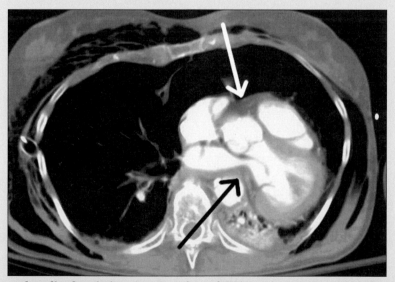

Figure 3. Pericardial rupture and cardiac herniation. Contrast-enhanced CT image in a trauma patient showing another cardiac "collar sign" (*arrows*) indicating a pericardial tear with concomitant cardiac herniation. Extensive soft tissue emphysema is additionally present. (*Courtesy of Dr. Steven L. Primack, Oregon Health and Science University, Portland, Oregon*)

Rollins M: Traumatic ventricular septal defect: Case review and review of the English literature since 1970. *J Trauma* 58:175-180, 2005.

RuDusky BM: Classification of myocardial contusion and blunt cardiac trauma. *Angiology* 58:610-613, 2007.

Wall M, Mattox KL, Wolf DA: The cardiac pendulum: Blunt rupture of the pericardium with strangulation of the heart. *J Trauma* 59:136-141, 2005.

Chest Wall and Vertebral Trauma

DEFINITION: Chest wall and vertebral trauma may lead to multiple rib, sternal, vertebral, clavicular, and scapular fractures.

IMAGING

Radiography
Findings
- Clavicle fractures occur.
- Rib fractures are evident.
- Scapular fracture may be seen.
- Peripheral opacities that parallel the chest wall represent extrapleural hematomas adjacent to rib fractures.
- Flail chest should be considered whenever a large extrapleural hematoma is seen.
- Extrapleural hematoma results from extrapleural bleeding from damaged intercostal vessels, muscles, and open fractures.
- Paraspinal hematoma and an indistinct/dense descending aorta are indirect signs of vertebral body injury.

Utility
- Frontal chest radiograph: initial screening test in thoracic trauma
- Of value in demonstrating evidence of mediastinal hematoma and in ruling out large pneumothorax

CT
Findings
- Scapular fractures
- Rib fractures
- Sternal fractures: not usually seen on frontal radiographs but like rib fractures are easily seen on CT
- Vertebral fracture

Utility
- Allows for evaluation of airways, pulmonary parenchyma, aorta, great vessels, pericardium, pleura, chest wall, diaphragm, and osseous structures.
- Far more sensitive in diagnosis of rib fractures than radiography.
- Multidetector CT with multiplanar reformatted images: modality of choice in diagnosis of vertebral and sternal fractures.
- 3D reformatted images: helpful in visualizing rib trauma in setting of flail chest and aid the surgeon in surgical planning.
- Modality of choice in assessment of patients with clinical/radiographic findings suggestive of vertebral fracture after blunt chest trauma.

DIAGNOSTIC PEARLS
- Multidetector CT with multiplanar reformatted images is the modality of choice in diagnosis of vertebral and sternal fractures.
- Segmental fracture of four or more contiguous ribs should alert to the possibility of flail chest.

CLINICAL PRESENTATION
- Flail chest is a clinical diagnosis in which mismatched inspiratory and expiratory mechanics impairs ventilation.

PATHOLOGY
- First, second, and third rib fractures along with scapular fractures are associated with significant mechanism of injury.
- Sternal fractures are seen predominately in restrained vehicular passengers and occur in 8% of those with significant mechanism of injury.
- Fractures of 10th, 11th, and 12th ribs are commonly associated with renal, splenic, and hepatic injuries.
- Posterior sternoclavicular dislocation is associated with an increased risk of tracheal, esophageal, and great vessel impingement/injury.
- Wedge compression and burst fractures secondary to hyperflexion and axial load mechanisms are predominant fracture types.

INCIDENCE/PREVALENCE AND EPIDEMIOLOGY
- Rib fractures occur in 60% of patients with blunt thoracic trauma.
- Rib fractures are more common in the elderly given the less elastic properties of their skeleton; mortality rate is higher in the pediatric population.
- Sternal fractures occur in 8% of those with significant mechanism of injury; 50% of patients have pneumothorax.

WHAT THE REFERRING PHYSICIAN NEEDS TO KNOW
- Segmental fracture of four or more contiguous ribs should alert clinician to the possibility of flail chest.
- Multidetector CT with multiplanar reformatted images is the modality of choice in diagnosis of vertebral and sternal fractures.

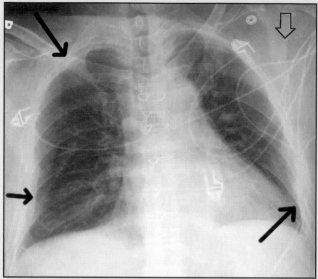

Figure 1. **Rib fractures and extrapleural hematoma.** Frontal chest radiograph in a trauma patient who has multiple bilateral rib fractures not easily appreciated on the radiograph. Note the isolated, peripheral opacities (*arrows*) that parallel the chest wall representing extrapleural hematomas adjacent to rib fractures. (*Courtesy of Dr. Steven L. Primack, Oregon Health and Science University, Portland, Oregon*)

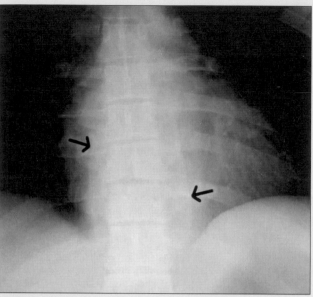

Figure 2. **Vertebral fractures and perivertebral hematoma.** Frontal radiograph in a 35-year-old man after a fall from 20 feet (6 meters) shows subtle irregularity of the inferior endplate of T10 and superior endplate of T11. There is an adjacent perivertebral hematoma (*arrows*). (*Courtesy of Dr. Steven L. Primack, Oregon Health and Science University, Portland, Oregon*)

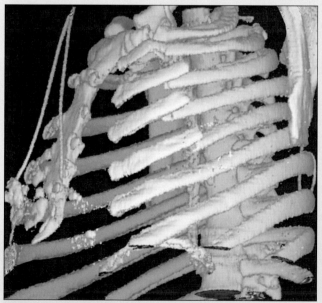

Figure 3. **Rib fractures.** 3D reformatted CT image in a trauma patient shows contiguous displaced rib fractures. This patient had a flail chest clinically. 3D reformatted images are useful to the surgeon for surgical planning. (*Courtesy of Dr. Steven L. Primack, Oregon Health and Science University, Portland, Oregon*)

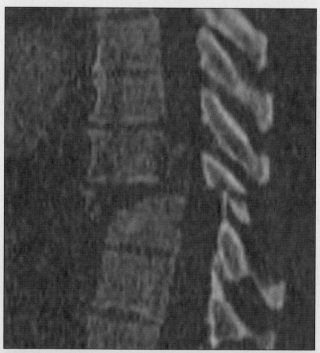

Figure 4. **Vertebral fractures and perivertebral hematoma.** Sagittal reformatted CT image demonstrates anterior displacement of T10 on T11 and endplate fractures at the same level. (*Courtesy of Dr. Steven L. Primack, Oregon Health and Science University, Portland, Oregon*)

■ Thoracic spine fractures occur in 3% of blunt trauma patients and are associated with a high percentage of secondary neurologic impairment.

■ Fourth through ninth ribs are most commonly fractured.

■ First, second, and third rib fractures are associated with aorta/great vessel injury in approximately 14% of cases and with tracheobronchial injuries in 2% of cases.

Suggested Readings

Collins J: Chest wall trauma. *J Thorac Imaging* 15:112-119, 2000.

Costantino M, Gosselin MV, Primack SL: The ABC's of thoracic trauma imaging. *Semin Roentgenol* 41:209-225, 2006.

Miller LA: Chest wall, lung, and pleural space trauma. *Radiol Clin North Am* 44:213-224, 2006.

Rivas LA, Fishman JE, Múnera F, Bajayo DE: Multislice CT in thoracic trauma. *Radiol Clin North Am* 41:599-616, 2003.

Van Hise ML, Primack SL, Israel RS, Müller N: CT in blunt chest trauma: Indications and limitations. *RadioGraphics* 18:1071-1084, 1998.

Traumatic Diaphragmatic Injury

DEFINITION: Traumatic diaphragmatic injury is a tear in the diaphragm resulting from penetrating or blunt injury.

IMAGING

Radiography

Findings
- Visualization of herniated stomach or bowel in chest
- Cephalad extension of nasogastric tube above level of diaphragm
- Irregularity of diaphragmatic contour
- Elevated hemidiaphragm in absence of atelectasis.
- Obscuration of hemidiaphragm
- Contralateral shift of mediastinum

Utility
- Frontal chest radiograph is often the initial screening test in thoracic trauma obtained in the emergency department.
- It is a useful screening tool but relatively insensitive in detection of diaphragmatic rupture.

CT

Findings
- Herniation of omental fat or abdominal viscera
- Waist-like narrowing of herniated viscera (collar sign)
- Lack of visualization of hemidiaphragm
- Thickening of diaphragm
- Dependent viscera sign: describes dependent position of stomach, spleen, and bowel that has herniated into thorax
- Direct discontinuity or focal defect of diaphragm
- Elevated abdominal organs

Utility
- Allows for evaluation of airways, pulmonary parenchyma, aorta, great vessels, pericardium, pleura, chest wall, diaphragm, and osseous structures.
- Imaging of choice in evaluation of patients with blunt chest trauma and suspected diaphragmatic injury.
- Thin collimation and thin reconstruction images recommended if diaphragmatic injury is suspected.
- Sagittal and coronal reformatted images shown to increase sensitivity and confidence of interpretation.
- Visualization of focal discontinuity of diaphragm: 73%-82% sensitivity and 90% specificity.
- Intrathoracic herniation: 55%-65% sensitivity and 100% specificity.

DIAGNOSTIC PEARLS

- Collar sign
- Dependent viscera sign
- Direct discontinuity or focal defect of the diaphragm
- Visualization of herniated stomach or bowel in chest

- Collar sign: 63% sensitivity and 100% specificity; dependent viscera sign: 55%-90% sensitivity.

MRI

Findings
- Tear: focal discontinuity with hypointensity on T1- and T2-weighted images.

Utility
- Cardiac and respiratory gated MRI: may be of use in stable patient if radiographic and CT findings nondiagnostic

CLINICAL PRESENTATION

- Seen mainly in patients with major blunt injury to the lower chest, abdomen, and pelvis and in patients with penetrating injuries to the upper abdomen or lower chest.
- Usually associated with other major traumatic injuries (pneumothorax, hepatic and splenic lacerations, pelvic fractures).

DIFFERENTIAL DIAGNOSIS

- Diaphragmatic eventration
- Bochdalek hernia
- Phrenic nerve palsy
- Normal variant

PATHOLOGY

- Penetrating diaphragmatic injury results from direct trauma and produces a small tear in the diaphragm usually <1 cm.

WHAT THE REFERRING PHYSICIAN NEEDS TO KNOW

- Detection of diaphragmatic injury requires a high index of suspicion.
- Masking of injury by pleural fluid or pulmonary contusion may delay diagnosis.
- Diaphragmatic injury is associated with other major traumatic injuries (pneumothorax, hepatic and splenic lacerations, pelvic fractures).
- Delay in diagnosis and treatment increases the potential for bowel strangulation and increases mortality.

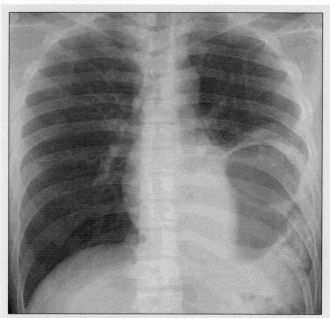

Figure 1. Traumatic diaphragmatic injury. Frontal chest radiograph in a male trauma patient shows a markedly elevated stomach in the lower left hemithorax. (*Courtesy of Dr. Steven L. Primack, Oregon Health and Science University, Portland, Oregon*)

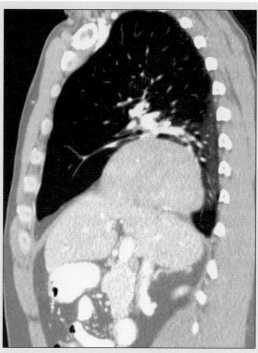

Figure 2. Traumatic diaphragamtic injury. Sagittal reformatted CT image through the right hemidiaphragm shows a collar sign of herniated liver into the right hemithorax. (*Courtesy of Dr. Steven L. Primack, Oregon Health and Science University, Portland, Oregon*)

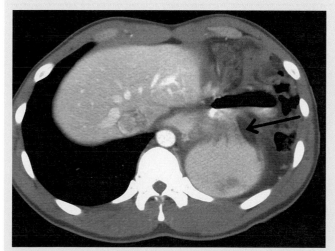

Figure 3. Traumatic diaphragmatic injury. CT image shows dependent viscera sign with the stomach layering posteriorly. Additionally, there is a collar sign with stomach herniating through the diaphragmatic defect (*arrow*). (*Courtesy of Dr. Steven L. Primack, Oregon Health and Science University, Portland, Oregon*)

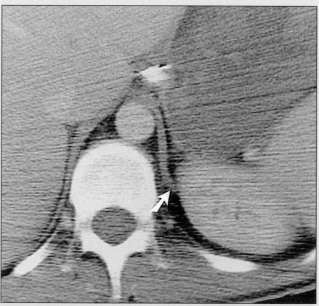

Figure 4. Traumatic rupture of the left hemidiaphragm. Contrast-enhanced CT scan shows abrupt discontinuity of the left hemidiaphragm (*arrow*) at the level of the medial arcuate ligament. The patient was a 24-year-old man being assessed 10 days after a motor vehicle accident for unresolving pulmonary contusions. The diagnosis of traumatic tear of the hemidiaphragm was confirmed at surgery. (*From Müller NL, Fraser RS, Colman NC, Paré PD: Radiologic Diagnosis of Diseases of the Chest. Philadelphia, WB Saunders, 2001.*)

- Penetrating injury results from shootings, stabbings, and, less commonly, iatrogenic causes such as a malpositioned chest tube.
- Blunt trauma causes an increase in intrathoracic pressure that ruptures diaphragm.
- Diaphragmatic tears associated with blunt trauma are usually ≥10 cm.
- Injury is most frequently left-sided owing to protective cushioning effect of liver.

INCIDENCE/PREVALENCE AND EPIDEMIOLOGY

- Penetrating diaphragmatic injury is twice as common as blunt injury.
- Diaphragmatic rupture occurs in 0.8%-8% of all patients with major blunt trauma.
- Diaphragmatic injury is associated with other major traumatic injuries (pneumothorax, hepatic and splenic lacerations, pelvic fractures).
- Injury is most frequently left sided (75%).
- Mortality from diaphragmatic rupture approaches 30%.

Suggested Readings

Bergin D, Ennis R, Keogh C, et al: The "dependent viscera" sign in CT diagnosis of blunt traumatic diaphragmatic rupture. *AJR Am J Roentgenol* 177:1137-1140, 2001.

Collins J: Chest wall trauma. *J Thorac Imaging* 15:112-119, 2000.

Costantino M, Gosselin MV, Primack SL: The ABC's of thoracic trauma imaging. *Semin Roentgenol* 41:209-225, 2006.

Killeen KL, Mirvis SE, Shanmuganathan K: Helical CT of diaphragmatic rupture caused by blunt trauma. *AJR Am J Roentgenol* 173:1611-1616, 1999.

Iochum S, Ludig T, Walter F, et al: Imaging of diaphragmatic injury: A diagnostic challenge? *RadioGraphics* 22:S103-S118, 2002.

Murray JG, Caoili E, Gruden JF, et al: Acute rupture of the diaphragm due to blunt trauma: Diagnostic sensitivity and specificity of CT. *AJR Am J Roentgenol* 166:1035-1039, 1996.

Nchimi A, Szapiro D, Ghaye B, et al: Helical CT of blunt diaphragmatic rupture. *AJR Am J Roentgenol* 184:24-30, 2005.

Rivas LA, Fishman JE, Múnera F, Bajayo DE: Multislice CT in thoracic trauma. *Radiol Clin North Am* 41:599-616, 2003.

Shackleton KL, Stewart ET, Taylor AJ: Traumatic diaphragmatic injuries: Spectrum of radiographic findings. *RadioGraphics* 18:49-59, 1998.

Van Hise ML, Primack SL, Israel RS, Müller NL: CT in blunt chest trauma: Indications and limitations. *RadioGraphics* 18:1071-1084, 1998.

Worthy SA, Kang EY, Hartman TE, et al: Diaphragmatic rupture: CT findings in 11 patients. *Radiology* 194:885-888, 1995.

Tracheobronchial Tears (Traumatic Airway Injury)

DEFINITION: Tracheobronchial tears refer to mucosal tears and complete transection of the airway.

IMAGING

Radiography
Findings
- Bronchial fracture: fallen-lung sign: lung "falling" dependently rather than collapsing centrally toward hilum in presence of pneumothorax.
- Double-wall sign: air is seen tracking within bronchial wall.
- Pneumomediastinum, pneumothorax, pneumoretroperitoneum, deep cervical emphysema, and subcutaneous emphysema.
- Tracheal injury indicated by extraluminal position of endotracheal tube and cuff overinflation.
- Persisting or increasing pneumothorax.

Utility
- Frontal chest radiograph: initial screening test
- Low sensitivity and specificity.

CT
Findings
- Bronchial tear
- Focal narrowing of main bronchus
- Focal collections of air within wall of bronchus
- Pneumothorax, pneumomediastinum

Utility
- Allows for evaluation of airways, pulmonary parenchyma, aorta, great vessels, pericardium, pleura, chest wall, diaphragm, and osseous structures.
- Has limited role in detection of tracheobronchial injuries.
- Direct visualization of tear difficult and best accomplished using thin (1-mm) collimation and multiplanar reformatted imaging.

DIAGNOSTIC PEARLS
- Fallen-lung sign (uncommon)
- Double-wall sign (uncommon)
- Extraluminal position of endotracheal tube and cuff overinflation (uncommon)
- Persistent or increasing pneumothorax
- Bronchial tear or focal narrowing on CT
- Majority of injuries occur within 2 cm of carina

CLINICAL PRESENTATION
- History of trauma
- Soft tissue emphysema or pneumothorax refractory to chest tube drainage

PATHOLOGY
- Tracheobronchial tears refers to mucosal tears and complete transection of airway.
- Deceleration injuries occur when shearing forces predominate because peripheral lung is more mobile than relatively fixed central bronchi and trachea.
- Crush injuries are also associated with airway damage.
- When glottis is closed, elevated pressure within airways can result in laceration of trachea or bronchi.
- Lungs deviate laterally when thoracic cavity is compressed, creating pulling force that can tear central airways.
- Iatrogenic injury can occur if endotracheal cuff is overinflated.

WHAT THE REFERRING PHYSICIAN NEEDS TO KNOW
- Tracheobronchial tear should be suspected particularly in patients with persistent or increasing pneumothorax despite continuous chest tube drainage.
- Injuries to trachea or proximal left main bronchus typically result in pneumomediastinum and not pneumothorax.
- Tear in mediastinal pleura may allow air to leak from mediastinum into pleural space, resulting in pneumothorax.
- Complications of tracheobronchial injury include bronchopleural fistula and, rarely, tracheoesophageal fistula.
- Undiagnosed, untreated tracheal and bronchial injuries may lead to stenosis; patient may develop postobstructive pneumonia and bronchiectasis.
- High index of suspicion and liberal use of bronchoscopy are important for prompt diagnosis of tracheobronchial injury.
- Treatment involves surgical repair and, in severe cases, lobectomy or pneumonectomy.

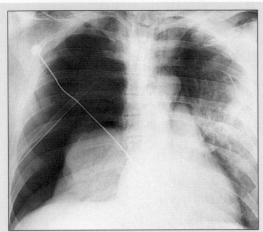

Figure 1. Fracture of the right main bronchus. Anteroposterior chest radiograph in a 24-year-old man after a motor vehicle accident shows large right and small left pneumothoraces, extensive pneumomediastinum, and multiple rib fractures. Despite the presence of a chest tube, the right lung is collapsed and displaced inferior to the right hilum (fallen-lung sign). A few air bronchograms still are visible within the collapsed lung. Complete transection of the right main bronchus was identified at surgery. (*From Müller NL, Fraser RS, Colman NC, Paré PD: Radiologic Diagnosis of Diseases of the Chest. Philadelphia, WB Saunders, 2001.*)

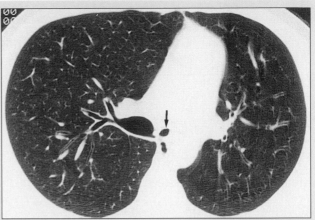

Figure 2. Fracture of the left main bronchus. High-resolution CT scan in a 26-year-old man shows focal narrowing of the left main bronchus (*straight arrow*). The patient presented with a history of cough and progressive shortness of breath 1 month after a motor vehicle accident. The diagnosis of fracture of the left main bronchus was confirmed bronchoscopically. (*From Müller NL, Fraser RS, Colman NC, Paré PD: Radiologic Diagnosis of Diseases of the Chest. Philadelphia, WB Saunders, 2001.*)

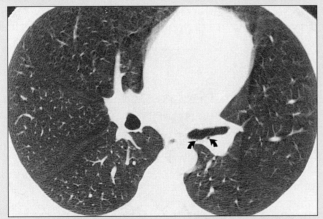

Figure 3. Fracture of the left main bronchus. High-resolution CT scan at a more caudad level than in Figure 2 shows focal collections of air within the wall of the left main and left upper lobe bronchus (*curved arrows*). The patient presented with a history of cough and progressive shortness of breath 1 month after a motor vehicle accident. The diagnosis of fracture of the left main bronchus was confirmed bronchoscopically. (*From Müller NL, Fraser RS, Colman NC, Paré PD: Radiologic Diagnosis of Diseases of the Chest. Philadelphia, WB Saunders, 2001.*)

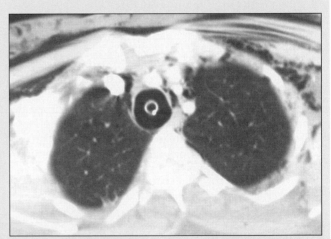

Figure 4. Airway injury and pneumomediastinum. CT image shows the abnormally enlarged endotracheal tube balloon, pneumomediastinum, and chest wall emphysema. The patient was found to have a 5-cm tear through the posterior membranous portion of the trachea that was believed to be secondary to traumatic intubation given the unusual location of injury (i.e., > 2 cm from the carina). (*Courtesy of Dr. Steven L. Primack, Oregon Health and Science University, Portland, Oregon*)

INCIDENCE/PREVALENCE AND EPIDEMIOLOGY

- Tracheobronchial tears are uncommon, occurring in 1%-3% of patients with blunt thoracic trauma.
- Approximately 75% of tracheobronchial injuries occur within 2 cm of carina.
- Right main bronchus is more frequently injured than either trachea or left main bronchus.

Suggested Readings

Cassada DC, Munyikwa MP, Moniz MP, et al: Acute injuries of the trachea and major bronchi: Importance of early diagnosis. *Ann Thoracic Surg* 69:1563-1567, 2000.

Kiser AC, O'Brien SM, Detterbeck FC: Blunt tracheobronchial injuries: Treatment and outcomes. *Ann Thorac Surg* 71:2059-2066, 2001.

Rivas LA, Fishman JE, Múnera F, Bajayo DE: Multislice CT in thoracic trauma. *Radiol Clin North Am* 41:599-616, 2003.

Unger JM, Schuchmann GG, Grossman JE, Pellett JR: Tears of the trachea and main bronchi caused by blunt trauma: Radiologic findings. *AJR Am J Roentgenol* 153:1175-1180, 1989.

Van Hise ML, Primack SL, Israel RS, Müller NL: CT in blunt chest trauma: Indications and limitations. *RadioGraphics* 18:1071-1084, 1998.

Thoracotomy (Including Pneumonectomy and Lobectomy)

DEFINITION: Postoperative complications include continuing air leaks, bronchopleural fistula, hemothorax, empyema, lung herniation, lobar torsion, postpneumonectomy syndrome, and wound infection.

IMAGING

Radiography

Findings

- Expected early postlobectomy changes: small fluid-filled intrapleural space, pneumothorax or hydrothorax, decreased lung density, widely spaced vascular markings (hyperinflation)
- Expected postpneumonectomy changes: intrapleural space completely filled with fluid in weeks or 3-7 months; ipsilateral mediastinal shift
- Decrease in air-fluid level >2 cm in postpneumonectomy space: sensitive indicator of bronchopleural fistula.
- Other indicators of bronchopleural fistula: new air-fluid level and expansion of loculated pleural air collection in postresection residual space
- Abnormal increase in the amount of fluid in the postpneumonectomy space suggests hemothorax or empyema
- Lung herniation: often not visible on frontal chest radiograph but appears as retrosternal lucency on lateral chest radiograph
- Lobar torsion: lobar atelectasis (earliest finding), lobar congestion (rapidly expanding consolidation/mass in affected lobe, hilar shift away from affected side)

Utility

- Radiography has low diagnostic accuracy in detection of postoperative complications.

CT

Findings

- Bronchopleural fistula: direct connection between central bronchus and pleura, parietal pleura enhancement after contrast, effacement of extrapleural fat.
- Postpneumonectomy syndrome: marked rightward, posterior displacement of mediastinum; counterclockwise rotation of heart and great vessels; and left lung hyperinflation and herniation; narrowing of bronchus.
- Lobar torsion: increased volume and consolidation and decreased attenuation because of poor arterial flow.

DIAGNOSTIC PEARLS

- Bronchopleural fistula: direct connection between central bronchus and pleura, parietal pleura enhancement after administration of a contrast agent, effacement of extrapleural fat.
- Postpneumonectomy syndrome: marked rightward, posterior displacement of mediastinum; counterclockwise rotation of heart and great vessels; and left lung hyperinflation and herniation.
- Lobar torsion: increased volume and consolidation and decreased attenuation because of poor arterial flow.
- Sensitive indicator of bronchopleural fistula: decrease in air-fluid level >2 cm in postpneumonectomy space.

- Additional findings of lobar torsion: tapering/obliteration of proximal pulmonary artery and associated bronchus and ground-glass attenuation in affected lobe.

Utility

- CT is best diagnostic technique to identify the pathologic process underlying abnormal mediastinal shifts.

CLINICAL PRESENTATION

- Chest pain, fever, cough, dyspnea

PATHOLOGY

- Wound infection occurs with increased frequency in chest wall reconstructions because prosthetic mesh is an excellent substrate for bacterial growth.
- Abnormal mediastinal shifts may be caused by restrictive or expansile lung process.
- Risk factors for bronchopleural fistula include inflammatory disease, preoperative irradiation, and resection involving the right lung.

WHAT THE REFERRING PHYSICIAN NEEDS TO KNOW

- Common complications after thoracotomy include hemorrhage at the surgical site, infection, and bronchopleural fistula.
- Bronchopleural fistula typically occurs within the first 2 weeks postoperatively.
- Postpneumonectomy syndrome typically occurs in children and young adults months to years after pneumonectomy and results in progressive narrowing of the contralateral main bronchus.

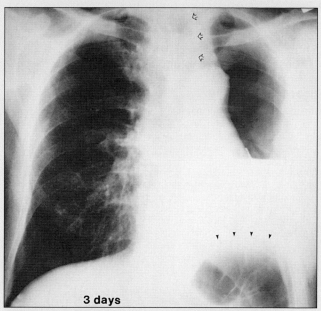

3 days

Figure 1. Postpneumonectomy course complicated by empyema. Three days after left pneumonectomy, the amount of fluid that has accumulated, the position of the left hemidiaphragm (*arrowheads*), and the shift of the tracheal air column to the left (*open arrows*) are all consistent with a normal postoperative course. (*From Müller NL, Fraser RS, Colman NC, Paré PD: Radiologic Diagnosis of Diseases of the Chest. Philadelphia, WB Saunders, 2001.*)

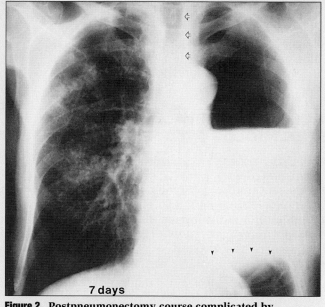

7 days

Figure 2. Postpneumonectomy course complicated by empyema. At 7 days, the left hemidiaphragm (*arrowheads*) has undergone some depression and the tracheal air column (*open arrows*) has returned to the midline. Such a change should suggest empyema, bronchopleural fistula, pleural hemorrhage, or (possibly) chylothorax. (*From Müller NL, Fraser RS, Colman NC, Paré PD: Radiologic Diagnosis of Diseases of the Chest. Philadelphia, WB Saunders, 2001.*)

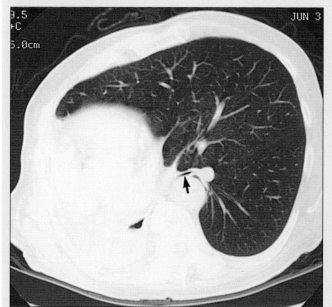

Figure 3. Postpneumonectomy syndrome. CT scan performed at end inspiration shows narrowing of the left lower lobe bronchus (*arrow*). (*Case courtesy of Dr. Fred Matzinger, Department of Radiology, The Ottawa Civic Hospital, Ottawa, Canada. From Müller NL, Fraser RS, Colman NC, Paré PD: Radiologic Diagnosis of Diseases of the Chest. Philadelphia, WB Saunders, 2001.*)

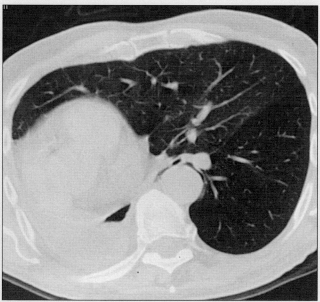

Figure 4. Postpneumonectomy syndrome. Expiratory CT scan shows decreased attenuation and vascularity in the left lower lobe as a result of air trapping. (*Case courtesy of Dr. Fred Matzinger, Department of Radiology, The Ottawa Civic Hospital, Ottawa, Canada. From Müller NL, Fraser RS, Colman NC, Paré PD: Radiologic Diagnosis of Diseases of the Chest. Philadelphia, WB Saunders, 2001.*)

- Postpneumonectomy syndrome results in compression of nonoperative main-stem bronchus leading to airway narrowing.
- Lobar torsion may result in pulmonary infarction and death; bronchial compression results in lobar atelectasis, and arterial compression causes lobar congestion.

INCIDENCE/PREVALENCE AND EPIDEMIOLOGY

- Wound infection occurs in almost 5% of chest wall reconstructions.
- Only one third of postpneumonectomy patients have complete pleural fluid resorption.
- Stump thrombosis occurs in approximately 10% of postoperative cases and is more common in the right pulmonary artery stump.
- Bronchopleural fistula incidence after pulmonary resection occurs in 5%-8%, 3%-6%, and 0.5%-1.0% after extrapleural pneumonectomy, pneumonectomy, and lobectomy, respectively.

- Postpneumonectomy syndrome almost exclusively follows right pneumonectomy and typically occurs in children and young adults months to years after pneumonectomy.
- Lobar torsion is uncommon.

Suggested Readings

Attili A, Kazerooni E: Postoperative cardiopulmonary thoracic imaging. *Radiol Clin North Am* 42:543-564, 2004.

Kim EA, Lee KS, Shim YM, et al: Radiographic and CT findings in complications following pulmonary resection. *RadioGraphics* 22:67-86, 2002.

Kim SH, Lee KS, Shim YM, et al: Esophageal resection: Indications, techniques, and radiologic assessment. *RadioGraphics* 21:1119-1137, 2001.

Konen E, Yellin A, Greenberg I, et al: Complications of tracheal and thoracic surgery: The role of multisection helical CT and computerized reformations. *Clin Radiol* 58:341-350, 2003.

Cardiovascular Surgery

DEFINITION: Complications can occur after coronary artery bypass grafting (CABG), cardiopulmonary bypass, aortic aneurysm repair, and aortic dissection surgery.

IMAGING

Radiography

Findings
- Saphenous vein graft aneurysm connecting to left anterior descending or left circumflex coronary artery: left upper cardiac border masses
- Saphenous graft aneurysm connecting to right coronary artery and left anterior descending artery: soft tissue at right and left lower cardiac borders
- Pneumopericardium: sharp outline of air contouring some or all of the heart
- Hemopericardium/pericardial effusion: loss of mediastinal contour detail, widened subcarinal angle, "differential density sign," increased pericardial stripe size > 2 mm
- Postpericardiotomy syndrome: most commonly presents as concomitant pericardial and bilateral pleural effusions, often with basilar opacities
- Aortic stent-graft complications: migration, kinking, and fracture; aortic perforation (rapidly enlarging periaortic hematoma or hemothorax)
- Post CABG: edema and bleeding (widened cardiomediastinal silhouette with loss of contour details), interstitial edema
- By third postoperative day: pulmonary edema beginning to resolve and cardiomediastinal silhouette beginning to return to its preoperative appearance
- Small pericardial effusion, pleural effusions, and atelectasis (commonly left sided): common in early postoperative period, often persists for weeks
- Transient phrenic nerve paresis (temporary hemidiaphragm elevation) may occur after cardiopulmonary bypass hypothermia with local ice-slush application

Utility
- Performed routinely
- Helpful in detecting most postoperative complications

CT

Findings
- Partial saphenous vein graft occlusion: vessel narrowing (from thrombosis, atherosclerotic plaque); complete occlusion: contrast within proximal graft segment, total graft absence

DIAGNOSTIC PEARLS

- Saphenous vein graft aneurysm: enhancing, round mass connected to graft lumen that contains variable amount of thrombus causing occlusion
- Constrictive pericarditis: pericardial calcification, narrowed tubular right ventricle, sigmoid-shaped ventricular septum, pericardial thickening ≥4 mm (hallmark sign)
- Pseudoaneurysm: enhancing outpouching from aortic anastomotic site, low-attenuation component (thrombosis); infected pseudoaneurysm demonstrating septa and fluid collections
- Graft infection: perigraft air; expanding, irregular, septated perigraft fluid/high-attenuation soft tissue; loss of perigraft fat attenuation
- Endoleak: appearance of contrast inside aneurysmal sac
- Enlarged pericardial space (> 2 mm) with water or blood attenuation for pericardial effusion and hemopericardium, respectively
- Postpericardiotomy syndrome: most commonly presents as concomitant pericardial and bilateral pleural effusions, often with basilar opacities

- Saphenous vein graft aneurysm: enhancing, round mass connected to graft lumen that contains variable amount of thrombus
- Enlarged pericardial space (>2 mm) with water or blood attenuation for pericardial effusion and hemopericardium, respectively
- Constrictive pericarditis: pericardial calcification, narrowed tubular right ventricle, sigmoid-shaped ventricular septum, pericardial thickening >4 mm (hallmark sign)
- Pseudoaneurysm: enhancing outpouching from aortic anastomotic site, low-attenuation component (thrombosis); infected pseudoaneurysm demonstrating septa and fluid collections
- Thrombotic graft occlusion: intraluminal low-attenuation mass; perigraft hematoma: homogeneous low-density collection, sharp margins, lacking septa and gas

---

WHAT THE REFERRING PHYSICIAN NEEDS TO KNOW

- Graft infection is a serious complication that can lead to complete graft failure.
- Normal postoperative changes often mimic a pathologic process.
- Differential diagnosis includes early postoperative changes (post-CABG edema and bleeding, interstitial edema, atelectasis, small pericardial/pleural effusions, perigraft air/fluid collections).
- Site of coronary artery reattachment to the graft often demonstrates contrast-enhancing bulge that can mimic a pseudoaneurysm.

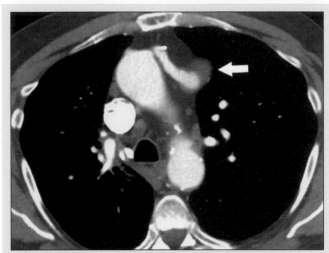

Figure 1. **Saphenous vein graft aneurysm in a 69-year-old man 2 years after coronary bypass graft surgery.** Contrast-enhanced chest CT shows dilatation and thrombosis in the proximal part of saphenous vein graft consistent with graft aneurysm (*arrow*). (*Courtesy of Dr. Charles S. White, University of Maryland, Baltimore*)

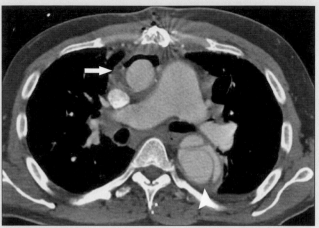

Figure 2. **Synthetic graft infection in a 42-year-old man after placement of a graft for aortic dissection.** Contrast-enhanced chest CT shows air and fluid anterior and lateral to ascending aorta consistent with a graft infection (*arrow*). Note also residual intimal flap in proximal descending aorta (*arrowhead*). (*Courtesy of Dr. Charles S. White, University of Maryland, Baltimore*)

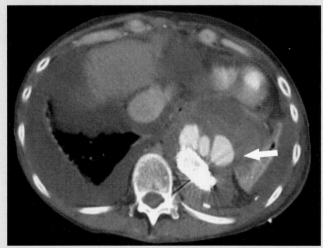

Figure 3. **Endoleak.** A 78-year-old man with stent-graft for aortic aneurysm repair presented with endoleak. Contrast-enhanced chest CT demonstrates a metallic stent with adjacent contrast extravasation and hematoma (*arrow*). (*Courtesy of Dr. Charles S. White, University of Maryland, Baltimore*)

- Graft infection: perigraft air; expanding, irregular, septated perigraft fluid/high attenuation soft tissue; loss of perigraft fat attenuation
- Endoleak: appearance of contrast medium inside aneurysmal sac

Utility

- Superior to radiograph in demonstrating postoperative complications.

Interventional Radiology
Utility

- Catheter angiography remains gold standard for post-CABG graft assessment

CLINICAL PRESENTATION

- Cardiac tamponade
- Postpericardiotomy syndrome from 2 weeks to 6 months after pericardiotomy
- Fever, chest pain

PATHOLOGY

- Complications after CABG include massive air embolism, sternal wound infection, hemomediastinum, and acute lung injury.
- Pericardial complications after CABG include pneumopericardium, hemopericardium, constrictive pericarditis, and postpericardiotomy syndrome.
- Pathologic mediastinal widening is caused by air, blood, and other fluids in pericardial sac; rapid and massive accumulation can cause cardiac tamponade.
- Postpericardiotomy syndrome is an autoimmune related disease occurring 2 weeks to 6 months after pericardiotomy.

- Important complications accompanying use of synthetic aortic grafts and stent-grafts are pseudoaneurysm, perigraft hematoma, aortic perforation, endoleak, and graft infection.
- Aortic perforation may occur either during stent-graft insertion or after erosion of aortic wall by stent-graft struts.
- Endoleak: connection between aneurysm sac and bloodstream through or around stent-graft is caused by stent-graft misplacement, lumen size mismatch, and incomplete expansion.

INCIDENCE/PREVALENCE AND EPIDEMIOLOGY

- Semicircular thin thrombi within inner circumference of the stent are seen in up to 19% of cases.
- Saphenous vein graft aneurysm is an infrequent complication after CABG and most common at the site of graft anastomosis.
- Thrombotic graft occlusion is rare.

Suggested Readings

Attili A, Kazerooni E: Postoperative cardiopulmonary thoracic imaging. *Radiol Clin North Am* 42:543-564, 2004.

Frazier AA, Qureshi F, Read KM, et al: Coronary artery bypass grafts: Assessment with multidetector CT in the early and late postoperative settings. *RadioGraphics* 25:881-896, 2005.

Garzón G, Fernández-Velilla M, Martí M, et al: Endovascular stent-graft treatment of thoracic aortic disease. *RadioGraphics* 25(Suppl 1): S229-S244, 2005.

Orton DF, LeVeen RF, Saigh JA, et al: Aortic prosthetic graft infections: Radiologic manifestations and implications for management. *RadioGraphics* 20:977-993, 2000.

Therasse E, Soulez G, Giroux MF, et al: Stent-graft placement for the treatment of thoracic aortic diseases. *RadioGraphics* 25:157-173, 2005.

Median Sternotomy

DEFINITION: Complications of median sternotomy include incisional dehiscence, wound infection, seroma, retrosternal abscess, mediastinitis, sternal osteomyelitis, sternal nonunion, and fistula formation.

IMAGING

Radiography

Findings
- Dehiscence: "midsternal stripe" may be identified as midline vertical radiolucency over sternum that may progressively widen over time.
- Reorientation of sternal wires (sternal wire displacement) is identified in patients with dehiscence.
- Mediastinal widening.

Utility
- "Midsternal stripe" sign is neither sensitive nor specific for dehiscence and occurs in up to 50% of all post-sternotomy patients.
- Sternal wire displacement is identified in 90% of patients with dehiscence, is considered the single best radiologic sign, and offers potential for early detection.
- Limited value in the diagnosis of retrosternal abscess and mediastinitis.

CT

Findings
- Sternal wire displacement in dehiscence.
- Parasternal soft tissue stranding, sinus tracts, and abscess formation.
- Large or enlarging retrosternal or mediastinal fluid collection in infection.
- High CT numbers (>30 HU) suggest hematoma.

Utility
- Superior to the radiograph in demonstrating postoperative complications
- Used almost routinely in patients with suspected retrosternal abscess or mediastinitis
- Used to determine sinus tract depth and reveal any mediastinal communication
- Osteomyelitis is difficult to differentiate from minor sternal irregularities caused by surgery and may not become fully apparent until reaching an advanced stage.

CLINICAL PRESENTATION

- Fever, chest pain, abnormal drainage from surgical wound

DIAGNOSTIC PEARLS

- Sternal wire displacement is the single best radiologic sign of dehiscence.
- Normal postoperative findings that may persist for 2-3 weeks after sternotomy include mild presternal and retrosternal soft tissue infiltration with edema fluid and blood, localized hematoma, postincisional bone defect, and mild pericardial thickening or effusion.
- Small localized collections of air may be present in the immediate postoperative period but usually resolve by 7 days after surgery.
- Enlarging retrosternal or mediastinal fluid collections are suggestive of infection.
- CT or ultrasound-guided needle aspiration can be helpful to determine if a fluid collection is infected.

PATHOLOGY

- Infectious complications of median sternotomy include retrosternal abscess, mediastinitis, sternal osteomyelitis, sternal nonunion, and fistula formation.

INCIDENCE/PREVALENCE AND EPIDEMIOLOGY

- The incidence of complications after median sternotomy is low (<5%).
- The three main complications are sternal dehiscence, mediastinitis, and osteomyelitis.
- Other complications include hematoma, abscess formation, empyema, pericardial effusion, and fracture of the first rib.

Suggested Readings

Attili A, Kazerooni E: Postoperative cardiopulmonary thoracic imaging. *Radiol Clin North Am* 42:543-564, 2004.

Konen E, Yellin A, Greenberg I, et al: Complications of tracheal and thoracic surgery: The role of multisection helical CT and computerized reformations. *Clin Radiol* 58:341-350, 2003.

Losanoff JE, Richman BW, Jones JW: Disruption and infection of median sternotomy: A comprehensive review. *Eur J Cardiothorac Surg* 21:831-839, 2002.

WHAT THE REFERRING PHYSICIAN NEEDS TO KNOW

- A 2- to 4-mm gap at the sternotomy site (the midsternal stripe) can be recognized in 30%-60% of patients sometime during the postoperative period and is of no diagnostic or prognostic significance.
- Sternal wire displacement is the single best radiologic sign of dehiscence and offers the potential for early detection.
- Fractured and displaced wires may extend into parasternal soft tissues or, rarely, migrate elsewhere in the thorax.

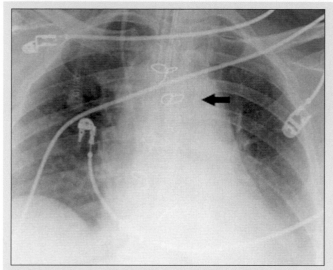

Figure 1. Frontal radiograph in a 71-year-old woman with sternal dehiscence after coronary bypass graft surgery demonstrates misaligned wires with leftward displacement of the second wire from top (*arrow*). (*Courtesy of Dr. Charles S. White, University of Maryland, Baltimore*)

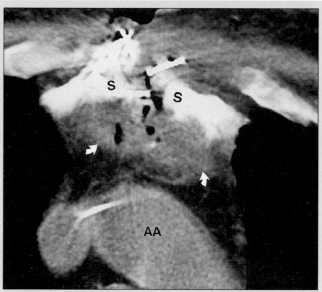

Figure 2. A 64-year-old patient presented with a persistent wound infection 5 weeks after coronary artery bypass surgery. The collection (see Fig. 3) extended cephalad to the level of the aortic arch (AA). Note sternal (S) dehiscence and broken sternal wires. The presence of a retrosternal abscess (*arrows*) was confirmed at surgery. Cultures grew *Staphylococcus aureus*. (*From Müller NL, Fraser RS, Colman NC, Paré PD: Radiologic Diagnosis of Diseases of the Chest. Philadelphia, WB Saunders, 2001.*)

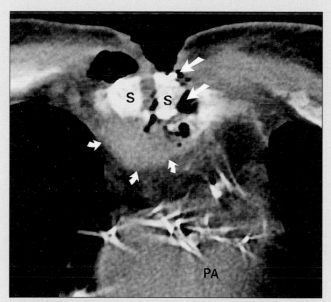

Figure 3. A 64-year-old patient presented with a persistent wound infection 5 weeks after coronary artery bypass surgery. CT scan at the level of the main pulmonary artery (PA) shows a draining sinus (*straight arrows*) communicating with a retrosternal collection (*curved arrows*). The collection extended cephalad to the level of the aortic arch. S, sternal dehiscence. (*From Müller NL, Fraser RS, Colman NC, Paré PD: Radiologic Diagnosis of Diseases of the Chest. Philadelphia, WB Saunders, 2001.*)

Pleural Disease

Spontaneous Pneumothorax

DEFINITION: Spontaneous pneumothorax occurs when air collects in the pleural space without preceding trauma or underlying lung disease.

IMAGING

Radiography

Findings
- Gas in pleural space.
- Thin white visceral pleural line (< 1 mm thick) parallel to chest wall with no lung markings projecting beyond it.
- Absence of lung markings beyond white line of pleura
- Deep sulcus sign: deep radiolucent costophrenic sulcus.
- Apical blebs or bullae may be seen.

Utility
- First and often only imaging modality used in patient assessment.
- Expiratory radiograph or lateral decubitus view may be helpful in demonstrating presence of pneumothorax.
- Supine view is less sensitive than upright radiograph or lateral view in demonstrating presence of pneumothorax.
- Apical bullae or blebs are seen on radiograph in approximately 40% of patients with primary spontaneous pneumothorax.

CT

Findings
- Gas in pleural space
- Thin white visceral pleural line readily seen
- Apical blebs or bullae

Utility
- High-resolution CT is the most reliable method of detecting bleb and bullae in spontaneous pneumothorax.
- Apical bullae or blebs are seen in high-resolution CT in 80% of patients with primary spontaneous pneumothorax.

DIAGNOSTIC PEARLS

- Thin white visceral pleural line
- Absence of lung markings beyond white line of pleura
- Deep sulcus sign on supine radiograph
- Apical blebs or bullae are evident on the radiograph in approximately 40% and on CT in 80% of patients with primary spontaneous pneumothorax

CLINICAL PRESENTATION

- Ipsilateral pleuritic chest pain minimal or severe, with acute dyspnea
- Occurs mostly with patient at rest; resolution of symptoms usually within 24 hours if pneumothorax is small

DIFFERENTIAL DIAGNOSIS

- Secondary pneumothorax
- Large bullae
- Skin fold
- Pneumomediastinum

PATHOLOGY

- Results from rupture of small, thin-walled air-containing spaces within visceral pleura into pleural cavity
- May also occur after pneumomediastinum with air tracking into pleural space; however, cause of primary spontaneous pneumothorax unclear

WHAT THE REFERRING PHYSICIAN NEEDS TO KNOW

- Most air-containing spaces associated with pneumothorax are, in fact, bullae.
- Apical bullae, or blebs, are seen on radiograph in approximately 40% of patients and on high-resolution CT in 80% of patients with spontaneous pneumothorax.
- Large pneumothoraces usually require chest tube drainage; small pneumothoraces may resolve spontaneously.
- Re-expansion pulmonary edema is an uncommon complication occurring in a collapsed lung rapidly re-expanded by air evacuation.

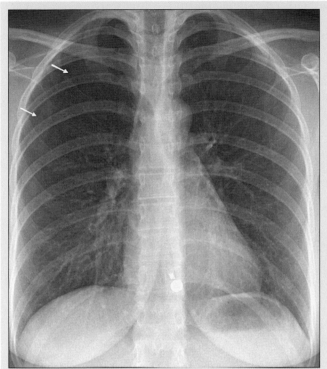

Figure 1. Right spontaneous pneumothorax. Posteroanterior chest radiograph in full inspiration demonstrates a thin white line of the visceral pleura (*arrow*) from a small right pneumothorax. The patient was a 32-year-old woman who was a lifetime nonsmoker. (*Courtesy of Dr. Jean M. Seely, University of Ottawa, Ottawa, Canada*)

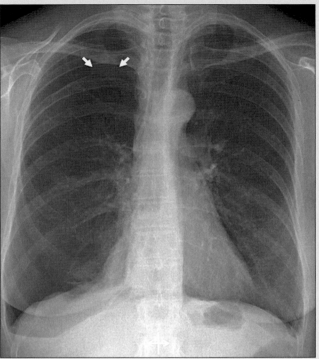

Figure 2. Bulla and right pneumothorax. Posteroanterior chest radiograph in inspiration demonstrates a moderate-sized right pneumothorax with apical bulla (*arrows*) outlined by air within the pleural space. A tiny right pleural effusion is seen in the costophrenic angle. (*Courtesy of Dr. Jean M. Seely, University of Ottawa, Ottawa, Canada*)

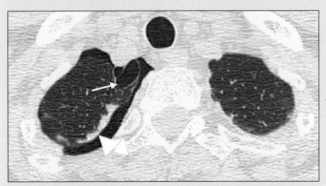

Figure 3. Bulla and right pneumothorax. High-resolution CT of the lung apices in another patient who presented with a recurrent spontaneous right pneumothorax shows a bulla (*thin arrow*) and the pneumothorax displacing thickened, fibrotic visceral pleura (*arrowhead*). (*Courtesy of Dr. Jean M. Seely, University of Ottawa, Ottawa, Canada*)

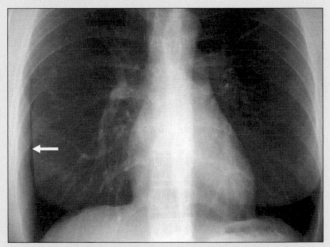

Figure 4. Skinfold. Magnified view from a chest radiograph shows a prominent skinfold (*arrow*) overlying the lower right hemithorax, creating a thick black Mach line, which is distinct from the white visceral pleural line of a pneumothorax. (*Courtesy of Dr. Jean M. Seely, University of Ottawa, Ottawa, Canada*)

INCIDENCE/PREVALENCE AND EPIDEMIOLOGY

- Primary spontaneous pneumothorax typically presents in a male smoker with a tall, thin, and asthenic body habitus.
- It occurs most commonly between 18-40 years of age; male-to-female ratio is 4:1 to 5:1.
- Incidence is 7.4-18.0/100,000 per year for men and 1.2-6.0/100,000 per year for women.
- Smoking is an important risk factor, with lifetime risk of developing pneumothorax 12%; in nonsmoking male it is 0.1%.
- Smoking increases relative risk of contracting first spontaneous pneumothorax approximately 9-fold among women and 22-fold among men.
- Over 10% of patients with primary spontaneous pneumothorax report a family history of the disease.
- Recurrence rates for all spontaneous pneumothoraces are high (30%).

Suggested Readings

Baumann MH: Management of spontaneous pneumothorax. *Clin Chest Med* 27:369-381, 2006.

Bense L, Eklund G, Wiman LG: Smoking and the increased risk of contracting spontaneous pneumothorax. *Chest* 92:1009-1012, 1987.

English JC, Leslie KO: Pathology of the pleura. *Clin Chest Med* 27:157-180, 2006.

Qureshi NR, Gleeson FV: Imaging of pleural disease. *Clin Chest Med* 27:193-213, 2006.

Sahn SA, Heffner JE: Spontaneous pneumothorax. *N Engl J Med* 342:868-874, 2000.

Secondary Pneumothorax

DEFINITION: Secondary pneumothorax is the presence of air in the pleural space due to underlying medical conditions or iatrogenic injury.

IMAGING

Radiography
Findings
- Thin white pleural line parallel to chest wall
- Air identified in pleural space, separating lung from chest wall
- Deep sulcus sign
- Underlying lung disease, including emphysema, interstitial lung disease, or pulmonary laceration

Utility
- Pleural line may be difficult to differentiate from wall of bulla.
- Diagnosis of pneumothorax in patients with cystic lung disease is difficult when relying on plain chest radiography alone.
- One study showed lateral decubitus film was most sensitive, followed by erect radiograph, with least sensitive being supine view.
- If only one chest radiograph is taken, it should be done with the patient upright, in inspiration.
- Potential pitfall: skinfold may mimic pneumothorax (skinfold typically has "black line" due to Mach effect); vessels can be seen beyond skinfold.

CT
Findings
- Air identified in pleural space, separating lung from chest wall
- Subpleural bullae or more extensive emphysema
- Lymphangioleiomyomatosis: thin-walled cysts scattered throughout both lungs
- Langerhans cell histiocytosis: cysts and nodules diffusely in upper and middle lung zones with relative sparing of the lung bases

Utility
- CT more sensitive than chest radiography for distinguishing apical bullae from pneumothorax.
- Diagnosis of interstitial lung disease is made with high-resolution CT.
- CT is useful in managing patients with pneumothorax recurrence, during management of persistent air leak, and planning for surgical intervention.

DIAGNOSTIC PEARLS
- Thin white pleural line parallel to the chest wall
- Deep sulcus sign on supine radiograph
- Evidence of underlying lung disease

Ultrasonography
Findings
- Absence of comet tail artifacts, which are normally seen when visceral and parietal pleura slide over each other with respiration

Utility
- Main advantage: portable and readily done at the bedside
- Superior to the supine chest radiograph in diagnosing pneumothorax
- Lower accuracy than upright chest radiograph or CT

CLINICAL PRESENTATION
- Dyspnea, ipsilateral chest pain
- Hypoxemia or hypotension, which can be life threatening
- Catamenial pneumothorax: shoulder/chest pain within 72 hours of onset of menses

DIFFERENTIAL DIAGNOSIS
- Spontaneous pneumothorax
- Bullae
- Skin fold

PATHOLOGY
- Association with formation of subpleural bullae or cystic spaces is related to emphysema or interstitial fibrosis.
- Rupture of bulla or cyst is considered likely cause of pneumothorax; mechanism of rupture is likely multifactorial.

WHAT THE REFERRING PHYSICIAN NEEDS TO KNOW
- Most common cause of pneumothorax is chronic obstructive pulmonary disease.
- Pneumothorax frequently leads to diagnosis of lymphangioleiomyomatosis in affected patients.
- Catamenial pneumothorax should be considered in women with recurrent pneumothorax; diagnosis is made by eliciting history of shoulder/chest pain within 72 hours of onset of menses.

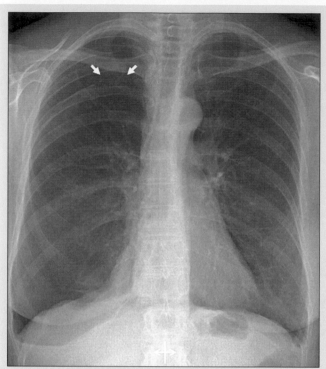

Figure 1. Bulla and right pneumothorax. Posteroanterior chest radiograph in inspiration demonstrates a moderate-sized right pneumothorax with apical bulla (*arrows*) outlined by air within the pleural space. A tiny right pleural effusion is seen in the costophrenic angle. (*Courtesy of Dr. Jean M. Seely, University of Ottawa, Ottawa, Canada*)

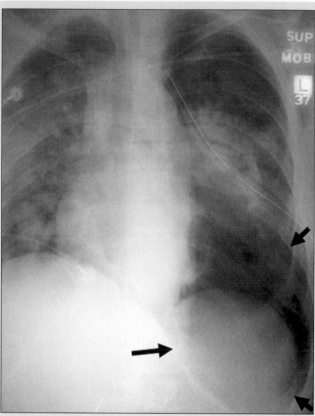

Figure 2. Pneumothorax: deep sulcus sign. Supine chest radiograph demonstrates a large anterior pneumothorax causing the deep sulcus sign (*arrows*). The left-sided chest tube was not functioning. (*Courtesy of Dr. Jean M. Seely, University of Ottawa, Ottawa, Canada*)

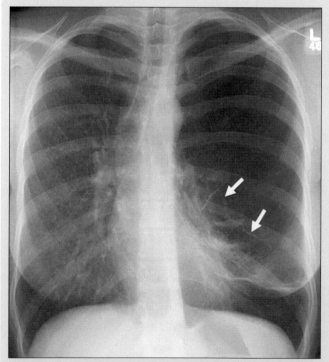

Figure 3. Giant bulla. Posteroanterior chest radiograph shows a hyperlucent left hemithorax. There is a faint white line (*arrows*) that is concave with respect to the chest wall, consistent with a large bulla, not a pneumothorax. (*Courtesy of Dr. Jean M. Seely, University of Ottawa, Ottawa, Canada*)

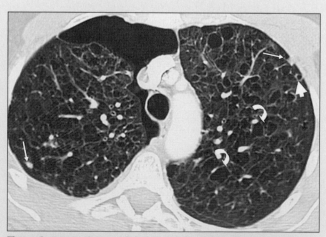

Figure 4. Langerhans cell histiocytosis. High-resolution CT demonstrates right pneumothorax, thin-walled cysts (*curved arrows*), several small nodules (*thin arrows*), and a thin-walled cavitary nodule (*thick arrow*). (*Courtesy of Dr. Jean M. Seely, University of Ottawa, Ottawa, Canada*)

- When alveolar pressure exceeds pressure of lung interstitium, alveolus ruptures and escaped air travels to hilum of ipsilateral lung.
- If rupture occurs at hilum, air moves through mediastinal pleura into pleural space and pneumothorax results (Macklin effect).
- Alternative mechanism is when air from ruptured alveolus moves directly into pleural space, resulting from lung necrosis.

INCIDENCE/PREVALENCE AND EPIDEMIOLOGY

- Annual incidence of secondary spontaneous pneumothorax is 6.3/100,000 population in males and 2.0/100,000 population in females.
- Most common cause of secondary pneumothorax is chronic obstructive pulmonary disease.
- Other common causes are acute respiratory distress syndrome, interstitial pulmonary fibrosis, Langerhans cell histiocytosis, lymphangioleiomyomatosis, chest trauma, *Pneumocystis* pneumonia, and iatrogenic causes (e.g., needle biopsy, bronchial biopsy, surgical procedure).

- In women, who are less commonly affected by secondary pneumothorax, specific causes are catamenial pneumothorax and pneumothorax from lymphangioleiomyomatosis; reported incidence of pneumothorax in women with lymphangioleiomyomatosis is 39%-76%.
- In pulmonary Langerhans cell histiocytosis, pneumothorax precedes or complicates clinical course of 25% of patients.
- Catamenial pneumothorax is uncommon, accounting for 1%-6% of cases of spontaneous pneumothorax.

Suggested Readings

Baumann MH, Strange C, Heffner JE, et al: Management of spontaneous pneumothorax: An American College of Chest Physicians Delphi consensus statement. *Chest* 119:590-602, 2001.

O'Connor AR, Morgan WE: Radiological review of pneumothorax. *BMJ* 330(7506):1493-1497, 2005.

Phillips GD, Trotman-Dickenson B, Hodson ME, Geddes DM: Role of CT in the management of pneumothorax in patients with complex cystic lung disease. *Chest* 112:275-278, 1997.

Tanaka F, Itoh M, Esaki H, et al: Secondary spontaneous pneumothorax. *Ann Thorac Surg* 55:372-376, 1993.

Tension Pneumothorax

DEFINITION: Tension pneumothorax is trapped air within the pleural space with increased intrapleural pressure that remains positive throughout the entire respiratory cycle.

IMAGING

Radiography

Findings
- Large right pneumothorax
- Marked mediastinal shift
- Ipsilateral flattening of heart border
- Hemidiaphragm depression
- Increased rib separation and increased thoracic volume

Utility
- Mild mediastinal shift may occur without tension pneumothorax.
- Chest radiograph is first test for tension pneumothorax in stable patient, but in hemodynamically unstable patient immediate chest decompression should precede chest radiography.
- Lateral costophrenic angles should be included on the radiograph.

CT

Findings
- Large right pneumothorax
- Marked mediastinal shift
- Ipsilateral flattening of heart border
- Hemidiaphragm depression

Utility
- May demonstrate focal tension pneumothorax not apparent on the radiograph.

CLINICAL PRESENTATION

- Sudden pleuritic chest pain, acute dyspnea
- Hemodynamically unstable
- Tachycardia, hypotension, and cyanosis suggestive features
- Hiss of air on thoracic needle decompression

DIFFERENTIAL DIAGNOSIS

- Large pneumothorax without tension
- Large bullae

DIAGNOSTIC PEARLS

- Trapped air within pleural space with hemodynamic compromise or increased intrapleural pressure
- Ipsilateral flattening of heart border, hemidiaphragm depression, and increased rib separation
- Hiss of air on thoracic needle decompression

PATHOLOGY

- Inspired air trapped in pleural space, presumably based on bronchopleural ball-valve mechanism, leading to tension pneumothorax
- Accumulation of intrapleural gas under pressure
- May be associated with considerable shift of the mediastinum and/or depression of the hemidiaphragm

INCIDENCE/PREVALENCE AND EPIDEMIOLOGY

- True clinical tension pneumothorax is an uncommon condition.
- In one series of 3500 autopsies, unsuspected tension pneumothorax was found in 12 cases.
- In a study of 63 major trauma patients, 5.4% were confirmed to have tension pneumothorax.

Suggested Readings

Coats TJ, Wilson AW, Xeropotamous N: Pre-hospital management of patients with severe thoracic injury. *Injury* 26:581-585, 1995.

de Jager CP, Trof RJ: Images in clinical medicine: Gastrothorax simulating acute tension pneumothorax. *N Engl J Med* 351: e5, 2004.

Leigh-Smith S, Harris T: Tension pneumothorax—time for a re-think? *Emerg Med J* 22:8-16, 2005.

Ludwig J, Kienzle GD: Pneumothorax in a large autopsy population: A study of 77 cases. *Am J Clin Pathol* 70:24-26, 1978.

Peatfield RC, Edwards PR, Johnson NM: Two unexpected deaths from pneumothorax. *Lancet* 1:356-358, 1979.

Rutherford RB, Hurt HH Jr, Brickman RD, Tubb JM: The pathophysiology of progressive, tension pneumothorax. *J Trauma* 8:212-227, 1968.

WHAT THE REFERRING PHYSICIAN NEEDS TO KNOW

- Immediate recognition of this complication is essential because affected patients rapidly become severely hypoxic and acidotic and often die.
- If patient is hemodynamically unstable, immediate chest decompression must always precede chest radiography.
- Re-expansion pulmonary edema is an uncommon complication that occurs when collapsed lung is rapidly re-expanded by evacuation of air or fluid.

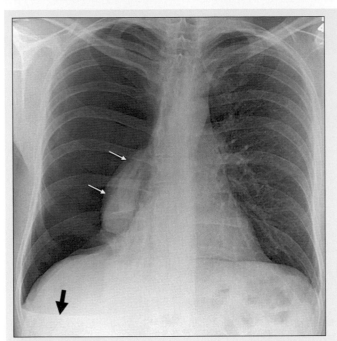

Figure 1. Large right pneumothorax. Posteroanterior chest radiograph in a 45-year-old man with sudden onset of chest pain and mild shortness of breath. The radiograph demonstrates a large right pneumothorax, with mediastinal shift and collapse of the entire right lung. Note the convex margins of the pleura (*white arrows*) outlining the collapsed lung. A small pleural effusion (hydropneumothorax) (*black arrow*) is also present. (*Courtesy of Dr. Jean M. Seely, University of Ottawa, Ottawa, Canada*)

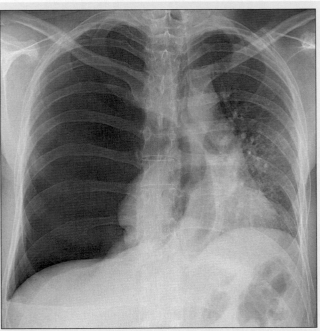

Figure 2. Large right pneumothorax. Expiratory chest radiograph demonstrates marked mediastinal shift, suggesting a tension pneumothorax; however, the patient was hemodynamically stable. A chest tube was placed subsequently. (*Courtesy of Dr. Jean M. Seely, University of Ottawa, Ottawa, Canada*)

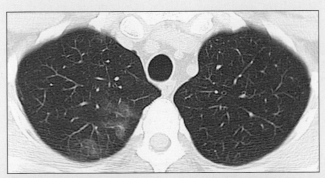

Figure 3. Re-expansion pulmonary edema. CT image at the level of the upper lobes obtained 48 hours after drainage of the right pneumothorax demonstrates patchy ground-glass opacities in the right upper lobe. The patient had increased dyspnea. (*Courtesy of Dr. Jean M. Seely, University of Ottawa, Ottawa, Canada*)

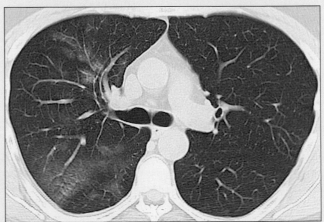

Figure 4. Re-expansion pulmonary edema. More caudad CT than in Figure 3 shows more extensive ground-glass opacification in the right upper and lower lobes, in keeping with re-expansion pulmonary edema. The edema resolved within 24 hours. (*Courtesy of Dr. Jean M. Seely, University of Ottawa, Ottawa, Canada*)

Pleural Effusion

DEFINITION: A pleural effusion is an accumulation of fluid in the pleural space due to disruption of homeostatic forces responsible for the movement of pleural fluid in and out of the space.

IMAGING

Radiography

Findings

- Pleural meniscus (appearance of fluid as homogeneous opacity with concave upper border, higher laterally than medially)
- Accumulation in subpulmonic region causing apparent flattening without significant blunting of costophrenic angles
- With subpulmonic effusion, apex of pseudodiaphragmatic contour more lateral than apex of normal diaphragm in half of cases
- Cap of pleural fluid on apex of lungs on supine view in about 50% of large effusions
- Hazy opacity of one hemithorax
- Loss of sharp silhouette of ipsilateral diaphragm
- Thickening of minor fissure

Utility

- Pleural effusions can be overlooked on supine radiographs or misdiagnosed as pulmonary consolidation.
- Lateral decubitus view is the most sensitive radiographic method for detecting small pleural effusions.

CT

Findings

- Free-flowing pleural effusion produces sickle-shaped opacity in most dependent part of thorax.
- Loculated effusions tend to have lenticular shape with smooth margins and relatively homogeneous attenuation.
- Pleural effusions have attenuation values between those of water (0 Hounsfield units [HU]) and soft tissue (100 HU) and typically are in the range of 10-20 HU.

DIAGNOSTIC PEARLS

- Blunting of costophrenic angle, pleural meniscus, flattening of diaphragm on radiograph
- Sickle-shaped opacity in most dependent part of thorax or lenticular shape with smooth margins, and homogeneous attenuation on CT
- Hypoechoic accumulation with sharp echogenic line that delineates visceral pleura and lung on ultrasonography

- Fluid may occur "outside" diaphragm (diaphragm sign).
- Pleural effusions displace crus anteriorly and laterally away from spine (displaced crus sign).
- There may be an indistinct interface between the pleural effusion and liver (interface sign).
- Fluid behind bare area of liver may be seen (bare area sign).

Utility

- CT is superior to the chest radiograph in detecting pleural effusion and associated parenchymal findings.
- CT scans for pleural effusion should be performed with contrast enhancement because pleural abnormalities will be better visualized.
- Distinction of small pleural effusions from ascites facilitated by four signs: diaphragm sign, displaced crus sign, interface sign, and bare area sign.

MRI

Findings

- Fluid collections in pleural cavity show low signal intensity on T1-weighted images and high signal intensity on T2-weighted images.

WHAT THE REFERRING PHYSICIAN NEEDS TO KNOW

- Pleural exudates have a protein level of >30 g/L and transudates <30 g/L.
- Left-sided heart failure accounts for most transudative pleural effusions; other causes include liver failure, hypoalbuminemia, nephrotic syndrome, constrictive pericarditis, and peritoneal dialysis.
- Pneumonia, malignancy, pulmonary thromboembolism, and connective tissue diseases account for most exudative effusions.
- CT density measurements alone are unreliable in differentiating transudates from exudates and in the diagnosis of chylous pleural effusions.
- Ultrasonography is a reliable method for detecting small pleural effusions and for guiding thoracentesis.
- Ultrasonography also has the added advantage of being portable, allowing bedside imaging with the patient sitting or recumbent.
- PET is often helpful in differentiating benign from malignant pleural effusions in patients with malignant disease, with sensitivity ranging between 88%-100% and specificity of 67%-94%.

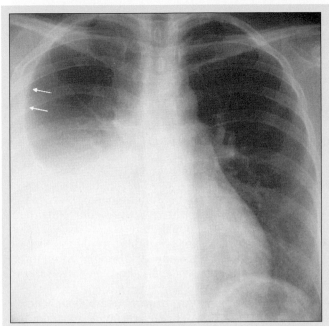

Figure 1. Free pleural effusion. Posteroanterior chest radiograph demonstrates the meniscus sign (*arrows*) in a large free right pleural effusion. (*Courtesy of Dr. Jean M. Seely, University of Ottawa, Ottawa, Canada*)

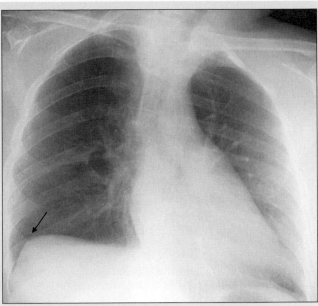

Figure 2. Subpulmonic effusion. Chest radiograph demonstrates that the crest of the pseudodiaphragmatic surface (*arrow*) lies more lateral than the expected location of the apex of an elevated hemidiaphragm. Note the nonvisualization of intrapulmonary blood vessels below the right hemidiaphragm. (*Courtesy of Dr. Jean M. Seely, University of Ottawa, Ottawa, Canada*)

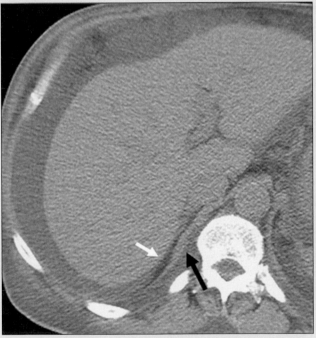

Figure 3. Displaced crus sign in pleural effusion. CT image reveals anterior and lateral displacement of the right diaphragmatic crus by the pleural fluid (*black arrow*) in a patient with bilateral effusions and ascites. Note that ascites does not extend behind the bare area of the liver (*white arrow*). (*Courtesy of Dr. Jean M. Seely, University of Ottawa, Ottawa, Canada*)

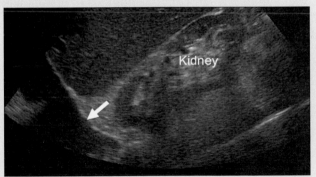

Figure 4. Right pleural effusion. Sagittal image of the right upper quadrant demonstrates an anechoic fluid collection above the right hemidiaphragm consistent with a pleural effusion (*arrow*). (*Courtesy of Dr. Jean M. Seely, University of Ottawa, Ottawa, Canada*)

- Subacute or chronic hemorrhage can be recognized by very high signal intensity on both T1- and T2- weighted images.

Utility

- Limited role in evaluation of pleural effusion

Ultrasonography

Findings

- Most pleural effusions, whether free flowing or loculated, are hypoechoic with sharp echogenic line that delineates visceral pleura and lung.
- Anechoic effusion can be transudate or exudate.
- Complex septated, complex nonseptated, or homogeneously echogenic effusions are always exudates.

Utility

- Reliable method for detecting small pleural effusions and for guiding thoracentesis
- Fibrinous septations better visualized with ultrasound than on CT
- Has added advantage of being portable, allowing bedside imaging with patient sitting or recumbent

Positron Emission Tomography

Findings

- Presence of concomitant pleural abnormalities is most accurate sign for malignancy when assessing nature of pleural effusion.
- Focal increased uptake within posterior portion of fluid is considered highly specific for malignancy.
- Negative PET result confirms absence of pleural metastatic disease.

Utility

- FDG-PET is helpful in differentiating benign from malignant pleural effusions.
- False-positive uptake of FDG by pleura can result from pleural infection or from inflammation after talc pleurodesis.

CLINICAL PRESENTATION

- Clinical presentation depends largely on underlying process.
- Symptoms include dyspnea, cough, and pleuritic chest pain.

DIFFERENTIAL DIAGNOSIS

- Pleural metastases
- Mesothelioma

- Left heart failure
- Pulmonary thromboembolism
- Connective tissue disease
- Pneumonia
- Tuberculosis
- Pulmonary carcinoma

PATHOLOGY

- Transudative effusions are caused by imbalance of hydrostatic and oncotic forces with low protein and low specific gravity.
- Left-sided heart failure accounts for majority of transudative pleural effusions; others include liver failure, hypoalbuminemia, nephrotic syndrome, constrictive pericarditis, and peritoneal dialysis.
- Exudative effusions are secondary to pleural diseases or adjacent lung injury and display high protein and lactate dehydrogenase levels and elevated specific gravity.
- Pneumonia, malignancy, thromboembolism, connective tissue diseases, and drugs account for most exudative effusions.

INCIDENCE/PREVALENCE AND EPIDEMIOLOGY

- About 1 million people develop pleural effusion each year in the United States.
- Pneumonia, malignancy, connective tissue disease, and drugs are the leading causes of exudative effusions.
- Transudative pleural effusions are common in patients with hydrostatic pulmonary edema caused by left-sided heart failure.

Suggested Readings

Andrews CO, Gora ML: Pleural effusions: Pathophysiology and management. *Ann Pharmacother* 28:894-903, 1994.

Light RW: The undiagnosed pleural effusion. *Clin Chest Med* 27:309-319, 2006.

Porcel JM, Light RW: Diagnostic approach to pleural effusion in adults. *Am Fam Physician* 73:1211-1220, 2006.

Qureshi NR, Gleeson FV: Imaging of pleural disease. *Clin Chest Med* 27:193-213, 2006.

Sahn SA: Pleural effusions of extravascular origin. *Clin Chest Med* 27:285-308, 2006.

Tarn AC, Lapworth R: BTS guidelines for investigation of unilateral pleural effusion in adults. *Thorax* 59:358-359, 2004; author reply 359.

Empyema

DEFINITION: An empyema is an accumulation of purulent pleural fluid.

IMAGING

Radiography

Findings
- Pleural effusion
- Loculated pleural effusion: major radiographic hallmark of parapneumonic effusion or empyema; shown by convex contour at upper margin of effusion

Utility
- Detection of pleural fluid affected by patient position, which alters pleural effusion distribution
- Chest radiograph of limited value in distinguishing empyema from other pleural effusions

Ultrasonography

Findings
- Complex septated effusions and regular pleural thickening

Utility
- Reliable method for detecting small pleural effusions and for guiding thoracentesis
- Useful for demonstrating early fibrin membranes and septations in pleural cavity in patients with empyema
- Use of transthoracic ultrasonography alone not effective in making confident distinction between uncomplicated parapneumonic effusion and infected effusion

CT

Findings
- Pleural effusion is present.
- Parietal and visceral pleural enhancement and thickening (split pleura sign) with increased attenuation of extrapleural fat is highly suggestive of an empyema.
- Loculated effusion often has an oval, lentiform shape.
- Presence of gas bubbles in pleural fluid in absence of recent thoracic surgery or drainage is highly suggestive of empyema.

Utility
- Should be performed with contrast enhancement
- Superior to chest radiography for differentiating pleural from parenchymal disease

MRI

Findings
- Demonstrates higher signal intensity on T1-weighted images for infected complex exudates when compared with transudates or simple exudates without malignant cells or infection

DIAGNOSTIC PEARLS
- Loculated pleural effusion: major radiographic hallmark of empyema
- Blunting of costophrenic sulcus, thickening of pleura, and hazy increased opacity
- Split pleura sign and oval, lentiform shape
- Obtuse angle with the adjacent lung
- Displacement of adjacent lung and airways from pleura

Utility
- Limited use in evaluating pleural infection

CLINICAL PRESENTATION
- Symptoms of empyema include fever, dyspnea, cough, pleuritic chest pain, and malaise.
- Pleural fluid usually has positive culture; neutrophils $> 10,000/\mu L$; pH < 7.20; glucose < 35 mg/dL; lactate dehydrogenase > 1000 IU/L.

DIFFERENTIAL DIAGNOSIS
- Chylothorax
- Hemothorax
- Pleural effusion
- Pneumonia
- Lung abscess

PATHOLOGY
- Parapneumonic effusion may be uncomplicated or effusions may be infected, mostly by bacteria.
- Common infecting organisms include *Staphylococcus aureus*, *Streptococcus pneumoniae*, and enteric gram-negative bacilli.
- Tuberculous effusion and empyema usually are due to rupture of subpleural Ghon focus into pleura.
- Empyema necessitatis is extension of empyema through parietal pleura into surrounding tissue and is most commonly seen in chronic empyema due to *Mycobacterium tuberculosis* or *Actinomyces israelii*.

WHAT THE REFERRING PHYSICIAN NEEDS TO KNOW
- Most empyemas occur as a complication of pneumonia or lung abscess, after thoracic surgery, or in association with an intra-abdominal infection.
- Empyema should be suspected in any patient with nonresolving pneumonia on antibiotic therapy.
- Contrast-enhanced CT is imaging modality of choice for assessment of patients with suspected empyema.
- Ultrasonography is a reliable method for detecting small pleural effusions and for guiding thoracentesis.

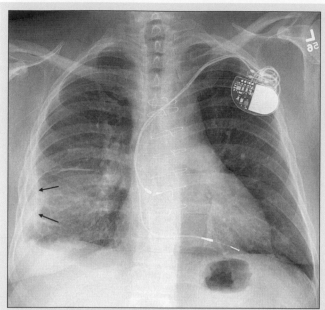

Figure 1. Empyema. Posteroanterior chest radiograph demonstrates blunting of the right costophrenic sulcus and thickening of the pleura laterally (*arrows*). A hazy increased opacity is seen overlying the lower lung suggestive of a loculated effusion. (*Courtesy of Dr. Jean M. Seely, University of Ottawa, Ottawa, Canada*)

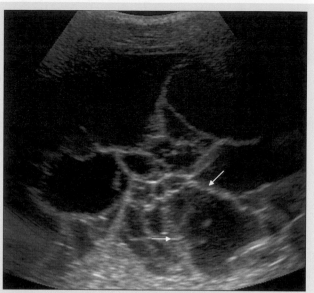

Figure 2. Empyema. Ultrasound image of a large parapneumonic effusion demonstrates thick septations (*arrows*) within the fluid in keeping with an exudate. Frank pus was aspirated during thoracentesis. (*Courtesy of Dr. Jean M. Seely, University of Ottawa, Ottawa, Canada*)

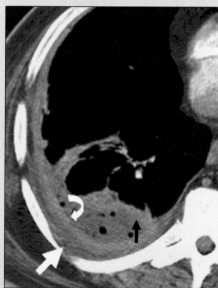

Figure 3. Empyema. Contrast-enhanced chest CT scan demonstrates the loculated fluid collection in the right pleural space containing multiple locules of air. The parietal (*curved arrow*) and visceral pleura (*black arrow*) show enhancement and thickening (split pleura sign). Note the stranding of the extra pleural fat (*large white arrow*), in keeping with an active inflammatory process. (*Courtesy of Dr. Jean M. Seely, University of Ottawa, Ottawa, Canada*)

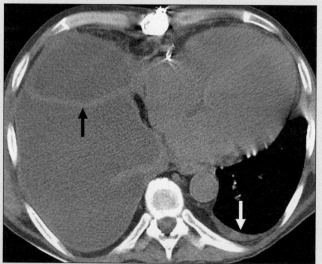

Figure 4. Contarini condition. Nonenhanced CT image illustrates a large loculated right pleural effusion displacing the heart contralaterally. Note the smooth costal pleural thickening and large pleural septation (*black arrow*) consistent with empyema. There is a small left-sided pleural effusion (*white arrow*) secondary to cardiac decompensation, consistent with Contarini condition. (*Courtesy of Dr. Jean M. Seely, University of Ottawa, Ottawa, Canada*)

INCIDENCE/PREVALENCE AND EPIDEMIOLOGY

- Most empyemas occur as a complication of pneumonia or lung abscess, after thoracic surgery, or in association with intra-abdominal infection.
- Empyema is usually due to bacterial infection; most common organisms are *Staphylococcus aureus, Streptococcus pneumoniae*, and enteric gram-negative bacilli.

Suggested Readings

Chae EJ, Seo JB, Kim SY, et al: Radiographic and CT findings of thoracic complications after pneumonectomy. *RadioGraphics* 26:1449-1468, 2006.

Light RW: Parapneumonic effusions and empyema. *Proc Am Thorac Soc* 3:75-80, 2006.

Kearney SE, Davies CW, Davies RJ, Gleeson FV: Computed tomography and ultrasound in parapneumonic effusions and empyema. *Clin Radiol* 55:542-547, 2000.

Kono SA, Nauser TD: Contemporary empyema necessitatis. *Am J Med* 120:303-305, 2007.

Qureshi NR, Gleeson FV: Imaging of pleural disease. *Clin Chest Med* 27:193-213, 2006.

Hemothorax

DEFINITION: Hemothorax is blood in the pleural space secondary to bleeding from systemic or pulmonary vessels.

IMAGING

Radiography

Findings
- Pleural effusion

Utility
- Detection of pleural fluid affected by patient position, which alters pleural effusion distribution
- Lateral decubitus view most sensitive for small pleural effusions

CT

Findings
- If acute, pleural hemorrhage is identified by presence of fluid-fluid level, increased density of pleural fluid, or presence of high-attenuation material.
- When blood in pleural space becomes defibrinated, fluid is radiologically indistinguishable from an effusion of any other cause.

Utility
- Superior to chest radiography for showing presence of pleural effusion and differentiating pleural from parenchymal disease

Ultrasonography

Findings
- Pleural effusion is seen.
- Acute hemothorax is associated with increased echogenicity.

Utility
- Reliable method for detecting small pleural effusions and for guiding thoracentesis
- More sensitive than chest radiography in detecting hemothorax after chest trauma

CLINICAL PRESENTATION

- History and signs of trauma
- Symptoms of dyspnea, cough, chest pain

DIFFERENTIAL DIAGNOSIS

- Chylothorax
- Empyema
- Pleural effusion

DIAGNOSTIC PEARLS

- Diagnosed by presence of fluid-fluid level or increased density of pleural fluid.
- When blood in pleural space becomes defibrinated, hemothorax becomes radiologically indistinguishable from an effusion of any other cause.

PATHOLOGY

- Hemothorax is presence of blood in pleural space secondary to bleeding from systemic or pulmonary vessels.
- Site of hemorrhage can impact the size of hemothorax.
- When bleeding occurs from systemic vessel the hemothorax tends to enlarge despite quantity of blood present.
- When it occurs from pulmonary vasculature, the expanding hemothorax compresses the lung and resultant pulmonary tamponade may produce hemostasis.

INCIDENCE/PREVALENCE AND EPIDEMIOLOGY

- Hemothorax is a common manifestation of both penetrating and nonpenetrating trauma.
- Occasionally, hemothorax may result from excessive anticoagulation, pulmonary infarction, arteriovenous malformation, asbestos-related pleural disease, or malignancy or may occur spontaneously without any apparent cause.
- Rarely, hemothorax may occur in association with endometriosis (catamenial hemothorax).

Suggested Readings

Hope-Gill B, Prathibha BV: Catamenial haemoptysis and clomiphene citrate therapy. *Thorax* 58:89-90, 2003.
McEwan K, Thompson P: Ultrasound to detect haemothorax after chest injury. *Emerg Med J* 24:581-582, 2007.
Meyer DM: Hemothorax related to trauma. *Thorac Surg Clin* 17:47-55, 2007.
Qureshi NR, Gleeson FV: Imaging of pleural disease. *Clin Chest Med* 27:193-213, 2006.
Shanmuganathan K, Matsumoto J: Imaging of penetrating chest trauma. *Radiol Clin North Am* 44:225-238, 2006:viii.

WHAT THE REFERRING PHYSICIAN NEEDS TO KNOW

- Acute hemothorax results in fluid-fluid level, increased attenuation of pleural fluid, or presence of high-attenuation pleural material on CT.
- When blood in the pleural space becomes defibrinated, fluid is radiologically indistinguishable from effusion of any other cause.

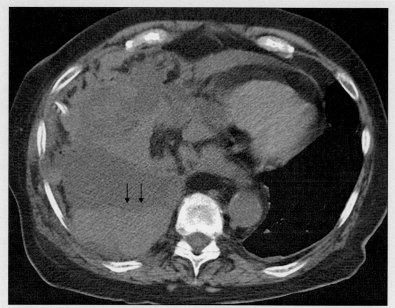

Figure 1. Hemothorax. Nonenhanced CT image demonstrates a multiloculated fluid collection with heterogeneous attenuation in the right pleural space. The effusion shows high density areas and fluid-fluid level (*arrows*), in keeping with a hemothorax. Note also cardiac displacement to the left side and a small pericardial effusion. The patient was the victim of a motor vehicle accident and had numerous right rib fractures superiorly (not shown). (*Courtesy of Dr. Jean M. Seely, University of Ottawa, Ottawa, Canada*)

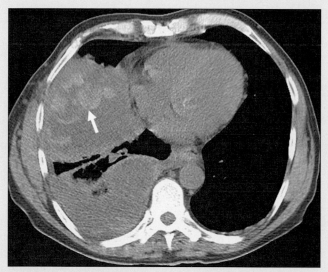

Figure 2. Pleural effusion caused by pulmonary thromboembolism. Nonenhanced CT image demonstrates a large right effusion, containing high-attenuation material (*arrow*) consistent with hemothorax. The patient had been excessively anticoagulated. (*Courtesy of Dr. Jean M. Seely, University of Ottawa, Ottawa, Canada*)

Chylothorax

DEFINITION: Chylothorax is leakage of chyle into the pleural space after obstruction or disruption of the thoracic duct or one of its major divisions.

IMAGING

Radiography
Findings
- Similar to those of pleural effusion of nonchylous etiology

Utility
- Detection of pleural fluid affected by patient position, which alters pleural effusion distribution
- Lateral decubitus view most sensitive for small pleural effusions and can differentiate it from pulmonary infiltrate and guide decision-making for thoracentesis

CT
Findings
- Similar to those of pleural effusion of nonchylous etiology
- Attenuation only occasionally low due to fat content of fluid; usually not low because of high protein content

Utility
- CT scans for pleural effusion should be performed with contrast enhancement.
- CT is superior to chest radiography for differentiating pleural from parenchymal disease.
- CT density measurements are unreliable in diagnosis of chylous pleural effusions.

Ultrasonography
Findings
- Hypoechoic or anechoic effusion

Utility
- More accurate than chest radiography in estimating pleural fluid volume
- Reliable method for detecting small pleural effusions and for guiding thoracentesis

Lymphangiography
Findings
- Leakage of contrast into pleural space on lymphangiography

Utility
- Lymphangiography: imaging modality of choice

DIAGNOSTIC PEARLS
- Presence of chyle in pleural space
- Chylothorax seldom has low attenuation suggestive of the diagnosis
- Leakage of contrast into pleural space on lymphangiography
- Presence of chylomicrons and high triglyceride level (> 1.24 mmol/L)

CLINICAL PRESENTATION
- History and signs of trauma (especially during surgery)
- Dyspnea, cough, chest pain

DIFFERENTIAL DIAGNOSIS
- Empyema
- Hemothorax
- Pleural effusion
- Trauma
- Lymphoma

PATHOLOGY
- Leakage of chyle occurs after disruption or obstruction of thoracic duct or its major divisions.
- Chyle is characteristically a milky, white, opalescent fluid.
- Gross appearance of pleural fluid can be misleading because milky effusions are not always chylous and not all chylous effusions are milky.
- Chylothorax is most commonly due to malignancy (lymphoma), trauma (especially during surgery), tuberculosis, sarcoidosis, and amyloidosis.
- Pseudochylothorax or chyliform effusion results from cholesterol crystal accumulation in chronic pleural effusion with milky appearance; associated with pleurisy.

WHAT THE REFERRING PHYSICIAN NEEDS TO KNOW
- If chylothorax or pseudochylothorax is suspected, pleural fluid should be analyzed for triglyceride/cholesterol levels, cholesterol crystals, and chylomicrons.
- Patients with cancer of middle third of esophagus are at risk for postoperative chylothorax.
- Chylothorax may be differentiated from pseudochylothorax by lipid analysis of fluid.
- CT density measurements alone are unreliable in differentiating transudates from exudates and in diagnosing chylous pleural effusions.
- Lymphangiography is the imaging procedure of choice to demonstrate leakage of contrast into pleural space.

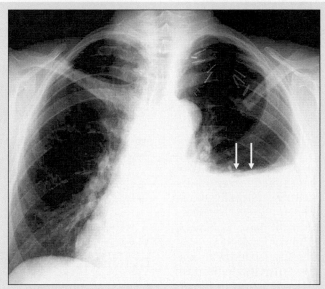

Figure 1. Chylothorax. Portable anteroposterior chest radiograph obtained 3 days after resection of fibrous dysplasia of the first left rib and medial half of the left clavicle demonstrates a moderate-sized left pleural effusion (*arrows*). (*Courtesy of Dr. Jean M. Seely, University of Ottawa, Ottawa, Canada*)

- Pseudochylothorax has no chylomicrons but very high cholesterol content (>5.18 mmol/L); entity has nothing to do with lymphatic vessels or chyle.
- Congenital chylothorax is more often due to malformation of thoracic duct than trauma at birth.

INCIDENCE/PREVALENCE AND EPIDEMIOLOGY

- Chylothorax is uncommon.
- Half of cases of chylothorax are due to malignancy, particularly lymphoma, and 25% are due to trauma usually discovered after surgery.
- Other causes include tuberculosis, sarcoidosis, and amyloidosis.

- It is a well-recognized complication of pleuropulmonary surgeries and the most common congenital pleural effusion (65%).

Suggested Readings

Andrews CO, Gora ML: Pleural effusions: Pathophysiology and management. *Ann Pharmacother* 28:894-903, 1994.

English JC, Leslie KO: Pathology of the pleura. *Clin Chest Med* 27:157-180, 2006.

Maskell NA, Butland RJ: BTS guidelines for the investigation of a unilateral pleural effusion in adults. *Thorax* 58(Suppl 2):i8-i17, 2003.

Nair SK, Petko M, Hayward MP: Aetiology and management of chylothorax in adults. *Eur J Cardiothorac Surg* 32:362-369, 2007.

Platis IE, Nwogu CE: Chylothorax. *Thorac Surg Clin* 16:209-214, 2006.

Qureshi NR, Gleeson FV: Imaging of pleural disease. *Clin Chest Med* 27:193-213, 2006.

Sahn SA: Pleural effusions of extravascular origin. *Clin Chest Med* 27:285-308, 2006.

Benign Pleural Thickening

DEFINITION: Benign pleural thickening is fibrosis of the pleura that may be focal or diffuse.

IMAGING

Radiography
Findings
- Apical cap shows thickening of pleural line over convexity of thorax and sharply marginated lower border that frequently is tented/undulating; normally thickness is < 5 mm.
- Pleural thickening may be focal or diffuse and may be associated with blunting of costophrenic angle.
- Diffuse pleural thickening is often associated with volume loss and may have focal or extensive calcification.
- Chronic fibrothorax occasionally may result in hypertrophy of adjacent ribs.

Utility
- First and often only imaging modality used for assessment

CT
Findings
- Apical cap shows thickening of pleural line over convexity of thorax commonly associated with extrapleural fat that is 3-20 mm thick.
- Apical pneumothorax can outline the apical cap.
- Pleural thickening may be focal or diffuse and may be associated with blunting of costophrenic angle.
- Diffuse thickening on CT is commonly defined as a continuous sheet of pleural thickening > 5 cm wide, > 8 cm in craniocaudal extent, and > 3 mm thick.
- Diffuse benign pleural thickening commonly results in ipsilateral volume loss.
- Diffuse benign pleural thickening commonly involves the costal and paravertebral regions but seldom involves the mediastinal pleura.
- Accumulation of extrapleural fat is commonly present on CT and suggestive of chronic pleural thickening.
- Chronic fibrothorax occasionally may be associated with hypertrophy of adjacent ribs.

Utility
- Superior to chest radiography in evaluating for diffuse pleural thickening and distinguishing benign from malignant pleural thickening

DIAGNOSTIC PEARLS
- Blunting or obliteration of costophrenic sulci
- Continuous pleural thickening of > 5 cm wide, 8 cm in height, 3 mm thick
- Typically located along posterolateral hemithorax
- Seldom involves mediastinal pleura
- Usually is smooth

CLINICAL PRESENTATION
- Often asymptomatic
- May present as dyspnea due to restrictive lung function

DIFFERENTIAL DIAGNOSIS
- Collagen vascular disease
- Previous empyema
- Previous hemothorax
- Previous thoracic surgery
- Asbestos related pleural disease
- Malignant mesothelioma
- Pleural metastases

PATHOLOGY
- Inflammation of pleural cavity is central to pathogenesis of pleural fibrosis.
- Diffuse pleural thickening results from thickening and fibrosis of visceral pleura with fusion to parietal pleura over a wide area.
- In asbestos exposure, diffuse pleural thickening is usually preceded by benign asbestos-related pleural effusion.

INCIDENCE/PREVALENCE AND EPIDEMIOLOGY
- Benign pleural thickening due to fibrosis is the second most common pleural abnormality.
- Most common causes of pleural fibrosis are collagen vascular diseases, asbestos exposure, and drugs, especially

---

WHAT THE REFERRING PHYSICIAN NEEDS TO KNOW
- Extrapleural fat may simulate diffuse pleural thickening on the radiograph.
- Diffuse pleural thickening is associated with significant restriction to lung function.
- Common causes include asbestos exposure, rheumatoid arthritis, hemothorax, tuberculosis, and previous surgery.
- Pleural thickening is almost always preceded by an exudative pleural effusion.

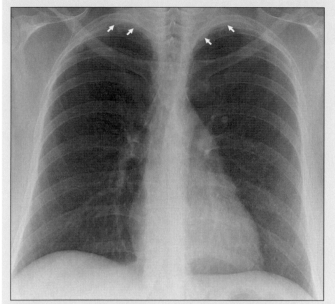

Figure 1. Apical caps. Posteroanterior chest radiograph demonstrates biapical pleural thickening (*arrows*), which has an undulating margin with the lung. This is symmetric bilaterally and measures < 5 mm in height. (*Courtesy of Dr. Jean M. Seely, University of Ottawa, Ottawa, Canada*)

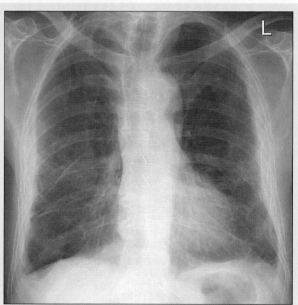

Figure 2. Diffuse pleural thickening. Posteroanterior chest radiograph in an asbestos-exposed male illustrates bilateral diffuse pleural thickening that is more than 50% of each hemithorax, is > 5 mm thick, and obliterates the costophrenic sulci. This meets all the International Labour Organization criteria for bilateral diffuse pleural thickening. (*Courtesy of Dr. Jean M. Seely, University of Ottawa, Ottawa, Canada*)

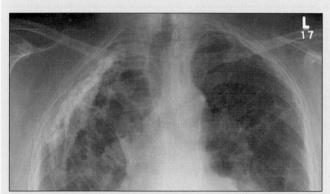

Figure 3. Fibrothorax. View from posteroanterior chest radiograph shows marked right pleural calcification along the upper eight ribs, associated with indrawing of the right ribs and ipsilateral shift of the mediastinum. (*Courtesy of Dr. Jean M. Seely, University of Ottawa, Ottawa, Canada*)

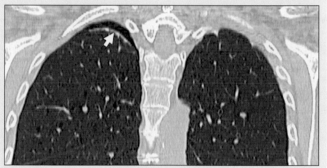

Figure 4. Apical cap and right pneumothorax. Coronal reconstruction of high-resolution CT shows a small right pneumothorax outlining the right apical pleural thickening (*arrow*). (*Courtesy of Dr. Jean M. Seely, University of Ottawa, Ottawa, Canada*)

methysergide, methotrexate, bromocriptine, practolol, and mitomycin.

■ Diffuse pleural fibrosis is caused by asbestos exposure, systemic lupus erythematosus, rheumatoid arthritis, tuberculous pleurisy, hemothorax, uremia, cryptogenic fibrosing pleuritis, drugs, thoracic irradiation, and previous surgery.

■ Prevalence of diffuse pleural thickening is unknown.

■ Diffuse pleural thickening occurs in 9%-22% of asbestos-exposed workers with pleural disease.

Suggested Readings

Huggins JT, Sahn SA: Causes and management of pleural fibrosis. *Respirology* 9:441-447, 2004.

Kim JS, Lynch DA: Imaging of nonmalignant occupational lung disease. *J Thorac Imaging* 17:238-260, 2002.

Qureshi NR, Gleeson FV: Imaging of pleural disease. *Clin Chest Med* 27:193-213, 2006.

Fibrous Tumor of the Pleura

DEFINITION: Fibrous tumor of the pleura is a collagenous tumor that arises from mesenchymal cells and is often solitary and well defined.

IMAGING

Radiography

Findings

- A peripheral solitary, smooth-walled, homogeneous rounded nodule or mass is seen.
- "Incomplete border" sign is when tapering margins form obtuse angles with the chest wall or mediastinum resulting in an ill-defined margin en face.
- When they are in contiguity with the diaphragm, they may simulate diaphragmatic eventration.
- Pedunculated tumors may be mobile, changing in position with respiration or posture.
- Pleural effusions, if large enough, may obscure mass.

Utility

- Main imaging modality used in initial assessment

CT

Findings

- A small tumor is typically a noninvasive, lobular, homogeneous, soft tissue mass that abuts the pleural surface and may form obtuse angles.
- If the tumor is large, areas of necrosis, hemorrhage, and cystic changes are typically identified within it.
- Mass effect on adjacent lung or mediastinum is common.
- Intermediate to high attenuation is seen on unenhanced CT scans.
- Contrast enhancement tends to be intense as a result of the rich vascularization of the tumor.
- Geographic, linear, or focal nonenhancing areas correspond to necrosis, myxoid degeneration, or hemorrhage within the tumor.

Utility

- For further evaluation and characterization of pleural lesion

DIAGNOSTIC PEARLS

- This is a solitary, well-defined, pleural-based lesion; calcification can occur in 25% of cases.
- Small lesions enhance homogeneously whereas large lesions enhance heterogeneously.
- Most are located in the lower hemithorax.
- Clubbing of fingers (hypertrophic osteoarthropathy) can occur in 4%-5% of cases.
- Symptomatic hypoglycemia is present in 4%-5% of cases and is more common in large tumors.

- Cannot differentiate benign from malignant pleural tumors unless there is local invasion of chest wall or diaphragm

MRI

Findings

- Low to intermediate signal intensity on T1- and T2-weighted images
- High heterogeneous T2-weighted signal intensity thought to relate to necrosis, cystic or myxoid degeneration, vascular structures, and high cellularity
- Low signal intensity septa
- Intense heterogeneous enhancement after intravenous injection of gadolinium

Utility

- MRI better characterizes fibrous tumors of pleura.
- Sagittal and coronal images permit tumor localization within chest and assessment of diaphragm.
- With large tumor, MRI is helpful to better define extent and relationship to mediastinum and diaphragm for surgical planning.
- MRI cannot differentiate benign from malignant pleural tumors unless there is local invasion of chest wall or diaphragm.

WHAT THE REFERRING PHYSICIAN NEEDS TO KNOW

- On CT, the differential diagnosis includes sarcomatoid mesothelioma, sarcoma, as well as epithelioid hemangiopericytoma.
- MRI is superior to CT in defining extent of large tumors.
- Histologically, differential diagnosis includes spindle cell carcinoma, spindle cell melanoma, sarcomatoid mesothelioma, and primary and metastatic soft tissue neoplasms.
- Immunohistochemical studies are helpful in excluding these other tumors.
- Four percent to 5% of cases are associated with hypertrophic osteoarthropathy and 4%-5% with symptomatic hypoglycemia.

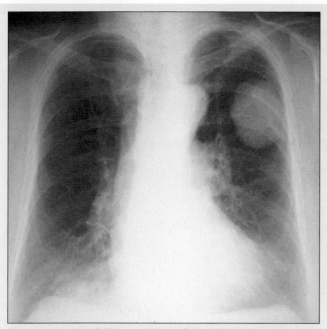

Figure 1. Localized fibrous tumor of the pleura. Posteroanterior chest radiograph demonstrates a large smoothly defined mass in the left upper hemithorax, abutting the pleura laterally. (*Courtesy of Dr. Jean M. Seely, University of Ottawa, Ottawa, Canada*)

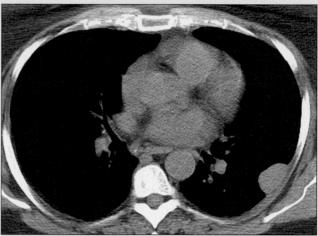

Figure 2. Localized fibrous tumor of the pleura. CT image without contrast depicts a small peripheral lesion that has obtuse angles with the pleura. Core needle biopsy confirmed a fibrous tumor of the pleura. (*Courtesy of Dr. Jean M. Seely, University of Ottawa, Ottawa, Canada*)

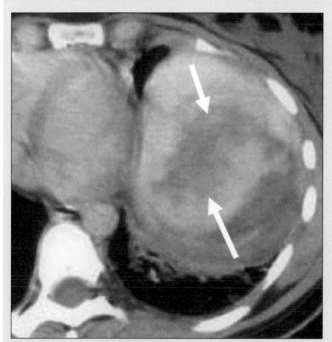

Figure 3. Localized malignant fibrous tumor of the pleura. Contrast-enhanced CT demonstrates a large left-sided mass, displacing the mediastinum contralaterally, which contains "geographic" areas of low attenuation (*arrows*) within a large malignant fibrous tumor of pleura. These areas correspond to necrosis. (*Courtesy of Dr. Jean M. Seely, University of Ottawa, Ottawa, Canada*)

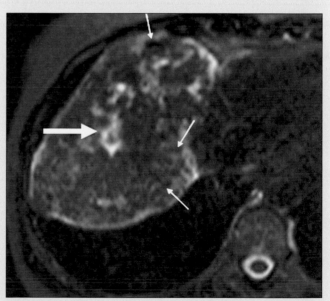

Figure 4. Localized fibrous tumor of the pleura. Cross-sectional MR image shows the tumor to be predominantly of low T2 signal intensity, containing a few high signal areas, which were thought to correspond with high cellularity (*thin arrows*) and necrosis (*thick arrow*). (*Courtesy of Dr. Jean M. Seely, University of Ottawa, Ottawa, Canada*)

CLINICAL PRESENTATION

- Approximately 50% of patients are symptomatic.
- Most frequent symptoms are dyspnea, cough, and chest pain and are present in 40% of patients.
- Clubbing of fingers (hypertrophic osteoarthropathy) occurs in 4%-5% of cases.
- Symptomatic hypoglycemia is present in 4%-5% of cases and more common with malignant tumors.
- Once the tumor is removed, symptoms of osteoarthropathy and hypoglycemia resolve.
- Hemoptysis and obstructive pneumonitis may rarely be observed, owing to airway obstruction.

DIFFERENTIAL DIAGNOSIS

- Malignant mesothelioma
- Pleural lymphoma
- Pleural metastases
- Lung cancer
- Pleural sarcoma

PATHOLOGY

- Tumor arises from mesenchymal cells; it commonly occurs in pleura but has also been described in other sites (e.g., pericardium, mediastinum).
- Etiology is unknown in vast majority of cases, and most tumors are benign, with about 12% being malignant.
- Tumors usually are well circumscribed, with size range from 1-38 cm; most originate in visceral pleura.
- Some fibrous tumors have been associated with the presence of insulin-like growth factor in tumor and serum.
- Tumors appear as low-grade neoplasms of variable cellularity; a "patternless pattern" with random intermingling of tumor cells and collagen is common.
- Sixty-five percent to 80% originate in the visceral pleura and 20%-35% from the parietal pleura.
- Calcification occurs in approximately 25% of cases.

INCIDENCE/PREVALENCE AND EPIDEMIOLOGY

- This relatively uncommon neoplasm accounts for 5%-10% of primary tumors of pleura.
- Prevalence is approximately 2.8 cases per 100,000 population.
- Men and women are equally affected.
- It may occur in all age groups (range: 5-87 years), with peak incidence in the sixth and seventh decades.

Suggested Readings

Bonomo L, Feragalli B, Sacco R, et al: Malignant pleural disease. *Eur J Radiol* 34:98-118, 2000.

Qureshi NR, Gleeson FV: Imaging of pleural disease. *Clin Chest Med* 27:193-213, 2006.

Robinson LA: Solitary fibrous tumor of the pleura. *Cancer Control* 13:264-269, 2006.

Rosado-de-Christenson ML, Abbott GF, McAdams HP, et al: From the archives of the AFIP: Localized fibrous tumor of the pleura. *RadioGraphics* 23:759-783, 2003.

Malignant Mesothelioma

DEFINITION: A malignant mesothelioma is a locally aggressive mesothelial tumor of the pleura that invades the chest wall and surrounding structures.

IMAGING

Radiography

Findings
- Normal in early disease to complete opacification of hemithorax
- Unilateral sheet-like or lobulated pleural thickening encasing entire lung
- Volume loss of affected hemithorax
- Nodular fissural thickening helpful in diagnosing pleural malignant disease
- Rib destruction and pneumothorax occasionally seen
- Unilateral pleural effusion without mediastinal shift or displacement toward or away from affected hemithorax

Utility
- Usually first imaging modality used

CT

Findings
- Unilateral pleural effusion, nodular pleural thickening, thickening of mediastinal pleura, and thickening of interlobar fissure.
- Extensive pleural thickening, which may encase lung with rind-like appearance.
- May start as one or two pleural nodules that later grow in size or number.
- Pleural plaques in 10%-50% of patients.
- Obliteration of extrapleural fat planes, invasion of intercostal muscles, displacement of ribs, or bone destruction seen in some patients.
- Nodular pericardial thickening or pericardial effusion
- Attenuation of pleura increased relative to fluid with strong postcontrast enhancement.

Utility
- CT is imaging modality of choice for evaluating mesothelioma.

DIAGNOSTIC PEARLS

- Mediastinal pleural thickening and nodular and circumferential pleural thickening are suggestive of pleural malignancy on CT.
- Pleural plaques are of limited help in distinguishing mesothelioma from metastatic pleural disease.
- Unilateral pleural effusion may be the only finding.

- Administration of contrast agent enables differentiation between thickened pleura and effusions as well as collapsed lung.
- Contrast-enhanced CT is ideally performed with 60-second delay, enabling optimal pleural and soft tissue enhancement.
- Use of narrow collimation allows for high-quality multiplanar reformatted images, which are helpful in visualizing involvement of interlobar fissure.
- CT helps in differentiation between benign and malignant pleural disease.
- It does not accurately stage local tumor extent.

MRI

Findings
- Relative to adjacent chest wall muscle, mesothelioma is isointense or slightly hyperintense on T1-weighted images.
- It is moderately hyperintense on proton-density–weighted and T2-weighted images.
- It enhances avidly after administration of a gadolinium-based contrast agent.
- Loss of normal fat planes, mediastinal fat extension, and tumoral encasement of >50% mediastinal structure circumference suggest tumor invasion.

WHAT THE REFERRING PHYSICIAN NEEDS TO KNOW

- Suggestive signs of pleural malignancy on CT include mediastinal pleural thickening and nodular and circumferential pleural thickening.
- Diagnostic procedure of choice is thoracoscopic surgery (91%-98% sensitivity) or image-guided needle biopsy as an alternative with high diagnostic accuracy.
- Overall prognosis is poor, which is related to tumor histology, nodal status, tumor stage, age, performance status, and other comorbidities.
- CT, MRI, and PET do not accurately stage local tumor extent; staging is better done surgically, with thoracoscopy, mediastinoscopy, and laparotomy.
- Mesothelioma has propensity to spread along chest tube tract, thoracoscopy trocars, and surgical incisions.
- Diagnostic dilemmas include adenocarcinoma vs. tubopapillary mesothelioma; reactive mesothelial hyperplasia vs. early mesothelioma; and desmoplastic mesothelioma vs. pleuritis vs. pleural plaque.
- Differential diagnosis includes parapneumonic effusion, empyema, and metastatic disease from another primary tumor (most commonly of the lung or breast).

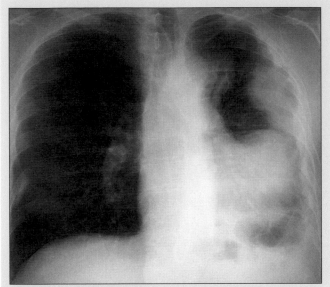

Figure 1. **Mesothelioma.** Chest radiograph demonstrates left nodular and circumferential pleural thickening, with associated volume loss of the left hemithorax, ipsilateral mediastinal shift, and elevation of the hemidiaphragm. (*Courtesy of Dr. Jean M. Seely, University of Ottawa, Ottawa, Canada*)

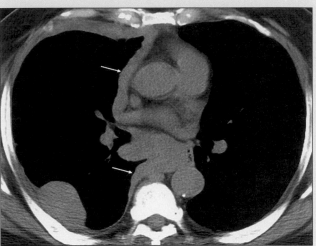

Figure 2. **Mesothelioma.** Nonenhanced CT shows nodular, circumferential, and mediastinal (*arrows*) pleural thickening of right hemithorax, in keeping with biopsy-proven mesothelioma. (*Courtesy of Dr. Jean M. Seely, University of Ottawa, Ottawa, Canada*)

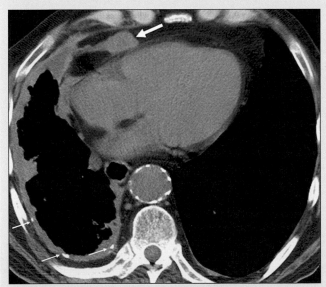

Figure 3. **Mesothelioma.** CT demonstrates circumferential, nodular right pleural thickening, along with contracted right hemithorax. A small pleural effusion is present, distinct from the thickened mediastinal pleura. Calcified pleural plaques (*thin arrows*) are present. Note mediastinal invasion by tumor (*thick arrow*). (*Courtesy of Dr. Jean M. Seely, University of Ottawa, Ottawa, Canada*)

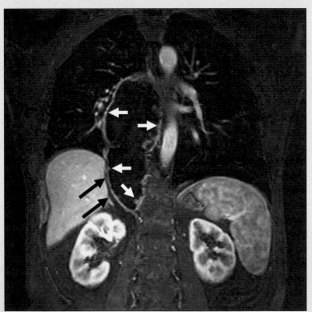

Figure 4. **Epithelial mesothelioma.** Coronal T1-weighted gadolinium-enhanced MR image depicts a loculated pleural effusion surrounded by nodular, enhancing, pleural thickening (*white arrows*) that extends to the right crus of the hemidiaphragm. Preservation of the fat plane between the crus and the liver (*black arrows*) is a helpful sign of lack of invasion by this mesothelioma, which was confirmed at surgery. (*Courtesy of Dr. Jean M. Seely, University of Ottawa, Ottawa, Canada*)

Utility

- Only performed in cases in which contrast-enhanced CT is contraindicated or when CT fails to adequately demonstrate extrapleural infiltration
- Excellent soft tissue contrast and multiplanar image acquisition, permitting ready assessment of chest wall and diaphragmatic invasion
- Can provide additional staging information
- Sensitivities and specificities equivalent to those of CT in differentiating benign and malignant pleural disease

Ultrasonography

Findings

- Pleural effusion
- Intrapleural nodules

Utility

- Useful in identifying pleural pathologic process
- Used for image-guided biopsy with reported accuracy of 80% in diagnosing mesothelioma
- Used for imaged-guided drainage of effusions

Positron Emission Tomography

Findings

- Semi-quantitative measure of metabolic activity of lesion is significantly higher in malignant than in benign pleural diseases.
- Elevated glucose metabolism of tumor cells suggests malignancy.
- Pleural thickening occurs.

Utility

- FDG-PET has been used for diagnosis of mesothelioma.
- Unsuspected distant metastases may be identified, which can preclude unnecessary surgery.
- PET does not accurately stage local tumor extent but has the ability to detect extrathoracic metastases.
- Sensitivity in pleural thickening is 97%, with positive predictive value of 94%.

CLINICAL PRESENTATION

- Most common first symptoms are dyspnea and chest pain, which is often vague, typically nonpleuritic, and may be referred to shoulder.
- Onset is often insidious; as disease progresses the patient may develop dry cough, fever, fatigue, and weight loss.
- Tumor may be asymptomatic, with presence of pleural effusion noted incidentally on physical examination or by chest radiography.
- Physical examination reveals finger clubbing; retraction and dullness on percussion of chest are common.
- Latency period is 35 to 40 years from time of exposure to development of mesothelioma.

DIFFERENTIAL DIAGNOSIS

- Benign pleural effusion
- Pleural metastases
- Pleural lymphoma
- Fibrous tumor of the pleura
- Benign pleural thickening
- Asbestos-related diffuse pleural thickening
- Lung cancer: Adenocarcinoma

PATHOLOGY

- Malignant mesothelioma develops in parietal pleura first, then spreads to visceral pleura, chest wall, mediastinum, diaphragm, and abdomen.
- It is usually due to the carcinogenic effect of asbestos via industrial or environmental exposure and classified into epithelial, sarcomatous, mixed epithelial and sarcomatous mesotheliomas.
- Epithelial forms are composed only of polygonal, rounded, cuboidal, or flattened epithelial cells arranged in papillary formations, sheets, or tubules.
- Sarcomatous mesotheliomas are usually composed of spindle cells, which may be relatively bland or high grade.
- Desmoplastic mesothelioma is a variant of sarcomatous mesothelioma in which malignant cells are embedded in a dense collagenous matrix.
- Mixed epithelial and sarcomatous mesotheliomas can show any combination of patterns seen in either form.

INCIDENCE/PREVALENCE AND EPIDEMIOLOGY

- Incidence has markedly increased in the past few decades in North America, Europe, the United States, Israel, New Zealand, Japan, and Denmark.
- There are 2000-3000 new cases per year reported in the United States.
- These tumors account for an estimated 20 deaths per million males per year in North America and Europe.
- Epithelial type is most common (50%-60%), then sarcomatous (35%) and mixed (15%) forms.
- Both men and women are affected, but overall incidence is much higher in men.
- Mean age at diagnosis is 63 years, with only 2%-5% estimated to appear in childhood or adolescence.
- Sex predominance is largely related to occupational asbestos exposure; at highest risk are plumbers, pipe fitters, and sheet-metal workers.
- Risk increases with prior radiation and chronic inflammation such as tuberculosis; simian virus SV40 association is estimated to account for 10%-20% of mesotheliomas.

Suggested Readings

Bonomo L, Feragalli B, Sacco R, et al: Malignant pleural disease. *Eur J Radiol* 34:98-118, 2000.

British Thoracic Society Standards of Care Committee: BTS statement on malignant mesothelioma in the UK, 2007. *Thorax* 62(Suppl 2): ii1-ii19, 2007.

Pistolesi M, Rusthoven J: Malignant pleural mesothelioma: Update, current management, and newer therapeutic strategies. *Chest* 126:1318-1329, 2004.

Qureshi NR, Gleeson FV: Imaging of pleural disease. *Clin Chest Med* 27:193-213, 2006.

Wang ZJ, Reddy GP, Gotway MB, et al: Malignant pleural mesothelioma: Evaluation with CT, MR imaging, and PET. *RadioGraphics* 24:105-119, 2004.

Yamamuro M, Gerbaudo VH, Gill RR, et al: Morphologic and functional imaging of malignant pleural mesothelioma. *Eur J Radiol* 64:356-366, 2007.

Pleural and Extrapleural Lipoma

DEFINITION: A lipoma is a benign soft tissue neoplasm of pleura that likely arises from submesothelial mesenchymal cells and has characteristic uniform fat density.

IMAGING

Radiography
Findings
- Tends to have tapered margins and form an obtuse angle with the chest wall and to have poorly defined margins when seen en face.

Utility
- Abnormality commonly seen incidentally on chest radiograph
- Limited value in differential diagnosis from other pleural or chest wall tumors

CT
Findings
- Uniform fat density (-50 to -120 Hounsfield units).

Utility
- Allows confident diagnosis of lipoma

MRI
Findings
- Mass with similar intensity to subcutaneous fat.
- Has no enhancement after contrast agent administration.

Utility
- Allows confident diagnosis of lipoma

CLINICAL PRESENTATION
- Usually asymptomatic

DIAGNOSTIC PEARLS
- Tumor with uniform fat density (-50 to -120 Hounsfield units) on CT.
- Smoothly marginated lesion of signal intensity similar to subcutaneuous fat on MR.
- No enhancement after contrast agent administration.

DIFFERENTIAL DIAGNOSIS
- Fibrous tumor of the pleura
- Neurogenic tumor
- Extrapleural fat

PATHOLOGY
- Benign soft tissue neoplasm of pleura that likely arises from submesothelial mesenchymal cells

INCIDENCE/PREVALENCE AND EPIDEMIOLOGY
- Benign lipoma is the most common soft tissue neoplasm of the pleura.

Suggested Reading
Qureshi NR, Gleeson FV: Imaging of pleural disease. *Clin Chest Med* 27:193-213, 2006.

WHAT THE REFERRING PHYSICIAN NEEDS TO KNOW
- Pleural lipomas are benign tumors usually found incidentally on the chest radiograph or CT.
- The CT findings are usually diagnostic.

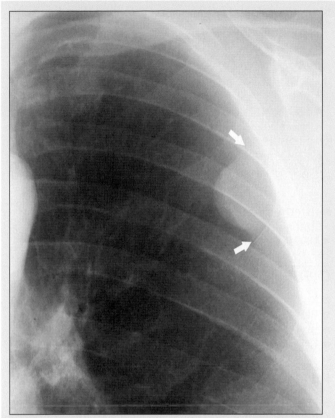

Figure 1. Pleural lipoma. Magnified view of the left upper lobe from a frontal chest radiograph shows a nodular opacity with tapered margins (*arrows*) that forms an obtuse angle with the chest wall. Note that the medial margins of the nodule are well defined, indicating contact with lung, whereas the outer margins are poorly defined, indicating contact with the pleura and chest wall.

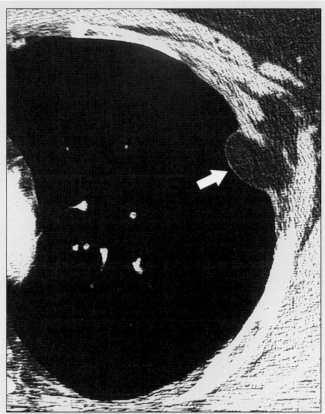

Figure 2. Pleural lipoma. Magnified view from a CT scan shows pleural and chest wall mass with homogeneous fat attenuation characteristic of lipoma (*arrow*). The patient was a 55-year-old man.

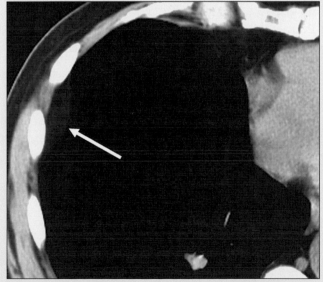

Figure 3. Pleural lipoma. Axial nonenhanced CT shows a pleural-based homogeneous fat attenuation lesion (*arrow*), consistent with a benign pleural lipoma. (*Courtesy of Dr. Jean M. Seely, University of Ottawa, Ottawa, Canada*)

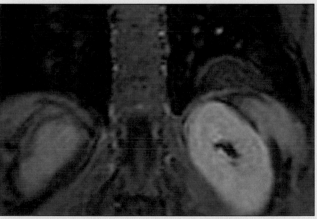

Figure 4. Pleural lipoma. Coronal, fat-saturated, T1-weighted MRI after gadolinium injection shows the lesion to be of low signal (fat suppressed) with no evidence of contrast enhancement. This is consistent with an incidental benign pleural lipoma. (*Courtesy of Dr. Jean M. Seely, University of Ottawa, Ottawa, Canada*)

Pleural Lymphoma

DEFINITION: A pleural lymphoma is a malignant proliferation of lymphocytes involving the pleura.

IMAGING

Radiography
Findings
- Pleural effusion
- Focal or diffuse, smooth or nodular pleural thickening

Utility
- Usually first imaging modality used for assessment

CT
Findings
- Pleural effusion
- Focal or diffuse, smooth or nodular pleural thickening
- Mediastinal and retrocrural lymphadenopathy common

Utility
- CT is superior to radiography in demonstrating pleural effusion and pleural thickening.

MRI
Findings
- Pleural effusion
- Focal or diffuse, smooth or nodular pleural thickening

Utility
- Comparable to CT for assessment of pleural lymphoma but seldom utilized in clinical practice
- Helpful in patients with contraindication to intravenous ionic contrast material

PET
Findings
- Increased uptake of FDG

Utility
- PET and PET/CT can be helpful in distinguishing lymphoma from benign pleural thickening.
- PET is superior to CT in the staging of lymphoma.

CLINICAL PRESENTATION

- Chest pain and fever
- Chest wall swelling

DIAGNOSTIC PEARLS

- Unilateral or bilateral pleural effusion, with or without pleural thickening
- Focal or diffuse or nodular or smooth pleural thickening
- Posterior mediastinal lymphadenopathy
- Pleural involvement usually associated with disseminated disease
- Increased uptake on FDG-PET imaging

- After tumor invasion of spinal cord, paralysis of lower limbs possible presenting feature
- Usually occurs as part of disseminated disease

DIFFERENTIAL DIAGNOSIS

- Malignant mesothelioma
- Pleural metastases
- Benign pleural thickening
- Benign pleural effusion

PATHOLOGY

- Lymphomatous deposits arise from lymphatic channels and lymphoid aggregates in subpleural connective tissue below visceral pleura.
- Pleural involvement occurs in both Hodgkin and non-Hodgkin lymphoma.

INCIDENCE/PREVALENCE AND EPIDEMIOLOGY

- Lymphoma constitutes 10% of secondary pleural tumors.
- Approximately 10% of malignant effusions are caused by pleural lymphoma.
- Prevalence of pleural disease in lymphoma is reported to be 26%-31%.
- Pleural lymphoma occurs in conjunction with mediastinal lymphadenopathy (70%) but may occur as extension of pulmonary lymphoma.

WHAT THE REFERRING PHYSICIAN NEEDS TO KNOW

- Secondary tumors account for about 90% of pleural neoplasms; they include metastases, lymphoma, and uncommon tumors such as thymoma.
- Approximately 80% of all malignant pleural effusions are caused by metastatic tumor from lung, breast, ovary, stomach, or lymphoma.
- Lymphoma constitutes 10% of secondary pleural tumors.
- Approximately 10% of malignant effusions are caused by pleural lymphoma.
- Prevalence of pleural disease in lymphoma is reported to be 26%-31%.
- Pleural lymphoma usually occurs as part of disseminated disease and most commonly in association with mediastinal lymphadenopathy.
- CT and PET are helpful in distinguishing benign from malignant pleural thickening.

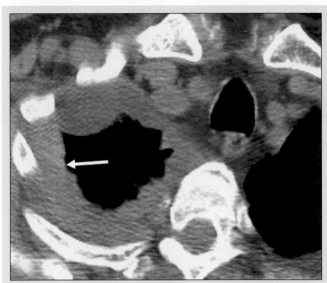

Figure 1. **Lymphoma.** CT image demonstrates thick, nodular, circumferential pleural thickening in the apical right hemithorax (*arrow*). (*Courtesy of Dr. Jean M. Seely, University of Ottawa, Ottawa, Canada*)

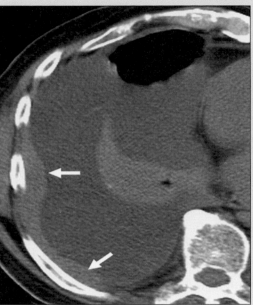

Figure 2. **Lymphoma.** CT image at the level of the lower hemithorax shows more nodular pleural thickening (*arrows*) in association with a large pleural effusion and right lower lobe atelectasis. The patient did not present with adenopathy elsewhere in the body, and biopsy of the pleural thickening was diagnostic for diffuse B-cell lymphoma. (*Courtesy of Dr. Jean M. Seely, University of Ottawa, Ottawa, Canada*)

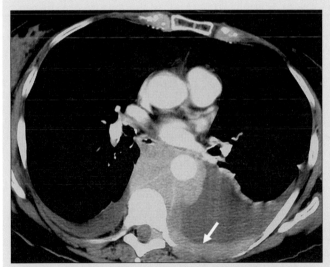

Figure 3. **Lymphoma.** Contrast-enhanced CT demonstrates a large enhancing periaortic mass that is contiguous with a smooth area of parietal pleural thickening (*arrow*) in the left hemithorax. Bilateral pleural effusions are present, typical for pleural involvement with lymphoma. The patient also had extensive retroperitoneal lymphadenopathy (not shown), and biopsy of the retrocrural mass was consistent with diffuse B-cell lymphoma. (*Courtesy of Dr. Jean M. Seely, University of Ottawa, Canada*)

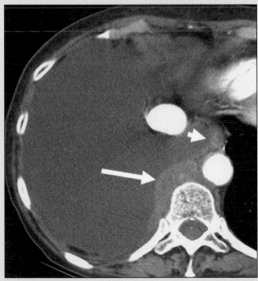

Figure 4. **Non-Hodgkin lymphoma.** Contrast-enhanced CT demonstrates smooth pleural thickening, contiguous with the retrocrural (*long arrow*) and posterior mediastinal lymphadenopathy (*short arrow*). The patient was known to have disseminated B-cell lymphoma. (*Courtesy of Dr. Jean M. Seely, University of Ottawa, Ottawa, Canada*)

Suggested Readings

Bonomo L, Ciccotosto C, Guidotti A, et al: Staging of thoracic lymphoma by radiological imaging. *Eur Radiol* 7:1179-1189, 1997.

Bonomo L, Feragalli B, Sacco R, et al: Malignant pleural disease. *Eur J Radiol* 34:98-118, 2000.

English JC, Leslie KO: Pathology of the pleura. *Clin Chest Med* 27:157-180, 2006.

Qureshi NR, Gleeson FV: Imaging of pleural disease. *Clin Chest Med* 27:193-213, 2006.

Pleural Metastases

DEFINITION: Metastases to the pleura occur most commonly in carcinoma of the lung, breast, ovary, and stomach.

IMAGING

Radiography
Findings
- Pleural effusion
- Focal or diffuse, smooth or nodular pleural thickening

Utility
- Usually first imaging modality
- Limited value in the diagnosis of pleural metastases

CT
Findings
- Pleural effusion
- Mediastinal pleural thickening, nodular pleural thickening, pleural nodule or mass, circumferential pleural thickening, and extension into adjacent soft tissues

Utility
- Superior to radiography in demonstrating pleural effusion and findings suggestive of pleural metastases

Positron Emission Tomography
Findings
- Increased FDG uptake

Utility
- Helpful in distinguishing benign from malignant pleural effusion and thickening

CLINICAL PRESENTATION

- Dyspnea, pleuritic chest pain, weight loss, malaise

DIFFERENTIAL DIAGNOSIS

- Malignant mesothelioma
- Pleural lymphoma
- Benign pleural effusion
- Benign pleural thickening

PATHOLOGY

- Mechanism is most often contiguous spread and invasion of tumor into pulmonary vasculature and lymphatics.
- Invasive thymoma can involve the pleura in a contiguous manner or with "drop metastases."

DIAGNOSTIC PEARLS

- Pleural effusion
- Circumferential pleural thickening
- Nodular pleural thickening
- Malignant pleural effusion shown by increased uptake on FDG-PET
- Bronchogenic carcinoma, breast cancer, lymphoma, and ovarian and gastric carcinoma account for the majority of metastases to the pleura.

- Adenocarcinoma of the lung involves the pleura because of its peripheral nature and its propensity to invade the vasculature.
- Metastatic carcinomas often have elevated levels of carcinoembryonic antigen.

INCIDENCE/PREVALENCE AND EPIDEMIOLOGY

- Approximately 80% of all malignant pleural effusions are caused by metastatic tumor from lung, breast, ovary, stomach, or lymphoma.
- Adenocarcinoma of the lung is most common cell type to involve the pleura.
- Secondary tumors account for about 90% of pleural neoplasms; they include metastases, lymphoma, and uncommon tumors such as thymoma.
- Approximately 25% of pleural effusions in older patients are malignant in origin.
- Most pleural metastases involve visceral pleura.

Suggested Readings

Aquino SL: Imaging of metastatic disease to the thorax. *Radiol Clin North Am* 43:481-495, 2005:vii.
Bonomo L, Feragalli B, Sacco R, et al: Malignant pleural disease. *Eur J Radiol* 34:98-118, 2000.
English JC, Leslie KO: Pathology of the pleura. *Clin Chest Med* 27(2):157-180, 2006.
Qureshi NR, Gleeson FV: Imaging of pleural disease. *Clin Chest Med* 27:193-213, 2006.

WHAT THE REFERRING PHYSICIAN NEEDS TO KNOW

- CT, MRI, and PET are helpful in distinguishing benign from malignant pleural thickening.
- It is often impossible radiologically to differentiate pleural metastases from mesothelioma.

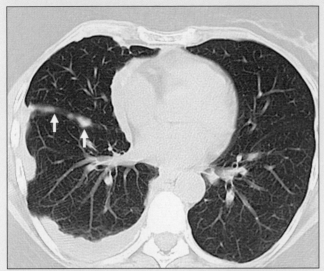

Figure 1. **Metastatic breast carcinoma.** CT image demonstrates nodular pleural thickening that involves the major fissure (*arrows*). The patient had a prior right mastectomy for breast cancer. (*Courtesy of Dr. Jean M. Seely, University of Ottawa, Ottawa, Canada*)

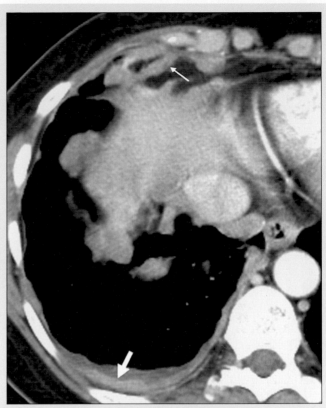

Figure 2. **Metastatic breast carcinoma.** Mediastinal windows show the enhancing parietal pleural thickening (*thick arrow*) and extension of pleural metastases into the anterior cardiophrenic angle (*thin arrow*). (*Courtesy of Dr. Jean M. Seely, University of Ottawa, Ottawa, Canada*)

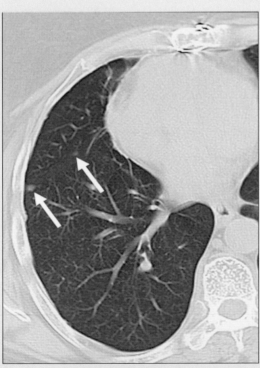

Figure 3. **Thymoma pleural metastases.** CT image shows two pleural nodules (*arrows*) in the major fissure in a man with prior sternotomy for resection of invasive thymoma. (*Courtesy of Dr. Jean M. Seely, University of Ottawa, Ottawa, Canada*)

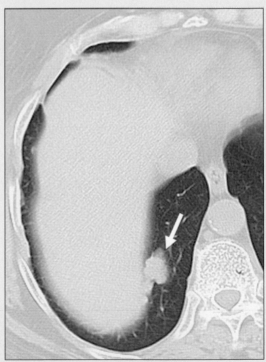

Figure 4. **Thymoma pleural metastases.** CT image at the level of the hemidiaphragm demonstrates a larger "drop metastasis" (*arrow*), which is pleural seeding from a thymoma. (*Courtesy of Dr. Jean M. Seely, University of Ottawa, Ottawa, Canada*)

Mediastinum

Pneumomediastinum

DEFINITION: Pneumomediastinum refers to the presence of air or other gas in the mediastinal space.

IMAGING

Radiography
Findings
- Increase in depth and lucency of retrosternal space in adults
- Gray-black density streaks separating portions of mediastinal pleura from contents
- Focal bubble-like/larger gas collections outlining mediastinal structures
- Vertical streaks of radiolucency adjacent within lateral borders of mediastinal shadow
- Loculated mediastinal air appearing as rounded hyperlucent cystic lesion adjacent/overlying mediastinum
- Continuous diaphragm sign
- V sign of Naclerio, ring-around-the-artery sign, thymic spinnaker-sail sign

Utility
- Often first imaging modality to show presence of pneumomediastinum
- Helpful in initial assessment and follow-up
- Lateral view more useful in showing streak-like areas produced by mediastinal air; may also identify pneumomediastinum not evident on a frontal view

CT
Findings
- Abnormal air collections within the various mediastinal compartments
- Abnormal air collections due to ruptured alveoli associated with acute respiratory distress syndrome/pulmonary fibrosis easily recognized on CT
- Pulmonary laceration in blunt chest trauma
- Periesophageal fluid and air collections suggestive of esophageal rupture

Utility
- Superior to radiography in demonstrating presence of pneumomediastinum and underlying cause

DIAGNOSTIC PEARLS
- Streaks of gray-black density separating portions of mediastinal pleura from mediastinal contents
- Focal bubble-like or larger collections of gas outlining the mediastinal structures
- Rounded hyperlucent paramediastinal lesions (loculated pneumomediastinum)
- Continuous diaphragm sign, V sign of Naclerio, ring-around-the artery sign, thymic spinnaker-sail sign

CLINICAL PRESENTATION
- May be asymptomatic or may present as variable degrees of chest discomfort
- Retrosternal chest pain aggravated by breathing and position changes, dyspnea, shortness of breath, dysphagia, and weakness
- Tension pneumomediastinum: acute diastolic dysfunction, cardiac tamponade, impaired venous return to heart, and airway distortion impeding air flow

DIFFERENTIAL DIAGNOSIS
- Mach effect
- Pneumothorax
- Pneumopericardium

PATHOLOGY
- Three-step pathophysiologic process (Macklin effect): traumatic alveolar rupture, air dissection along bronchovascular sheaths, and spread of pulmonary interstitial emphysema into mediastinum

---

WHAT THE REFERRING PHYSICIAN NEEDS TO KNOW
- Diagnosis of pneumomediastinum is made by chest radiography in most cases.
- Radiographic distinction between pneumomediastinum and pneumopericardium is that pneumopericardium does not extend above aortic arch or into superior mediastinum.
- Clinical correlation is essential and dictates further evaluation and type of examination needed.
- Main conditions to exclude are trauma, mediastinitis, and perforated esophagus.
- Boerhaave syndrome is considered in a patient with history of vomiting followed by chest pain and pneumomediastinum.
- Patients with suspected esophageal perforation require contrast-enhanced swallow testing and esophagoscopy for further evaluation.

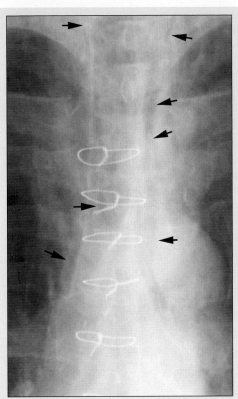

Figure 1. Postsurgical pneumomediastinum. Close-up view from a posteroanterior chest radiograph in a 46-year-old man shows multiple streaks of air outlining the mediastinal structures (*arrows*). (*Courtesy of Dr. Tomás Franquet, Universitat Autónoma de Barcelona, Barcelona, Spain*)

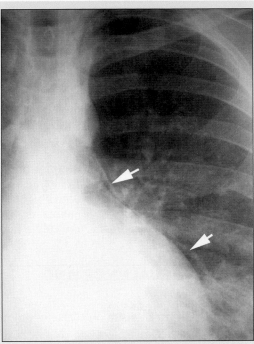

Figure 2. Pneumomediastinum after strenuous exercise. Close-up view of the chest from a posteroanterior chest radiograph in a 21-year-old man shows a long linear opacity along the left-sided heart border (*arrows*). (*Courtesy of Dr. Tomás Franquet, Universitat Autónoma de Barcelona, Barcelona, Spain*)

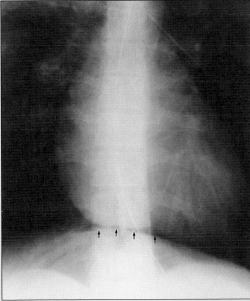

Figure 3. Pneumomediastinum with continuous diaphragm sign. Anteroposterior chest radiograph in a 58-year-old woman shows pneumomediastinum outlining the central portion of the diaphragm (*arrows*), a finding known as the continuous diaphragm sign. The pneumomediastinum was secondary to barotrauma related to mechanical ventilation instituted for adult respiratory distress syndrome. (*From Müller NL, Fraser RS, Colman NC, Paré PD: Radiologic Diagnosis of Diseases of the Chest. Philadelphia, WB Saunders, 2001.*)

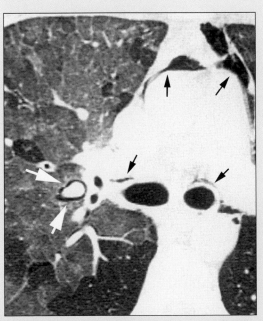

Figure 4. Interstitial emphysema and pneumomediastinum in a young man with AIDS and *Pneumocystis* pneumonia. Close-up view from a CT scan shows gas in the anterior mediastinum and surrounding the main bronchi (*black arrows*). Air is also seen surrounding the intrapulmonary vessels (*white arrows*). Interstitial emphysema leads directly to pneumomediastinum (Macklin effect). (*Courtesy of Dr. Tomás Franquet, Universitat Autónoma de Barcelona, Barcelona, Spain*)

- Alterations in breathing pattern causing spontaneous pneumothorax: asthma, violent coughing, vomiting, athletic competition, seizure, croup, marijuana/crack smoking, pneumonia
- Idiopathic "spontaneous" pneumomediastinum (Hamman syndrome) in patients without history of predisposing cause and normal lung parenchyma
- Mechanical ventilation with positive end-expiratory pressure (tracheostomy, endotracheal intubation) a traumatic source of pneumomediastinum in intensive care unit patients
- Air tracking from neck into mediastinum from surgical procedures involving upper respiratory tract
- Dissection of air into mediastinum after perforation of hollow viscus, ulcerative colitis, sigmoid diverticulitis, pneumatosis cystoides intestinalis, and colon procedures

INCIDENCE/PREVALENCE AND EPIDEMIOLOGY

- Rupture of alveoli most common cause of pneumomediastinum

- Other conditions associated with spontaneous pneumomediastinum: seizures, croup, marijuana/crack cocaine, pneumonia, diabetic ketoacidosis, and diffuse interstitial pulmonary fibrosis
- Mechanical ventilation with positive end-expiratory pressure recognized as traumatic source of pneumomediastinum in intensive care unit patients
- Most common cause of admission of young, healthy individuals experiencing sudden chest pain or shortness of breath
- Pneumomediastinum associated with mediastinitis more commonly due to communication with gastrointestinal tract or respiratory tract/head and neck soft tissue infection

Suggested Readings

Bejvan SM, Godwin JD: Pneumomediastinum: Old signs and new signs. *AJR Am J Roentgenol* 166:1041-1048, 1996.
Zylak CM, Standen JR, Barnes GR, Zylak CJ: Pneumomediastinum revisited. *RadioGraphics* 20:1043-1057, 2000.

Acute Mediastinitis

DEFINITION: Acute mediastinitis is focal or diffuse acute inflammation of tissues located in the middle chest cavity.

IMAGING

Radiography

Findings

- Widening and poor definition of margins of superior mediastinum
- Air may also be seen in soft tissues of neck (subcutaneous emphysema)
- Pneumomediastinum: visualization of pleura as white line adjacent to mediastinum, linear streaks of radiolucency in mediastinum, cervical soft tissues, focal retrosternal air collections, "continuous diaphragm," V sign of Naclerio

Utility

- Main role of imaging in diagnosis of acute mediastinitis is confirmation of mediastinal abnormalities consistent with clinical diagnosis.
- Radiographic finding of widened mediastinum in clinical setting of fever and pleuritic chest pain strongly suggests acute mediastinitis.

CT

Findings

- Soft tissue infiltration of mediastinal fat, obliteration of fat planes, localized fluid collections, mediastinal widening, and lymphadenopathy
- Gas bubbles associated with fluid collections in up to 50% of cases
- Low attenuation areas with rim enhancement after administration of a contrast agent suggestive of abscess formation
- Pericardial effusion, pleural effusion
- Esophageal perforation: esophageal thickening, extraluminal gas, extravasation of oral contrast material, pleural effusion
- Late complications resulting from esophageal perforation: esophagocutaneous, esophagopleural, and esophagobronchial fistulas

DIAGNOSTIC PEARLS

- Esophageal perforation, pleural effusion, pneumomediastinum
- Mediastinal abscess
- Proper clinical setting

Utility

- CT is imaging modality of choice in evaluation of patients with suspected acute mediastinitis and mediastinal abscess.
- Normal post-sternotomy findings are difficult to distinguish from mediastinitis on CT performed within first few days after surgery; CT is most helpful 2 weeks or more after surgery.
- Percutaneous catheter aspiration and drainage of mediastinal fluid collections, under CT guidance, can be useful as diagnostic and therapeutic approach.

Fluoroscopy

Findings

- Extravasation of oral contrast material into mediastinum or into pleural cavity is unequivocal sign of perforation on esophagography.

Utility

- Esophagography is superior to CT in demonstrating esophageal perforation.

CLINICAL PRESENTATION

- Characteristic clinical findings of sudden onset with chills, high fever, tachycardia, tachypnea, and prostration
- Retrosternal pain, worsened by breathing or coughing, common; radiation to the neck and ear possible

---

WHAT THE REFERRING PHYSICIAN NEEDS TO KNOW

- In majority of patients with acute mediastinitis confident diagnosis can be made based on clinical and CT findings.
- Esophagography with water-soluble contrast agent such as Gastrografin or barium is superior to CT in demonstrating esophageal perforation but is not 100% accurate.
- Cross-sectional imaging techniques are generally required for diagnosis and evaluation of site and extent of mediastinal involvement.
- Acute mediastinitis is potentially life-threatening condition that necessitates aggressive medical and surgical intervention.

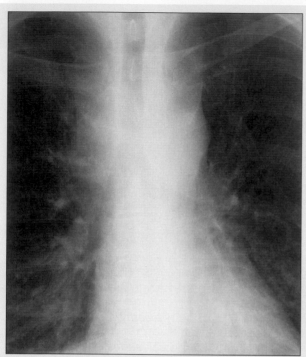

Figure 1. Acute mediastinitis secondary to retropharyngeal abscess. A 47-year-old man presented with acute dysphagia and high fever. Clinical examination showed a retropharyngeal abscess. Close-up view from posteroanterior chest radiograph shows smooth widening of the upper mediastinum. (*From Müller NL, Fraser RS, Colman NC, Paré PD: Radiologic Diagnosis of Diseases of the Chest. Philadelphia, WB Saunders, 2001.*)

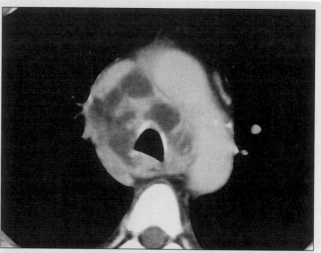

Figure 2. Acute mediastinitis secondary to retropharyngeal abscess. A 47-year-old man presented with acute dysphagia and high fever. Clinical examination showed a retropharyngeal abscess. CT scan at the level of the aortic arch shows localized areas of low attenuation consistent with abscess formation anterior and lateral to the trachea. (*From Müller NL, Fraser RS, Colman NC, Paré PD: Radiologic Diagnosis of Diseases of the Chest. Philadelphia, WB Saunders, 2001.*)

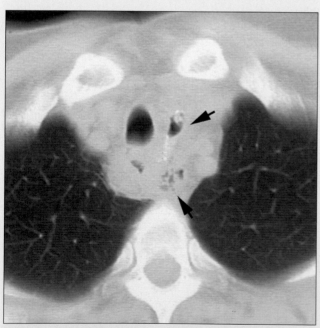

Figure 3. Acute mediastinitis secondary to esophageal perforation in a 54-year-old man. CT scan shows multiple bubbles of air in the superior mediastinum (*arrows*). (*Courtesy of Dr. Tomàs Franquet, Universitat Autànoma de Barcelona, Barcelona, Spain*)

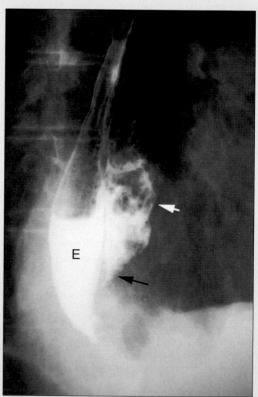

Figure 4. Spontaneous perforation of the esophagus (Boerhaave syndrome) with mediastinal abscess in a 58-year-old man with burning substernal pain. Esophagogram shows a massive leak of barium to the mediastinum (*arrows*). E, esophagus. (*From Giménez A, Franquet T, Erasmus JJ, et al: Thoracic complications of esophageal disorders. RadioGraphics 22:S247-S258, 2002, with permission.*)

- Boerhaave syndrome: esophageal perforation in association with vomiting, chest pain, fever, subcutaneous emphysema, and hematemesis

DIFFERENTIAL DIAGNOSIS

- Aortic dissection
- Acute pulmonary embolism

PATHOLOGY

- Focal or diffuse acute inflammation.
- Esophageal perforation occurs secondary to diagnostic and therapeutic procedures, as well as carcinoma, irradiation, and forceful vomiting.
- Hemorrhagic mediastinitis occurs with inhalational anthrax related to bioterrorism.
- Pancreatitis can extend from retroperitoneum into mediastinum and present as mediastinitis.
- Descending necrotizing mediastinitis is complication of oropharyngeal infections spreading to mediastinum through anatomic fascial planes and cervical spaces.
- Occasionally, osteomyelitis of spine and ribs may lead to mediastinitis.

INCIDENCE/PREVALENCE AND EPIDEMIOLOGY

- One of the most common causes of acute mediastinitis is iatrogenic esophageal perforation during diagnostic or therapeutic endoscopic procedures.
- Boerhaave syndrome affects approximately 1 in 6000 patients.
- Postoperative acute mediastinitis occurs in 0.5%-1.0% of patients who undergo median sternotomy for cardiothoracic surgery.
- Organisms commonly isolated include *Staphylococcus epidermidis* and *Staphylococcus aureus,* various gram-negative organisms, fungi, and atypical mycobacteria.
- Risk of infection is increased with obesity, insulin-dependent diabetes, internal mammary artery grafting (especially bilaterally), and reoperation.

Suggested Readings

Akman C, Kantarci F, Cetinkaya S: Imaging in mediastinitis: A systematic review based on aetiology. *Clin Radiol* 59:573-585, 2004.

Exarhos DN, Malagari K, Tsatalou EG, et al: Acute mediastinitis: Spectrum of computed tomography findings. *Eur Radiol* 15:1569-1574, 2005.

Gimenez A, Franquet T, Erasmus JJ, et al: Thoracic complications of esophageal disorders. *RadioGraphics* 22(Spec No):S247-S258, 2002.

Fibrosing Mediastinitis

DEFINITION: Fibrosing mediastinitis is an excessive fibrotic reaction within the mediastinum usually caused by granulomatous infection.

IMAGING

Radiography
Findings
- Granulomatous infection: localized calcified mass, usually in right paratracheal region
- Widening of mediastinum with distortion and obliteration of normally recognizable mediastinal interfaces or lines
- Superior vena cava obstruction: prominent aortic nipple
- Parenchymal opacities
- Airway narrowing
- Findings of pulmonary venous hypertension: septal thickening and pulmonary edema
- Pleural effusion

Utility
- Usually nonspecific; frequently underestimates the extent of mediastinal disease

CT
Findings
- Increased soft tissue with obliteration of fat planes in mediastinum or large infiltrative mass
- Idiopathic form usually diffuse; post-granulomatous form more commonly focal and mass-like
- Foci of calcification in localized form related to previous granulomatous infection
- Bronchial narrowing
- Obstruction or narrowing of pulmonary artery and superior vena cava.
- Multiple collateral veins
- Enlarged left superior intercostal vein
- Parenchymal opacities: septal lines; pulmonary edema

Utility
- Excellent evaluation of extent of mediastinal soft tissue infiltration and calcification
- Identifies location and degree of narrowing of tracheobronchial tree
- Properly assesses involvement of blood vessels through intravenous contrast and multiplanar reformatted imaging

MRI
Findings
- Typically shows heterogeneous signal intensity on T1- and T2-weighted images

DIAGNOSTIC PEARLS
- Calcified mass, usually in paratracheal region
- Widened mediastinum
- Compression of mediastinal structures, particularly vessels and bronchi

Utility
- Superior to CT in assessment of vascular involvement
- Does not allow confident assessment of calcification, a finding highly suggestive of previous histoplasmosis or tuberculosis

Positron Emission Tomography
Findings
- Preliminary reports suggest that fibrosing mediastinitis often has no uptake on FDG-PET; cases with increased uptake have also been described.

Utility
- Helpful in distinguishing fibrosing mediastinitis from malignancy when CT findings are nonspecific and PET shows no uptake

CLINICAL PRESENTATION
- Involvement of central airways: dyspnea, cough, and hemoptysis
- Recurrent laryngeal nerve involvement: hoarseness; involvement of phrenic nerves: diaphragmatic paralysis; impingement on autonomic nerves/ganglia: Horner syndrome
- Esophageal involvement: dysphagia and chest pain; thoracic duct involvement: chylothorax and chylopericardium
- Superior vena cava syndrome: face or neck swelling, upper extremity swelling, dyspnea, cough
- Pulmonary hypertension, cor pulmonale, refractory right-sided heart failure due to obstruction of pulmonary arteries

DIFFERENTIAL DIAGNOSIS
- Lymphoma
- Pulmonary carcinoma
- Mediastinal lymphadenopathy

WHAT THE REFERRING PHYSICIAN NEEDS TO KNOW
- CT is imaging modality of choice in evaluating presence and extent of mediastinitis.
- Localized mediastinal soft tissue mass with calcification is virtually diagnostic if correlated clinically.
- In noncalcified mass or with evidence of disease progression, biopsy is required to exclude neoplasm.
- Most common causes of chronic (fibrosing) mediastinitis are histoplasmosis and tuberculosis.

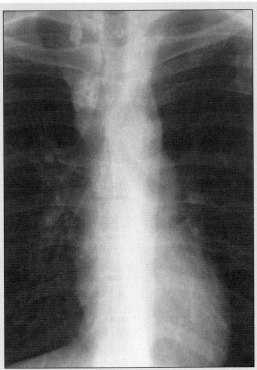

Figure 1. Fibrosing mediastinitis related to histoplasmosis. Close-up view of the chest from posteroanterior radiograph shows enlarged and calcified right paratracheal lymph nodes. The patient presented with superior vena cava syndrome. (*Courtesy of Dr. Robert Tarver, Indiana University Medical Center, Indianapolis, IN. From Müller NL, Fraser RS, Colman NC, Paré PD: Radiologic Diagnosis of Diseases of the Chest. Philadelphia, WB Saunders, 2001.*)

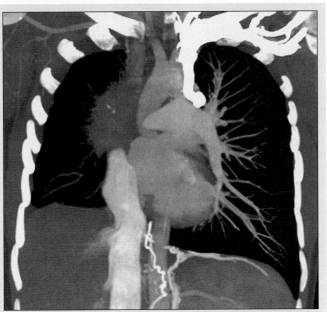

Figure 2. Focal fibrosing mediastinitis due to histoplasmosis in a 37-year-old woman. Coronal maximum intensity projection reformatted image from a multidetector CT scan shows right mediastinal mass and prominent venous collateral circulation. (*Courtesy of Dr. Renata Romano, CDPI, Rio de Janeiro, Brazil.*)

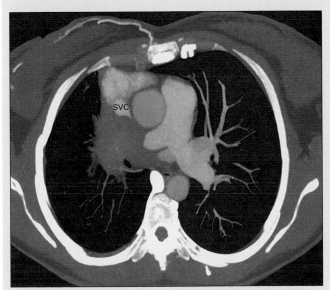

Figure 3. Focal fibrosing mediastinitis due to histoplasmosis in a 37-year-old woman. Axial maximal intensity projection reformatted image demonstrates that the right mediastinal mass obstructs the superior vena cava (SVC) and narrows the bronchus intermedius. (*Courtesy of Dr. Renata Romano, CDPI, Rio de Janeiro, Brazil.*)

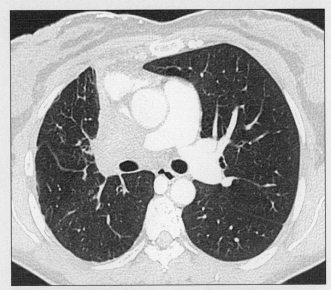

Figure 4. Focal fibrosing mediastinitis due to histoplasmosis in a 37-year-old woman. CT image photographed at lung window shows right upper lobe volume loss and septal lines secondary to pulmonary venous obstruction. The patient had been treated for histoplasmosis 2 years previously. (*Courtesy of Dr. Renata Romano, CDPI, Rio de Janeiro, Brazil.*)

PATHOLOGY

- Benign disorder caused by proliferation of acellular collagen and fibrous tissue within mediastinum obstructing vital structures
- Idiopathic form: tends to be diffuse and not associated with foci of calcification
- Secondary form: necrotizing granulomatous inflammation due to histoplasmosis or tuberculosis that tends to be focal and frequently has foci of dystrophic calcification
- Compression of mediastinal structures
- Narrowing or occlusion of superior vena cava, pulmonary arteries and veins, and major airways

INCIDENCE/PREVALENCE AND EPIDEMIOLOGY

- Rare
- Granulomatous mediastinitis: most cases due to histoplasmosis (especially in North America) or tuberculosis
- Typically affects young adults

Suggested Readings

Akman C, Kantarci F, Cetinkaya S: Imaging in mediastinitis: A systematic review based on aetiology. *Clin Radiol* 59:573-585, 2004.

Atasoy C, Fitoz S, Erguvan B, Akyar S: Tuberculous fibrosing mediastinitis: CT and MRI findings. *J Thorac Imaging* 16:191-193, 2001.

Chong S, Kim TS, Kim BT, Cho EY: Fibrosing mediastinitis mimicking malignancy at CT: Negative FDG uptake in integrated FDG PET/CT imaging. *Eur Radiol* 17:1644-1646, 2007.

Rossi SE, McAdams HP, Rosado-de-Christenson ML, et al: Fibrosing mediastinitis. *RadioGraphics* 21:737-757, 2001.

Takalkar AM, Bruno GL, Makanjoula AJ, et al: A Potential role for F-18 FDG PET/CT in evaluation and management of fibrosing mediastinitis. *Clin Nucl Med* 32:703-706, 2007.

Superior Vena Cava Syndrome

DEFINITION: Superior vena cava syndrome is the name given to the clinical symptoms and signs that occur when there is partial or complete obstruction of the superior vena cava.

IMAGING

Radiography

Findings
- Diffuse mediastinal widening
- Obstruction of the SVC frequently resulting in prominent aortic nipple from dilated left superior intercostal vein
- Enlarged and calcified right paratracheal lymph nodes in fibrosing mediastinitis related to previous histoplasmosis or tuberculosis

Utility
- Often first imaging modality
- Limited value in the diagnosis

CT

Findings
- Narrowing or complete obstruction of the SVC
- Collateral circulation systemic veins
- Paratracheal lymphadenopathy, mass, or calcified nodes

Utility
- Contrast-enhanced CT imaging modality of choice
- Allows assessment of site of obstruction and cause
- Coronal images particularly helpful in assessment of tumor extension into subcarinal region, aortopulmonary window, and SVC

MRI

Findings
- Narrowing or complete obstruction of the SVC
- Collateral circulation systemic veins
- Mediastinal mass

Utility
- Can accurately assess vascular abnormalities
- Allows assessment of vascular abnormalities without ionizing radiation and without intravenous contrast

DIAGNOSTIC PEARLS

- Obstruction of the SVC
- May result from intraluminal thrombosis, neoplastic infiltration, or fibrosing mediastinitis
- The most common cause is bronchogenic carcinoma
- Collateral circulation systemic veins

- Main disadvantages: limited availability and lower spatial resolution than CT
- Recommended in young patients and in follow-up of patients who require repeated examinations

Angiography

Findings
- Marked stenosis or complete obstruction of SVC seen on angiography

Utility
- Angiography useful in selected cases
- Performed before stenting of SVC

CLINICAL PRESENTATION

- Face or neck swelling
- Upper extremity swelling
- Dyspnea
- Cough
- Dilated chest vein collaterals
- Chest pain

PATHOLOGY

- Obstruction of SVC may result from intraluminal thrombosis, neoplastic infiltration, or fibrosing mediastinitis.

WHAT THE REFERRING PHYSICIAN NEEDS TO KNOW

- Contrast-enhanced CT is the imaging modality of choice in the assessment of patients with SVC syndrome.
- Vascular abnormalities can usually be accurately assessed with contrast-enhanced CT or MRI.
- MRI allows assessment of vascular abnormalities without ionizing radiation and without use of an intravenous contrast agent.
- Main disadvantages of MRI are limited availability and lower spatial resolution than CT.
- MRI is particularly recommended in young patients and in follow-up of patients who require repeated examinations.

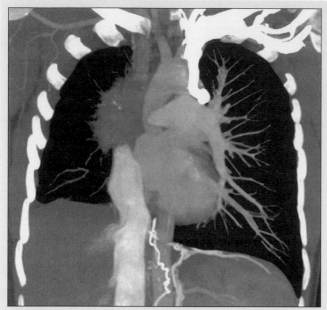

Figure 1. Focal fibrosing mediastinitis due to histoplasmosis in a 37-year-old woman. Coronal maximum intensity projection reformatted image from a multidetector CT scan shows right mediastinal mass and prominent venous collateral circulation. The patient had been treated for histoplasmosis 2 years earlier. (*Courtesy of Dr. Renata Romano, CDPI, Rio de Janeiro, Brazil.*)

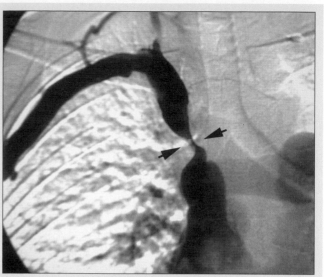

Figure 2. Fibrosing mediastinitis secondary to tuberculosis in a 62-year-old man presenting with SVC syndrome. Angiogram confirms marked stenosis of SVC (*arrows*). (*Courtesy of Dr. Tomás Franquet, Universitant Autónoma de Barcelona, Barcelona, Spain*)

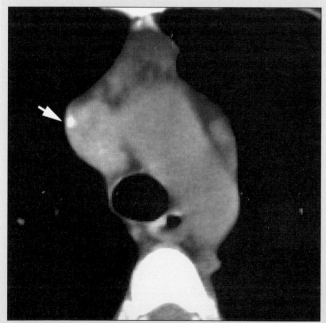

Figure 3. Fibrosing mediastinitis secondary to tuberculosis in a 62-year-old man presenting with SVC syndrome. Nonenhanced CT scan shows a mediastinal mass (*arrow*). Note small punctate calcification adjacent to the mediastinal mass. (*Courtesy of Dr. Tomás Franquet, Universitant Autónoma de Barcelona, Barcelona, Spain*)

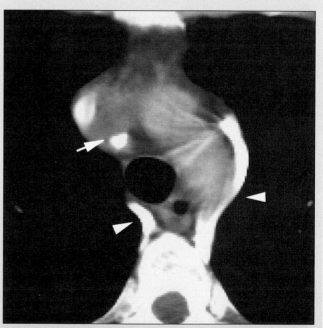

Figure 4. Fibrosing mediastinitis secondary to tuberculosis in a 62-year-old man presenting with SVC syndrome. Contrast-enhanced CT scan at same level as Figure 2 shows displacement and narrowing of the superior vena cava (*arrow*). Note dilation of the azygos and left superior intercostal veins (*arrowheads*). (*Courtesy of Dr. Tomás Franquet, Universitant Autónoma de Barcelona, Barcelona, Spain*)

- Obstruction develops gradually; collateral veins tend to divert much of venous flow.
- Fibrosing mediastinitis is a rare benign disorder; proliferation of acellular collagen and fibrous tissue within mediastinum encases and obstructs vital structures.

INCIDENCE/PREVALENCE AND EPIDEMIOLOGY

- Bronchogenic carcinoma is the most common cause of SVC syndrome (80%-85%).
- Most common benign SVC obstruction causes include fibrosing mediastinitis and iatrogenic causes (e.g., sclerosis, obstruction caused by pacemakers and central venous catheters)

Suggested Readings

Burney K, Young H, Barnard SA, et al: CT appearances of congenital and acquired abnormalities of the superior vena cava. *Clin Radiol* 62:837-842, 2007.

Lawler LP, Corl FM, Fishman EK: Multi-detector row and volume-rendered CT of the normal and accessory flow pathways of the thoracic systemic and pulmonary veins. *RadioGraphics* 22(Spec No):S45-S60, 2002.

Rice TW, Rodriguez RM, Light RW: The superior vena cava syndrome: Clinical characteristics and evolving etiology. *Medicine* (Baltimore): 85:37-42, 2006.

Wilson LD, Detterbeck FC, Yahalom J: Clinical practice: Superior vena cava syndrome with malignant causes. *N Engl J Med* 356:1862-1869, 2007.

Normal Thymus

DEFINITION: The thymus is a normal soft tissue structure in the anterior mediastinum.

IMAGING

CT
Findings
- Bilobed structure with homogeneous soft tissue attenuation in prevascular space, at aortic arch level, or at origin of great vessels
- Fatty infiltration: lobular and speckled appearance
- Two separate lobes (two thirds of patients) or bilobed arrowhead/triangle appearance
- Lobes ovoid, elliptical, triangular, or semilunar
- Thymic lobe thickness measured perpendicular to longest axis of gland
- Left lobe slightly larger than right
- Maximal normal thickness: <20 years old, 18 mm; > 20 years old, 13 mm

Utility
- Most common imaging modality for assessment of normal and abnormal thymus in adults

MRI
Findings
- Same shape and location as on CT
- Homogeneous signal greater than muscle but less than fat on both T1- and T2-weighted images in patients <19 years of age
- Fatty infiltration in older patients
- On chemical shift imaging, homogeneously decreased signal intensity on opposed-phase images due to diffuse fatty infiltration

Utility
- Imaging modality of choice to assess thymus in children and young adults
- Thickness values slightly greater than in CT (15-20 mm for age 20-70 years)

CLINICAL PRESENTATION

- Asymptomatic

DIFFERENTIAL DIAGNOSIS

- Thymic hyperplasia
- Thymoma

DIAGNOSTIC PEARLS

- Bilobed or triangular anterior mediastinal structure
- Homogeneous soft tissue attenuation
- Fatty infiltration in older patients

- Thymic carcinoma
- Thymic carcinoid

PATHOLOGY

- Normal thymus.
- The thymus arises bilaterally from the third and fourth branchial pouches, which contain elements from all three germinal layers.
- By the 8th embryonic week, thymic primordia have migrated caudad, fused in midline, and reached their final position within the anterosuperior mediastinum.
- After birth, the thymus is a bilobed, triangular gland that occupies the thyropericardiac space of the anterior mediastinum and extends caudad.

INCIDENCE/PREVALENCE AND EPIDEMIOLOGY

- Normal thymus is well seen on CT and MRI.

Suggested Readings

Baron RL, Lee JK, Sagel SS, Peterson RR: Computed tomography of the normal thymus. *Radiology* 142:121-125, 1982.
Bogot NR, Quint LE: Imaging of thymic disorders. *Cancer Imaging* 5:139-149, 2005.
De Geer G, Webb WR, Gamsu G: Normal thymus: Assessment with MR and CT. *Radiology* 158:313-317, 1986.
Mendelson DS: Imaging of the thymus. *Chest Surg Clin North Am* 11:269-293, 2001.
Siegel MJ, Glazer HS, Wiener JI, Molina PL: Normal and abnormal thymus in childhood: MR imaging. *Radiology* 172:367-371, 1989.

WHAT THE REFERRING PHYSICIAN NEEDS TO KNOW

- CT is most important imaging modality in assessing anterior mediastinal masses.
- Because of the lack of radiation exposure, MRI is recommended over CT in children and young adults.

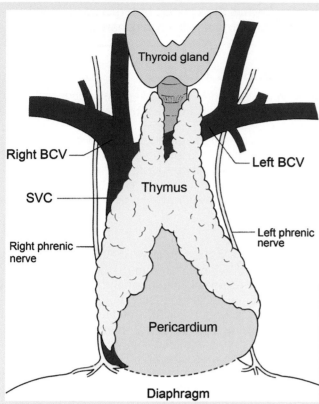

Figure 1. Schematic drawing of normal thymus. BCV, brachiocephalic vein; SVC, superior vena cava. (*Modified by Dr. C. Isabela S. Silva.*)

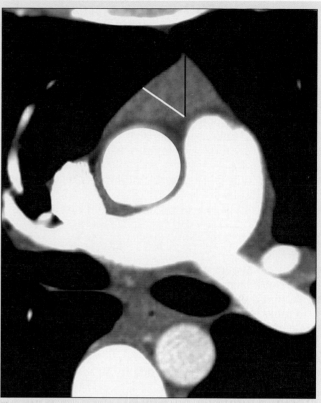

Figure 2. Measurement of thymic size. The thymus typically has a triangular or arrowhead shape. For measurement purposes, the thymus is divided in half by a line through the anterior apex of the gland and perpendicular to it (*black line*). The thickness of each thymic lobe corresponds to the short-axis diameter of the lobe (*white line*). The maximal normal thickness of the thymus is 1.8 cm in patients younger than the age of 20 and 1.3 cm in older patients.

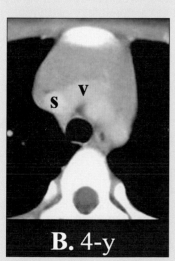

Figure 3. Variations (age-related change) in size, shape, and attenuation of the normal thymus on CT. Four-year-old boy. Right lobe: thickness = 1.7 cm; left lobe: thickness = 1.9 cm. s, superior vena cava; v, brachiocephalic vein. (*Courtesy of Dr. Kiminori Fujimoto, Kurume, Fukuoka, Japan*)

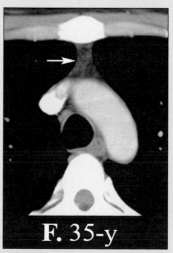

Figure 4. Variations (age-related change) in size, shape, and attenuation of the normal thymus on CT. A 35-year-old man. Fatty infiltration within triangular thymus (*arrow*). Right lobe: thickness = 0.6 cm; left lobe: thickness = 0.7 cm. (*Courtesy of Dr. Kiminori Fujimoto, Kurume, Fukuoka, Japan*)

Thymic Hyperplasia

DEFINITION: Thymic hyperplasia can involve the entire thymus (true thymic hyperplasia, rebound hyperplasia) or be limited to the lymphoid germinal centers (thymic lymphoid hyperplasia).

IMAGING

Radiography
Findings
- True thymic hyperplasia or rebound hyperplasia: generalized increase in thymic size
- Lymphoid hyperplasia: thymus usually normal in size

Utility
- Rebound hyperplasia more evident on CT or MRI than on radiography
- Lymphoid hyperplasia seldom evident on radiography

CT
Findings
- Rebound hyperplasia: initial thymic atrophy followed by generalized enlargement on serial studies
- Lymphoid hyperplasia: normal or diffusely enlarged thymus, less commonly focal mass
- Maximal normal thickness of thymus on CT is: < 20 years old, 18 mm; > 20 years old, 13 mm

Utility
- Most important imaging modality in assessing anterior mediastinal masses
- Limited value in thymic lymphoid hyperplasia, usually showing a normal appearing thymus.
- Increase in thymus volume more readily evident on CT or MRI than on radiography
- Maximal normal thymus thickness on CT: < 20 years, 18 mm; > 20 years, 13 mm

MRI
Findings
- Lymphoid hyperplasia: normal or diffusely enlarged thymus, less commonly a focal mass.
- Lymphoid hyperplasia: soft tissue with heterogeneous low signal intensity slightly greater than muscle but less than fat.
- On chemical shift imaging, lymphoid hyperplasia shown as homogeneously decreased signal intensity on opposed-phase images due to diffuse fatty infiltration.
- Signal changes between in-phase and opposed-phase images strongly suggest that lesion contains adipose tissue, consistent with thymic hyperplasia.

Utility
- Standard MRI is of limited value in diagnosis of lymphoid hyperplasia; lesion may be indistinguishable from thymoma.

DIAGNOSTIC PEARLS
- Thymic rebound hyperplasia: generalized increase in size of thymus after atrophy caused by corticosteroids or chemotherapy.
- Thymic lymphoid hyperplasia is most commonly associated with myasthenia gravis.
- Thymic lymphoid hyperplasia may be present in a normal-sized thymus or, less commonly, manifest as diffuse thymic enlargement or a focal mass.

- Chemical shift MRI is potentially helpful in distinguishing lymphoid hyperplasia from thymoma.
- Lymphoid hyperplasia and normal thymus show same findings on chemical shift imaging.
- Thymus thickness is slightly greater on MRI (15-20 mm between ages 20-70 years) than on CT.
- Increase in thymus volume is more readily evident on CT or MRI than on radiography.

Positron Emission Tomography
Utility
- Cannot easily differentiate between thymic hyperplasia and thymic involvement by malignancy because thymus demonstrates normal physiologic uptake

SPECT
Findings
- At 15 minutes after administration of thallium-201, lymphoid hyperplasia has less intense uptake than thymoma.
- At 180 minutes after thallium-201 imaging, lymphoid hyperplasia has same uptake as thymoma but less than normal.

Utility
- Potentially helpful in distinguishing lymphoid hyperplasia from thymoma.
- In difficult cases, findings should be correlated with those of CT or MRI.

CLINICAL PRESENTATION
- Anterior mediastinal mass
- Asymptomatic
- Rebound hyperplasia: occurs several months after resolution of cause of atrophy

---

WHAT THE REFERRING PHYSICIAN NEEDS TO KNOW
- CT is the most important imaging modality in assessing anterior mediastinal masses.
- CT and MRI are of limited value in the diagnosis of thymic lymphoid hyperplasia.

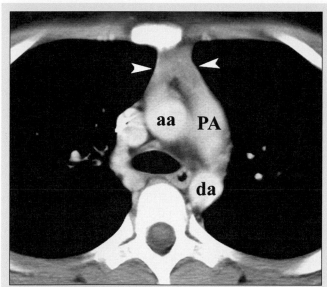

Figure 1. Thymic "rebound" hyperplasia. Contrast-enhanced CT scan in an 11-year old boy with pulmonary metastasis (not shown) from retroperitoneal neuroblastoma demonstrates the normal thymus (*arrowheads*) before chemotherapy. PA, pulmonary artery; aa, ascending aorta; da, descending aorta. The patient underwent successful chemotherapy. (*Courtesy of Dr. Kiminori Fujimoto, Kurume, Fukuoka, Japan*)

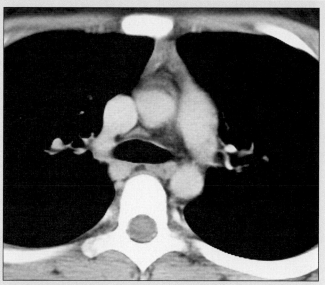

Figure 2. Thymic atrophy. CT scan performed 4 months after completion of chemotherapy in same patient as in Figure 1 shows decrease in the thymic volume (atrophic change). (*Courtesy of Dr. Kiminori Fujimoto, Kurume, Fukuoka, Japan*)

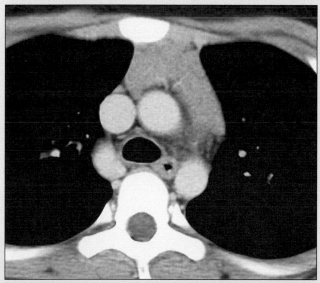

Figure 3. Thymic "rebound" hyperplasia. CT scan performed 1 year after the initial scan (see Fig.1) demonstrates increase in thymic size with homogeneous attenuation, representing "rebound" thymic hyperplasia. There was no evidence of tumor recurrence. (*Courtesy of Dr. Kiminori Fujimoto, Kurume, Fukuoka, Japan*)

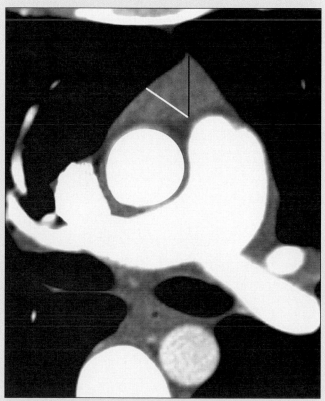

Figure 4. Measurement of thymic size. The thymus typically has a triangular or arrowhead shape. For measurement purposes, the thymus is divided in half by a line through the anterior apex of the gland and perpendicular to it (*black line*). The thickness of each thymic lobe corresponds to the short-axis diameter of the lobe (*white line*). The maximal normal thickness of the thymus is 1.8 cm in patients younger than the age of 20 and 1.3 cm in older patients.

- Lymphoid hyperplasia: usually associated with myasthenia gravis and other immunologically mediated disease

DIFFERENTIAL DIAGNOSIS

- Normal thymus
- Thymic hyperplasia
- Thymoma

PATHOLOGY

- Rebound hyperplasia is an increase in thymic size after atrophy caused by corticosteroids or chemotherapy.
- Lymphoid hyperplasia is hyperplasia of germinal centers.
- Thymus usually involutes during periods of stress and slowly returns to its premorbid size after stress resolution.
- True thymus hyperplasia is known as thymic hyperplasia or thymic rebound, and hyperplasia limited to thymic medulla lymphoid germinal center is referred to as lymphoid hyperplasia.
- Thymic hyperplasia is an increase in thymus size and weight beyond normal upper limit for patient's age but normal appearance of the gland.
- Thymic hyperplasia typically occurs as rebound phenomenon after atrophy caused by some recent stress (e.g., chemotherapy, radiotherapy).

INCIDENCE/PREVALENCE AND EPIDEMIOLOGY

- Rebound hyperplasia occurs in 12%-25% of patients after chemotherapy.
- Lymphoid hyperplasia is most commonly associated with myasthenia gravis, being seen in 60%-80% of cases.
- Lymphoid hyperplasia is associated with systemic lupus erythematosus, rheumatoid arthritis, scleroderma, thyrotoxicosis, and Graves disease.
- True thymic hyperplasia has no gender predominance; lymphoid hyperplasia has male predominance.
- Mean age at occurrence for true thymic hyperplasia is 20 years old; for lymphoid hyperplasia it is 40 years old.

Suggested Readings

de Kraker M, Kluin J, Renken N, et al: CT and myasthenia gravis: Correlation between mediastinal imaging and histopathological findings. *Interact Cardiovasc Thorac Surg* 4:267-271, 2005.

Higuchi T, Taki J, Kinuya S, et al: Thymic lesions in patients with myasthenia gravis: Characterization with thallium 201 scintigraphy. *Radiology* 221:201-206, 2001.

Inaoka T, Takahashi K, Mineta M, et al: Thymic hyperplasia and thymus gland tumors: Differentiation with chemical shift MR imaging. *Radiology* 243:869-876, 2007.

Kissin CM, Husband JE, Nicholas D, Eversman W: Benign thymic enlargement in adults after chemotherapy: CT demonstration. *Radiology* 163:67-70, 1987.

Nicolaou S, Müller NL, Li DKB, Oger JJF: Thymus in myasthenia gravis: Comparison CT and pathologic findings and clinical outcome after thymectomy. *Radiology* 201:471-474, 1996.

Takahashi K, Inaoka T, Murakami N, et al: Characterization of the normal and hyperplastic thymus on chemical-shift MR imaging. *AJR Am J Roentgenol* 180:1265-1269, 2003.

Thymic Carcinoid

DEFINITION: A thymic carcinoid is a malignant neuroendocrine tumor of the thymus.

IMAGING

Radiography
Findings
- Well-circumscribed or ill-defined anterior mediastinal mass

Utility
- Chest radiograph initial imaging modality for evaluation of paraneoplastic syndromes

CT
Findings
- Heterogeneous well-circumscribed or ill-defined anterior mediastinal mass
- Frequently contains areas of necrosis
- May contain cystic areas or calcification
- Heterogeneous contrast enhancement
- May have evidence of lymphadenopathy and vascular or pleural involvement

Utility
- Superior to radiography for diagnosis and assessment of extent
- Superior to MRI in demonstrating calcifications
- Used to rule out carcinoid in patients presenting with Cushing syndrome
- Used to distinguish low-grade tumors from aggressive tumors and thymic carcinoma

MRI
Findings
- Ill-defined or well-circumscribed mass of mixed signal intensity
- Characteristically bright on T2-weighted images
- Focal areas of hemorrhage or necrosis
- Heterogeneous contrast enhancement
- May have evidence of lymphadenopathy, vascular invasion, or metastases

Utility
- Superior to CT in assessment of tumor capsule, intratumoral fibrous septa, and hemorrhage
- Used to distinguish low-grade tumors from aggressive tumors and thymic carcinoma

DIAGNOSTIC PEARLS
- Ill-defined, heterogeneously enhancing anterior mediastinal mass
- Characteristic high T2 signal
- Heterogeneous uptake with standardized uptake value on FDG-PET > 5.0
- May be associated with Cushing syndrome or, occasionally, carcinoid syndrome

Positron Emission Tomography
Findings
- Heterogeneous uptake with standardized uptake value > 5.0

Utility
- FDG-PET helpful in differential diagnosis of thymic masses
- Integrate with CT findings to improve depiction of tumor and nodal metastases

CLINICAL PRESENTATION
- Chest pain, cough, dyspnea, superior vena cava syndrome
- Occasional clubbing and hypertrophic osteoarthropathy
- Most frequent paraneoplastic syndrome: Cushing syndrome
- Carcinoid syndrome rare (< 1%)

DIFFERENTIAL DIAGNOSIS
- Thymoma
- Germ cell tumor
- Thymic carcinoma
- Lymphoma

PATHOLOGY
- Thymic epithelial tumors predominantly composed of neuroendocrine cells

---

WHAT THE REFERRING PHYSICIAN NEEDS TO KNOW
- Anterior mediastinal carcinoid tumors may result in Cushing syndrome.
- CT is most important imaging modality in assessment of anterior mediastinal masses.
- MRI is helpful for evaluation of local invasion.
- Diagnosis can be confirmed by either CT-guided needle biopsy or surgical biopsy.
- PET/CT is particularly helpful in follow-up of malignant anterior mediastinal tumors.
- Carcinoid is included in thymic carcinoma category of thymic epithelial tumors in 2004 World Health Organization classification.

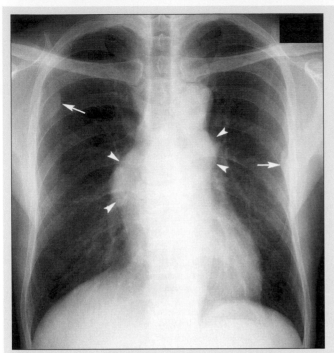

Figure 1.   Thymic well-differentiated neuroendocrine carcinoma (typical carcinoid). Posteroanterior chest radiograph in a 58-year-old man demonstrates an anterior mediastinal mass widening both sides of the mediastinum (*arrowheads*). Pleural nodules are seen bilaterally (*arrows*). (*Courtesy of Dr. Kiminori Fujimoto, Kurume, Fukuoka, Japan*)

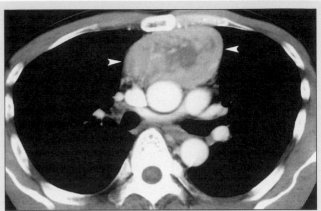

Figure 2.   Thymic well-differentiated neuroendocrine carcinoma (typical carcinoid) in a 58-year-old man. Contrast-enhanced CT image shows anterior mediastinal mass with relatively smooth margins (*arrowheads*) and heterogeneous enhancement. (*Courtesy of Dr. Kiminori Fujimoto, Kurume, Fukuoka, Japan*)

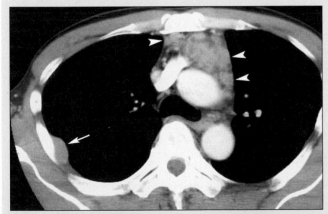

Figure 3.   Thymic well-differentiated neuroendocrine carcinoma (typical carcinoid) in a 58-year-old man. Contrast-enhanced CT image in the same patient and slightly cephalad to Figure 2 shows lymphadenopathy (*arrowheads*). Note pleural metastasis (*arrow*). (*Courtesy of Dr. Kiminori Fujimoto, Kurume, Fukuoka, Japan*)

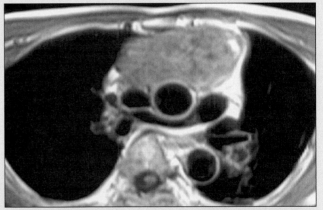

Figure 4.   Thymic well-differentiated neuroendocrine carcinoma (typical carcinoid) in a 58-year-old man. The mass has relatively heterogeneous low signal intensity on a T1-weighted MR image. (*Courtesy of Dr. Kiminori Fujimoto, Kurume, Fukuoka, Japan*)

- Well-differentiated (typical [classic] and atypical carcinoids) and poorly differentiated (small cell and large cell) subtypes
- Typical carcinoid: composed of polygonal cells with granular cytoplasm arranged in ribbons, festoons, solid nests, and rosette-like glands; < 2 mitoses/2 mm^2 (10 HPF) without necrosis
- Atypical carcinoid: carcinoid tumor with architectural features of typical type but exhibiting greater degree of mitotic activity; 2-10 mitoses/2 mm^2 (10 HPF) and/or foci of necrosis
- Cushing syndrome: due to adrenocorticotropic hormone (ACTH) production
- Aggressive tumors: spread to regional lymph nodes, invasion of adjacent structures, source of metastases

INCIDENCE/PREVALENCE AND EPIDEMIOLOGY

- Rare, constitutes 2%-7% of all thymic epithelial tumors
- Twenty-five percent of patients with positive family history of multiple endocrine neoplasia type 1
- Typical tumor: any age

- Atypical tumor: mean age 48-55 years with male-to-female ratio of 1:2-7
- Small cell: slightly younger average age, no gender predominance
- Large cell: rare, 55-75 years of age

Suggested Readings

Groves AM, Mohan HK, Wegner EA, et al: Positron emission tomography with FDG to show thymic carcinoid. *AJR Am J Roentgenol* 182:511-513, 2004.

Pathology and genetics of tumours of the lung, pleura, thymus, and heart. In Travis WD, Brambilla E, Müller-Hermelink HK, Harris CC, editors: *World Health Organization Classification of Tumours*, Lyon, 2004, IARCPress.

Quint LE: Imaging of anterior mediastinal masses. *Cancer Imaging* 7(Spec No A):S56-S62, 2007.

Rosado de Christenson ML, Abbott GF, Kirejczyk WM, et al: Thoracic carcinoids: Radiologic-pathologic correlation. *RadioGraphics* 19:707-736, 1999.

Sadohara J, Fujimoto K, Müller NL, et al: Thymic epithelial tumors: Comparison of CT and MR imaging findings of low-risk thymomas, high-risk thymomas, and thymic carcinomas. *Eur J Radiol* 60:70-79, 2006.

Soga J, Yakuwa Y, Osaka M: Evaluation of 342 cases of mediastinal/thymic carcinoids collected from literature: A comparative study between typical carcinoids and atypical varieties. Review. *Ann Thorac Cardiovasc Surg* 5:285-292, 1999.

Thymic Carcinoma

DEFINITION: Thymic carcinoma is a malignant tumor of the thymus with squamous differentiation.

IMAGING

Radiography
Findings
- Large and poorly defined anterior mediastinal mass
- Widened mediastinum

Utility
- Usually initial imaging modality for evaluation of suspected mediastinal tumors

CT
Findings
- Heterogeneous anterior mediastinal mass with irregular or lobulated contour
- Frequently contains areas of necrosis
- May contain cystic areas or calcification
- Heterogeneous contrast enhancement
- Evidence of lymphadenopathy or vascular invasion

Utility
- Superior to radiography for diagnosis and assessment of extent
- Superior to MRI in demonstrating calcifications

MRI
Findings
- Ill-defined mass of mixed signal intensity with irregular contour
- Focal areas of hemorrhage or necrosis
- Heterogeneous contrast enhancement
- Evidence of lymphadenopathy, vascular invasion, metastases

Utility
- Superior to CT in assessment of tumor capsule, intratumoral fibrous septa, and hemorrhage

Positron Emission Tomography
Findings
- Heterogeneous FDG uptake with standardized uptake value > 5.0

Utility
- FDG-PET helpful in differential diagnosis of thymic masses
- Integrate with CT findings to improve depiction of tumor and nodal metastases
- Reasonably accurate in differentiating thymic carcinomas from thymomas

DIAGNOSTIC PEARLS
- Ill-defined heterogeneously enhancing anterior mediastinal mass
- Regional lymphadenopathy or local invasion
- Heterogeneous uptake with standardized uptake value on FDG-PET > 5.0

CLINICAL PRESENTATION
- Chest pain, cough, fatigue, fever, anorexia, superior vena cava syndrome
- Paraneoplastic polymyositis

DIFFERENTIAL DIAGNOSIS
- Thymic carcinoid
- Thymoma
- Nonseminomatous malignant germ cell tumor
- Seminoma
- Lymphoma

PATHOLOGY
- Neoplasm with histologic features of squamous differentiation with or without keratinization, mature T lymphocytes
- Invasion of adjacent structures, with spread to pleura, pericardium, and abdomen

INCIDENCE/PREVALENCE AND EPIDEMIOLOGY
- Uncommon; annual incidence: 1-5/million population
- Thymic epithelial tumors 50% of anterior mediastinal masses
- 15%-20% of all thymic epithelial tumors
- Occurs in middle age with male-to-female ratio of 1:1 to 2.3:1
- 5-Year survival rates of 20%-40%

WHAT THE REFERRING PHYSICIAN NEEDS TO KNOW
- CT most important imaging modality in assessment of anterior mediastinal masses
- MRI helpful for evaluation of local invasion
- Diagnosis confirmed by either CT-guided needle biopsy or surgical biopsy
- PET/CT particularly helpful in follow-up of malignant anterior mediastinal tumors
- Included in thymic carcinoma category of thymic epithelial tumors in 2004 World Health Organization classification
- Aggressive tumor with poor prognosis

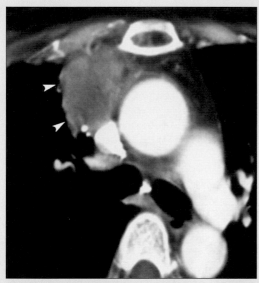

Figure 1. **Thymic squamous cell carcinoma.** Contrast-enhanced CT scan demonstrates anterior mediastinal mass with heterogeneous enhancement suggestive of extensive necrosis and irregular margins with the right lung (*arrowheads*). Surgery confirmed the presence of a thymic carcinoma. The tumor did not invade the lung. (*Courtesy of Dr. Kiminori Fujimoto, Kurume, Fukuoka, Japan*)

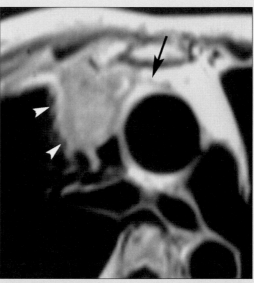

Figure 2. **Thymic squamous cell carcinoma.** T1-weighted MR image shows the fat plane between the lung and the anterior mediastinal tumor (*arrowheads*). Also noted is residual thymic tissue (*arrow*) adjacent to the tumor. Surgery confirmed the presence of a thymic carcinoma. The tumor did not invade the lung. (*Courtesy of Dr. Kiminori Fujimoto, Kurume, Fukuoka, Japan*)

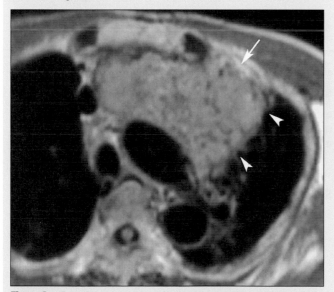

Figure 3. **Thymic squamous cell carcinoma.** T1-weighted image in a 70-year-old man shows an anterior mediastinal mass with heterogeneous signal intensities invading the anterior chest wall (*arrow*), left lung (*arrowheads*), and ascending aorta. The tumor insinuates between the superior vena cava and the aortic arch. (*Courtesy of Dr. Kiminori Fujimoto, Kurume, Fukuoka, Japan*)

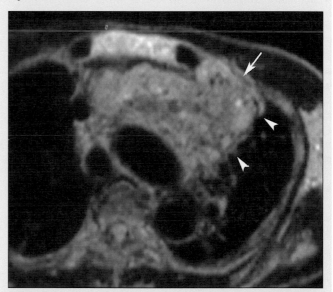

Figure 4. **Thymic squamous cell carcinoma.** T2-weighted image in a 70-year-old man shows an anterior mediastinal mass with heterogeneous signal intensities invading the anterior chest wall (*arrow*), left lung (*arrowheads*), and ascending aorta. The tumor insinuates between the superior vena cava and the aortic arch. (*Courtesy of Dr. Kiminori Fujimoto, Kurume, Fukuoka, Japan*)

Suggested Readings

Inoue A, Tomiyama N, Fujimoto K, et al: MR imaging of thymic epithelial tumors: Correlation with World Health Organization classification. *Radiat Med* 24:171-181, 2006.

Jeong SM, Lee KY, Shin D, et al: Does CT of thymic epithelial tumors enable us to differentiate histologic subtypes and predict prognosis? *AJR Am J Roentgenol* 183:283-289, 2004.

Jung KJ, Lee KS, Han J, et al: Malignant thymic epithelial tumors: CT-pathologic correlation. *AJR Am J Roentgenol* 176:433-439, 2001.

Pathology and genetics of tumours of the lung, pleura, thymus, and heart. In Travis WD, Brambilla E, Müller-Hermelink HK, Harris CC, editors: *World Health Organization Classification of Tumours.* Lyon, 2004, IARC Press.

Sadohara J, Fujimoto K, Müller NL, et al: Thymic epithelial tumors: Comparison of CT and MR imaging findings of low-risk thymomas, high-risk thymomas, and thymic carcinomas. *Eur J Radiol* 60:70-79, 2006.

Thymolipoma

DEFINITION: A thymolipoma is a mesenchymal tumor in the mediastinum consisting of adipose and thymic tissue.

IMAGING

Radiography
Findings
- Large anterior mediastinal mass that may extend to inferior hemithorax on one or both sides of midline.
- Mimics cardiomegaly or elevated hemidiaphragm.
- Low density of mass may be appreciated
- May change shape or position on decubitus view

Utility
- Majority found incidentally on chest radiography

CT
Findings
- Anterior mediastinal mass with smooth margins
- Predominant fat attenuation or equivalent fat and soft tissue attenuation

Utility
- Useful in detecting connection to thymus
- Attenuation dependent on relative amounts of adipose tissue and thymus
- Accurate diagnosis achieved in most cases owing to characteristic findings

MRI
Findings
- Anterior mediastinal mass with smooth margins
- High signal intensity on T1-weighted imaging (fat) with areas of intermediate signal (soft tissue)
- Loss of fat signal on fat-suppressed imaging

Utility
- Useful in detecting connection to thymus
- Signal intensity dependent on relative amounts of adipose tissue and thymus
- Fat suppression or chemical shift imaging helpful in assessing fat content
- Accurate diagnosis achieved in most cases owing to characteristic findings

CLINICAL PRESENTATION

- Mostly asymptomatic, found incidentally on radiography
- Association with myasthenia gravis (7%)

DIAGNOSTIC PEARLS

- Low-density mediastinal mass that changes with position
- Areas of fat and soft tissue attenuation on CT
- May be associated with myasthenia gravis

DIFFERENTIAL DIAGNOSIS

- Teratoma
- Thymoma
- Thymic carcinoma
- Mediastinal lipomatosis

PATHOLOGY

- Benign mesenchymal tumor consisting of mature adipose tissue with areas of non-neoplastic thymic tissue
- Range from 4-30 cm in diameter; most weigh >500 g

INCIDENCE/PREVALENCE AND EPIDEMIOLOGY

- Uncommon, <200 reported cases
- Most common in young adults (mean age, 30 years)
- Approximately 7% of cases associated with myasthenia gravis

Suggested Readings

Damadoglu E, Salturk C, Takir HB, et al: Mediastinal thymolipoma: An analysis of 10 cases. *Respirology* 12:924-927, 2007.

Gamanagatti S, Sharma R, Hatimota P, et al: Giant thymolipoma. *AJR Am J Roentgenol* 185:283-284, 2005.

Moran CA, Rosado-de-Christenson M, Suster S: Thymolipoma: Clinicopathologic review of 33 cases. *Mod Pathol* 8:741-744, 1995.

Otto HF, Löning TH, Lachenmayer L, et al: Thymolipoma in association with myasthenia gravis. *Cancer* 50:1623-1628, 1982.

Rosado de Christenson ML, Pugatch RD, Moran CA: Thymolipoma: Analysis of 27 cases. *Radiology* 193:121-126, 1994.

WHAT THE REFERRING PHYSICIAN NEEDS TO KNOW

- CT most important imaging modality in assessment of anterior mediastinal masses
- Thymolipoma may be associated with myasthenia gravis

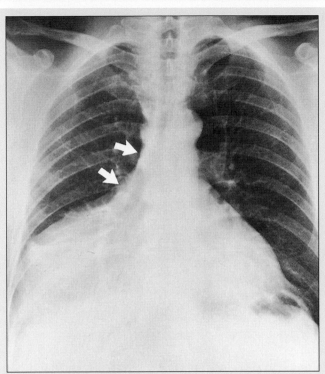

Figure 1. Thymolipoma. Posteroanterior radiograph shows a large mass situated in the lower half of the right hemithorax. The obtuse angle the mass creates with the mediastinum (*arrows*) indicates its origin from that structure. (*Courtesy of Dr. R. Hedvigi, Montreal Chest Institute. From Müller NL, Fraser RS, Colman NC, Paré PD: Radiologic Diagnosis of Diseases of the Chest. Philadelphia, WB Saunders, 2001.*)

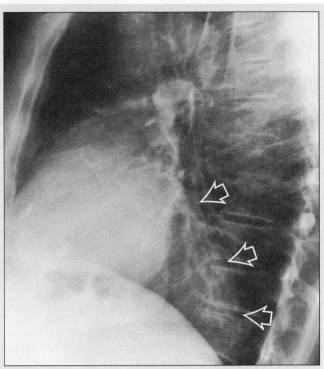

Figure 2. Thymolipoma. Lateral radiograph shows a large mass situated in the lower half of the right hemithorax. The mass extends almost the whole anteroposterior depth of the thorax, obscuring most of the right hemidiaphragm (the posterior margin of the mass is indicated by *arrows*). The anterior mediastinum looks empty. (*Courtesy of Dr. R. Hedvigi, Montreal Chest Institute. From Müller NL, Fraser RS, Colman NC, Paré PD: Radiologic Diagnosis of Diseases of the Chest. Philadelphia, WB Saunders, 2001.*)

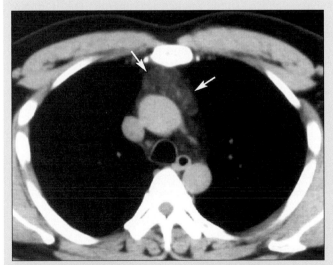

Figure 3. Thymolipoma in a 38-year-old man with myasthenia gravis. CT image demonstrates heterogeneous anterior mediastinal mass (*arrows*) with soft tissue and fat density. (*Courtesy of Dr. Kiminori Fujimoto, Kurume, Fukuoka, Japan*)

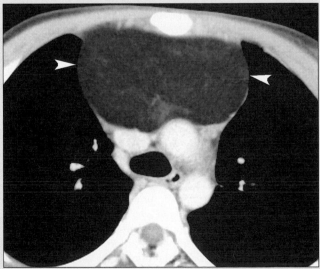

Figure 4. Thymolipoma without myasthenia gravis. Contrast-enhanced CT scan in an asymptomatic 14-year-old girl reveals an anterior mediastinal mass (*arrowheads*) with smooth margins, fat-attenuation (0-15 Hounsfield units) and soft tissue strands. Thymolipoma was proven histologically. (*Courtesy of Dr. Noriyuki Tomiyama, Osaka University Graduate School of Medicine, Suita, Japan.*)

Thymoma

DEFINITION: A thymoma is a thymic tumor that consists of thymic epithelial cells and lymphocytes.

IMAGING

Radiography

Findings
- Two- to 10-cm diameter anterior mediastinal mass near junction of heart and great vessels
- Well-circumscribed, round or oval mass with smooth or lobulated margins
- Widened mediastinum
- May displace heart and great vessels posterolaterally

Utility
- Initial modality for evaluation of paraneoplastic syndromes
- One third of masses detected incidentally on chest radiography

CT

Findings
- Well-defined round or oval masses with sharply demarcated margins or lobulated contours
- Usually homogeneous soft tissue attenuation and enhancement
- Heterogeneous: cysts or focal low-attenuation areas representing hemorrhage or necrosis
- Punctate, linear, or ring-like capsular or internal calcifications
- Invasion: irregular margins, vascular or chest wall invasion, encasement of mediastinal structures, irregular lung interface
- Pleural or pericardial nodules or diffuse smooth or nodular thickening
- Gravitation of metastases to abdominal cavity

Utility
- Superior to radiography for diagnosis and assessment of extent
- Superior to MRI in demonstrating calcifications
- Useful in assessing tumor margins for features suggestive of invasion (capsular or extracapsular)
- Used to distinguish low-grade tumors from aggressive tumors and thymic carcinoma

DIAGNOSTIC PEARLS

- Well-circumscribed anterior mediastinal mass with smooth or lobulated contour
- Homogeneous contrast enhancement with septa and capsule
- Heterogeneous uptake with standardized uptake value on FDG-PET < 5.0
- Paraneoplastic syndromes: myasthenia gravis (40%), pure red cell aplasia, hypogammaglobulincmia, stiff person syndrome
- Patients are usually > 40 years of age

MRI

Findings
- Well-circumscribed anterior mediastinal mass of low to intermediate signal intensity on T1-weighted images and intermediate to high signal intensity on T2-weighted images
- Intratumoral cystic degeneration and necrosis: areas of low signal intensity on T1-weighted images and high signal intensity on T2-weighted images
- Hemorrhage of high signal intensity on both T1- and T2-weighted images, with hemosiderin ring or fluid-fluid levels seen
- Fibrous septa seen as low signal lines or network patterns on both T1- and T2-weighted imaging
- Homogeneous enhancement but heterogeneous if with septa, cystic or necrotic components, and/or hemorrhage
- May exhibit evidence of capsular and extracapsular extension
- No change in signal intensity on chemical shift imaging

Utility
- Superior to CT in assessment of tumor capsule, intratumoral fibrous septa, and hemorrhage
- Used to distinguish low-grade tumors from aggressive tumors and thymic carcinoma
- Chemical shift MRI potentially helpful in distinguishing from thymic hyperplasia

---

WHAT THE REFERRING PHYSICIAN NEEDS TO KNOW

- Patients with thymoma are usually > 40 years of age.
- Paraneoplastic syndromes associated with thymoma include myasthenia gravis (40%), pure red cell aplasia, hypogammaglobulinemia, and stiff person syndrome.
- Eighty percent of patients with thymoma and myasthenia gravis have positive serum anti-acetylcholine receptor binding antibody with specificity of 98%.
- CT is most important imaging modality in assessment of anterior mediastinal masses; MRI is helpful for evaluation of local invasion.
- Diagnosis can be confirmed by either CT-guided needle biopsy or surgical biopsy.
- World Health Organization Classification includes thymomas and thymic carcinomas together under thymic epithelial tumors.

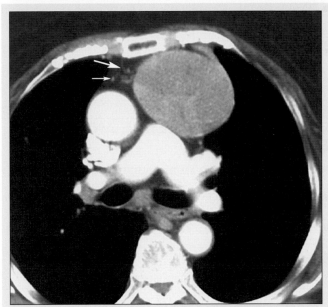

Figure 1. Type AB thymoma in a 70-year-old woman. Contrast-enhanced CT demonstrates a smoothly marginated mass with relatively homogeneous enhancement and linear areas of low attenuation. Thymic vein (*small arrow*) and dilated feeders (*large arrow*) are seen in the adjacent mediastinum. (*Courtesy of Dr. Kiminori Fujimoto, Kurume, Fukuoka, Japan*)

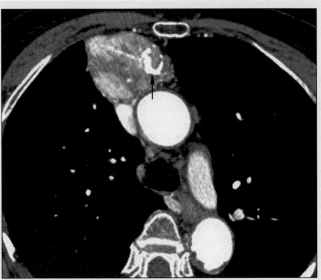

Figure 2. Type B3 thymoma. Contrast-enhanced CT image demonstrates a heterogeneous enhancing mass with partially spiculated margins and with ring-like (*black arrow*) and punctate calcifications. (*Courtesy of Dr. Kiminori Fujimoto, Kurume, Fukuoka, Japan*)

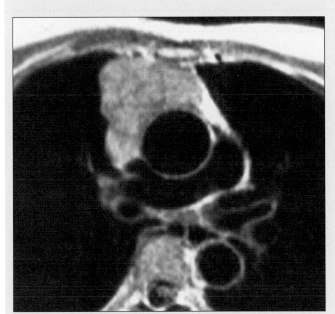

Figure 3. Type B2 thymoma in a 56-year-old woman. T1-weighted image demonstrates a lobulated-contour mass adhering tightly to the right lung (Masaoka stage III). Low signal intensity lines subdivide the mass into lobules. Histologically the tumor was shown to be a type B2 thymoma. (*Courtesy of Dr. Kiminori Fujimoto, Kurume, Fukuoka, Japan*)

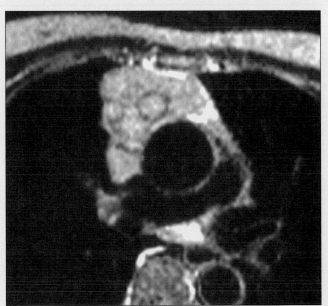

Figure 4. Type B2 thymoma in a 56-year-old woman. T2-weighted image demonstrates a lobulated-contour mass adhering tightly to the right lung (Masaoka stage III). Low signal intensity lines subdivide the mass into lobules. Histologically the tumor was shown to be a type B2 thymoma. (*Courtesy of Dr. Kiminori Fujimoto, Kurume, Fukuoka, Japan*)

Positron Emission Tomography

Findings

- Heterogeneous FDG uptake with standardized uptake value < 5.0

Utility

- FDG-PET helpful in differential diagnosis of thymic masses
- Integrate with CT findings to improve depiction of tumor and nodal metastases
- Reasonably accurate in differentiating thymic carcinomas from thymomas

CLINICAL PRESENTATION

- Often asymptomatic
- Chest pain, dyspnea, superior vena cava syndrome
- Paraneoplastic syndromes: myasthenia gravis (40%), pure red cell aplasia, hypogammaglobulinemia, stiff person syndrome

DIFFERENTIAL DIAGNOSIS

- Thymic carcinoma
- Thymic carcinoid
- Nonseminomatous malignant germ cell tumor
- Seminoma
- Teratoma
- Lymphoma

PATHOLOGY

- Tumors contain thymic epithelial cells and lymphocytes without apparent cellular atypia

- World Health Organization classification: spectrum from low-risk organotypic (types A, AB, B1) to high-risk (types B2, B3)
- Aggressive tumors: invade capsule, extend to adjacent structures, and spread to pleura, pericardium, and abdomen

INCIDENCE/PREVALENCE AND EPIDEMIOLOGY

- Thymic epithelial tumors comprise 50% of anterior mediastinal masses.
- Thymoma occurs in persons 50-65 years of age; there is no gender predilection.
- An increased risk of a second malignancy is associated.

Suggested Readings

Maher MM, Shepard JAO: Imaging of thymoma. *Semin Thorac Cardiovasc Surg* 17:12-19, 2005.

Pathology and genetics of tumours of the lung, pleura, thymus, and heart. In Travis WD, Brambilla E, Müller-Hermelink HK, Harris CC, editors: *World Health Organization Classification of Tumours*, Lyon, 2004, IARC Press.

Rosado-de-Christenson ML, Galobardes J, Moran CA: Thymoma, radiologic-pathologic correlation. *RadioGraphics* 12:151-168, 1992.

Sadohara J, Fujimoto K, Müller NL, et al: Thymic epithelial tumors: Comparison of CT and MR imaging findings of low-risk thymomas, high-risk thymomas, and thymic carcinomas. *Eur J Radiol* 60:70-79, 2006.

Tomiyama N, Müller NL, Ellis SJ, et al: Invasive and noninvasive thymoma: Distinctive CT features. *J Comput Assist Tomogr* 25:388-393, 2001.

Nonseminomatous Malignant Germ Cell Tumor

DEFINITION: Malignant nonseminomatous mediastinal germ cell tumors include embryonal carcinoma, yolk sac tumor, choriocarcinoma, and mixed germ cell tumors.

IMAGING

Radiography
Findings
- Large anterior mediastinal mass with smooth, lobulated, or irregular margins
- Evidence of pulmonary metastases

Utility
- May be found incidentally on chest radiograph

CT
Findings
- Heterogeneous anterior mediastinal mass; usually poorly marginated
- Intratumoral areas of hemorrhage, necrosis, or focal calcification
- Peripheral or heterogeneous contrast enhancement
- May have direct chest wall invasion, regional lymph nodes, pulmonary and distant metastases, and pleural and/or pericardial effusions

Utility
- Superior to radiography for diagnosis and assessment of extent

MRI
Findings
- Heterogeneous, poorly marginated anterior mediastinal mass
- Intratumoral areas of hemorrhage, necrosis, or focal calcification
- Distant metastases (central nervous system, bone)

Utility
- More sensitive in depicting local invasion and distant metastases

Positron Emission Tomography
Findings
- Positive uptake of FDG

Utility
- Helpful in differentiating viable tumor from necrotic masses after chemotherapy

DIAGNOSTIC PEARLS
- Virtually all patients are male
- Large, heterogeneous, poorly marginated anterior mediastinal mass
- Areas of necrosis, hemorrhage, or calcification
- Evidence of local invasion or metastases
- Elevated serum α-fetoprotein and/or serum β-hCG levels

CLINICAL PRESENTATION
- Thoracic or shoulder pain; shortness of breath
- Less commonly, hoarseness, cough, superior vena cava syndrome
- Elevated serum α-fetoprotein level (yolk sac tumor component), elevated serum β-hCG level (choriocarcinoma component)

DIFFERENTIAL DIAGNOSIS
- Thymoma
- Thymic carcinoma
- Thymic carcinoid
- Thyroid masses
- Teratoma
- Seminoma

PATHOLOGY
- Malignant nonseminomatous germ cell tumors: embryonal carcinoma, yolk sac tumor, choriocarcinoma, and mixed germ cell tumors
- Embryonal carcinoma: germ cell tumor composed of large primitive cells of epithelial appearance with abundant clear or granular cytoplasm

WHAT THE REFERRING PHYSICIAN NEEDS TO KNOW
- CT most important imaging modality in assessment of anterior mediastinal masses
- MRI helpful for evaluation of local invasion
- Malignant nonseminomatous germ cell tumors: embryonal carcinoma, yolk sac tumor, choriocarcinoma, and mixed germ cell tumors
- Diagnosis confirmed by either CT-guided needle biopsy or surgical biopsy
- Tumor commonly associated with elevated serum α-fetoprotein and β-hCG levels
- Serum tumor markers helpful in assessment of response to therapy or tumor recurrence

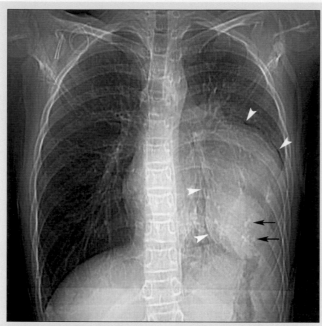

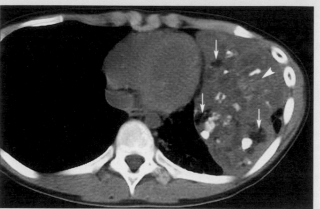

Figure 1. **Mixed germ cell tumor (immature teratoma containing yolk sac tumor component) in a 14-year-old boy.** Chest radiograph demonstrates a large mass (*white arrowheads*) occupying most of the left hemithorax. Note presence of foci of calcification (*black arrows*). The serum α-fetoprotein in this patient was markedly elevated (70,000 ng/mL). (*Courtesy of Dr. Kiminori Fujimoto, Kurume, Fukuoka, Japan*)

Figure 2. **Mixed germ cell tumor (immature teratoma containing yolk sac tumor component) in a 14-year-old boy.** CT image without contrast shows a large mass compressing and adhering to the left lung with heterogeneous attenuation containing foci of very high attenuation (calcifications), areas of slightly increased attenuation (hemorrhage, *arrowhead*), foci of low attenuation (fat, *arrows*), and areas of soft tissue to water attenuation. (*Courtesy of Dr. Kiminori Fujimoto, Kurume, Fukuoka, Japan*)

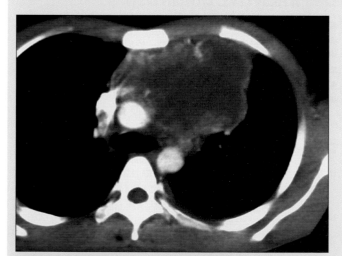

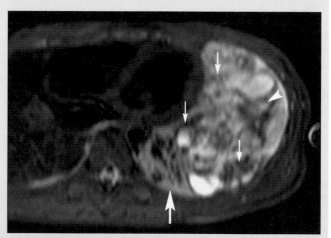

Figure 3. **Choriocarcinoma in a 25-year-old man.** Contrast-enhanced CT shows anterior mediastinal mass with irregular contours and invasion into the left lung. The tumor has large areas of low attenuation due to necrosis and irregular peripheral enhancement. (*Courtesy of Dr. Kiminori Fujimoto, Kurume, Fukuoka, Japan*)

Figure 4. **Mixed germ cell tumor (immature teratoma containing yolk sac tumor component) in a 14-year-old boy.** Short tau inversion recovery (STIR) image shows markedly heterogeneous signal intensities suggestive of areas of hemorrhage (*arrowhead*), foci of fat (*small arrows*), and soft tissue. Note collapse with bronchiectasis in compressed left lung (*large arrow*). (*Courtesy of Dr. Kiminori Fujimoto, Kurume, Fukuoka, Japan*)

- Yolk sac tumor/endodermal sinus tumor: tumor characterized by numerous patterns that recapitulate the yolk sac, allantois, and extraembryonic mesenchyme
- Choriocarcinoma: highly malignant neoplasm displaying trophoblastic differentiation composed of syncytiotrophoblast, cytotrophoblast, and variably intermediate trophoblast cells
- Mixed germ cell tumor: neoplasm composed of two or more types of germ cell tumors

INCIDENCE/PREVALENCE AND EPIDEMIOLOGY

- Mediastinal germ cell tumors account for 15% of mediastinal neoplasms in adults and 19%-25% in children.
- Mean age at presentation is 27 years (range: 18-67 years).

- Virtually all patients are male.
- Adjacent structures are frequently invaded, with hematogenous metastases to lungs, liver, brain, and bones (50%).

Suggested Readings

Drevelegas A, Palladas P, Scordalaki A: Mediastinal germ cell tumors: A radiologic-pathologic review. *Eur Radiol* 11:1925-1932, 2001.

Lee KS, Im JG, Han CH, et al: Malignant primary germ cell tumors of the mediastinum: CT features. *AJR Am J Roentgenol* 153:947-951, 1989.

Moran CA, Suster S, Koss MN: Primary germ cell tumors of the mediastinum: III. Yolk sac tumor, embryonal carcinoma, choriocarcinoma, and combined nonteratomatous germ cell tumors of the mediastinum—a clinicopathologic and immunohistochemical study of 64 cases. *Cancer* 80:699-707, 1997.

Strollo DC, Rosado-de-Christenson ML: Primary mediastinal malignant germ cell neoplasms: Imaging features. *Chest Surg Clin North Am* 12:645-658, 2002.

Germ Cell Tumor: Seminoma

DEFINITION: A malignant anterior mediastinal tumor composed of primordial germ cell types is a seminoma.

IMAGING

Radiography
Findings
- Large, central, lobulated, well-marginated anterior mediastinal mass; typically grows to both sides of midline

Utility
- May be found incidentally on chest radiograph

CT
Findings
- Large anterior mediastinal mass with sharply demarcated borders, irregular if invasive
- Homogeneous soft tissue attenuation; occasional areas of low attenuation.
- Rarely, necrosis with cystic changes or calcification
- Slight contrast enhancement

Utility
- Superior to radiography for diagnosis and assessment of extent

MRI
Findings
- Large anterior mediastinal mass with lobulated or irregular margins
- Heterogeneous mixed signal on T1-weighted, T2-weighted, and contrast-enhanced images

Utility
- Superior to CT in depiction of soft tissues

Positron Emission Tomography
Findings
- Positive uptake of FDG

Utility
- Helpful in differentiating viable tumor from necrotic masses after chemotherapy

CLINICAL PRESENTATION

- Twenty percent to 30% of patients asymptomatic at time of diagnosis
- Chest pain, shortness of breath, superior vena cava (SVC) syndrome (10%), gynecomastia

DIAGNOSTIC PEARLS

- Large, relatively homogeneous anterior mediastinal mass
- Evidence of local invasion
- Necrosis and calcifications rare
- Occurs almost exclusively in males
- Elevated serum β-hCG

- Lymph node metastases most commonly in cervical (25%) and abdominal (8%) lymph nodes
- Elevated serum β-hCG; normal serum α-fetoprotein

DIFFERENTIAL DIAGNOSIS

- Thymoma
- Thymic carcinoma
- Thymic carcinoid
- Nonseminomatous malignant germ cell tumor
- Teratoma

PATHOLOGY

- Anterior mediastinal mass, usually large with lobulated or irregular margins
- Primitive germ cell tumor composed of uniform cells with clear to eosinophilic, glycogen-rich cytoplasm, distinct cell borders, and round nucleus with one or more nucleoli

INCIDENCE/PREVALENCE AND EPIDEMIOLOGY

- Eight percent of extragonadal germ cell tumors
- Ten percent of mediastinal germ cell tumors
- Pure seminomas: 1.6% of all mediastinal neoplasms
- Occurs almost exclusively in males
- Age range at presentation: 13-79 years; approximately two thirds in patients age 20-40 years

---

WHAT THE REFERRING PHYSICIAN NEEDS TO KNOW
- CT most important imaging modality in assessment of anterior mediastinal masses
- MRI helpful for evaluation of local invasion
- Diagnosed with either CT-guided needle biopsy or surgical biopsy
- Elevated serum β-hCG; normal serum α-fetoprotein
- Post-chemotherapy residual necrotic masses detectable on CT and MRI
- PET helpful in differentiating viable tumor from necrotic masses after chemotherapy

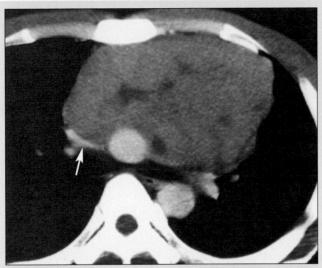

Figure 1. **Seminoma in a 25-year-old man.** Contrast-enhanced CT scan demonstrates a large anterior mediastinal tumor with heterogeneous enhancement, irregular bands, and small foci of low attenuation. The superior vena cava (*arrow*) is stretched by tumor compression, but blood flow is maintained. (*Courtesy of Dr. Kiminori Fujimoto, Kurume, Fukuoka, Japan*)

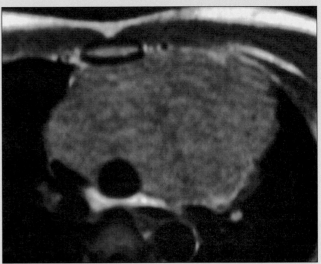

Figure 2. **Seminoma in a 25-year-old man.** T1-weighted MR image shows heterogeneous mixed signal intensities and irregular boundaries between the tumor and left lung. (*Courtesy of Dr. Kiminori Fujimoto, Kurume, Fukuoka, Japan*)

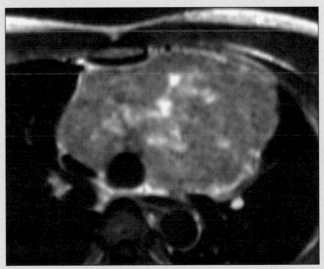

Figure 3. **Seminoma in a 25-year-old man.** Contrast-enhanced T1-weighted MR image shows heterogeneously enhancing tumor. (*Courtesy of Dr. Kiminori Fujimoto, Kurume, Fukuoka, Japan*)

Suggested Readings

De Santis M, Bokemeyer C, Becherer A, et al: Predictive impact of 2-18fluoro-2-deoxy-d-glucose positron emission tomography for residual postchemotherapy masses in patients with bulky seminoma. *J Clin Oncol* 19:3740-3744, 2001; erratum *J Clin Oncol* 19:4355, 2001.

Drevelegas A, Palladas P, Scordalaki A: Mediastinal germ cell tumors: A radiologic-pathologic review. *Eur Radiol* 11:1925-1932, 2001.

Lee KS, Im JG, Han CH, et al: Malignant primary germ cell tumors of the mediastinum: CT features. *AJR Am J Roentgenol* 153:947-951, 1989.

Moran CA, Suster S, Przygodzki RM, Koss MN: Primary germ cell tumors of the mediastinum: II. Mediastinal seminomas—a clinico-pathologic and immunohistochemical study of 120 cases. *Cancer* 80:691-698, 1997.

Strollo DC, Rosado-de-Christenson ML: Primary mediastinal malignant germ cell neoplasms: Imaging features. *Chest Surg Clin North Am* 12:645-658, 2002.

Germ Cell Tumor: Teratoma

DEFINITION: A teratoma is a benign mediastinal germ cell tumor composed of tissues derived from two or three germinal layers.

IMAGING

Radiography
Findings
- Well-circumscribed, rounded or lobulated masses widening the mediastinum
- Calcifications common, either of tumor wall, bone, or teeth or nonspecific
- Rupture: margins irregular or ill defined, with pleural effusion

Utility
- May be found incidentally on chest radiograph

CT
Findings
- Heterogeneous well-circumscribed anterior mediastinal mass most commonly including soft tissue and fluid
- Foci of fat attenuation 50%-70%
- Calcification curvilinear, flocculent, or punctate or osseous/dental in approximately 50%
- Rupture: inhomogeneity of internal components with changes in adjacent structures

Utility
- Superior to radiography for diagnosis and assessment of extent

MRI
Findings
- Multiloculated anterior mediastinal mass with markedly heterogeneous or mixed signal intensity
- Signal characteristic of soft tissue, fluid, and fat

Utility
- Inferior to CT in the diagnosis of mediastinal teratomas

CLINICAL PRESENTATION

- Often asymptomatic, incidental on radiograph
- Cough, dyspnea, or chest, back, or shoulder pain
- Recurrent pneumonia, superior vena cava syndrome, Horner syndrome, pneumothorax, trichoptysis
- Hyperinsulinism and hypoglycemia if with mature pancreatic tissue
- Rupture or hemorrhage: severe acute retrosternal pain, large pleural effusions, cardiac tamponade

DIAGNOSTIC PEARLS

- Multiloculated anterior mediastinal mass
- Heterogeneous enhancement with areas of fat
- Calcifications curvilinear, flocculent, or punctate or osseous/dental in approximately 50%

DIFFERENTIAL DIAGNOSIS

- Thymoma
- Thymic carcinoma
- Thymic carcinoid
- Nonseminomatous malignant germ cell tumor
- Seminoma

PATHOLOGY

- Encapsulated 3- to 25- cm multilocular tumors
- Mostly benign tumors with tissue from all three germ cell layers
- Types: mature (including dermoid cyst) and immature
- Haphazard admixture of well-differentiated adult-type tissues; ectodermal elements predominate
- May contain pancreatic (60%), bronchial, neural, gastrointestinal, smooth muscle, and adipose tissues
- Complications: intracystic hemorrhage and inflammation; rupture
- Cystic spaces contain fluid, ectodermal derivatives, and mature tissues.

INCIDENCE/PREVALENCE AND EPIDEMIOLOGY

- Fifty percent to 70% percent of mediastinal germ cell tumors
- Seven percent to 9% percent of mediastinal tumors
- Mature, male-to-female ratio of 1:1.4; immature, usually males
- Mean adult age: 28 years (18-60 years)

WHAT THE REFERRING PHYSICIAN NEEDS TO KNOW
- CT is most important imaging modality in assessment of anterior mediastinal masses.
- MRI is helpful for evaluation of local invasion.
- Diagnosis can be confirmed by either CT-guided needle biopsy or surgical biopsy.
- Mature teratomas occasionally undergo malignant transformation with poor prognosis.
- Course may be complicated by synchronous or subsequent leukemia.

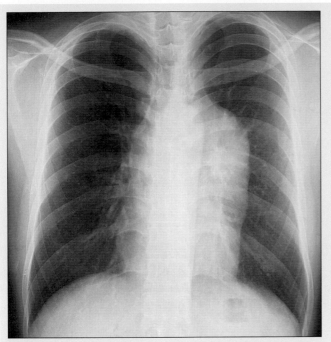

Figure 1. Mature teratoma in a 28-year-old man. A posteroanterior chest radiograph shows a smoothly margined mediastinal mass with positive hilum overlay sign (*Courtesy of Dr. Kiminori Fujimoto, Kurume, Fukuoka, Japan*).

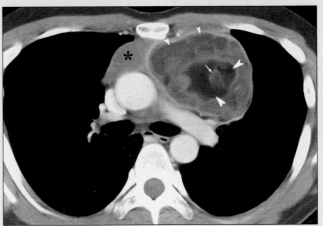

Figure 2. Mature teratoma in a 28-year-old man. Contrast-enhanced CT scan demonstrates a heterogeneous mass with enhancing wall. The mass contains foci of fat density (− 30 to − 100 Hounsfield units [HU]) (*large arrowheads*), small focus of calcification (200 to 300 HU) (*arrow*), weakly enhancing areas (20 to 40 HU) (*small arrowheads*), high-attenuation areas within the tumor, and foci of water density area (*asterisk*). (*Courtesy of Dr. Kiminori Fujimoto, Kurume, Fukuoka, Japan*)

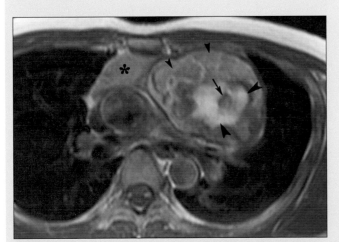

Figure 3. Mature teratoma in a 28-year-old man. T1-weighted image shows a mass with heterogeneous signal intensities. Areas with low signal intensity on T1-weighted images, with high signal intensity on T2-weighted images, and with very high signal intensity on STIR images suggest water/fluid (*asterisk*); areas with high signal intensity on both T1- and T2-weighted images and low signal intensity (signal suppression) on STIR image suggest fat (*large arrowheads*); areas with low signal intensity on all images suggest calcifications (*arrow*) or fibrous tissue (*small arrowheads*). (*Courtesy of Dr. Kiminori Fujimoto, Kurume, Fukuoka, Japan*)

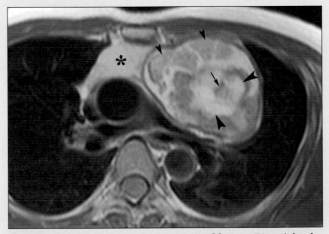

Figure 4. Mature teratoma in a 28-year-old man. T2-weighted image shows a mass with heterogeneous signal intensities. Areas with low signal intensity on T1-weighted images, high signal intensity on T2-weighted images, and very high signal intensity on STIR images suggest water-fluid (*asterisk*); areas with high signal intensity on both T1- and T2-weighted images and low signal intensity (signal suppression) on STIR image suggest fat (*large arrowheads*); areas with low signal intensity on all images suggest calcifications (*arrow*) or fibrous tissue (*small arrowheads*). (*Courtesy of Dr. Kiminori Fujimoto, Kurume, Fukuoka, Japan*)

Suggested Readings

Choi SJ, Lee JS, Song KS, Lim TH: Mediastinal teratoma: CT differentiation of ruptured and unruptured tumors. *AJR Am J Roentgenol* 171:591-594, 1998.

Drevelegas A, Palladas P, Scordalaki A: Mediastinal germ cell tumors: A radiologic-pathologic review. *Eur Radiol* 11:1925-1932, 2001.

Jeung MY, Gasser B, Gangi A, et al: Imaging of cystic masses of the mediastinum. *RadioGraphics* 22(Spec No):S79-S93, 2002.

Moeller KH, Rosado-de Christenson ML, Templeton PA: Mediastinal mature teratoma: Imaging features. *AJR Am J Roentgenol* 169:985-990, 1997.

Tomiyama N, Honda O, Tsubamoto M, et al: Anterior mediastinal tumors: Diagnostic accuracy of CT and MRI. *Eur J Radiol* 69:280-288, 2009.

Anterior Mediastinal Cysts and Cystic Neoplasms

DEFINITION: Lesions that are predominantly cystic in the anterior mediastinum can be benign or malignant.

IMAGING

Radiography

Findings
- Mediastinal cysts and cystic neoplasms: mediastinal mass of variable appearance, usually sharply marginated
- Pericardial cyst: focal opacity that obscures inferior cardiac border

Utility
- Initial modality for evaluation; may be found incidentally
- Limited value in the differential diagnosis

CT

Findings
- Thymic cyst: smoothly marginated homogeneous water-attenuation density; may be unilocular or contain thin or thick septa
- Benign cysts: contents do not enhance; walls may enhance
- Cystic degeneration of neoplasms: fluid-filled portions within enhancing mass
- Bronchogenic cyst: solitary, smooth, round/oval mass with imperceptible wall and uniform attenuation
- Bronchogenic cyst: approximately 50% have water attenuation and 50% have soft tissue attenuation
- Pericardial cyst: well-circumscribed; unilocular; uniform water attenuation; nonenhancing
- Pericardial cysts usually occur in the cardiophrenic angle

Utility
- Superior to radiography for diagnosis
- Most important imaging modality in anterior mediastinal mass assessment
- Contrast useful for differentiating problematic soft tissue attenuation cysts from mediastinal neoplasia

MRI

Findings
- Homogeneous water-containing cysts of low T1 signal intensity and high T2 signal intensity
- T1 signal intensity may be variable in hemorrhage or increased intracystic protein
- High signal on diffusion-weighted images and diffusion coefficient equal to water

DIAGNOSTIC PEARLS

- Thymic cysts account for 1%-2% of all anterior mediastinal masses.
- Thymic cysts are congenital, have smooth margins, thin walls, and homogeneous water attenuation.
- Pericardial cysts usually are located in the region of the cardiophrenic angle and have uniform water attenuation.
- Cystic degeneration resulting in fluid-filled portions within the mass may occur in thymomas, germ cell tumors, lymphomas, and neurogenic tumors.

- Congenital thymic cyst: low signal intensities on T1-weighted images and high signal intensities on T2-weighted images
- Intracystic hemorrhage: increased signal on T1-weighted images due to T1 shortening effect of methemoglobin
- Bronchogenic cyst: high signal intensity on T2-weighted images; variable patterns of signal intensity on T1-weighted images
- Pericardial cyst: homogeneous low signal intensity on T1-weighted images; high signal intensity on T2-weighted images

Utility
- Useful for differentiating problematic soft tissue attenuation cysts from mediastinal neoplasia
- Helpful for local invasion evaluation

CLINICAL PRESENTATION

- Variable
- May be asymptomatic
- Symptoms, when present, nonspecific: mainly chest discomfort and cough

DIFFERENTIAL DIAGNOSIS

- Thymic cyst
- Pericardial cyst
- Bronchogenic cyst
- Thymoma

WHAT THE REFERRING PHYSICIAN NEEDS TO KNOW

- CT most important imaging modality in assessment of anterior mediastinal masses
- MRI helpful for evaluation of local invasion
- Diagnosis confirmed by either CT-guided needle biopsy or surgical biopsy

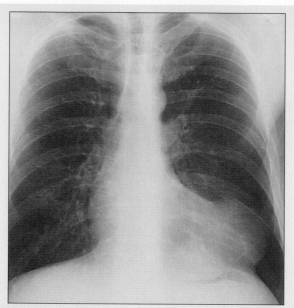

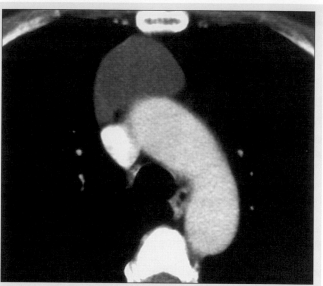

Figure 1. Pericardial cyst. Posteroanterior chest radiograph in a 46-year-old man shows smoothly marginated increased opacity in the left cardiophrenic angle. The diagnosis was confirmed at thoracotomy. *(From Müller NL, Fraser RS, Colman NC, Paré PD: Radiologic Diagnosis of Diseases of the Chest. Philadelphia, WB Saunders, 2001.)*

Figure 2. Thymic cyst in a 54-year-old woman. Contrast-enhanced CT demonstrates a well-circumscribed anterior mediastinal soft cystic mass with homogeneous fluid density (0-10 Hounsfield units). *(Courtesy of Dr. Kiminori Fujimoto, Kurume, Fukuoka, Japan)*

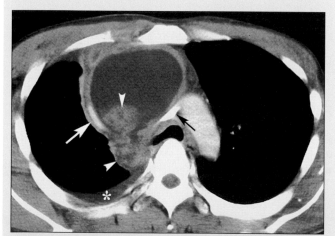

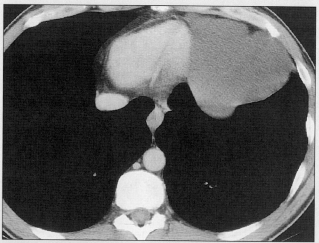

Figure 3. Spontaneous rupture of mature teratoma. A 20-year-old man presented with severe chest pain and dyspnea. Contrast-enhanced CT scan at the level of the aortic arch shows cystic mass with enhancing thick walls. The mass has ruptured posteriorly and intratumoral solid soft tissue lesions (*white arrowheads*) have burst out. Superior vena cava (*white arrow*) and left brachiocephalic vein (*black arrow*) are stretched by tumor compression. Right pleural effusion (*asterisk*) has high attenuation, suggestive of hemorrhage. *(Courtesy of Dr. Kiminori Fujimoto, Kurume, Fukuoka, Japan)*

Figure 4. Pericardial cyst in a 46-year-old man. Contrast-enhanced CT scan shows a water-density cyst in the region of the left cardiophrenic angle. The diagnosis was confirmed at thoracotomy. *(From Müller NL, Fraser RS, Colman NC, Paré PD: Radiologic Diagnosis of Diseases of the Chest. Philadelphia, WB Saunders, 2001.)*

- Thymic carcinoma
- Thymic carcinoid
- Teratoma
- Lymphangioma
- Hodgkin lymphoma
- Non-Hodgkin lymphoma

PATHOLOGY

- Congenital thymic cyst: derived from remnants of fetal thymopharyngeal duct; unilocular; contains serous or hemorrhagic fluid
- Multilocular thymic cyst: acquired, induced by presence of inflammatory lymphoid infiltrate; contains turbid fluid/gelatinous material; thick fibrous walls; inflammation/fibrosis
- Bronchogenic cyst: cyst wall lined by pseudostratified columnar respiratory epithelium; usually contains cartilage, smooth muscle, and mucus glands
- Congenital bronchogenic cysts of mediastinum classified into five subtypes depending on their sites of origin
- Cystic degeneration of neoplasms (thymic epithelial tumors, germ cell tumors, lymphoma, lymph node metastases, neurogenic tumors)
- May be associated with immune-mediated systemic diseases, radiation, surgical trauma, thymic neoplasia

INCIDENCE/PREVALENCE AND EPIDEMIOLOGY

- Primary tumors and cysts in mediastinum are uncommon and represent approximately 3% of chest tumors.
- Thymic cysts comprise 1%-2% of all anterior mediastinal masses.
- Most thymic cysts are congenital.

Suggested Readings

Bogot NR, Quint LE: Imaging of thymic disorders. *Cancer Imaging* 5:139-149, 2005.

Jeung MY, Gasser B, Gangi A, et al: Imaging of cystic masses of the mediastinum. *RadioGraphics* 22(Spec No):S79-S93, 2002.

Kim JH, Goo JM, Lee HJ, et al: Cystic tumors in the anterior mediastinum: Radiologic-pathological correlation. *J Comput Assist Tomogr* 27:714-723, 2003.

Murayama S, Murakami J, Watanabe H, et al: Signal intensity characteristics of mediastinal cystic masses on T1-weighted MRI. *J Comput Assist Tomogr* 19:188-191, 1995.

Wang ZJ, Reddy GP, Gotway MB, et al: CT and MR imaging of pericardial disease. *RadioGraphics* 23(Spec No):S167-S180, 2003.

Lymphangioma

DEFINITION: A lymphangioma is a benign cystic lymphatic tumor that may occur in the mediastinum, axilla, or neck.

IMAGING

Radiography
Findings
- Sharply defined, smooth, rounded, or lobulated mass
- Frequently displaces adjacent mediastinal structures
- Widened mediastinum

Utility
- May be initial imaging modality for evaluation

CT
Findings
- Smoothly marginated cystic mass with homogeneous water density (60%)
- Sometimes multilocular cystic masses with minimally enhancing septa (cavernous type)

Utility
- Superior to radiography for diagnosis and assessment of extent

MRI
Findings
- Homogeneous water-containing cysts (cystic or unilocular type) with low signal intensity on T1-weighted images and high signal intensity on T2-weighted images
- Cavernous: enhancing multiseptated/multicystic mass

Utility
- Nonspecific findings

DIFFERENTIAL DIAGNOSIS

- Thymoma
- Teratoma
- Bronchogenic cyst
- Thymic cyst

DIAGNOSTIC PEARLS

- Well-defined unilocular or multilocular cystic mass in neck or axilla with mediastinal extension
- Minimally enhancing septa
- Homogeneous water attenuation

PATHOLOGY

- Thin-walled vascular spaces lined by endothelial cells, with wall composed of connective tissue with variable amount of lymphoid tissue
- Types: cystic (unilocular), cavernous, mixed

INCIDENCE/PREVALENCE AND EPIDEMIOLOGY

- Rare
- Typically found in children or young adults
- Present at birth in 50%, with 90% discovered by 2 years of age
- Involvement of neck or axilla in 95%, with 10% extending into superior aspect of anterior mediastinum or middle mediastinal compartment

Suggested Readings

Charruau L, Parrens M, Jougon J, et al: Mediastinal lymphangioma in adults: CT and MR imaging features. *Eur Radiol* 10:1310-1314, 2000.

Park JG, Aubry MC, Godfrey JA, Midthun DE: Mediastinal lymphangioma: Mayo Clinic experience of 25 cases. *Mayo Clin Proc* 81:1197-1203, 2006.

Scalzetti EM, Heitzman ER, Groskin SA, et al: Developmental lymphatic disorders of the thorax. *RadioGraphics* 11:1069-1085, 1991.

Shaffer K, Rosado-de-Christenson ML, Patz EF Jr, et al: Thoracic lymphangioma in adults: CT and MR imaging features. *AJR Am J Roentgenol* 162:283-289, 1994.

WHAT THE REFERRING PHYSICIAN NEEDS TO KNOW

- CT most important imaging modality in assessment of anterior mediastinal masses
- MRI helpful for evaluation of local invasion
- Diagnosis confirmed by either CT-guided needle biopsy or surgical biopsy

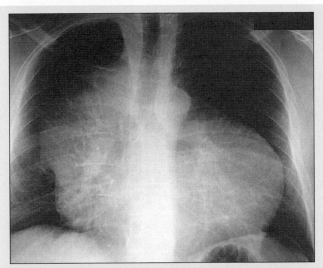

Figure 1. Lymphangioma in a 37-year-old man. Posteroanterior chest radiograph shows diffuse mediastinal widening. (*From Müller NL, Fraser RS, Colman NC, Paré PD: Radiologic Diagnosis of Diseases of the Chest. Philadelphia, WB Saunders, 2001.*)

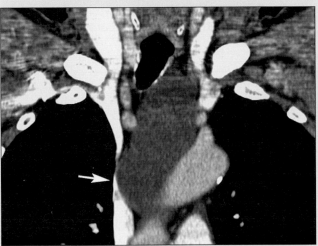

Figure 2. Cystic lymphangioma in a 58-year-old man. Coronal reformatted image obtained from a contrast-enhanced multidetector CT scan demonstrates a well-circumscribed, large cystic mass with homogeneous water density extending from the neck into superior aspect of mediastinum. The mass compresses the superior vena cava (*arrow*). (*Courtesy of Dr. Noriyuki Tomiyama, Osaka University Graduate School of Medicine, Suita, Japan.*)

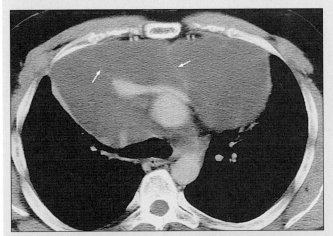

Figure 3. Lymphangioma in a 37-year-old man. Contrast-enhanced CT scan at the level of the brachiocephalic veins shows a predominantly anterior mediastinal cystic mass. The mass has homogeneous water attenuation and contains a few soft tissue septations (*arrows*). (*From Müller NL, Fraser RS, Colman NC, Paré PD: Radiologic Diagnosis of Diseases of the Chest. Philadelphia, WB Saunders, 2001.*)

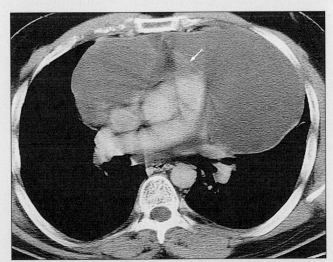

Figure 4. Lymphangioma in a 37-year-old man. Contrast-enhanced CT scan at the level of the main pulmonary artery shows a predominantly anterior mediastinal cystic mass. The mass has homogeneous water attenuation and contains a few soft tissue septations (*arrow*). (*From Müller NL, Fraser RS, Colman NC, Paré PD: Radiologic Diagnosis of Diseases of the Chest. Philadelphia, WB Saunders, 2001.*)

Parathyroid Adenoma

DEFINITION: A parathyroid adenoma is a benign tumor that may occur in an ectopic parathyroid gland situated in the anterior mediastinum or, less commoly, in the aortopulmonary window or paraesophageal region.

IMAGING

Radiography
Findings
- Usually normal

Utility
- Most lesions radiographically invisible

CT
Findings
- Usually range from 0.3-3.0 cm in diameter
- Homogeneous attenuation
- Minimal enhancement after intravenous administration of a contrast agent
- In upper anterior mediastinum, paraesophageal region, or aortopulmonary window

Utility
- May resemble a lymph node

MRI
Findings
- Hypointense or isointense relative to muscle on T1-weighted images and of high signal intensity on T2-weighted images
- Enhances after intravenous administration of gadolinium-based contrast agents

Utility
- Superior to CT in demonstrating parathyroid adenomas

Nuclear Medicine
Findings
- Positive uptake on technetium-99m sestamibi scintigraphy

Utility
- Optimally, technetium-99m sestamibi is combined with single-photon emission computed tomography (SPECT).
- One may include fast spin-echo MRI with sestamibi SPECT scintigraphy to improve spatial resolution.

CLINICAL PRESENTATION

- Hyperparathyroidism signs and symptoms: anorexia, weakness, fatigue, nausea, vomiting, constipation, and hypotonicity of muscles

DIAGNOSTIC PEARLS

- Small minimally enhancing anterior mediastinal nodule
- Hypointense or isointense to muscle on T1-weighted images and of high signal intensity on T2-weighted images
- Hyperparathyroidism signs and symptoms: anorexia, weakness, fatigue, nausea, vomiting, constipation, hypotonicity of muscles

DIFFERENTIAL DIAGNOSIS

- Anterior mediastinal lymph node
- Thymoma

PATHOLOGY

- Parathyroid glands migrate with thymus into mediastinum during embryonic development
- May be located in anterior mediastinum, aortopulmonary window, or paraesophageal region
- Nodule usually composed of a single cell type, most commonly chief cells, surrounded by fibrous capsule

INCIDENCE/PREVALENCE AND EPIDEMIOLOGY

- Approximately 10% of parathyroid glands ectopic
- Rare cause of anterior mediastinal mass
- Parathyroid adenoma usually suspected clinically

Suggested Readings

Lee VS, Spritzer CE, Coleman RE, et al: The complementary roles of fast spin-echo MR imaging and double-phase 99m Tc-sestamibi scintigraphy for localization of hyperfunctioning parathyroid glands. *AJR Am J Roentgenol* 167:1555-1562, 1996.

Seelos KC, DeMarco R, Clark OH, Higgins CB: Persistent and recurrent hyperparathyroidism: Assessment with gadopentetate dimeglumine-enhanced MR imaging. *Radiology* 177:373-378, 1990.

Smith JR, Oates ME: Radionuclide imaging of the parathyroid glands: Patterns, pearls, and pitfalls. *RadioGraphics* 24:1101-1115, 2004.

Udelsman R: Parathyroid imaging: The myth and the reality. *Radiology* 201:317-318, 1996.

WHAT THE REFERRING PHYSICIAN NEEDS TO KNOW

- Diagnosis can usually be made on basis of clinical and laboratory findings.
- Parathyroid adenomas may mimic lymph nodes on CT and MRI.
- Technetium-99m sestamibi scintigraphy and MRI are the imaging modalities of choice.

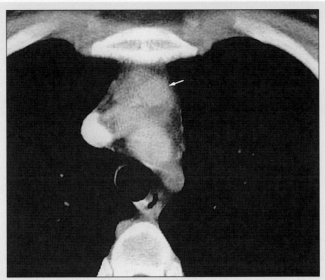

Figure 1. Mediastinal parathyroid adenoma. CT scan performed during intravenous administration of contrast material shows a poorly defined nodule (*arrow*) immediately anterior to the lower margin of the left brachiocephalic vein. (Contrast material can be seen in the right brachiocephalic vein.) The patient was a 30-year-old woman who had hyperparathyroidism. Surgical excision confirmed the lesion to be a parathyroid adenoma. (*From Müller NL, Fraser RS, Colman NC, Paré PD: Radiologic Diagnosis of Diseases of the Chest. Philadelphia, WB Saunders, 2001.*)

Pericardial Cyst

DEFINITION: A pericardial cyst is a mesothelial-lined cyst of the pericardium.

IMAGING

Radiography
Findings
- Focal opacity that obscures inferior cardiac border (cardiophrenic angle)

Utility
- Usually initial imaging modality used; lesion may be found incidentally
- If in unusual location, may be indistinguishable from bronchogenic or thymic cyst

Ultrasonography
Findings
- Characteristic appearance is usually of echo-free fluid with increased through-transmission.
- Occasionally, the presence of proteinaceous material may result in increased echogenicity.

Utility
- 2D and transesophageal echocardiography helpful in diagnosis

CT
Findings
- Well-circumscribed, nonenhancing, unilocular, uniform fluid-attenuation (0-20 Hounsfield units) mass
- Wall calcification seen rarely

Utility
- CT is most important imaging modality in assessment of anterior mediastinal masses.
- Diagnosis is usually readily made by characteristic fluid-filled cyst in cardiophrenic angle.
- Pericardial cyst in unusual location may be indistinguishable from bronchogenic cyst or thymic cyst.

MRI
Findings
- Homogeneous low signal intensity on T1-weighted images and high signal intensity on T2-weighted images

Utility
- Comparable to CT in the diagnosis of pericardial cysts

CLINICAL PRESENTATION

- Usually asymptomatic; found incidentally on chest radiograph or CT scan
- May result in atypical chest pain, dyspnea and cough.

DIAGNOSTIC PEARLS

- Cardiophrenic angle mass
- Uniformly homogeneous fluid attenuation
- Homogeneous cysts of low T1 signal intensity and high T2 signal intensity

DIFFERENTIAL DIAGNOSIS

- Thymic cyst
- Bronchogenic cyst
- Hydatid cyst

PATHOLOGY

- Congenital aberrant fusion of anterior pericardial recesses during early development
- May be acquired after cardiothoracic surgery
- Usually have thin smooth walls and no internal septa
- Cystic walls composed of connective tissue and single layer of mesothelial cells
- Contains serous fluid
- Occurs most commonly in the right cardiophrenic angle but may occur anywhere in the mediastinum

INCIDENCE/PREVALENCE AND EPIDEMIOLOGY

- Rare congenital abnormality of pericardium
- Approximately 1 per 100,000 persons

Suggested Readings

Patel J, Park C, Michaels J, et al: Pericardial cyst: Case reports and a literature review. *Echocardiography* 21:269-272, 2004.
Wang ZJ, Reddy GP, Gotway MB, et al: CT and MR imaging of pericardial disease. *RadioGraphics* 23(Spec No):S167-S180, 2003.

WHAT THE REFERRING PHYSICIAN NEEDS TO KNOW

- Confident diagnosis can usually be made on CT and MRI

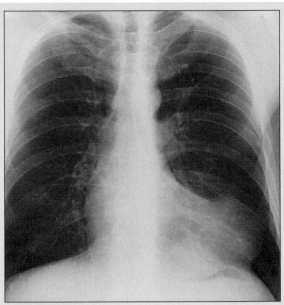

Figure 1. Pericardial cyst in a 46-year-old man. Posteroanterior chest radiograph shows smoothly marginated increased opacity in the left cardiophrenic angle. The diagnosis was confirmed at thoracotomy. (*From Müller NL, Fraser RS, Colman NC, Paré PD:* Radiologic Diagnosis of Diseases of the Chest. *Philadelphia, WB Saunders, 2001.*)

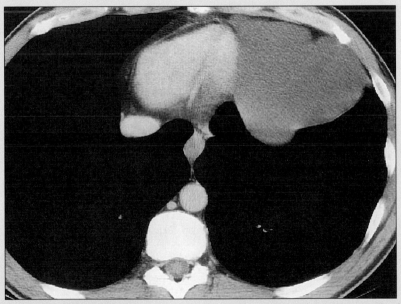

Figure 2. Pericardial cyst in a 46-year-old man. Contrast-enhanced CT scan shows a water-density cyst. The diagnosis was confirmed at thoracotomy. (*From Müller NL, Fraser RS, Colman NC, Paré PD:* Radiologic Diagnosis of Diseases of the Chest. *Philadelphia, WB Saunders, 2001.*)

Thyroid Masses

DEFINITION: Thyroid masses may extend into the anterior, middle, or posterior mediastinum.

IMAGING

Radiography
Findings
- Sharply defined neck or superior mediastinal mass
- Tracheal displacement and narrowing
- Middle mediastinal goiters: trachea displaced laterally, usually to the left
- Posterior mediastinal goiters: trachea displaced anteriorly

Utility
- May be found incidentally on chest radiography

CT
Findings
- Continuity with cervical thyroid
- Often containing foci of calcification
- Attenuation value of intrathoracic thyroid often greater than 100 Hounsfield units before administration of contrast material
- Enhances intensely and for prolonged period (> 2 minutes) after intravenous injection of a contrast agent
- Intense prolonged contrast enhancement
- Focal nonenhancing areas of low attenuation secondary to hemorrhage or cyst formation
- Most common cause: goiter, typically with sharply defined smooth margins
- Carcinoma: may have homogeneous or inhomogeneous attenuation and well-defined or poorly defined margins
- Cervical or mediastinal lymphadenopathy

Utility
- Superior to radiography for diagnosis and assessment of extent
- Thyroid carcinoma likely if evidence of spread into adjacent tissue or lymphadenopathy

Ultrasonography
Findings
- Enlarged thyroid gland or focal mass
- Increased or decreased echogenicity compared with the normal gland
- Cervical lymphadenopathy

Utility
- Important in workup of thyroid nodules and masses
- Imaging modality of choice to guide needle biopsy of thyroid lesions

Nuclear Medicine
Findings
- Increased uptake of iodine on ^{131}I scintigraphy

Utility
- Helpful in the staging of thyroid cancer and in the assessment of tumor recurrence

Positron Emission Tomography
Findings
- Increased uptake of FDG on PET in patients with thyroid cancer

Utility
- PET-CT helpful in staging of thyroid carcinoma and assessment of tumor recurrence
- Helpful mainly in patients with negative ^{131}I scintigraphy

CLINICAL PRESENTATION
- Intrathoracic goiter usually asymptomatic
- May have respiratory distress (worsened by certain neck movements)
- Hoarseness

DIFFERENTIAL DIAGNOSIS
- Thymoma
- Germ cell tumor: Teratoma
- Thymic carcinoma
- Lymphoma

PATHOLOGY
- Multinodular goiter, thyroiditis, or thyroid carcinoma
- Arise from lower pole or isthmus and extend into anterior or middle mediastinum (80%)

WHAT THE REFERRING PHYSICIAN NEEDS TO KNOW
- CT is most important imaging modality in assessment of mediastinal masses.
- Ultrasonography is the imaging modality of choice to guide needle biopsy of thyroid lesions

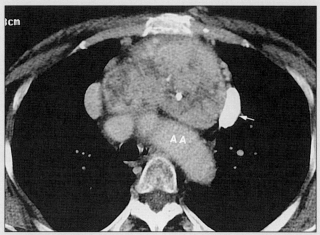

Figure 1. Multinodular goiter. CT scan performed during intravenous administration of contrast material shows a large anterior mediastinal mass that has inhomogeneous attenuation and contains small foci of calcification. The mass lies anterior to the aortic arch (AA) and innominate artery and displaces the left brachiocephalic vein (*arrow*). The patient was a 67-year-old woman with long-standing multinodular goiter. (*From Müller NL, Fraser RS, Colman NC, Paré PD:* Radiologic Diagnosis of Diseases of the Chest. *Philadelphia, WB Saunders, 2001.*)

- Remainder arise from posterior aspect of either thyroid lobe and extend into posterior aspect of mediastinum behind the trachea

INCIDENCE/PREVALENCE AND EPIDEMIOLOGY

- Most common mediastinal thyroid mass is multinodular goiter.
- Diagnosis noted most commonly in women in their 40s.
- Approximately 80% of mediastinal thyroid tumors arise from lower pole or isthmus and extend into anterior or middle mediastinum.

Suggested Readings

Hegedüs L: Clinical practice: The thyroid nodule. *N Engl J Med* 351:1764-1771, 2004.

Hoang JK, Lee WK, Lee M, et al: US Features of thyroid malignancy: Pearls and pitfalls. *RadioGraphics* 27:847-860, 2007; discussion 861–865.

Imhof H, Czerny C, Hörmann M, Krestan C: Tumors and tumor-like lesions of the neck: From childhood to adult. *Eur Radiol* 14(Suppl 4):L155-L165, 2004.

Wang TS, Cheng DW, Udelsman R: Contemporary imaging for thyroid cancer. *Surg Oncol Clin North Am* 16:431-445, 2007.

Weber AL, Randolph G, Aksoy FG: The thyroid and parathyroid glands: CT and MR imaging and correlation with pathology and clinical findings. *Radiol Clin North Am* 38:1105-1129, 2000.

Part 63

MIDDLE AND POSTERIOR MEDIASTINAL MASSES

Unilateral Hilar Lymphadenopathy

DEFINITION: Unilateral lymph node enlargement exists when these nodes have a short-axis diameter >10 mm.

IMAGING

Radiography
Findings
- Unilateral hilar lymphadenopathy
- Increased size and opacity of the hilum and a lobulated contour

Utility
- First and often only imaging modality used

CT
Findings
- Unilateral hilar lymphadenopathy is evident.
- Enlarged nodes may have homogeneous or inhomogeneous appearance and be hypoattenuating or show diffuse or rim enhancement after intravenous administration of a contrast agent.
- Rim enhancement and a low-attenuation center are seen most commonly in patients with tuberculosis.
- The hilar lymph nodes include the peribronchial and bronchopulmonary lymph nodes (stations 10 and 11 in the American Thoracic Society classification)

Utility
- Superior to radiography in demonstrating presence of lymphadenopathy and associated findings
- Hilar nodes best seen after intravenous administration of a contrast agent

MRI
Findings
- Unilateral hilar lymphadenopathy

Utility
- Similar to CT in demonstrating presence of enlarged hilar nodes
- Advantage over CT: lack of radiation or need for a contrast agent

DIAGNOSTIC PEARLS

- Increased size and opacity of the hilum
- Lobulated contour of the hilum
- Short-axis diameter greater than 10 mm on CT
- Common causes: pulmonary carcinoma, tuberculosis, bacterial pneumonia, lymphoma

Positron Emission Tomography
Findings
- Increased FDG uptake

Utility
- Superior to CT and MRI in distinguishing benign from malignant lymphadenopathy
- Limited specificity

CLINICAL PRESENTATION

- The condition is asymptomatic, or symptoms related to an underlying cause are noted.
- Weight loss, cough, and hemoptysis are suggestive of pulmonary carcinoma.
- Fever and night sweats are suggestive of infection (tuberculosis, histoplasmosis, coccidioidomycosis).

PATHOLOGY

- Mediastinal and hilar lymph nodes are considered enlarged when their short-axis diameter is > 10 mm.
- Neoplastic causes include pulmonary carcinoma, lymphoma, metastasis from kidney, breast, head and neck tumor.
- Infectious causes include tuberculosis, histoplasmosis, coccidioidomycosis, and bacterial pneumonia.

WHAT THE REFERRING PHYSICIAN NEEDS TO KNOW

- Once mediastinal or hilar abnormality is detected or suspected on the chest radiograph, cross-sectional imaging is performed.
- Contrast-enhanced CT is the imaging modality of choice in the assessment of hilar lymphadenopathy and associated findings in adults.
- Unilateral hilar lymphadenopathy is most commonly due to neoplasm (pulmonary carcinoma, lymphoma, or metastasis from kidney, breast, or head and neck tumor).
- Association is also common with infection (e.g., tuberculosis, histoplasmosis, coccidioidomycosis, bacterial pneumonia, lung abscess).

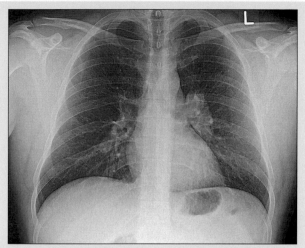

Figure 1. **Chest radiograph shows increased size and lobulated contour of the left hilum.** The patients was a 33-year-old man with primary tuberculosis.

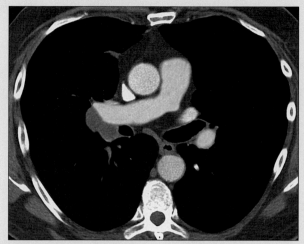

Figure 2. **Contrast-enhanced CT demonstrates enlarged right hilar lymph nodes.** The patient was a 64-year-old man with pulmonary carcinoma.

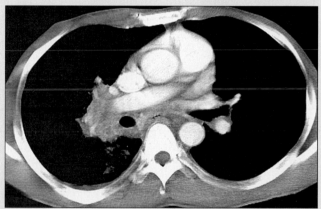

Figure 3. **Unilateral hilar lymphadenopathy in a patient with AIDS and tuberculosis.** Contrast-enhanced CT image shows hypodense right hilar lymphadenopathy. (*Courtesy of Dr. Joel E. Fishman University of Miami, Miami, Florida*)

- Infectious granulomas: lymphadenopathy tends to be unilateral.
- Tuberculosis: lymph node enlargement is on side of lung disease, but involvement of contralateral nodes is not rare.

INCIDENCE/PREVALENCE AND EPIDEMIOLOGY

- Unilateral hilar lymphadenopathy is most commonly due to neoplasm (pulmonary carcinoma, lymphoma, or metastasis from kidney, breast, or head and neck tumor).
- Association is also common with infection (e.g., tuberculosis, histoplasmosis, coccidioidomycosis, bacterial pneumonia, lung abscess).

- Unilateral hilar lymphadenopathy is particularly common in primary tuberculosis and tuberculosis associated with AIDS.

Suggested Readings

Boiselle PM, Patz EF Jr, Vining DJ, et al: Imaging of mediastinal lymph nodes: CT, MR, and FDG PET. *RadioGraphics* 18:1061-1069, 1998.

Müller NL, Webb WR: Radiographic imaging of the pulmonary hila. *Invest Radiol* 20:661-671, 1985.

Sharma A, Fidias P, Hayman LA, et al: Patterns of lymphadenopathy in thoracic malignancies. *RadioGraphics* 24:419-434, 2004.

Bilateral Hilar Lymphadenopathy

DEFINITION: Bilateral hilar lymphadenopathy exists when these lymph nodes have a short-axis diameter >10 mm.

IMAGING

Radiography
Findings
- Bilateral symmetric or asymmetric hilar lymph node enlargement is evident.
- Enlarged nodes result in lobulation and increased size and opacity of the hila.
- Symmetric hilar lymphadenopathy in a patient without systemic symptoms is most suggestive of sarcoidosis.
- Asymmetric hilar lymphadenopathy or presence of systemic symptoms (fever, night sweats) should raise the suspicion of lymphoma or another neoplasm.
- Stage I sarcoidosis is symmetric bilateral hilar and mediastinal lymph node enlargement without parenchymal abnormality.
- Stage II sarcoidosis is symmetric bilateral hilar and mediastinal lymph node enlargement plus parenchymal abnormality.
Utility
- Usually first imaging modality used

CT
Findings
- Bilateral symmetric or asymmetric hilar lymph node enlargement
- Mediastinal lymph node enlargement commonly present
- Short-axis diameter > 10 mm
- The hilar lymph nodes include the peribronchial and bronchopulmonary lymph nodes (stations 10 and 11 in the American Thoracic Society classification)
Utility
- CT is superior to radiography in demonstrating presence of hilar lymphadenopathy and associated findings.
- Slightly enlarged nodes are best seen after intravenous contrast agent administration.

DIAGNOSTIC PEARLS
- Sarcoidosis: symmetric bilateral hilar and mediastinal lymphadenopathy in young adults with no systemic symptoms
- Common causes of bilateral symmetric hilar lymphadenopathy: sarcoidosis, lymphoma, metastases (renal cell carcinoma, testicular tumor), and silicosis
- Common causes of bilateral asymmetric hilar lymphadenophathy: lymphoma, sarcoidosis, and metastases (renal cell carcinoma, testicular tumor, breast cancer, pulmonary carcinoma)

MRI
Findings
- Bilateral hilar lymph node enlargement
Utility
- Comparable to CT in the assessment of hilar and mediastinal lymphadenopathy

Positron Emission Tomography
Findings
- Increased FDG uptake
Utility
- Superior to CT and MRI in distinguishing benign from malignant lymphadenopathy

CLINICAL PRESENTATION

- Thirty percent to 50% of patients with sarcoidosis are asymptomatic, with sarcoidosis being first suspected based on the presence of bilateral hilar lymphadenopathy on routine chest radiographs.
- Common symptoms in sarcoidosis include dyspnea, cough, and chest pain.
- Patients with lymphoma usually present with systemic symptoms, including fever, night sweats, and weight loss.

WHAT THE REFERRING PHYSICIAN NEEDS TO KNOW
- Symmetric hilar lymphadenopathy in patient without systemic symptoms is most suggestive of sarcoidosis.
- Asymmetric hilar lymphadenopathy or presence of systemic symptoms (fever, night sweats) should raise suspicion of lymphoma or another neoplasm or infection.
- CT and MRI are comparable in the assessment of hilar and mediastinal lymphadenopathy.
- In clinical practice, contrast-enhanced CT is usually performed to further evaluate presence and extent of lymphadenopathy.
- PET, particularly when combined with CT (PET-CT), is superior to CT and MRI in the staging of carcinoma and lymphoma.

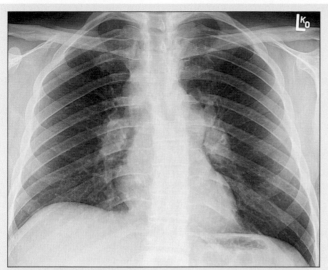

Figure 1. **Stage I sarcoidosis.** Posteroanterior chest radiograph in a 33-year-old man with sarcoidosis shows right paratracheal, aortopulmonary window, and symmetric bilateral hilar lymph node enlargement.

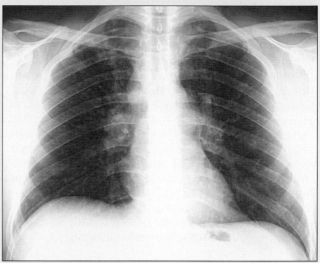

Figure 2. **Stage II sarcoidosis.** Posteroanterior chest radiograph in a 35-year-old man with sarcoidosis demonstrates right paratracheal, aortopulmonary window, and symmetric bilateral hilar lymph node enlargement and small round and irregular opacities in the upper zones. Note medial deviation of the gastric bubble due to splenomegaly.

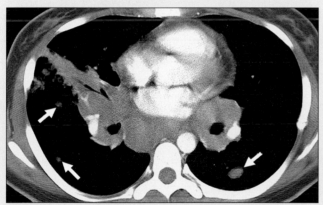

Figure 3. **Mixed cellularity Hodgkin disease in a 20-year-old woman.** CT scan obtained at level of basal trunk demonstrates extensive bilateral hilar nodal enlargement. Also note multiple pulmonary nodules (*arrows*) and right middle lobe consolidation. (*Courtesy of Dr. Kyung Soo Lee, Seoul, Korea*)

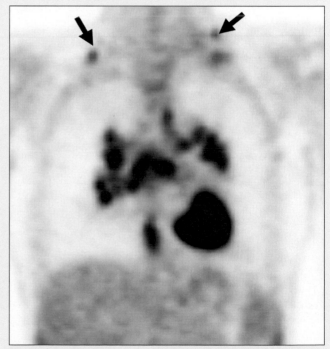

Figure 4. **Nodular sclerosing Hodgkin disease in a 25-year-old woman.** PET scan demonstrates increased FDG uptake in mediastinal and hilar nodes bilaterally. Also note FDG uptake in bilateral supraclavicular and left lower neck nodes (*arrows*), which were not identified on conventional staging methods. (*Courtesy of Dr. Kyung Soo Lee, Seoul, Korea*)

PATHOLOGY

- Most common cause of bilateral symmetric hilar lymphadenopathy is sarcoidosis.
- Other causes include Hodgkin and non-Hodgkin lymphoma, metastases (renal cell carcinoma, testicular tumor, breast cancer), cystic fibrosis, and silicosis.
- Common causes of bilateral asymmetric lymphadenopathy include Hodgkin and non-Hodgkin lymphoma, sarcoidosis, and metastases (pulmonary carcinoma, renal cell carcinoma, testicular tumor, breast cancer).
- Less common causes of bilateral hilar lymphadenopathy include leukemia, multicentric giant lymph node hyperplasia (Castleman disease), granulomatous infection (tuberculosis, histoplasmosis), and Löfgren syndrome (triad of bilateral hilar lymphadenopathy, erythema nodosum, polyarticular arthralgia).

INCIDENCE/PREVALENCE AND EPIDEMIOLOGY

- Most common cause of bilateral symmetric hilar lymphadenopathy is sarcoidosis.

- Common causes of bilateral asymmetric lymphadenopathy include Hodgkin and non-Hodgkin lymphoma, leukemia, sarcoidosis, and metastases (pulmonary carcinoma, renal cell carcinoma, testicular tumor, breast cancer).
- Less common causes of bilateral hilar lymphadenopathy include leukemia, multicentric giant lymph node hyperplasia (Castleman disease), and granulomatous infection (tuberculosis, histoplasmosis)

Suggested Readings

Boiselle PM, Patz EF Jr, Vining DJ, et al: Imaging of mediastinal lymph nodes: CT, MR, and FDG PET. *RadioGraphics* 18:1061-1069, 1998.

Müller NL, Webb WR: Radiographic imaging of the pulmonary hila. *Invest Radiol* 20:661-671, 1985.

Nunes H, Brillet PY, Valeyre D, et al: Imaging in sarcoidosis. *Semin Respir Crit Care Med* 28:102-120, 2007.

Sharma A, Fidias P, Hayman LA, et al: Patterns of lymphadenopathy in thoracic malignancies. *RadioGraphics* 24:419-434, 2004.

Mediastinal Lymphadenopathy

DEFINITION: Mediastinal lymphadenopathy exists when mediastinal lymph nodes have a short-axis diameter >10 mm.

IMAGING

Radiography

Findings
- Widening of paratracheal stripe
- Increased opacity and a convexity in the region of superior vena cava
- Increased opacity and a convexity in the region of aortopulmonary window
- Increased opacity and a convexity in the subcarinal region
- Mediastinal widening

Utility
- Radiography is often the initial imaging modality performed in patients with suspected hilar or mediastinal lymphadenopathy, although it is of limited accuracy in the diagnosis of mediastinal lymphadenopathy.
- Symmetric bilateral hilar and mediastinal lymphadenopathy in young adults with no systemic symptoms is suggestive of sarcoidosis.
- Asymmetric bilateral hilar and mediastinal lymphadenopathy in patients with systemic symptoms is suggestive of lymphoma or metastases.

CT

Findings
- Enlarged mediastinal nodes, short-axis diameter > 10 mm
- Sarcoidosis: symmetric bilateral hilar and mediastinal lymphadenopathy
- Lymphoma or metastasis: asymmetric lymphadenopathy
- Severe infection, fibrosing mediastinitis, aggressive neoplasm: poor definition of lymph node margins and obscuration of adjacent fat
- Granulomatous infections: foci of necrosis or calcification
- Tuberculosis, fungal infection, metastasis from bronchogenic carcinoma, lymphoma: low attenuation after intravenous administration of a contrast agent
- Giant lymph node hyperplasia (Castleman disease): marked enhancement of single enlarged mediastinal lymph node group

Utility
- Once mediastinal or hilar abnormality is detected/suspected on chest radiograph, cross-sectional imaging is usually performed.
- CT is used to assess the location and extent of the findings.

DIAGNOSTIC PEARLS

- Enlarged mediastinal lymph nodes
- Sarcoidosis: symmetric bilateral hilar and mediastinal lymphadenopathy in young adults with no systemic symptoms
- Lymphoma or metastasis: asymmetric lymphadenopathy with systemic symptoms
- Severe infection, fibrosing mediastinitis, aggressive neoplasm: poor definition of lymph node margins and obscuration of adjacent fat

- Symmetric bilateral hilar and mediastinal lymphadenopathy in young adults with no systemic symptoms is suggestive of sarcoidosis.
- Asymmetric bilateral hilar and mediastinal lymphadenopathy in patients with systemic symptoms is suggestive of lymphoma or metastases.

MRI

Findings
- Enlarged mediastinal lymph nodes

Utility
- Used to assess the location and extent of the findings
- Comparable to CT in the assessment of mediastinal lymphadenopathy

Positron Emission Tomography

Findings
- Increased uptake on FDG-PET

Utility
- FDG-PET relies on increased metabolic rate of neoplastic cells and is superior to CT and MRI in distinguishing malignant from benign nodes.
- Increased uptake (false-positive diagnosis) may also occur with active inflammation or infection.
- False-negative diagnosis occurs mainly in small nodes.
- Integrated PET/CT is superior to CT or PET.

CLINICAL PRESENTATION

- Asymptomatic or nonspecific symptoms of fever, malaise, and weight loss

---

WHAT THE REFERRING PHYSICIAN NEEDS TO KNOW

- CT is the imaging modality of choice to assess the presence and extent of mediastinal lymphadenopathy.
- Mediastinal lymph nodes are considered enlarged when their short-axis diameter is > 10 mm on CT.
- CT and MRI assess mainly lymph node size; they are of limited value in distinguishing malignant from benign lymph node enlargement.
- Integrated PET/CT is superior to CT or MRI in distinguishing benign from malignant lymph nodes.
- PET/CT is of limited value in distinguishing enlarged lymph nodes due to active infection from malignancy.

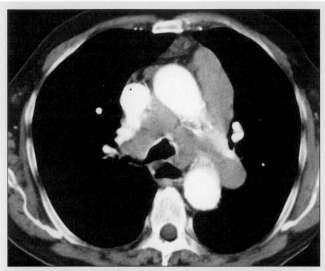

Figure 1. Middle and posterior mediastinal lymphadenopathy. Contrast-enhanced CT image shows enlarged lymph nodes in the paratracheal, prevascular, and subcarinal spaces. Hilar nodes are also evident. The patient was a 67-year-old woman with chronic lymphocytic leukemia.

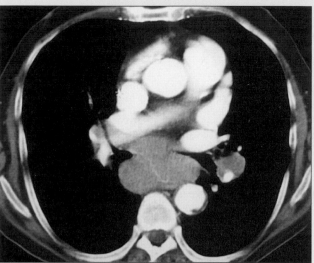

Figure 2. Middle and posterior mediastinal lymphadenopathy. Same patient as in Figure 1. Contrast-enhanced CT image shows enlarged lymph nodes in the paratracheal, prevascular, and subcarinal spaces. Hilar nodes are also evident. The patient was a 67-year-old woman with chronic lymphocytic leukemia.

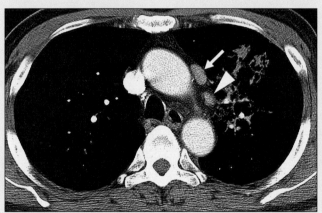

Figure 3. True positive integrated PET/CT in a 70-year-old man with adenocarcinoma of lung. Contrast-enhanced CT scan shows enlarged lymph nodes in para-aortic (station 6, *arrow*) and subaortic (station 5, *arrowhead*) areas. Also note obstructive atelectasis in left upper lobe. (*Courtesy of Dr. Kyung Soo Lee, Seoul, Korea*)

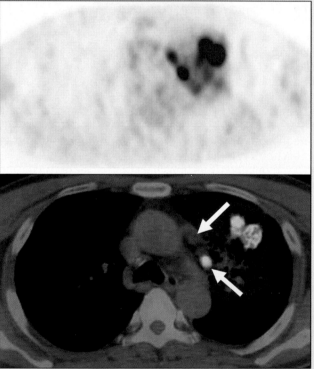

Figure 4. True positive integrated PET/CT in a 70-year-old man with adenocarcinoma of lung. Same patient as in Figure 3. PET and integrated PET/CT show increased FDG uptake (maximum standardized uptake value, 11.5) in enlarged nodes (*arrows*) as well as primary lung cancer. The patient had surgically confirmed lymph node metastases. (*Courtesy of Dr. Kyung Soo Lee, Seoul, Korea*)

PATHOLOGY

- Mediastinal lymph nodes are considered enlarged when their short-axis diameter is > 10 mm.
- Common causes of enlarged mediastinal lymph nodes include lymphoma, metastases, granulomatous infections, and sarcoidosis.
- Mediastinal lymph nodes can also be involved in patients with leukemia, particularly lymphocytic leukemia.
- Primary malignancies that commonly metastasize to intrathoracic lymph nodes include tumors of head and neck, genitourinary tract, and breast and malignant melanoma.
- Metastases are frequently accompanied by lymphangitic or hematogenous spread to the lungs.
- Involvement of the anterior and posterior mediastinal lymph nodes is unusual in the absence of middle mediastinal lymphadenopathy.
- Lymph nodes may be separated by fat or may conglomerate into multiple large masses.

INCIDENCE/PREVALENCE AND EPIDEMIOLOGY

- Enlarged lymph nodes are one of the most frequent causes of mediastinal masses.

- Up to 85% of patients with Hodgkin lymphoma present with mediastinal lymph node enlargement (prevascular, paratracheal, hilar, subcarinal node groups).
- Extension of the nodal disease to the lungs occurs in approximately 10% of patients.
- Involvement of a single lymph node group, usually the prevascular and/or pretracheal, is much more common in patients with non-Hodgkin lymphoma.
- Mediastinal lymph nodes are involved in 60%-90% of patients with sarcoidosis.

Suggested Readings

Boiselle PM, Patz EF Jr, Vining DJ, et al: Imaging of mediastinal lymph nodes: CT, MR, and FDG PET. *RadioGraphics* 18:1061-1069, 1998.

de Langen AJ, Raijmakers P, Riphagen I, et al: The size of mediastinal lymph nodes and its relation with metastatic involvement: A meta-analysis. *Eur J Cardiothorac Surg* 29:26-29, 2006.

Dooms C, Vansteenkiste J: Positron emission tomography in non–small cell lung cancer. *Curr Opin Pulm Med* 13:256-260, 2007.

Schrevens L, Lorent N, Dooms C, Vansteenkiste J: The role of PET scan in diagnosis, staging, and management of non-small cell lung cancer. *Oncologist* 9:633-643, 2004.

Sharma A, Fidias P, Hayman LA, et al: Patterns of lymphadenopathy in thoracic malignancies. *RadioGraphics* 24:419-434, 2004.

Azygos and Hemiazygos Veins: Normal and Abnormal Findings

DEFINITION: The azygos and hemiazygos veins may become dilated in heart failure, obstruction of the superior vena cava, interruption of the inferior vena cava, and portal hypertension.

IMAGING

Radiography
Findings
- Azygos vein is normally seen as an elliptical opacity in the region of the right tracheobronchial angle.
- Transverse diameter of azygos vein at right tracheobronchial angle level is normally < 10 mm in upright position and < 15 mm in supine position.
- Dilation of the azygos vein results in increased diameter of opacity in right tracheobronchial angle.

Utility
- Abnormality often first seen on chest radiograph

CT
Findings
- Dilation of azygos vein
- Enlargement of arch of azygos vein
- Enlargement of paraspinal portions of azygos and hemiazygos veins
- Enlargement of retrocrural portions of these veins in absence of definable inferior vena cava

Utility
- Superior to radiograph in demonstrating dilation of azygos and hemiazygos vein and underlying cause

CLINICAL PRESENTATION

- May be asymptomatic
- If symptoms are present, these are related to the underlying cause, including heart failure, portal hypertension, and obstruction of superior vena cava

PATHOLOGY

- Dilation of azygos and hemiazygos veins is classically associated with anomalies of the inferior vena cava.
- Inferior vena cava interruption is evident with azygos and hemiazygos continuation.

DIAGNOSTIC PEARLS

- Round mass along right mediastinal border just above the hilum on the radiograph
- Enlargement of the arch of the azygos vein
- Enlargement of the paraspinal portions of the azygos and hemiazygos veins
- Associated abnormalities such as left heart failure, obstruction of the superior vena cava, interruption of the inferior vena cava, or portal hypertension

- Heart failure, portal hypertension, and obstruction of superior vena cava are other causes of hemiazygos and azygos veins dilation.

INCIDENCE/PREVALENCE AND EPIDEMIOLOGY

- Most common cause: heart failure
- Other causes: interruption of the inferior vena cava with azygos and hemiazygos continuation, portal hypertension, obstruction of the superior vena cava

Suggested Readings

Bass JE, Redwine MD, Kramer LA, et al: Spectrum of congenital anomalies of the inferior vena cava: Cross-sectional imaging findings. *RadioGraphics* 20:639-652, 2000.
Lawler LP, Corl FM, Fishman EK: Multi-detector row and volume-rendered CT of the normal and accessory flow pathways of the thoracic systemic and pulmonary veins. *RadioGraphics* 22(Spec No):S45-S60, 2002.
McComb BL: The chest in profile. *J Thorac Imaging* 17:58-69, 2002.
Ravenel JG, Erasmus JJ: Azygoesophageal recess. *J Thorac Imaging* 17:219-226, 2002.

WHAT THE REFERRING PHYSICIAN NEEDS TO KNOW

- Dilation of the azygos vein is a common finding in right-sided heart failure.
- Other causes: interruption of the inferior vena cava with azygos and hemiazygos continuation, portal hypertension, obstruction of the superior vena cava.

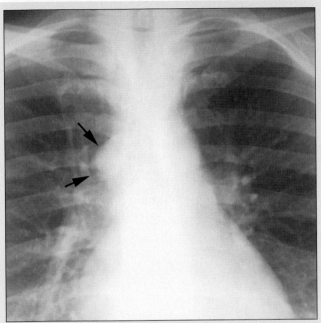

Figure 1. Azygos continuation of the inferior vena cava. A close-up view of the chest from a posteroanterior radiograph shows dilation of the azygos vein (*arrows*). The patient was an asymptomatic 48-year-old man. (*Courtesy of Dr. Tomás Franquet, Barcelona, Spain*)

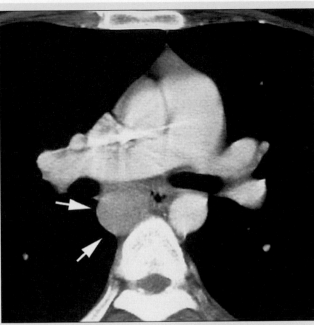

Figure 2. Azygos continuation of the inferior vena cava. In the same patient, CT image at the level of right pulmonary artery shows markedly dilated azygos vein (*arrows*). The patient was an asymptomatic 48-year-old man. (*Courtesy of Dr. Tomás Franquet, Barcelona, Spain*)

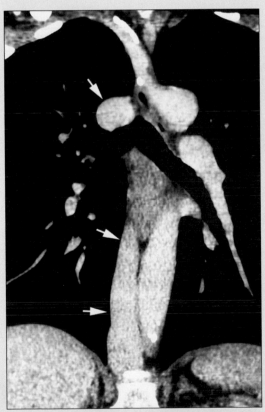

Figure 3. Azygos continuation of the inferior vena cava. In the same patient, coronal reformatted image of a contrast-enhanced CT scan shows a dilated azygos vein (*arrows*). Note that the azygos vein is as large as the descending aorta. The patient was an asymptomatic 48-year-old man. (*Courtesy of Dr. Tomás Franquet, Barcelona, Spain*)

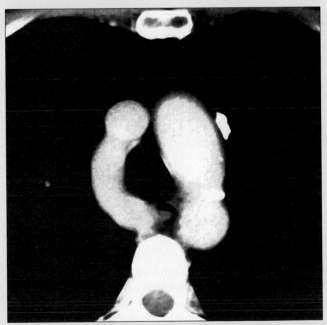

Figure 4. Azygos continuation of the inferior vena cava. In the same patient, contrast-enhanced CT scan shows enlargement of the azygos arch. The patient was an asymptomatic 48-year-old man. (*Courtesy of Dr. Tomás Franquet, Barcelona, Spain*)

Congenital Anomalies of Aorta

DEFINITION: Anomalous development of the aortic arch can result in a variety of anatomic variations that encircle the trachea or esophagus.

IMAGING

Radiography

Findings

- Aberrant right subclavian artery may result in obliquely oriented soft tissue density extending superiorly to right from superior margin of aortic arch.
- Proximal portion of aberrant artery frequently is dilated (diverticulum of Kommerell).
- Absence of left aortic arch and well-defined soft tissue opacity in right paratracheal region is consistent with right aortic arch.
- Focal opacity in retrotracheal space can obscure upper aspect of aortic arch.
- Double aortic arch results in a right paratracheal mass-like opacity with focal tracheal impression.

Utility

- Congenital anomalies of aorta in adults are often first suspected because of abnormal findings on radiography.
- Radiography often allows confident diagnosis of right aortic arch but is of limited value in diagnosis of other aortic and great vessel anomalies.

CT Angiography

Findings

- Congenital anomalies and associated anomalies of the great vessels
- Aberrant right subclavian artery
- Anomalous left subclavian artery
- Right-sided aortic arch

Utility

- Useful in confirming diagnosis and identifying associated abnormalities or complications

MRI

Findings

- Congenital anomalies and associated anomalies of the great vessels
- Right and left aortic arches

Utility

- Useful in confirming diagnosis and identifying associated abnormalities or complications
- Recommended over CT in younger patients because of lack of radiation

DIAGNOSTIC PEARLS

- Double aortic arch: right paratracheal mass-like opacity with focal tracheal impression on radiograph
- Absence of left aortic arch and well-defined soft tissue opacity in right paratracheal region consistent with right aortic arch on radiograph
- Proximal portion of the aberrant artery frequently dilated (diverticulum of Kommerell)
- Diagnosis can be confirmed with CT or MRI

Ultrasonography

Findings

- Double aortic arch

Utility

- Surface echocardiography is diagnostic imaging modality of choice in infancy and childhood for double aortic arch.

CLINICAL PRESENTATION

- Congenital anomalies of the aorta seen in adults are often asymptomatic.
- Vascular rings can produce symptoms (stridor, wheezing, dysphagia) due to tracheal or esophageal compression.
- Double aortic arch manifests in infancy as respiratory distress of difficulty in feeding due to esophageal and tracheal compression.

DIFFERENTIAL DIAGNOSIS

- Mediastinal mass
- Lymphadenopathy

PATHOLOGY

- Aberrant right subclavian artery arises from posterior portion of aortic arch and crosses mediastinum obliquely from left to right, posterior to esophagus and trachea.
- Right-sided aortic arch with an aberrant left subclavian artery is seldom associated with congenital heart disease.

WHAT THE REFERRING PHYSICIAN NEEDS TO KNOW

- Most congenital anomalies of the aorta seen in adults are asymptomatic.
- Diagnosis can be confirmed with CT or MRI.
- MRI is recommended particularly in young adults and children because radiation exposure is avoided.

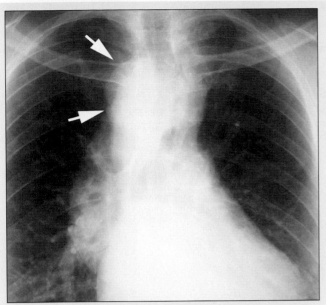

Figure 1. **Right-sided aortic arch with aberrant left subclavian artery in a 58-year-old man.** Posteroanterior chest radiograph shows a right-sided thoracic aorta (*arrows*). *(From Franquet T, Erasmus JJ, Giménez A, et al: The retrotracheal space:Normal anatomic and pathologic appearances. RadioGraphics 22:S231-S246, 2002.)*

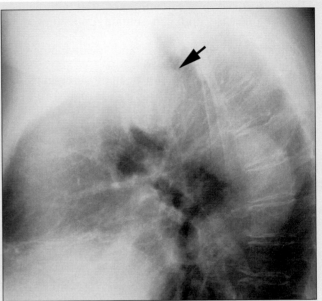

Figure 2. **Right-sided aortic arch with aberrant left subclavian artery in a 58-year-old man.** In the same patient as Figure 1, lateral chest radiograph shows an aberrant left subclavian artery as a mass-like area of increased opacity in the retrotracheal space (*arrow*). *(From Franquet T, Erasmus JJ, Giménez A, et al: The retrotracheal space: Normal anatomic and pathologic appearances. RadioGraphics 22:S231-S246, 2002.)*

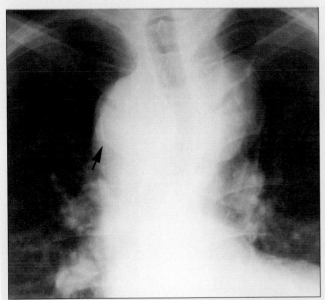

Figure 3. **Double aortic arch incidentally discovered in an asymptomatic 58-year-old man.** Frontal chest radiograph reveals bilateral paratracheal masses that represent the double aortic arch. Note focal wall calcification in the right-sided aortic arch (*arrow*). *(From Franquet T, Erasmus JJ, Giménez A, et al: The retrotracheal space: Normal anatomic and pathologic appearances. RadioGraphics 22:S231-S246, 2002.)*

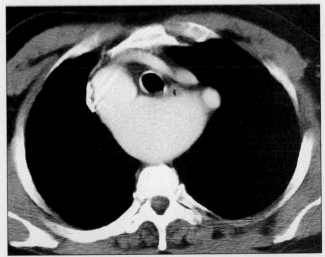

Figure 4. **Right-sided aortic arch with aberrant left subclavian artery in a 58-year-old man.** In the same patient as Figure 1, contrast-enhanced CT reveals the origin of the anomalous left subclavian artery. *(From Franquet T, Erasmus JJ, Giménez A, et al: The retrotracheal space: Normal anatomic and pathologic appearances. RadioGraphics 22:S231-S246, 2002.)*

- Double aortic arch is seldom associated with congenital heart disease and can remain undiagnosed into adulthood.
- Right arch is usually larger and located higher and more posteriorly than left arch.
- Arches join posteriorly to form single descending aorta that is typically left sided.
- Aneurysmal dilation of vascular rings may occur in adults.

INCIDENCE/PREVALENCE AND EPIDEMIOLOGY

- Most common aortic arch anomaly is right subclavian artery originating from an otherwise normal left-sided aortic arch.
- Left aortic arch with an aberrant right subclavian artery occurs in approximately 1% of the population.

- Most common right-sided aortic arch anomaly is right aortic arch with an aberrant left subclavian artery, with an incidence of 0.05%.
- Double aortic arch is one of the most common symptomatic arch anomalies.

Suggested Readings

Bisset GS 3rd, Strife JL, Kirks DR, Bailey WW: Vascular rings: MR imaging. *AJR Am J Roentgenol* 149:251-256, 1987.

Lowe GM, Donaldson JS, Backer CL: Vascular rings: 10-year review of imaging. *RadioGraphics* 11:637-646, 1991.

Steiner RM, Gross GW, Flicker S, et al: Congenital heart disease in the adult patient: The value of plain film chest radiology. *J Thorac Imaging* 10:1-25, 1995.

VanDyke CW, White RD: Congenital abnormalities of the thoracic aorta presenting in the adult. *J Thorac Imaging* 9:230-245, 1994.

Aortic Aneurysm

DEFINITION: Irreversible dilation of the aorta that involves all three wall layers.

IMAGING

Radiography
Findings
- Aneurysms of ascending aorta and proximal aortic arch project anteriorly and to the right.
- Aneurysms of distal arch and descending aorta project posteriorly and to the left.
- Mass that is contiguous with any part of aorta is suggestive of an aneurysm.

Utility
- Differentiation of elongated and tortuous aorta from aneurysm is not always possible by chest radiography.

CT
Findings
- Focal or diffuse dilation of aorta

Utility
- CT is the most commonly used technique to diagnose aortic aneurysms and usually the only imaging modality required before surgery.
- Contrast-enhanced CT allows accurate assessment of presence and extent of aneurysm, its relationship to adjacent structures, and presence of complications.

MRI
Findings
- Dilation of aorta
- Aneurysm

Utility
- Comparable to CT in diagnosis of aortic aneurysms

CLINICAL PRESENTATION

- Aortic aneurysm is often asymptomatic.
- Clinical presentation of aortic disease varies according to size of aneurysms and part of involved aorta.
- Most common presenting complaint is chest pain.
- Symptoms of aneurysms of transverse arch result from compression of superior vena cava, recurrent laryngeal nerve, or tracheobronchial tree.

DIAGNOSTIC PEARLS

- On the chest radiograph, aneurysms of ascending aorta and proximal aortic arch project anteriorly and to the right.
- On the chest radiograph, aneurysms of distal arch and descending aorta project posteriorly and to the left.
- The diameter of the aorta increases with age. Therefore, a 4.2 cm ascending aorta in a 35-year-old is aneurysmal but normal in an 80-year-old.
- Range of normal diameters: ascending aorta 2.4-4.7 cm, proximal descending aorta 1.6-3.7 cm, distal descending aorta 1.4-3.3 cm

- Aneurysms of descending aorta may cause bony erosion, leading to severe pain.
- Most serious complication of aneurysm of thoracic aorta is death from rupture.

DIFFERENTIAL DIAGNOSIS

- Aortitis
- Aortic dissection
- Congenital anomalies of aorta
- Atherosclerosis
- Cystic medial necrosis
- Trauma

PATHOLOGY

- Irreversible dilation of aorta involves all three wall layers.
- It may result from atherosclerosis, cystic medial necrosis, or, rarely, infection (mycotic aneurysm).
- Cystic medial degeneration can be idiopathic or associated with connective tissue disorder such as Marfan syndrome or Ehlers-Danlos syndrome.
- Risk of rupture rises with increasing aneurysm size.

WHAT THE REFERRING PHYSICIAN NEEDS TO KNOW

- Aortic aneurysm should be considered in the differential diagnosis for any mass that is contiguous with any part of aorta.
- Aneurysms of aorta may result in anterior, middle, or posterior mediastinal mass-like opacities on chest radiography.
- Diagnosis can be readily made on CT or MRI.
- Because of the variable size of the aorta and because surgery is seldom contemplated for aortas of smaller size, for practical purposes aortic aneurysm may be considered present when the aorta measures ≥ 5 cm in diameter.

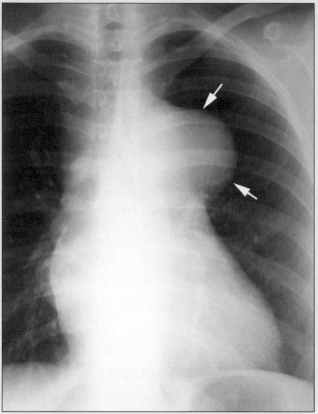

Figure 1. Aortic aneurysm in a 45-year-old man with Takayasu arteritis. Posteroanterior chest radiograph shows a large well-defined mass in the aortopulmonary window (*arrows*). (*Courtesy of Dr. Tomas Franquet, Barcelona, Spain*)

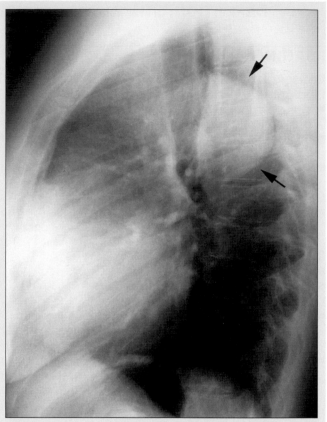

Figure 2. Aortic aneurysm in a 45-year-old man with Takayasu arteritis. In the same patient, on the lateral chest radiograph the mass projects posteriorly (*arrows*). (*Courtesy of Dr. Tomas Franquet, Barcelona, Spain*)

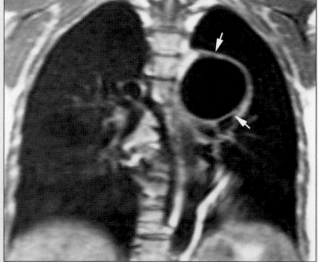

Figure 3. Aortic aneurysm in a 45-year-old man with Takayasu arteritis. In the same patient, coronal cardiac gated T1-weighted black blood MR image shows a large aneurysm of the aortic arch (*arrows*). (*Courtesy of Dr. Tomas Franquet, Barcelona, Spain*)

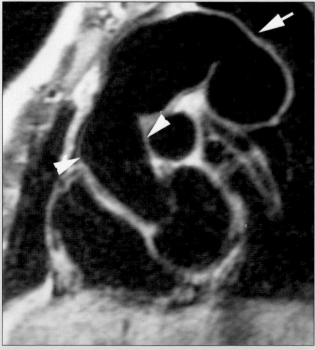

Figure 4. Aortic aneurysm in a 45-year-old man with Takayasu arteritis. In the same patient, sagittal cardiac gated T1-weighted black blood MR image shows a slight dilation of the aortic root (*arrowheads*) and a tortuous aneurysmatic aortic arch (*arrow*). (*Courtesy of Dr. Tomas Franquet, Barcelona, Spain*)

INCIDENCE/PREVALENCE AND EPIDEMIOLOGY

- Aortic aneurysm occurs most commonly in elderly persons.
- Approximately 50% originate in ascending aorta, 10% in aortic arch, and 40% in descending aorta.
- By far the most common cause of aortic aneurysm is atherosclerosis.
- Other causes include cystic medial necrosis (as seen in Marfan syndrome and Ehlers-Danlos syndrome), aortitis (infective and inflammatory), and hemodynamic alterations (e.g., aortic stenosis or regurgitation).
- Although trauma can result in true aneurysms, usually it results in pseudoaneurysm formation.

Suggested Readings

Castañer E, Andreu M, Gallardo X, et al: CT in nontraumatic acute thoracic aortic disease: Typical and atypical features and complications. *RadioGraphics* 23(Spec No):S93-S110, 2003.

Fann JI: Descending thoracic and thoracoabdominal aortic aneurysms. *Coron Artery Dis* 13:93-102, 2002.

Posniak HV, Olson MC, Demos TC, et al: CT of thoracic aortic aneurysms. *RadioGraphics* 10:839-855, 1990.

Tatli S, Yucel EK, Lipton MJ: CT and MR imaging of the thoracic aorta: Current techniques and clinical applications. *Radiol Clin North Am* 42:565-585, vi, 2004.

Aortic Dissection

DEFINITION: Aortic dissection is a cardiovascular emergency that arises after intimal tear of the aorta, with blood dissecting the aortic media to form true and false lumens.

IMAGING

Radiography
Findings
- May be normal or show dilation of the aorta

Utility
- Limited value in the diagnosis

CT Angiography
Findings
- True and false lumens are separated by intimal flap that projects into the opacified lumen.
- In the majority of cases the true lumen can be identified by its continuity with the lumen of the aorta proximal or distal to the dissection.
- "Beak sign:" acute angle between the dissection flap and the outer wall identifies the false lumen.
- False lumen may contain contrast-enhanced blood or low-attenuation material (hematoma).

Utility
- CT angiography using spiral acquisitions with multidetector arrays is modality of choice in evaluating aorta.
- Motion artifacts of aorta may simulate dissection on spiral CT.
- Despite artifacts, CT angiography has high accuracy as imaging of choice for diagnosis of aortic dissection.

MRI
Findings
- True and false lumens separated by intimal flap

Utility
- Accuracy similar to that of CT in diagnosis of aortic dissection
- Limited sensitivity in detection of intramural hematoma
- Most often used in follow-up of patients with aortic dissection

CLINICAL PRESENTATION

- Most common symptom is sudden onset of severe chest pain, which is slightly more common in type A than type B dissections.
- Other manifestations include back pain, pulse deficits, and syncope.

DIAGNOSTIC PEARLS

- Intimal flap
- Blood flow within true and false lumen
- "Beak sign": when intimal flap creates acute angle with outer wall on false lumen side
- Type A dissection involves the ascending aorta
- Type B dissection starts distal to the left subclavian artery

- Majority of deaths from dissection occur in first 2 weeks.
- Dissections are classified into acute (<2 weeks old) and chronic (>2 weeks old).
- Type A dissection has higher complication rates and may lead to life-threatening rupture into pericardium, causing tamponade and death.
- Type B dissections are frequently stable lesions, with 60% being reported to have a benign course.

DIFFERENTIAL DIAGNOSIS

- Primary intramural hematoma of aorta
- Aneurysm

PATHOLOGY

- The aortic media is separated (between the middle and outer third) by a stream of blood (false lumen).
- Inner two thirds of the media and the intima remain contiguous, forming the intimal flap that separates the true from the false lumen.
- Usual cause is tear of the intima with blood dissecting into aortic media; less commonly, the cause is bleeding from the vasa vasorum into the aortic media.
- There are two main forms: Stanford A, which involves ascending aorta, and Stanford B, which begins distal to the left subclavian artery and therefore does not involve ascending aorta.

WHAT THE REFERRING PHYSICIAN NEEDS TO KNOW

- Majority of deaths from dissection occur in the first 2 weeks.
- Type A dissection has higher complication rates and may lead to life-threatening rupture into pericardium causing tamponade and death and requires surgical repair.
- Intramural hematoma is clinically indistinguishable variant of aortic dissection.
- No discrete intimal flap is identified and no flowing blood is observed within false channel in intramural hematoma.

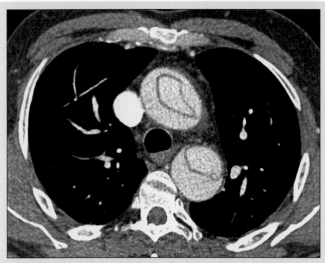

Figure 1. Acute Stanford type A dissection. Contrast-enhanced CT image obtained in a multidetector CT scanner shows an intimal flap within slightly dilated ascending and descending aorta consistent with Stanford type A dissection. (*Courtesy of Dr. Jorge I. Kavakama, São Paulo, Brazil.*)

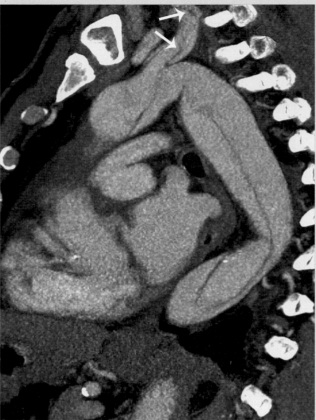

Figure 2. Acute Stanford type A dissection. In the same patient, sagittal maximum intensity projection image better demonstrates the extent of the aortic dissection shown in Figure 1. Also noted is an intimal flap in the left subclavian artery (*arrows*). (*Courtesy of Dr. Jorge I. Kavakama, São Paulo, Brazil.*)

INCIDENCE/PREVALENCE AND EPIDEMIOLOGY

- Incidence: approximately 3 cases per 100,000 persons/year
- More common in males (approximately 2:1)
- Predisposing factors: hypertension, trauma, prior aortic surgery, hereditary and congenital disorders (Marfan syndrome, Ehlers-Danlos), aortic valve disease, coarctation, arteritis

Suggested Readings

Castaner E, Andreu M, Gallardo X, et al: CT in nontraumatic acute thoracic aortic disease: Typical and atypical features and complications. *RadioGraphics* 23(Spec No):S93-S110, 2003.

Hartnell GG: Imaging of aortic aneurysms and dissection: CT and MRI. *J Thorac Imaging* 16:35-46, 2001.

Jeudy J, White CS: Evaluation of acute chest pain in the emergency department: Utility of multidetector computed tomography. *Semin Ultrasound CT MR* 28:109-114, 2007.

Khan IA, Nair CK: Clinical, diagnostic, and management perspectives of aortic dissection. *Chest* 122:311-328, 2002.

Liu Q, Lu JP, Wang F, et al: Three-dimensional contrast-enhanced MR angiography of aortic dissection: A pictorial essay. *RadioGraphics* 27:1311-1321, 2007.

Shiga T, Wajima Z, Apfel CC, et al: Diagnostic accuracy of transesophageal echocardiography, helical computed tomography, and magnetic resonance imaging for suspected thoracic aortic dissection: Systematic review and meta-analysis. *Arch Intern Med* 166:1350-1356, 2006.

Penetrating Aortic Ulcer

DEFINITION: Penetrating aortic ulcer is an ulcer of the aorta that penetrates the internal elastic lamina and extends into the aortic media.

IMAGING

CT
Findings
- Penetrating aortic ulcer manifests on contrast-enhanced CT as collection of contrast material visible outside the aortic lumen.
- Frequently associated with intramural hemorrhage and pseudoaneurysm formation.

Utility
- Blood vessels can usually be accurately assessed with contrast-enhanced CT.

MR Angiography
Findings
- Ulcer-like projection of contrast on MR angiography

Utility
- Requires combination of MR angiography and black blood imaging

CLINICAL PRESENTATION

- Patients are often asymptomatic, with ulcer detected incidentally on CT.
- Chest pain and back pain resemble that of aortic dissection.

DIFFERENTIAL DIAGNOSIS

- Aortic dissection
- Intramural hematoma
- Aortic aneurysm

PATHOLOGY

- Ulceration of atheromatous plaque that extends deeply through the intima and into the aortic media

DIAGNOSTIC PEARLS

- Aortic ulcer manifests on contrast-enhanced CT as a collection of contrast material visible outside the aortic lumen.
- Often associated is thickening of the aortic wall, which appears enhanced.
- Frequently associated with intramural hemorrhage and pseudoaneurysm formation.
- Patients may be asymptomatic or present with chest pain and back pain similiar to aortic dissection.

INCIDENCE/PREVALENCE AND EPIDEMIOLOGY

- Seen mainly in elderly patients with extensive atherosclerosis of the aorta
- Frequently associated with intramural hemorrhage and pseudoaneurysm formation and occasionally with rupture

Suggested Readings

Castañer E, Andreu M, Gallardo X, et al: CT in nontraumatic acute thoracic aortic disease: Typical and atypical features and complications. *RadioGraphics* 23(Spec No):S93-S110, 2003.

Macura KJ, Szarf G, Fishman EK, Bluemke DA: Role of computed tomography and magnetic resonance imaging in assessment of acute aortic syndromes. *Semin Ultrasound CT MR* 24:232-254, 2003.

Sundt TM: Intramural hematoma and penetrating aortic ulcer. *Curr Opin Cardiol* 22:504-509, 2007.

Quint LE, Williams DM, Francis IR, et al: Ulcerlike lesions of the aorta: Imaging features and natural history. *Radiology* 218: 719-723, 2001.

WHAT THE REFERRING PHYSICIAN NEEDS TO KNOW

- Contrast-enhanced CT (CT angiography) is imaging modality of choice in the assessment of aortic ulcers.
- Patients may be asymptomatic or have symptoms similar to those of aortic dissection.
- Ulcers may increase in size, result in aortic pseudoaneurysm or aneurysm, and, occasionally, rupture.

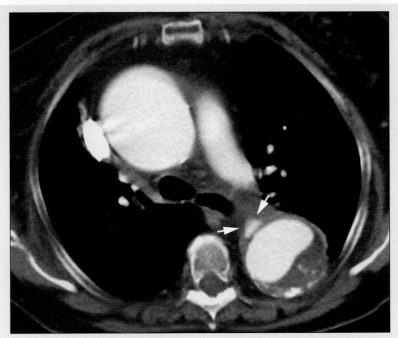

Figure 1. **Penetrating atherosclerotic ulcer in a 78-year-old woman.** Contrast-enhanced CT scan shows a penetrating ulcer (*arrows*) in the anterior aspect of the descending aorta. (*Courtesy of Dr. Tomás Franquet, Barcelona, Spain*)

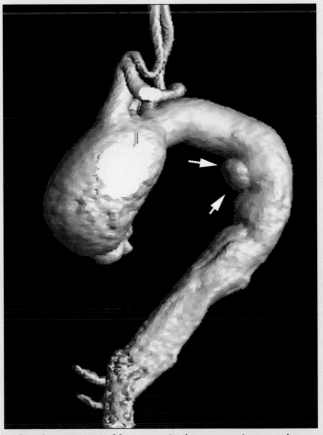

Figure 2. **Penetrating atherosclerotic ulcer in a 78-year-old woman.** In the same patient, a volume-rendered reformatted image of a contrast-enhanced CT scan also demonstrates the ulcer (*arrows*). (*Courtesy of Dr. Tomás Franquet, Barcelona, Spain*)

Achalasia

DEFINITION: Achalasia is a motor disorder of the esophagus resulting in esophageal dilation due to aperistalsis and inadequate relaxation of the lower esophageal sphincter.

IMAGING

Radiography

Findings

- Marked dilation of esophagus
- Anterior displacement and bowing of trachea by fluid-filled esophagus
- Frequently manifests as abnormality in retrotracheal space or as posterior mediastinal mass
- Aspiration pneumonia possibly evident

Utility

- Limited sensitivity in the detection of esophageal abnormalities

Fluoroscopy

Utility

- Barium esophagography used to evaluate dilation, peristalsis, and lower esophageal sphincter relaxation
- Superior to CT in demonstrating functional abnormalities of the esophagus

CT

Utility

- Abnormally dilated esophagus readily recognized on CT

CLINICAL PRESENTATION

- Dysphagia
- Regurgitation of food
- Chest pain, which may increase after eating

DIFFERENTIAL DIAGNOSIS

- Esophageal carcinoma
- Esophageal leiomyoma

DIAGNOSTIC PEARLS

- Dilation of esophagus
- Retained fluid, food debris, air-fluid level common
- Anterior displacement and bowing of trachea by fluid/food-filled esophagus

- Distal esophageal stricture
- Scleroderma

PATHOLOGY

- Aperistalsis of lower esophagus
- Inadequate relaxation of lower esophageal sphincter

INCIDENCE/PREVALENCE AND EPIDEMIOLOGY

- Uncommon
- Affects equally both genders and all ages
- Usually idiopathic
- Occasionally seen in association with Chagas disease, vagotomy, or diabetic neuropathy

Suggested Readings

Pohl D, Tutuian R: Achalasia: An overview of diagnosis and treatment. *J Gastrointestin Liver Dis* 16:297-303, 2007.
Whitten CR, Khan S, Munneke GJ, Grubnic S: A diagnostic approach to mediastinal abnormalities. *RadioGraphics* 27:657-671, 2007.

WHAT THE REFERRING PHYSICIAN NEEDS TO KNOW

- Diagnosis is based on clinical findings, results of barium esophagography, and esophageal motility testing (esophageal manometry).
- Megaesophagus can also be due to result of distal obstruction (carcinoma, stricture, or extrinsic compression).
- Endoscopy is necessary to rule out malignancy.
- Megaesophagus can occur secondary to other motility disorders (post-vagotomy syndrome, Chagas disease, scleroderma, systemic lupus erythematosus, presbyesophagus, diabetic neuropathy, esophagitis).

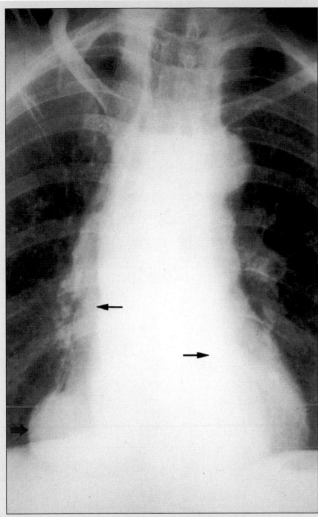

Figure 1. Achalasia in a 47-year-old woman with chest pain. A posteroanterior chest radiograph shows marked dilation of the esophagus (*thin arrows*) and a rounded opacity in the right cardiophrenic region (*thick arrow*). (*Courtesy of Dr. Tomás Franquet, Barcelona, Spain*)

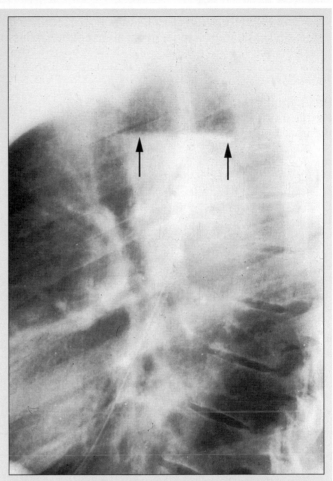

Figure 2. Achalasia in a 47-year-old woman with chest pain. Close-up view of the lateral chest radiograph shows anterior displacement and bowing of the trachea by the fluid-filled esophagus. Note air-fluid level (*arrows*). (*Courtesy of Dr. Tomás Franquet, Barcelona, Spain*)

Esophageal Carcinoma

DEFINITION: Esophageal carcinoma manifests radiologically as concentric or eccentric thickening of esophagus, a focal mass, or esophageal obstruction.

IMAGING

Radiography
Findings
- Abnormality or mass in middle or posterior mediastinum
- Widening of posterior tracheal/tracheoesophageal stripe on lateral radiograph
- Esophageal air-fluid level

Utility
- Of limited value in differential diagnosis of mediastinal masses

CT
Findings
- Concentric or eccentric thickening of the esophagus (usually > 5 mm)
- Narrowing of esophageal lumen
- Dilation above obstructing tumor
- Focal intraluminal mass
- Obscuration of periesophageal fat planes with or without evidence of invasion of adjacent structures such as trachea
- Periesophageal, paratracheal, aortopulmonary window, cervical, and upper abdominal lymphadenopathy

Utility
- CT with oral and intravenous contrast is imaging modality of choice for assessment of esophageal masses.

Positron Emission Tomography
Findings
- Increased uptake on FDG-PET

Utility
- PET, particularly PET/CT, is superior to CT in the staging of esophageal carcinoma.

CLINICAL PRESENTATION

- Dysphagia
- Anorexia, weight loss

DIAGNOSTIC PEARLS

- Paratracheal, paraesophageal lymphatic engorgement due to obstruction or direct invasion by tumor
- Retained secretions caused by tumor occluding esophagus at lower level
- Esophageal air-fluid level
- Widening of posterior tracheal/tracheoesophageal stripe on lateral radiograph

DIFFERENTIAL DIAGNOSIS

- Esophageal leiomyoma
- Esophagitis
- Esophageal stricture
- Achalasia

PATHOLOGY

- Majority of esophageal carcinomas are squamous cell carcinomas.
- Approximately 20% of esophageal carcinomas are adenocarcinomas; the latter typically involve the distal esophagus.
- Most esophageal carcinomas present at an advanced stage.

INCIDENCE/PREVALENCE AND EPIDEMIOLOGY

- Diseases of esophagus are one of most common causes of posterior/middle mediastinal abnormalities.
- Esophageal carcinoma accounts for approximately 10% of carcinomas of the gastrointestinal tract.

WHAT THE REFERRING PHYSICIAN NEEDS TO KNOW

- Esophageal wall thickening is an early but nonspecific manifestation of esophageal carcinoma; it may also occur with benign processes such as esophagitis and reflux.
- CT is currently the most commonly used imaging modality in the staging of esophageal carcinoma and has a relatively high accuracy in the diagnosis of periesophageal extension of tumor and invasion of adjacent organs.
- FDG-PET is superior to CT in the diagnosis of regional lymph node and distal metastases.

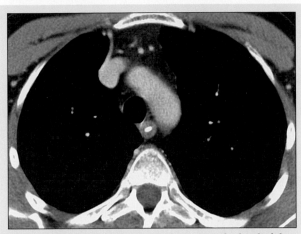

Figure 1. **Esophageal carcinoma.** CT image at the level of the aortic arch shows normal esophagus. The patient was a 38-year-old man with distal esophageal carcinoma.

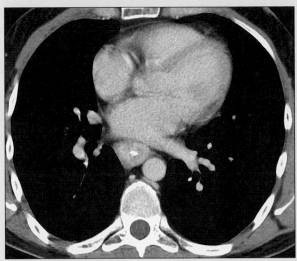

Figure 2. **Esophageal carcinoma.** In the same patient, CT image at the level of the left inferior pulmonary vein demonstrates circumferential thickening of the esophageal wall. The patient was a 38-year-old man with esophageal carcinoma.

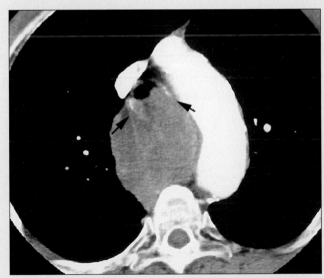

Figure 3. **Advanced esophageal squamous carcinoma with tracheal invasion in a 68-year-old man.** Contrast-enhanced CT scan shows a large esophageal mass with tracheal invasion (*arrows*). (*Courtesy of Dr. Tomás Franquet, Barcelona, Spain*)

Suggested Readings

Bruzzi JF, Truong MT, Macapinlac H, et al: Integrated CT-PET imaging of esophageal cancer: Unexpected and unusual distribution of distant organ metastases. *Curr Probl Diagn Radiol* 36:21-29, 2007.

Gibbs JM, Chandrasekhar CA, Ferguson EC, Oldham SA: Lines and stripes: Where did they go?—From conventional radiography to CT. *RadioGraphics* 27:33-48, 2007.

Korst RJ, Altorki NK: Imaging for esophageal tumors. *Thorac Surg Clin* 14:61-69, 2004.

Plukker JT, van Westreenen HL: Staging in oesophageal cancer. *Best Pract Res Clin Gastroenterol* 20:877-891, 2006.

Esophageal Diverticula

DEFINITION: An esophageal diverticulum is a focal outpouching of the esophagus that may contain all layers of the esophageal wall (true diverticulum) or only the mucosa (false diverticulum).

IMAGING

Radiography
Findings
- Zenker diverticulum usually extends dorsally into the postcricoid area; if large, it can be detected in the retrotracheal space as an air-filled or fluid-filled mass-like lesion.
- Traction diverticula occur at the level of the middle esophagus.
- Epiphrenic diverticula occur at the level of the lower esophagus on the right side.

Utility
- Often first imaging modality used in the diagnosis
- Limited sensitivity and specificity

CT
Findings
- Zenker diverticulum: pulsion diverticulum at the level of the pharyngoesophageal junction and typically projecting posteriorly
- Traction diverticula owing to granulomatous infection located at middle esophagus; calcified nodes commonly present
- Epiphrenic diverticula located at lower esophagus, usually on right side

Utility
- Esophageal diverticula are usually readily identified on CT.

Barium Esophagography
Findings
- Filling of the diverticulum with barium
Utility
- Best imaging modality to show presence of esophageal diverticula

CLINICAL PRESENTATION

- Zenker diverticulum may present as dysphagia, cough, and recurrent aspiration pneumonia.

DIAGNOSTIC PEARLS

- Zenker diverticulum projects posteriorly from pharyngoesophageal junction.
- Traction diverticula owing to granulomatous infection are located at middle esophagus.
- Epiphrenic diverticula are located at lower esophagus on the right side.

PATHOLOGY

- Esophageal diverticula may be formed by pulsion (increased intraluminal esophageal pressure) or by traction (fibrosis in adjacent periesophageal tissue).
- Pulsion diverticula usually contain only mucosa, whereas traction diverticula contain all layers of the esophageal wall.
- Zenker diverticulum is a pulsion diverticulum at the pharyngoesophageal junction.
- Epiphrenic diverticulum is a pulsion diverticulum located at lower esophagus on right side.
- Traction diverticulum is located at the middle esophagus and usually due to previous granulomatous infection.

INCIDENCE/PREVALENCE AND EPIDEMIOLOGY

- Uncommon

Suggested Readings

Cassivi SD, Deschamps C, Nichols FC 3rd, et al: Diverticula of the esophagus. *Surg Clin North Am* 85:495-503, ix, 2005.
Gibbs JM, Chandrasekhar CA, Ferguson EC, Oldham SA: Lines and stripes: Where did they go?—From conventional radiography to CT. *RadioGraphics* 27:33-48, 2007.
Jang KM, Lee KS, Lee SJ, et al: The spectrum of benign esophageal lesions: Imaging findings. *Korean J Radiol* 3:199-210, 2002.

WHAT THE REFERRING PHYSICIAN NEEDS TO KNOW

- Zenker diverticulum is a pulsion diverticulum at the level of the pharyngoesophageal junction.
- Traction diverticula owing to granulomatous infection are located at middle esophagus.
- Epiphrenic diverticula are located at lower esophagus on the right side.

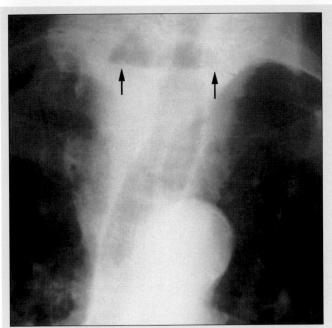

Figure 1. Zenker diverticulum in a 54-year-old man with dysphagia and cough. Posteroanterior chest film shows abnormal widening of the superior mediastinum. An air-fluid level is also seen (*arrows*). (*Courtesy of Dr. Tomás Franquet, Barcelona, Spain*)

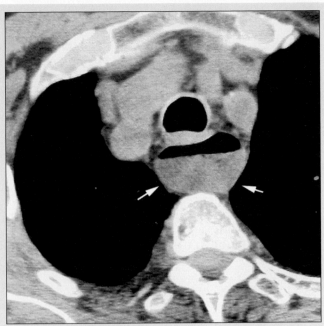

Figure 2. Zenker diverticulum in a 54-year-old man with dysphagia and cough. CT scan shows a large retrotracheal diverticulum with an air-fluid level due to retained alimentary content (*arrows*). (*Courtesy of Dr. Tomás Franquet, Barcelona, Spain*)

Aorticopulmonary Paraganglioma (Chemodectoma)

DEFINITION: An aorticopulmonary paraganglioma is a neuroendocrine tumor that originates from paraganglia such as carotid body, glomus jugulare, or Zuckerkandl's body located in the perivascular adventitial tissue and bounded by the aorta superiorly, pulmonary artery inferiorly, and ligamentum arteriosum and right pulmonary artery on either side.

IMAGING

Radiography
Findings
- Round, well-circumscribed mediastinal mass; ranges from 1.2-7.0 cm in diameter; in close relation to base of heart and aortic arch
- Occasionally located in subcarinal region or posterior mediastinum

Utility
- Has limited value in differential diagnosis of mediastinal masses

CT
Findings
- Round mass in region of aorticopulmonary window.
- Homogeneous attenuation or large central areas of low attenuation as a result of necrosis are seen.
- After intravenous administration of a contrast agent, tumors usually show dense enhancement.

Utility
- Of limited value in differential diagnosis from other mediastinal masses

MRI
Findings
- Hypointense or isointense compared with skeletal muscle on T1-weighted images
- Hyperintense on T2-weighted images

Utility
- Of limited value in differential diagnosis from other mediastinal masses
- Useful screening for patients at high risk for extra-adrenal paragangliomas

CLINICAL PRESENTATION

- Usually asymptomatic at the time of diagnosis
- Sometimes compresses or invades local structures, causing hoarseness, dysphagia, chest pain, hemoptysis, and occasionally superior vena cava syndrome

DIAGNOSTIC PEARLS

- Well-circumscribed mediastinal mass
- Usually homogeneous on noncontrast CT; may contain large areas of necrosis
- Hypointense or isointense compared with skeletal muscle on T1-weighted MR images
- Hyperintense on T2-weighted MR sequences

PATHOLOGY

- Paragangliomas: neuroendocrine tumors that originate from paraganglia, such as carotid body, glomus jugulare, or Zuckerkandl's body
- Location: perivascular adventitial tissue bounded by aorta superiorly, pulmonary artery inferiorly, and ligamentum arteriosum and right pulmonary artery on either side
- Indolent and slow-growing tumor

INCIDENCE/PREVALENCE AND EPIDEMIOLOGY

- These tumors are uncommon.
- They occur in all age groups, but mean age at time of diagnosis is 45-50 years.
- Women are affected more often than men.
- Approximately 10% are malignant.
- Local recurrence is reported in 55% of cases after surgery.
- Metastasis is documented in approximately 25% of patients.

Suggested Readings

Dajee A, Dajee H, Hinrichs S, Lillington G: Pulmonary chondroma, extra-adrenal paraganglioma, and gastric leiomyosarcoma: Carney's triad. *J Thorac Cardiovasc Surg* 84:377-381, 1982.

Moran CA, Suster S, Fishback N, Koss MN: Mediastinal paragangliomas: A clinicopathologic and immunohistochemical study of 16 cases. *Cancer* 72:2358-2364, 1993.

Somasundar P, Krouse R, Hostetter R, et al: Paragangliomas—a decade of clinical experience. *J Surg Oncol* 74:286-290, 2000.

WHAT THE REFERRING PHYSICIAN NEEDS TO KNOW

- Chest radiography is of limited value in assessment of mediastinal masses.
- CT and MRI accurately depict the location of the tumor but do not allow distinction of paragangliomas from other mediastinal masses.

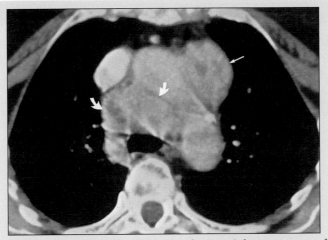

Figure 1. **Aorticopulmonary paraganglioma.** Contrast-enhanced CT scan shows an inhomogeneous soft tissue mass involving the aorticopulmonary window (*straight arrow*) and paratracheal region (*curved arrows*). The patient was a 68-year-old woman who had surgically proven mediastinal paraganglioma. (*From Müller NL, Fraser RS, Colman NC, Paré PD:* Radiologic Diagnosis of Diseases of the Chest. *Philadelphia, WB Saunders, 2001.*)

Giant Lymph Node Hyperplasia (Castleman Disease)

DEFINITION: Giant lymph node hyperplasia is a benign lymphoproliferative disorder characterized by a large number of germinal centers interspersed with lymphocytes and multiple capillaries (hyaline vascular type) or plasma cells (plasma cell type).

IMAGING

Radiography

Findings

- Localized hyaline vascular form is a focal, well-defined, smooth or lobulated mass most commonly situated in the hila or middle mediastinum.
- Occasionally lesion is found at other sites, including aorticopulmonary window, posterior mediastinum, and chest wall.
- Multicentric plasma cell variety involves multiple mediastinal compartments and manifests as diffuse mediastinal widening.
- Diffuse lung involvement may also occur and is usually due to lymphoid interstitial pneumonia.

Utility

- Usually first imaging modality used
- Has limited value in differential diagnosis of other causes of lymphadenopathy

CT

Findings

- Localized hyaline vascular form presents as a mass of enlarged lymph nodes of homogeneous soft tissue attenuation; it may contain coarse and central calcifications.
- Enlarged lymph nodes of hyaline vascular type show marked homogeneous enhancement after contrast medium injection because of their highly vascular nature.
- Multicentric form is characterized by multiple slightly enlarged mediastinal and hilar lymph nodes with homogeneous attenuation that usually show little enhancement after intravenous administration of a contrast agent.
- Pulmonary manifestations of multicentric Castleman disease are typically those of lymphoid interstitial pneumonia.

DIAGNOSTIC PEARLS

- Homogeneous soft tissue attenuation
- Hyaline vascular: focal, well-defined, smooth or lobulated mass most commonly situated in the hila or middle posterior mediastinum
- Plasma cell type: mediastinal, hilar, cervical, and abdominal lymphadenopathy; multicentric disease

- On high-resolution CT there are poorly defined centrilobular nodules, thin-walled cysts, and thickening of bronchovascular bundles and septa.
- Less common findings are subpleural nodules, groundglass opacities, airspace consolidation, and bronchiectasis.

Utility

- Used to assess location and extent of findings
- In multicentric plasma cell variety, characteristic findings of lymphoid interstitial pneumonia evident on high-resolution CT

MRI

Findings

- Hypointense signal compared with that characteristic of mediastinal fat
- Hyperintense signal compared with that of skeletal muscle on T1- and T2-weighted sequences
- Diffuse enhancement after administration of gadolinium-based contrast medium in localized form because of hypervascularity of lesions
- Lymph node enhancement not a prominent finding in multifocal form but can occur

Utility

- Used to assess location and extent of findings
- Has limited value in the diagnosis

WHAT THE REFERRING PHYSICIAN NEEDS TO KNOW

- There are two histologic types: hyaline vascular and plasma cell.
- Localized or hyaline vascular form is associated with good prognosis after surgical resection.
- Hyaline vascular type is characterized by a focal, well-defined, smooth or lobulated mass commonly situated in the hila or middle posterior mediastinum and with marked enhancement after contrast agent administration.
- Plasma cell type is characterized by mediastinal, hilar, cervical, and abdominal lymphadenopathy; multicentric disease; usually little enhancement; and possible involvement of lungs with lymphoid interstitial pneumonia pattern.
- High-resolution CT findings of lymphoid interstitial pneumonia are often characteristic enough to allow diagnosis in the proper clinical context.

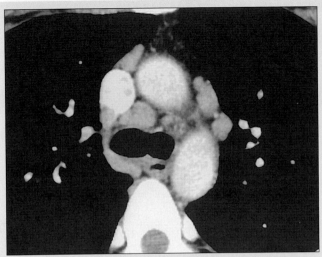

Figure 1. Multicentric Castleman's disease. Contrast-enhanced CT scan from a 44-year-old woman shows enlarged mediastinal and bilateral hilar lymph nodes. The diagnosis of Castleman disease was proved by lymph node biopsy. (*Courtesy of Dr. Takeshi Johkoh, Department of Radiology, Osaka University Medical School, Osaka, Japan. From Müller NL, Fraser RS, Colman NC, Paré PD: Radiologic Diagnosis of Diseases of the Chest. Philadelphia, WB Saunders, 2001.*)

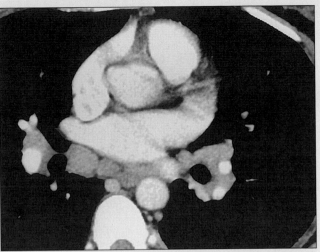

Figure 2. Multicentric Castleman's disease. Contrast-enhanced CT scan from a 44-year-old woman shows enlarged mediastinal and bilateral hilar lymph nodes. The diagnosis of Castleman disease was proved by lymph node biopsy. (*Courtesy of Dr. Takeshi Johkoh, Department of Radiology, Osaka University Medical School, Osaka, Japan. From Müller NL, Fraser RS, Colman NC, Paré PD: Radiologic Diagnosis of Diseases of the Chest. Philadelphia, WB Saunders, 2001.*)

CLINICAL PRESENTATION

- Multicentric or plasma cell variety typically presents as a multicentric process that is associated with generalized lymphadenopathy.
- Multicentric or plasma cell variety is associated with evidence of systemic disease characterized by fever, sweating, fatigue, anemia, lymphadenopathy, and hepatosplenomegaly.

DIFFERENTIAL DIAGNOSIS

- Non-Hodgkin lymphoma
- Hodgkin lymphoma
- Sarcoidosis

PATHOLOGY

- Form of benign lymphoproliferative disorder of unknown etiology and pathogenesis
- Affects mediastinal lymph nodes but has also been reported in lung, pleura, and chest wall
- Multiple extrathoracic locations: cervical, mesenteric, and retroperitoneal nodes and spleen
- Represents an unusual form of lymphoid reaction to an unknown agent, probably of viral nature
- Hyaline vascular type: large number of germinal centers interspersed in lymphocytes and multiple capillaries surrounded by hyaline sheets
- Germinal centers surrounded by concentric cuffs of lymphocytes arranged in onionskin pattern and by hypoplastic postcapillary venules

- Plasma cell type: large sheets of mature/immature plasma cells admixed with immunoblasts, lymphocytes, and macrophages between germinal centers

INCIDENCE/PREVALENCE AND EPIDEMIOLOGY

- Uncommon
- Affects patients of all ages
- No sex predilection
- Hyaline vascular type most common (90%); occurs in young adults
- Multicentric or plasma cell variety less frequent (10% of cases); affects persons older than those who have isolated form

Suggested Readings

Ferrozzi F, Tognini G, Spaggiari E, Pavone P: Focal Castleman disease of the lung: MRI findings. *Clin Imaging* 25:400-402, 2001.

Johkoh T, Müller NL, Ichikado K, et al: Intrathoracic multicentric Castleman disease: CT findings in 12 patients. *Radiology* 209:477-481, 1998.

Kim JH, Jun TG, Sung SW, et al: Giant lymph node hyperplasia (Castleman's disease) in the chest. *Ann Thorac Surg* 59:1162-1165, 1995.

McAdams HP, Rosado-de-Christenson M, Fishback NF, Templeton PA: Castleman disease of the thorax: Radiologic features with clinical and histopathologic correlation. *Radiology* 209:221-228, 1998.

Moon WK, Im JG, Han MC: Castleman's disease of the mediastinum: MR imaging features. *Clin Radiol* 49:466-468, 1994.

Moon WK, Im JG, Kim JS, et al: Mediastinal Castleman disease: CT findings. *J Comput Assist Tomogr* 18:43-46, 1994.

Nerve Sheath Tumors (Neurilemoma, Neurofibroma, and Malignant Nerve Sheath Tumor)

DEFINITION: Nerve sheath tumors are neoplasms of the peripheral nerves and include neurilemoma, neurofibroma, and malignant tumor of nerve sheath origin.

IMAGING

Radiography

Findings

- Neurilemoma: smoothly rounded or oval mass, occasionally lobulated mass
- Adjacent bone changes such as erosion, splaying of ribs, or enlargement of intervertebral foramen
- Neurofibromas: smooth rounded masses

Utility

- Often first imaging modality to demonstrate abnormality
- Of limited value in differential diagnosis

CT

Findings

- Neurilemomas: well-demarcated round or oval mass with homogeneous attenuation; homogeneous or heterogeneous enhancement after contrast agent administration
- Neurofibromas: smooth margins, round or ellipsoid shape, and homogeneous attenuation; early central blush after contrast agent administration
- Neurilemomas and neurofibromas: grow through adjacent intervertebral foramen and extend into spinal canal, resulting in "dumbbell" or "hourglass" configuration
- Malignant nerve sheath tumor: lesions > 5 cm in diameter, low-attenuation areas within primary tumor, irregular/ill-defined margins, adjacent structure compression/destruction
- Pleural abnormalities (e.g., pleural effusion or pleural nodules, presence of metastatic pulmonary nodules)

Utility

- Often allows diagnosis of nerve sheath tumor

MRI

Findings

- Neurilemomas: low-intermediate signal intensity on T1-weighted images; areas of intermediate-high signal intensity on T2-weighted sequences

DIAGNOSTIC PEARLS

- Neurilemoma and neurofibroma: well-demarcated round or elliptical masses with smooth margins; may have "dumbbell" or "hourglass" configuration
- Malignant nerve sheath tumor: lesions > 5 cm in diameter, irregular/ill-defined margins, adjacent structure compression/destruction

- Very high signal intensity areas on T2-weighted images corresponding pathologically to areas of cystic degeneration
- Gadolinium-enhanced MR images with contrast enhancement in peripheral portion of tumor and no enhancement in areas of cystic degeneration
- Neurofibromas: homogeneous low-intermediate signal intensity on T1-weighted MR images; target appearance on T2-weighted sequence

Utility

- Should be performed preoperatively in all patients with suspicious neurogenic tumors to definitely exclude intraspinal tumor extension

CLINICAL PRESENTATION

- Often asymptomatic
- Pain and neurologic symptoms

DIFFERENTIAL DIAGNOSIS

- Mesenchymal tumor
- Fibrous tumor of the pleura
- Duplication cysts
- Meningocele
- Pulmonary carcinoma

WHAT THE REFERRING PHYSICIAN NEEDS TO KNOW

- Prognosis of neurilemoma is excellent, and recurrence is rarely reported after surgical resection.
- Recurrences in neurofibromas are rare after surgical resection.
- Recurrences in malignant nerve sheath tumor are common even after surgical resection.
- Majority of paravertebral masses in adults are benign.

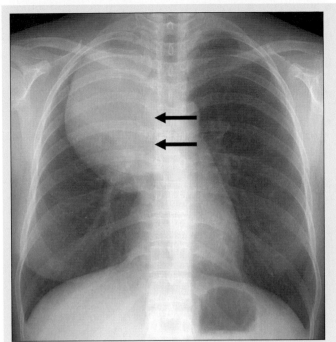

Figure 1. Schwannoma in a 31-year-old woman. Chest radiograph shows large well-defined soft tissue mass in right upper and middle lung zones with its broad base in the mediastinum. Also note widening of intercostal spaces (*arrows*), especially between right fifth and sixth ribs. (*Courtesy of Dr. Kyung Soo Lee, Seoul, Korea*)

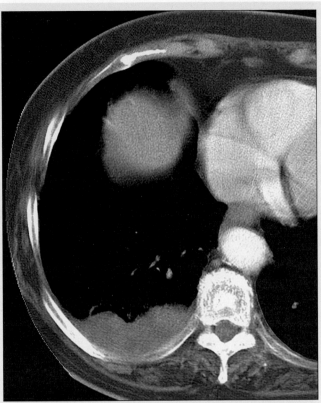

Figure 2. Cellular schwannoma in a 70-year-old woman. Contrast-enhanced CT image obtained at level of liver dome shows dumbbell-shaped soft tissue mass along course of intercostal nerve. (*Courtesy of Dr. Kyung Soo Lee, Seoul, Korea*)

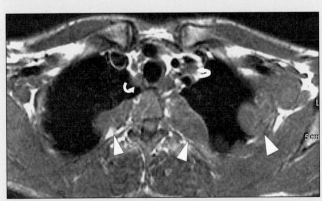

Figure 3. Neurofibromas in a 20-year-old man with neurofibromatosis. Unenhanced T1-weighted MR image obtained at level of great vessels shows soft tissue masses with globular enhancing portion in bilateral paraspinal areas and left axilla and along the course of left intercostal (*arrowheads*) and bilateral vagus (*curved arrows*) nerves. (*Courtesy of Dr. Kyung Soo Lee, Seoul, Korea*)

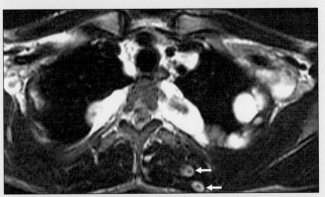

Figure 4. Neurofibromas in a 20-year-old man with neurofibromatosis. In the same patient as Figure 3, T2-weighted MR image shows slightly heterogeneous, but mainly high signal intensity lesions at same sites on previous image (see Fig. 3). Also note small neurofibromas (*arrows*) in the posterior chest wall. Some lesions in left paraspinal region and left chest wall show target sign (peripheral high and central low signal intensity). (*Courtesy of Dr. Kyung Soo Lee, Seoul, Korea*)

PATHOLOGY

- Neurilemomas grow by formation of lateral mass on parent nerve, compressing it; they are encapsulated with nerve fibers stretched around the tumor.
- Histologically, they consist of two components: highly ordered cellular component (Antoni type A) and loose myxoid component (Antoni type B).
- They occur in the paravertebral region, along vagus/phrenic nerve, along a rib, in the anterior mediastinum, and in the brachial plexus.
- Neurofibromas are tumors of cranial, spinal, or peripheral nerves, which are intimately continuous with the nerve proper.
- Affected nerve is circumferentially compressed or diffusely penetrated by elements of tumor.
- Proliferation of nerve sheath cells interspersed with thick wavy collagen bundles occurs, and there may be variable degrees of myxoid degeneration.

INCIDENCE/PREVALENCE AND EPIDEMIOLOGY

- Over 90% of peripheral nerve tumors are benign; benign lesions are identified in young and middle-aged adults.

- Neurilemoma has equal frequency in men and women and affects all ages (mean age, 41 years).
- Neurofibroma is more frequent in men, usually second to fourth decades of age at diagnosis
- Malignant nerve sheath tumors account for up to 15% of nerve sheath tumors.
- Incidence of sarcomatous degeneration in patients with neurofibromatosis is approximately 5%.
- Malignant nerve sheath tumors have equal involvement in men and women; they are common in persons 20-50 years of age.

Suggested Readings

Ko SF, Lee TY, Lin JW, et al: Thoracic neurilemomas: An analysis of computed tomography findings in 36 patients. *J Thorac Imaging* 13:21-26, 1998.

Lee JY, Lee KS, Han J, et al: Spectrum of neurogenic tumors in the thorax: CT and pathologic findings. *J Comput Assist Tomogr* 23:399-406, 1999.

Tanaka O, Kiryu T, Hirose Y, et al: Neurogenic tumors of the mediastinum and chest wall: MR imaging appearance. *J Thorac Imaging* 20:316-320, 2005.

Sympathetic Ganglia Tumors (Ganglioneuromas, Ganglioneuroblastomas, and Neuroblastomas)

DEFINITION: Tumors of the sympathetic ganglia include ganglioneuromas, ganglioneuroblastomas, and neuroblastomas.

IMAGING

Radiography
Findings
- Ganglioneuromas and ganglioneuroblastomas are elongated and oriented in a vertical axis following direction of sympathetic chain
- Ganglioneuroma: well-defined, oval lesion with little mass effect relative to size of tumor
- Ganglioneuroblastoma: well-defined, oval lesion usually oriented in vertical axis following sympathetic chain direction
- Neuroblastoma: paravertebral in location; contains calcification (10%); results in rib and vertebral erosion

Utility
- Usually initial modality in the assessment of patients with suspected mediastinal or paravertebral abnormality

CT
Findings
- Ganglioneuroma: low attenuatison (unenhanced CT); mild/moderate enhancement after intravenous administration of a contrast agent
- Calcification pattern: discrete and punctate (ganglioneuroma); amorphous and coarse (neuroblastoma)
- Ganglioneuroblastoma: variable, ranging from homogeneous solid mass to predominantly cystic mass with few thin strands of soft tissue attenuation
- Neuroblastoma: lobulated contour, lacks a capsule, inhomogeneous attenuation due to tumor necrosis

Utility
- Superior to chest radiography in demonstrating presence and extent of paravertebral masses
- Foci of calcification seen in approximately 20% of patients

MRI
Findings
- Ganglioneuroma: homogeneous lesion of intermediate signal intensity on both T1- and T2-weighted sequences

DIAGNOSTIC PEARLS
- Ganglioneuroma/ganglioneuroblastoma: elongated oval tumors typically oriented along the sympathetic chain
- Ganglioneuroblastoma: ranging from homogeneous solid mass to predominantly cystic mass with a few thin strands of soft tissue
- Neuroblastoma: inhomogeneous attenuation due to tumor necrosis
- Neuroblastomas and ganglioneuroblastomas occur in infants and young children
- Ganglioneuromas occur in older children and young adults

- Whorled appearance caused by curvilinear/nodular bands of low signal intensity on T1-weighted images; heterogeneous high signal intensity on T2-weighted images
- Variable enhancement with gadolinium
- Neuroblastoma: homogeneous or heterogeneous signal intensity on all sequences and variable enhancement after gadolinium administration

Utility
- Best imaging modality for assessment of tumor extension into spinal canal

CLINICAL PRESENTATION
- Signs and symptoms include fatigue, loss of appetite, weight loss, and chest discomfort.
- Large tumors may result in dyspnea.

PATHOLOGY
- Ganglioneuromas are encapsulated benign tumors, attached to either sympathetic or intercostal nerve trunk; they arise anywhere along paravertebral sympathetic plexus and adrenal medulla and are composed of large ganglion cells, nerve sheath cells, and nerve fibers.

WHAT THE REFERRING PHYSICIAN NEEDS TO KNOW
- Ganglioneuromas: prognosis is excellent and recurrences are rare after surgical resection.
- Ganglioneuroblastoma: response to therapy and prognosis are significantly more favorable than those of neuroblastomas.
- Neuroblastomas: there is a wide spectrum of clinical behavior ranging from spontaneous regression to aggressive disease with metastatic dissemination leading to death.

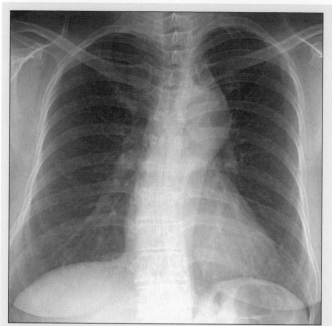

Figure 1. Ganglioneuroma in a 14-year-old girl. Chest radiograph shows vertically oriented, well-defined soft tissue mass in the medial aspect of the left upper lung zone with its broad base in the mediastinal side. (*Courtesy of Dr. Kyung Soo Lee, Seoul, Korea*)

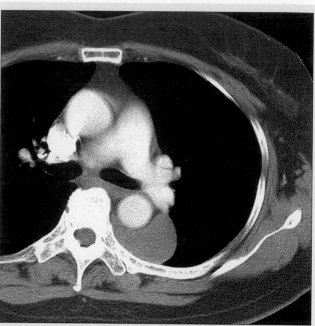

Figure 2. Ganglioneuroma in a 14-year-old girl. In the same patient as Figure 1, close-up view from contrast-enhanced CT scan obtained at level of distal main bronchi shows pear-shaped, homogeneous, low-attenuation, soft tissue mass in left paraspinal area. (*Courtesy of Dr. Kyung Soo Lee, Seoul, Korea*)

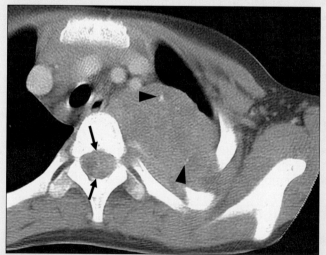

Figure 3. Neuroblastoma in a 6-year-old boy. Contrast-enhanced CT scan obtained at level of great vessels shows inhomogeneously enhancing soft tissue mass occupying left paraspinal area. Mass extends into spinal canal (*arrows*). Also note calcifications (*arrowheads*) within mass lesion. (*Courtesy of Dr. Kyung Soo Lee, Seoul, Korea*)

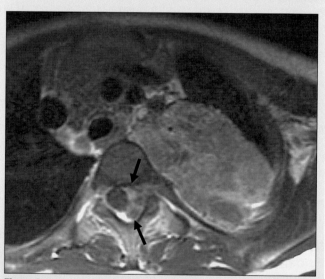

Figure 4. Neuroblastoma in a 6-year-old boy. In the same patient as Figure 3, gadolinium-enhanced T1-weighted MR image shows heterogeneously enhancing mass. Also note intraspinal component (*arrows*) of tumor. (*Courtesy of Dr. Kyung Soo Lee, Seoul, Korea*)

- Ganglioneuroblastomas are transitional tumors containing elements of both malignant neuroblastoma and benign ganglioneuroma; they may be partially or totally encapsulated and frequently contain granular calcification.
- Neuroblastomas are of neural crest origin and usually arise in adrenal glands; they are composed of small, dark neuroepithelial cells showing glial/ganglionic differentiation and contain primitive round cells with dark-staining nuclei and scanty cytoplasm and may show gross or microscopic calcification but lack any capsular structures.

INCIDENCE/PREVALENCE AND EPIDEMIOLOGY

- These tumors occur predominantly in infants and children.
- Malignant tumors are noted in younger patients, and benign lesions are observed in older children or adolescents.
- Neuroblastoma accounts for approximately 10% of pediatric cancers and 15% of cancer deaths in children.

- Ganglioneuromas occur in all age groups, but 60% are seen in patients < age 20 years; males are more frequently affected.
- Ganglioneuroblastomas are seen in young children but are rare after age of 10; there is an equal frequency in boys and girls.
- Neuroblastomas are childhood neoplasms; boys are affected more than girls, and 90% are diagnosed in the first 8 years of life.
- Overall 2-year survival for mediastinal primary neuroblastoma is >60%.
- Primary intrathoracic neuroblastomas comprise 14% of all neuroblastomas.

Suggested Readings

Ichikawa T, Ohtomo K, Araki T, et al: Ganglioneuroma: Computed tomography and magnetic resonance features. *Br J Radiol* 69:114-121, 1996.

Lonergan GJ, Schwab CM, Suarez ES, Carlson CL: Neuroblastoma, ganglioneuroblastoma, and ganglioneuroma: Radiologic-pathologic correlation. *RadioGraphics* 22:911-934, 2002.

Extramedullary Hematopoiesis

DEFINITION: Extramedullary hematopoiesis is a compensatory phenomenon in various diseases in which there is inadequate production or excessive destruction of blood cells.

IMAGING

Radiography
Findings
- One or several smooth, lobulated masses in lower chest
- Masses at multiple levels or involving entire paravertebral region

Utility
- Often first and only imaging modality used

CT
Findings
- Homogeneous soft tissue attenuation
- Large fatty component occasionally evident
- Widening of ribs as a result of expansion of medullary cavity
- Lacy appearance of vertebrae
- Absence of bone erosion

Utility
- Superior to radiography in demonstrating presence of paravertebral masses consistent with extramedullary hematopoiesis

Nuclear Medicine
Findings
- Uptake within mass in majority of cases on bone marrow scintigraphy

Utility
- Specific diagnosis can often be made on bone marrow scintigraphy

CLINICAL PRESENTATION

- Congenital hemolytic anemia (usually hereditary spherocytosis) or thalassemia (thalassemia major or intermedia)

PATHOLOGY

- Compensatory phenomenon in various diseases in which there is inadequate production or excessive destruction of blood cells

DIAGNOSTIC PEARLS

- Smooth, lobulated masses situated in the lower chest
- Homogeneous soft tissue attenuation
- Large fatty component
- Patient with congenital hemolytic anemia or thalassemia

- Associated with congenital hemolytic anemia (usually hereditary spherocytosis) or thalassemia (thalassemia major or intermedia)
- Fatty replacement as result of adipocytic metaplasia after resolution of underlying hemolytic disorder

INCIDENCE/PREVALENCE AND EPIDEMIOLOGY

- Most common sites of extramedullary hematopoiesis are liver and spleen.
- Seldom evident in paravertebral region.

Suggested Readings

Castelli R, Graziadei G, Karimi M, Cappellini MD: Intrathoracic masses due to extramedullary hematopoiesis. *Am J Med Sci* 328:299-303, 2004.

Hennessy OF, Salanitri JC: Computed tomography of intrathoracic extramedullary haematopoiesis occurring as a complication of osteopetrosis. *Australas Radiol* 49:430-432, 2005.

Kakite S, Tanabe Y, Kinoshita F, et al: Clinical usefulness of In-111 chloride and Tc-99m Sn colloid scintigraphy in the diagnosis of intrathoracic extramedullary hematopoiesis. *Ann Nucl Med* 19:317-320, 2005.

Martin J, Palacio A, Petiti J, Martin C: Fatty transformation of thoracic extramedullary hematopoiesis following splenectomy: CT features. *J Comput Assist Tomogr* 14:477-478, 1990.

Psichoglou H, Malagarl K, Spanomichos G: Mediastinal extramedullary hematopoiesis in hemolytic anemia. *JBR-BTR* 87:150-151, 2004.

WHAT THE REFERRING PHYSICIAN NEEDS TO KNOW

- Associated with congenital hemolytic anemia (usually hereditary spherocytosis) or thalassemia (thalassemia major or intermedia)
- Specific diagnosis can often be made on bone marrow scintigraphy

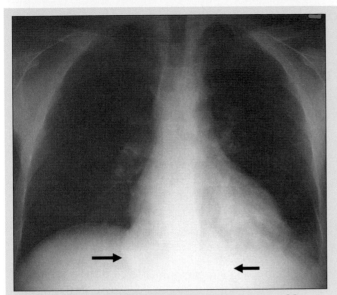

Figure 1. Extramedullary hematopoiesis in a 39-year-old man. Posteroanterior chest radiograph shows displacement of paraspinal interfaces (*arrows*).

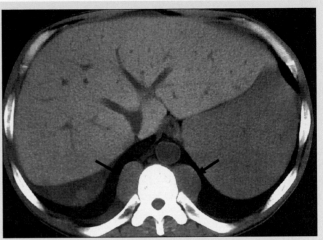

Figure 2. Extramedullary hematopoiesis in a 39-year-old man. Transverse unenhanced CT scan obtained at level of liver dome shows bilateral, homogeneous, isoattenuation, paravertebral, soft tissue lesions (*arrows*). Also note bilateral pleural effusions and increased attenuation in liver due to hemosiderosis and splenomegaly.

Meningocele or Meningomyelocele

DEFINITION: Meningocele and meningomyelocele are rare anomalies that consist of herniation of the leptomeninges through an intervertebral foramen.

IMAGING

Radiography
Findings
- Well-demarcated mass, with round or elliptical, smooth margins.

Utility
- Abnormality often first detected on the radiograph
- Radiographic findings similar to those of neurogenic tumor

CT
Findings
- Continuity between cerebrospinal fluid in thecal sac and meningocele
- Kyphoscoliosis and meningocele usually at apex of curvature on its convex side
- Enlargement of intervertebral foramen
- Associated vertebral and rib anomalies common

Utility
- CT usually diagnostic

MRI
Findings
- Continuity between cerebrospinal fluid in thecal sac and meningocele

Utility
- Diagnostic method of choice; provides best visualization of spinal cord, meninges, and adjacent structures

CLINICAL PRESENTATION

- Pain and neurologic symptoms

DIFFERENTIAL DIAGNOSIS

- Nerve sheath tumors (neurilemoma, neurofibroma, and malignant nerve sheath tumor)
- Sympathetic ganglia tumors (ganglioneuromas, ganglioneuroblastomas, and neuroblastomas)

DIAGNOSTIC PEARLS

- Continuity between the cerebrospinal fluid in the thecal sac and the meningocele
- Enlargement of the intervertebral foramen
- Meningocele: contains cerebrospinal fluid only
- Meningomyelocele: contains neural tissue
- Majority of patients have neurofibromatosis

PATHOLOGY

- Meningocele and meningomyelocele are rare anomalies that consist of herniation of leptomeninges through an intervertebral foramen.
- Meningocele contains cerebrospinal fluid only, whereas meningomyelocele also contains neural tissue.
- Abnormalities occur slightly more often on right side than on the left and are situated anywhere between thoracic inlet and diaphragm.

INCIDENCE/PREVALENCE AND EPIDEMIOLOGY

- Approximately 75% of patients present between ages of 30-60 years.
- Sixty percent to 80% of patients have neurofibromatosis.

Suggested Readings

Cabooter M, Bogaerts Y, Javaheri S, et al: Intrathoracic meningocele. *Eur J Respir Dis* 63:347-350, 1982.
Glazer HS, Siegel MJ, Sagel SS: Low-attenuation mediastinal masses on CT. *AJR Am J Roentgenol* 152:1173-1177, 1989.
Rainov NG, Heidecke V, Burkert W: Thoracic and lumbar meningocele in neurofibromatosis type 1: Report of two cases and review of the literature. *Neurosurg Rev* 18:127-134, 1995.
Strollo DC, Rosado-de-Christenson ML, Jett JR: Primary mediastinal tumors: II. Tumors of the middle and posterior mediastinum. *Chest* 112:1344-1357, 1997.

WHAT THE REFERRING PHYSICIAN NEEDS TO KNOW

- Association with vertebral and rib anomalies is common and should suggest the diagnosis.
- Majority of patients have neurofibromatosis.
- MRI is the diagnostic method of choice.

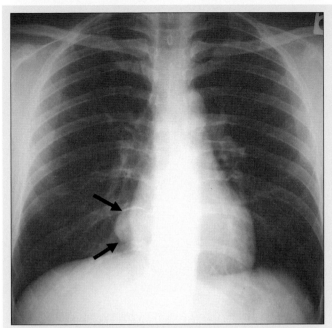

Figure 1. **Meningocele in a 29-year-old man.** Posteroanterior chest radiograph shows paraspinal mass (*arrows*) at level of T10.

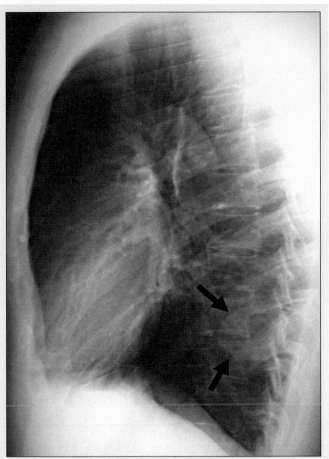

Figure 2. **Meningocele in a 29-year-old man.** Lateral chest radiograph shows paraspinal mass (*arrows*) at level of T10.

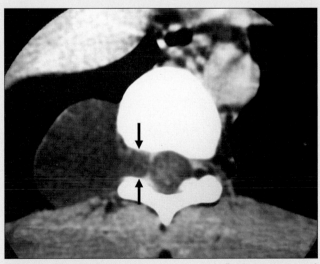

Figure 3. **Meningocele in a 29-year-old man.** CT scan demonstrates characteristic fluid attenuation of meningocele, which communicates with the thecal sac (*arrows*).

Diaphragm and Chest Wall

Bilateral Elevation of the Diaphragm

DEFINITION: Both hemidiaphragms may become elevated.

IMAGING

Radiography
Findings
- Bilateral elevation of diaphragm
- May show likely cause, including pleural disease, obesity, and hepatosplenomegaly

Utility
- Chest radiograph is first imaging modality used.
- Poor inspiratory effort or expiratory radiograph may mimic bilateral elevation of diaphragm.

Fluoroscopy
Findings
- Bilateral elevation of diaphragm
- Bilateral phrenic nerve palsy: paradoxical upward motion of both hemidiaphragms during inspiratory effort or sniff usually observed on fluoroscopic examination
- Cephalad movement of paralyzed diaphragm during inspiration accompanied by outward chest wall and inward abdominal wall motion ("thoracoabdominal paradox")

Utility
- Cephalad movement of ribs in response to accessory muscles contraction may give false appearance of caudad displacement of diaphragm.
- Despite this potential pitfall, fluoroscopy can be effectively used to evaluate condition.

CT
Findings
- Bilateral elevation of diaphragm
- May show causes, including pleural disease, obesity, hepatosplenomegaly, ascites, abdominal neoplasm, and bilateral subphrenic abscess

Utility
- Superior to radiography in demonstrating underlying causes

DIAGNOSTIC PEARLS

- Bilateral elevation of diaphragm
- Paradoxical upward motion of both hemidiaphragms during an inspiratory effort or sniff
- Characteristic findings: cephalad movement of paralyzed diaphragm during inspiration
- Elevated diaphragm with normal diaphragmatic motion possibly due to obesity, bilateral fibrothorax, hepatosplenomegaly, ascites, abdominal neoplasm, bilateral subphrenic abscess, or pregnancy

MRI
Findings
- Bilateral elevation of diaphragm
- Abnormal diaphragmatic motion

Utility
- Can assess normal and abnormal diaphragmatic motion and diaphragmatic paralysis
- Seldom used in evaluation of patients

Ultrasonography
Findings
- Bilateral elevation of diaphragm
- Abnormal diaphragmatic motion
- May show causes, including hepatosplenomegaly, ascites, abdominal neoplasm, and bilateral subphrenic abscess

Utility
- Can assess normal and abnormal diaphragmatic motion and diaphragmatic paralysis
- Has ability to assess diaphragmatic thickness and changing thickness with respiration, which makes it possibly superior to fluoroscopy

---

WHAT THE REFERRING PHYSICIAN NEEDS TO KNOW
- Common causes are spinal cord injury and generalized neuromuscular syndromes.
- Radiologic and fluoroscopic findings show elevation of both hemidiaphragms with paradoxical motion on sniff test.
- Causes of bilateral elevation of normal diaphragm include poor inspiratory effort, obesity, bilateral fibrothorax, hepatosplenomegaly, ascites, abdominal neoplasm, and bilateral subphrenic abscess.

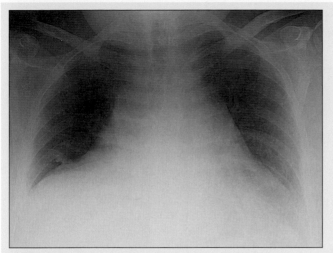

Figure 1. Bilateral elevation of diaphragm in obesity.
Anteroposterior chest radiograph in a patient on long-term corticosteroid therapy shows bilateral elevation of the diaphragm, widening of the mediastinum, and apparent enlargement of the cardiopericardial silhouette.

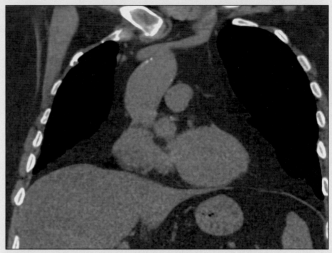

Figure 2. Bilateral elevation of diaphragm in obesity. Coronal reformatted image from a multidetector CT scan in the same patient as in Figure 1 demonstrates extensive mediastinal lipomatosis and increased size of the cardiophrenic fat pads. The heart size is within normal limits.

CLINICAL PRESENTATION

- Patients usually have respiratory symptoms consisting mainly of dyspnea and orthopnea.

DIFFERENTIAL DIAGNOSIS

- Spinal cord injury
- Bilateral fibrothorax
- Ascites
- Hepatosplenomegaly
- Abdominal neoplasm
- Systemic lupus erythematosus
- Pregnancy
- Obesity

PATHOLOGY

- Bilateral diaphragmatic palsy causes bilateral diaphragm elevation, which is, in turn, caused by spinal cord injury and generalized neuromuscular syndromes.
- Causes of bilateral elevation of normal diaphragm include poor inspiratory effort, obesity, bilateral fibrothorax, hepatosplenomegaly, ascites, abdominal neoplasm, bilateral subphrenic abscess, and pregnancy.

INCIDENCE/PREVALENCE AND EPIDEMIOLOGY

- Bilateral elevation of diaphragm is uncommon.
- Most common cause of bilateral phrenic nerve palsy is spinal cord injury.

Suggested Readings

Celli BR: Respiratory management of diaphragm paralysis. *Semin Respir Crit Care Med* 23:275-281, 2002.

Eren S, Ciris F: Diaphragmatic hernia: Diagnostic approaches with review of the literature. *Eur J Radiol* 54:448-459, 2005.

Gierada DS, Slone RM, Fleishman MJ: Imaging evaluation of the diaphragm. *Chest Surg Clin North Am* 8:237-280, 1998.

Mirvis SE: Imaging of acute thoracic injury: The advent of MDCT screening. *Semin Ultrasound CT MR* 26:305-331, 2005.

Sliker CW: Imaging of diaphragm injuries. *Radiol Clin North Am* 44:199-211, 2006.

Unilateral Elevation of the Diaphragm

DEFINITION: Unilateral elevation of the diaphragm may be due to phrenic nerve palsy, diaphragmatic eventration, or due to intrathoracic or intra-abdominal abnormalities.

IMAGING

Radiography
Findings
- With paralysis or eventration the hemidiaphragm is elevated, with accentuated dome configuration in both posteroanterior and lateral projections.
- Partial eventration usually involves anteromedial portion of right hemidiaphragm.

Utility
- Tumor invasion or compression of phrenic nerve may be suspected on radiography but usually requires confirmation with CT.
- Mimics of elevated hemidiaphragm on the radiograph include subpulmonic effusion and diaphragmatic hernia.

Fluoroscopy
Findings
- Phrenic nerve palsy: paradoxical upward motion of affected side consisting of reverse excursion of at least 2 cm indicates phrenic nerve palsy
- Eventration: initial inspiratory lag or small paradoxical motion (but downward motion later in inspiration)

Utility
- Most reliable maneuver for detecting hemidiaphragmatic paralysis is sniff test performed while visualizing the diaphragm with fluoroscopy or ultrasonography.
- Sniff test is positive in over 90% of patients with unilateral phrenic nerve palsy.
- False-negative results can occur if patient uses abdominal musculature to elevate diaphragm during expiratory phase of breathing.

CT
Findings
- Hemidiaphragm is elevated.
- In eventration, a thin diaphragm is seen as a continuous layer above elevated abdominal viscera and retroperitoneal or omental fat.

DIAGNOSTIC PEARLS

- Paralyzed hemidiaphragm is elevated and has an accentuated dome configuration in both posteroanterior and lateral projections.
- With unilateral diaphragmatic paralysis there is paradoxical upward motion of the affected side.
- Elevated normal diaphragm occurs secondary to decreased lung volume, splinting of diaphragm, or intra-abdominal contents (e.g., an abdominal mass) pushing hemidiaphragm upward.

- Tumor, lymph node, or another mass may be compressing the phrenic nerve or the diaphragm.

Utility
- Helpful in differentiating diaphragmatic paralysis or eventration from other causes of elevation of hemidiaphragm (e.g., abdominal mass or cyst)

MRI
Findings
- Elevation of hemidiaphragm

Utility
- Seldom indicated
- Detects normal and abnormal motion and paralysis of diaphragm

Ultrasonography
Findings
- Phrenic nerve palsy: paradoxical upward motion of affected side consisting of reverse excursion of at least 2 cm
- Eventration: initial inspiratory lag or small paradoxical motion (but downward motion later in inspiration)

Utility
- Can assess normal and abnormal diaphragmatic motion and diaphragmatic paralysis

---

WHAT THE REFERRING PHYSICIAN NEEDS TO KNOW

- Common causes: invasion of phrenic nerve by tumor or trauma
- Most reliable maneuver for detecting hemidiaphragmatic paralysis: sniff test done while visualizing diaphragm with fluoroscopy or ultrasonography.
- Thoracic causes of elevation of normal hemidiaphragm: atelectasis, splinting of diaphragm due to acute process (e.g., fractured rib, pleurisy, pneumonia) or after surgery (e.g., lobectomy, pneumonectomy)
- Abdominal causes of elevation of normal hemidiaphragm: distended stomach, interposition of colon between liver and right hemidiaphragm (Chilaiditi syndrome), subphrenic abscess, hepatomegaly, and abdominal neoplasm

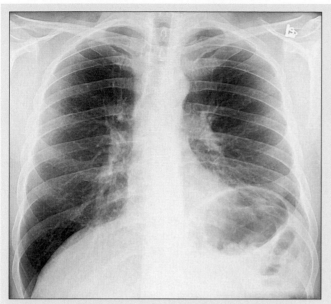

Figure 1. **Posteroanterior chest radiograph shows marked elevation of the left hemidiaphragm.** Minimal linear atelectasis is also present in the left lung base. Note that costophrenic and costovertebral sulci are deepened, narrowed, and sharpened, a feature best seen on the frontal view. Fluoroscopy demonstrated paradoxical motion of the left hemidiaphragm. The patient was a 44-year-old man with idiopathic left phrenic nerve palsy.

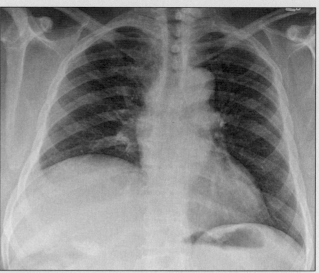

Figure 2. **Eventration of right hemidiaphragm.** Chest radiograph shows marked elevation of the right hemidiaphragm. The appearance is indistinguishable from phrenic nerve palsy. The patient was a 65-year-old man.

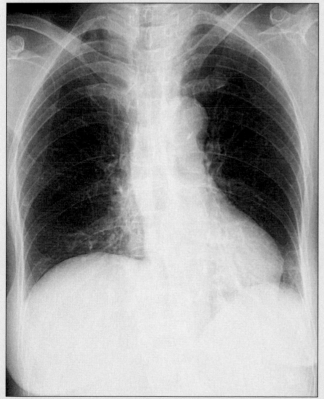

Figure 3. **Elevation of hemidiaphragm due to abdominal lesion.** Chest radiograph shows elevation of the right hemidiaphragm. The patient was an 82-year-old woman with liver cyst.

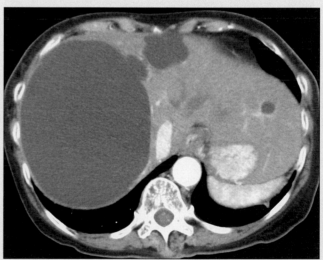

Figure 4. **Elevation of hemidiaphragm due to abdominal abnormality.** In the same patient as Figure 3, CT image demonstrates liver cysts resulting in increased size of the liver and elevation of the right hemidiaphragm. The patient was an 82-year-old woman.

- Has ability to assess diaphragmatic thickness and changing thickness with respiration, which makes it possibly superior to fluoroscopy

CLINICAL PRESENTATION

- Patients are usually asymptomatic.
- Abnormality is usually found as incidental finding in patients undergoing chest radiography for other reasons.
- Dyspnea with mild to moderate effort may develop in patients with underlying lung disease.

DIFFERENTIAL DIAGNOSIS

- Phrenic nerve palsy
- Diaphragmatic eventration
- Hepatomegaly
- Pleurisy
- Lobectomy
- Pneumonectomy
- Abdominal neoplasm
- Distended stomach

PATHOLOGY

- Most common cause of phrenic nerve palsy is compression or invasion of nerve by neoplasm.
- Other causes include trauma (natural or surgical) and phrenic "frostbite" after cardiac surgery.
- Herpes zoster, cervical spondylosis, poliomyelitis, and pneumonia may also be causative.
- Eventration may occur.

- Thoracic causes of elevation of normal hemidiaphragm include atelectasis, splinting of diaphragm due to acute process (e.g., fractured rib, pleurisy, pneumonia) or after surgery (e.g., lobectomy, pneumonectomy).
- Abdominal causes of elevation of normal hemidiaphragm include distended stomach, interposition of colon between liver and right hemidiaphragm (Chilaiditi syndrome), subphrenic abscess, hepatomegaly, and abdominal neoplasm.

INCIDENCE/PREVALENCE AND EPIDEMIOLOGY

- Most common cause of phrenic nerve palsy is compression or invasion of nerve by neoplasm, which accounts for approximately 30% of cases.
- Other common causes include trauma (natural or surgical) and phrenic "frostbite" after cardiac surgery.
- Less common causes include herpes zoster, cervical spondylosis, poliomyelitis, and pneumonia.
- However, in many cases of phrenic nerve palsy, etiology is unknown.
- Unilateral diaphragmatic elevation may also be due to eventration of diaphragm.

Suggested Readings

Celli BR: Respiratory management of diaphragm paralysis. *Semin Respir Crit Care Med* 23:275-281, 2002.
Eren S, Ciris F: Diaphragmatic hernia: Diagnostic approaches with review of the literature. *Eur J Radiol* 54:448-459, 2005.
Gierada DS, Slone RM, Fleishman MJ: Imaging evaluation of the diaphragm. *Chest Surg Clin N Am* 8:237-280, 1998.
Mirvis SE: Imaging of acute thoracic injury: The advent of MDCT screening. *Semin Ultrasound CT MR* 26:305-331, 2005.
Sliker CW: Imaging of diaphragm injuries. *Radiol Clin North Am* 44:199-211, 2006.

Phrenic Nerve Palsy

DEFINITION: Phrenic nerve palsy may be due to injury, invasion, or compression of the phrenic nerve and results in paralysis of the ipsilateral hemidiaphragm.

IMAGING

Radiography

Findings

- Paralyzed hemidiaphragm is elevated, with accentuated dome configuration in both posteroanterior and lateral projections.
- Costophrenic and costovertebral sulci tend to be deepened, narrowed, and sharpened.
- With left-sided paralysis, stomach and splenic flexure of colon relate to hemidiaphragm and contain more gas than normal.

Utility

- Tumor invasion or compression of phrenic nerve may be suspected on radiography but usually requires confirmation with CT.

Fluoroscopy

Findings

- Paradoxical upward motion of affected side consisting of reverse excursion of at least 2 cm during deep inspiration and sniff test.

Utility

- Most reliable maneuver for detecting hemidiaphragmatic paralysis is sniff test performed while visualizing diaphragm with fluoroscopy or ultrasonography.
- Sniff test is positive in over 90% of patients with unilateral phrenic nerve palsy.
- False-negative results can occur if patient uses abdominal musculature to elevate diaphragm during expiratory phase of breathing.

CT

Findings

- Elevation of diaphragm

Utility

- Used to rule out tumor, lymph node, or other mass that may be compressing the phrenic nerve
- Helpful in differentiating diaphragmatic paralysis or eventration from other causes of hemidiaphragm elevation such as abdominal mass or cyst

MRI

Findings

- Elevation of diaphragm

DIAGNOSTIC PEARLS

- Paralyzed hemidiaphragm is elevated and with an accentuated dome configuration in posteroanterior and lateral projections.
- With unilateral diaphragmatic paralysis there is paradoxical upward motion of the affected side.
- Paradoxical motion should consist of a reverse excursion of at least 2 cm to be consistent with diaphragmatic paralysis.

Utility

- Seldom indicated
- Detects normal and abnormal motion and paralysis of diaphragm

Ultrasonography

Findings

- Paradoxical upward motion of affected side consisting of reverse excursion of at least 2 cm

Utility

- Assesses normal and abnormal diaphragmatic motion and diaphragmatic paralysis
- Has ability to assess diaphragmatic thickness and changing thickness with respiration, possibly making it superior to fluoroscopy

CLINICAL PRESENTATION

- With unilateral phrenic nerve palsy, patients are usually asymptomatic.
- Abnormality is usually found as an incidental finding in patients undergoing chest radiography for other reasons.
- Dyspnea with mild to moderate effort may develop in patients with underlying lung disease.
- With bilateral phrenic nerve palsy, patients usually have severe respiratory symptoms consisting mainly of dyspnea and orthopnea.

WHAT THE REFERRING PHYSICIAN NEEDS TO KNOW

- Common causes include invasion of phrenic nerve by tumor, trauma, or spinal cord injury.
- Radiologic findings include elevation of the hemidiaphragm or hemidiaphragms.
- Paradoxical motion on sniff test is performed while visualizing the diaphragm with fluoroscopy or ultrasonography.
- Positive sniff test requires reverse excursion of at least 2 cm.

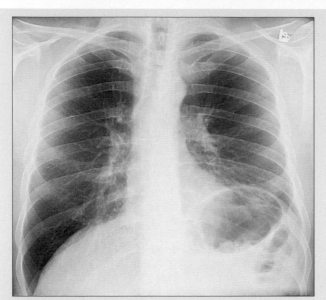

Figure 1. Phrenic nerve palsy. Posteroanterior chest radiograph shows marked elevation of the left hemidiaphragm. Minimal linear atelectasis is also present in the left lung base. Note that costophrenic and costovertebral sulci are deepened, narrowed, and sharpened, a feature best seen on the frontal view. Fluoroscopy demonstrated paradoxical motion of the left hemidiaphragm. The patient was a 44-year-old man with idiopathic left phrenic nerve palsy.

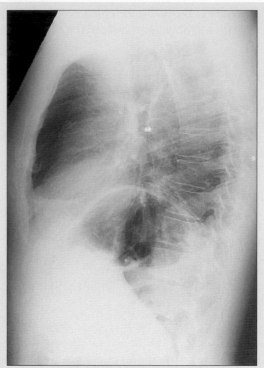

Figure 2. Phrenic nerve palsy. Lateral chest radiograph shows marked elevation of the left hemidiaphragm. Minimal linear atelectasis is also present in the left lung base. Note that costophrenic and costovertebral sulci are deepened, narrowed, and sharpened, a feature best seen on the frontal view (see Fig. 1). Fluoroscopy demonstrated paradoxical motion of the left hemidiaphragm. The patient was a 44-year-old man with idiopathic left phrenic nerve palsy.

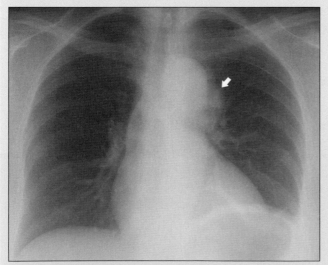

Figure 3. Phrenic nerve palsy due to lung cancer. Chest radiograph shows elevation of the left hemidiaphragm and mass (*arrow*) adjacent to the aorticopulmonary window. The patient was a 54-year-old woman with phrenic nerve palsy due to lung cancer.

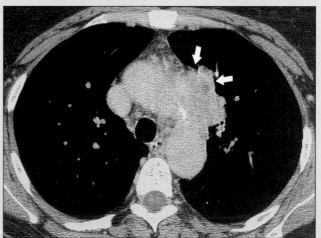

Figure 4. Phrenic nerve palsy due to lung cancer. In the same patient as Figure 3, CT image demonstrates mass (*arrows*) invading the mediastinum at the region of the phrenic nerve and aorticopulmonary window. The patient was a 54-year-old woman with phrenic nerve palsy due to lung cancer.

DIFFERENTIAL DIAGNOSIS

- Diaphragmatic eventration
- Diaphragmatic hernia
- Hepatomegaly
- Fibrothorax
- Subpulmonic pleural effusion

PATHOLOGY

- Caused by compression or invasion of nerve by neoplasm
- Other causes include trauma (natural or surgical) and phrenic "frostbite" after cardiac surgery
- May also be due to herpes zoster, cervical spondylosis, poliomyelitis, and pneumonia

INCIDENCE/PREVALENCE AND EPIDEMIOLOGY

- Most common cause is compression or invasion of nerve by neoplasm, which accounts for approximately 30% of cases.

- Other common causes include trauma (natural or surgical) and phrenic "frostbite" after cardiac surgery.
- Less common causes include herpes zoster, cervical spondylosis, poliomyelitis, and pneumonia.
- However, in many cases the etiology is unknown.
- For bilateral phrenic nerve palsy, the most common cause is spinal cord injury.

Suggested Readings

Celli BR: Respiratory management of diaphragm paralysis. *Semin Respir Crit Care Med* 23:275-281, 2002.

Gierada DS, Slone RM, Fleishman MJ: Imaging evaluation of the diaphragm. *Chest Surg Clin North Am* 8:237-280, 1998.

Diaphragmatic Eventration

DEFINITION: Diaphragmatic eventration is failure of muscular development of part or all of one or both hemidiaphragms.

IMAGING

Radiography
Findings
- Elevation of hemidiaphragm is evident.
- With partial eventration, affected hemidiaphragm shows smaller than normal inspiratory excursion/
- Usually the anteromedial portion of the right hemidiaphragm is involved.

Utility
- Eventration is usually first detected by radiography.

Fluoroscopy
Findings
- Initial inspiratory lag or small paradoxical motion can be seen; however, later in inspiration it has a downward motion.

Utility
- Helpful in distinguishing eventration from diaphragmatic paralysis

Ultrasonography
Findings
- Diaphragm may show an initial inspiratory lag or small paradoxical motion; however, later in inspiration it has a downward motion.

Utility
- Ability of ultrasonography to assess diaphragmatic thickness and changing thickness with respiration makes it possibly superior to fluoroscopy.

CT
Findings
- Thin diaphragm is seen as continuous layer above elevated abdominal viscera and retroperitoneal or omental fat.

Utility
- Main role in partial eventration is distinguishing abnormality from focal bulge in diaphragmatic contour caused by tumor or hernia.

CLINICAL PRESENTATION
- Eventration is typically asymptomatic.
- Symptoms may be present in obese patients as a result of raised intra-abdominal pressure.

DIAGNOSTIC PEARLS
- Radiologic signs of complete eventration of a hemidiaphragm are identical to those of diaphragmatic paralysis consisting of elevation of hemidiaphragm.
- With partial eventration, affected hemidiaphragm shows a smaller than normal inspiratory excursion.
- On fluoroscopy, there may be an initial inspiratory lag or small paradoxical motion; however, later in inspiration there is downward motion.

DIFFERENTIAL DIAGNOSIS
- Diaphragmatic palsy
- Diaphragmatic hernia
- Hepatomegaly
- Subpulmonic pleural effusion

PATHOLOGY
- There is congenital failure of muscular development of part or all of one or both hemidiaphragms.
- Totally eventrated hemidiaphragm consists of membranous sheet attached peripherally to normal muscle at points of origin from rib cage.
- Total eventration occurs almost exclusively on left side.
- Partial eventration is usually present in anteromedial portion of right hemidiaphragm.
- Partial eventration rarely occurs on the left and occasionally in central portion of either cupola.

INCIDENCE/PREVALENCE AND EPIDEMIOLOGY
- Complete eventration of hemidiaphragm is always congenital.
- Partial eventration is more common than total form, seen in patients older than age 60 years, and may be acquired.
- Partial eventration occurs with equal frequency in men and women.

WHAT THE REFERRING PHYSICIAN NEEDS TO KNOW
- Unilateral and partial eventration when seen in adults typically involves the anteromedial portion of the right hemidiaphragm.
- Radiologically, complete eventration of hemidiaphragm is identical to diaphragmatic paralysis and consists of elevation of the hemidiaphragm.
- Distinction of eventration from diaphragmatic paralysis can usually be made during fluoroscopy ("sniff test") or ultrasonography.

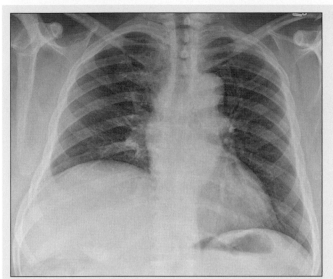

Figure 1. Eventration of right hemidiaphragm. Chest radiograph shows marked elevation of the right hemidiaphragm. The appearance is indistinguishable from phrenic nerve palsy. The patient was a 65-year-old man.

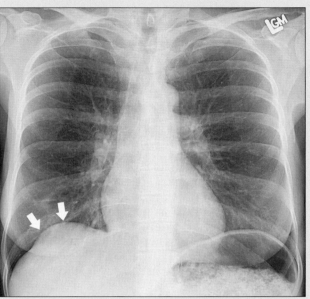

Figure 2. Partial eventration of the right hemidiaphragm. Posteroanterior chest radiograph demonstrates focal elevation (*arrows*) of the anteromedial portion of the right hemidiaphragm characteristic of partial eventration. The patient was a 51-year-old woman.

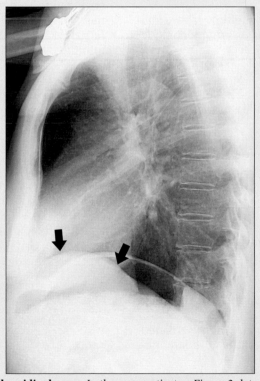

Figure 3. Partial eventration of the right hemidiaphragm. In the same patient as Figure 2, lateral chest radiograph demonstrates focal elevation (*arrows*) of the anteromedial portion of the right hemidiaphragm characteristic of partial eventration. The patient was a 51-year-old woman.

Suggested Readings

Deslauriers J: Eventration of the diaphragm. *Chest Surg Clin North Am* 8:315-330, 1998.

Gierada DS, Slone RM, Fleishman MJ: Imaging evaluation of the diaphragm. *Chest Surg Clin North Am* 8:237-280, 1998.

Verhey PT, Gosselin MV, Primack SL, et al: Differentiating diaphragmatic paralysis and eventration. *Acad Radiol* 14:420-425, 2007.

Hiatal Hernia

DEFINITION: A hiatal hernia is a hernia through the esophageal hiatus of the diaphragm into the thorax.

IMAGING

Radiography
Findings
- Hiatal hernia typically manifests radiographically as a retrocardiac mass, usually containing air or air-fluid level.
- A large mass may contain a double air-fluid level.
- In cases in which most of stomach has herniated through hiatus, the stomach may undergo volvulus.
- Other structures, such as portion of transverse colon, omentum, or liver, may also be seen.
- Signs of strangulation of herniated contents are evident.

Utility
- Large hiatus hernias can usually be readily recognized.

CT
Findings
- Widening of esophageal hiatus allows stomach and omentum to protrude into chest
- Normally, esophageal hiatus is elliptical and measures ≤15 mm in width

Utility
- Multidetector CT with coronal and sagittal reformatted images is most effective and useful imaging technique in assessing diaphragmatic hernias.

MRI
Findings
- Widening of esophageal hiatus allows stomach and omentum to protrude into chest.

Utility
- Diagnosis can be readily made with MRI, but use of this modality is rarely indicated.

CLINICAL PRESENTATION

- Most diaphragmatic hernias do not give rise to symptoms.
- Patients with symptomatic hiatal hernia may present with heartburn and regurgitation.
- Occasionally, chronic reflux may result in scarring and narrowing of lower esophagus and symptoms of esophageal obstruction.
- In cases in which most of stomach has herniated through hiatus, it may undergo volvulus and strangulation may occur.

DIAGNOSTIC PEARLS

- Hiatal hernia typically manifests radiographically as a retrocardiac mass, usually containing air or an air-fluid level.
- Esophageal hernias usually result from widening of esophageal hiatus, allowing stomach and omentum to protrude into chest.
- Other structures, such as portion of transverse colon, omentum, or liver, may also be seen.
- Esophageal hernias are evident on CT in 5% of individuals younger than 40 years, 30% of those aged 40-49, and 65% of those aged 60-79.

PATHOLOGY

- Herniation of diaphragm occurs through esophageal hiatus into thorax.
- Hiatal hernias may be sliding or paraesophageal.
- Sliding hernias are the most common; the hernia slides back and forth between the abdominal and chest cavities.
- In paraesophageal hernias part of the stomach bulges into the thorax and remains there.

INCIDENCE/PREVALENCE AND EPIDEMIOLOGY

- Prevalence of esophageal hiatal hernias increases with age.
- They are evident on CT in approximately 5% of individuals younger than 40 years, 30% of those aged 40-59, and 65% of those aged 60-79.

Suggested Readings

Abbara S, Kalan MM, Lewicki AM: Intrathoracic stomach revisited. *AJR Am J Roentgenol* 181:403-414, 2003.
Canon CL, Morgan DE, Einstein DM, et al: Surgical approach to gastroesophageal reflux disease: What the radiologist needs to know. *RadioGraphics* 25:1485-1499, 2005.
Eren S, Ciris F: Diaphragmatic hernia: Diagnostic approaches with review of the literature. *Eur J Radiol* 54:448-459, 2005.

WHAT THE REFERRING PHYSICIAN NEEDS TO KNOW
- Prevalence increases with age.
- Patients are usually asymptomatic.
- Strangulation of hernial contents may occur.

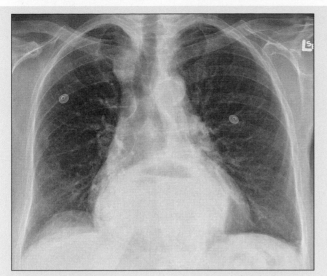

Figure 1. Hiatal hernia. Posteroanterior chest radiograph demonstrates large retrocardiac mass with fluid level. The appearance is characteristic of a hiatal hernia. The patient was an 85-year-old woman.

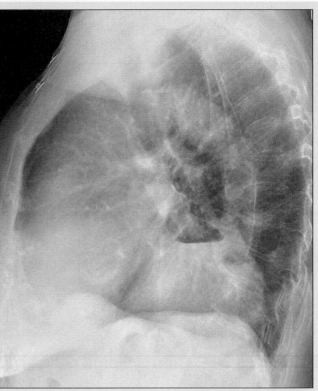

Figure 2. Hiatal hernia. In the same patient as Figure 1, lateral chest radiograph demonstrates large retrocardiac mass with fluid level. The appearance is characteristic of a hiatal hernia. The patient was an 85-year-old woman.

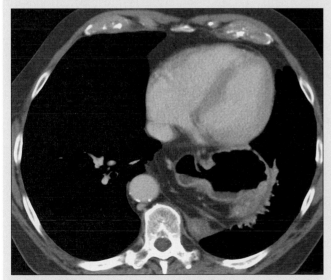

Figure 3. Hiatal hernia. CT image shows herniation of stomach and omentum into the retrocardiac region. The patient was a 79-year-old man.

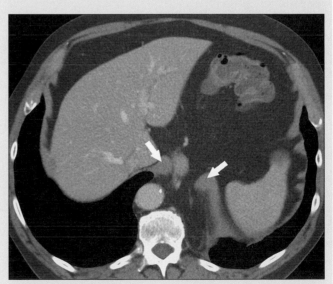

Figure 4. Hiatal hernia. In the same patient as Figure 3, CT image at the level of the esophageal hiatus shows widening of the space between the right and left crura (*arrows*) and hiatal hernia. The patient was a 79-year-old man.

Bochdalek Hernia

DEFINITION: A Bochdalek hernia is herniation of omentum and abdominal viscera into the chest through a defect in the posterolateral aspect of the diaphragm.

IMAGING

Radiography
Findings
- These lesions manifest as a focal bulge in the hemidiaphragm or as a mass adjacent to the posteromedial aspect of either hemidiaphragm.
- Prevalence increases with age; they may manifest in patients with previously normal radiographs.

Utility
- Diagnosis can often be suspected on radiography by typical location and by lower density than soft tissue of mass.
- Appearance can mimic that of pulmonary, mediastinal, or paravertebral masses.

CT
Findings
- In adults, results from herniation through posterior diaphragmatic defect lateral to crura.
- Occasionally may be large and contain portions of kidney and, rarely, stomach and small bowel

Utility
- Diagnosis is readily made on CT.
- Multidetector CT with coronal and sagittal reformatted images is most effective and useful imaging technique in assessing diaphragmatic hernias.

MRI
Utility
- Diagnosis of diaphragmatic hernias can be readily made.

CLINICAL PRESENTATION

- In infants this hernia is associated with severe respiratory distress.
- Adult patients with Bochdalek hernias are usually asymptomatic.
- Occasionally patients may complain of epigastric or lower sternal pressure and discomfort and sometimes cardiorespiratory and gastrointestinal symptoms.

PATHOLOGY

- When hernia is large, almost entire abdominal contents may be in left hemithorax, interfering with normal lung development.

DIAGNOSTIC PEARLS

- Manifests as a focal bulge in hemidiaphragm or as a mass adjacent to posteromedial aspect of either hemidiaphragm
- May manifest in patients with previously normal radiographs
- Occasionally may be large and contain portions of kidney and, rarely, stomach and small bowel
- Prevalence increases with age
- Adult Bochdalek hernias are usually small and asymptomatic

- Congenital Bochdalek hernias are frequently associated with pulmonary hypoplasia.
- Most large hernias have no peritoneal sac, so communication between pleural and peritoneal cavities is wide open.
- Adult Bochdalek hernias are presumably acquired defects.

INCIDENCE/PREVALENCE AND EPIDEMIOLOGY

- In infants, Bochdalek hernia is most common form of diaphragmatic hernia, with incidence of 1:2000 births.
- In adults, small hernias are more common than in infants; they are seen on CT in 5%-10% of adults.
- Incidence of adult Bochdalek hernia increases with age, suggesting that they are acquired.
- Most cases are left sided.
- These hernias are rare in adult patients younger than 40; they are seen in approximately 5% of patients aged 40-49 years, 15% of patients aged 50-69 years, and 35% of older patients.

Suggested Readings

Eren S, Ciris F: Diaphragmatic hernia: Diagnostic approaches with review of the literature. *Eur J Radiol* 54:448-459, 2005.
Mullins ME, Stein J, Saini SS, et al: Prevalence of incidental Bochdalek's hernia in a large adult population. *AJR Am J Roentgenol* 177:363-366, 2001.

WHAT THE REFERRING PHYSICIAN NEEDS TO KNOW
- May be congenital or acquired
- Manifests on radiographs as a focal bulge in the hemidiaphragm or as a mass adjacent to the posteromedial aspect of either hemidiaphragm

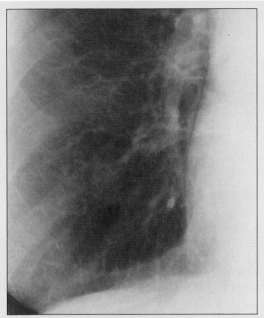

Figure 1. Development of a Bochdalek hernia in an elderly patient. A view of the right lower chest from a posteroanterior radiograph in a 78-year-old woman is unremarkable. (*From Müller NL, Fraser RS, Colman NC, Paré PD:* Radiologic Diagnosis of Diseases of the Chest. *Philadelphia, WB Saunders, 2001.*)

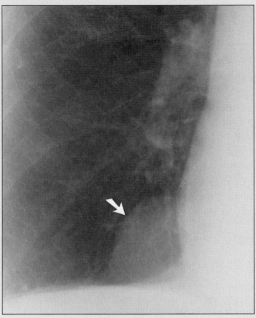

Figure 2. Development of a Bochdalek hernia in an elderly patient. View from posteroanterior radiograph performed 5 years later than in Figure 1 demonstrates a large mass adjacent to the posteromedial aspect of the right hemidiaphragm (*arrow*). The mass has lower opacity than the heart and soft tissues of the abdomen, consistent with fat. The patient had no symptoms related to the hernia. (*From Müller NL, Fraser RS, Colman NC, Paré PD:* Radiologic Diagnosis of Diseases of the Chest. *Philadelphia, WB Saunders, 2001.*)

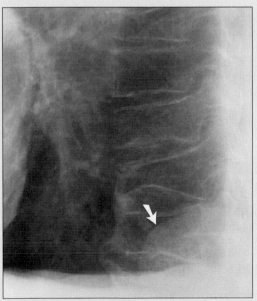

Figure 3. Development of a Bochdalek hernia in an elderly patient. View from lateral radiograph performed 5 years later than in Figure 1 demonstrates a large mass adjacent to the posteromedial aspect of the right hemidiaphragm (*arrow*). The mass has lower opacity than the heart and soft tissues of the abdomen, consistent with fat. The patient had no symptoms related to the hernia. (*From Müller NL, Fraser RS, Colman NC, Paré PD:* Radiologic Diagnosis of Diseases of the Chest. *Philadelphia, WB Saunders, 2001.*)

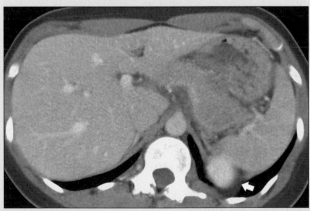

Figure 4. Bochdalek hernia. CT image shows focal discontinuity of the left hemidiaphragm and herniation of omental fat and part of the left kidney. The patient was a 36-year-old woman with no symptoms related to the small Bochdalek hernia.

Morgagni Hernia

DEFINITION: A Morgagni hernia is a herniation through the parasternal hiatus of the diaphragm.

IMAGING

Radiography
Findings
- A smooth, well-defined homogeneous opacity is seen in the right cardiophrenic angle.
- Occasionally, this opacity is inhomogeneous owing to either air-containing loops of bowel or fatty nature of hernial contents.
- In rare cases when the hernia penetrates into the pericardial sac, loops of air-containing bowel are identified anterior to the cardiac shadow.
Utility
- Often first detected incidentally on chest radiograph

CT
Findings
- Herniation of abdominal contents between costal and sternal attachments of diaphragm
- Anteromedial in location and usually occurs on right side
- Majority containing only omentum, which is seen as a mass with fat attenuation
- Transverse colon situated high in abdomen, with peak situated anteriorly and superiorly—a location that is virtually diagnostic
Utility
- Multidetector CT with coronal and sagittal reformatted images is most effective and useful imaging technique in assessing diaphragmatic hernias.

MRI
Findings
- Herniation of abdominal contents between costal and sternal attachments of diaphragm
- Anteromedial in location and usually occurs on right side
Utility
- Diagnosis of diaphragmatic hernias can be readily made on MRI, although use of this modality is seldom indicated.

CLINICAL PRESENTATION

- Adult patients with Morgagni hernia are often asymptomatic.

DIAGNOSTIC PEARLS

- Smooth, well-defined, homogeneous, occasionally inhomogeneous, opacity in right cardiophrenic angle
- Anteromedial in location and occurs on the right side
- Transverse colon situated high in abdomen, with peak situated anteriorly and superiorly—a finding that is virtually diagnostic

- Some patients may complain of epigastric or lower sternal pressure and discomfort and sometimes cardiorespiratory and gastrointestinal symptoms.
- Occasionally, stomach or colon may become incarcerated or strangulated, resulting in pain and vomiting.

DIFFERENTIAL DIAGNOSIS

- Pericardial fat pad
- Pericardial cyst
- Diaphragmatic lipoma

PATHOLOGY

- Hernia may be developmental in origin or post-traumatic.
- In contrast to Bochdalek hernia, peritoneal sac is present in most cases.
- Hernial sac may include, in order of decreasing frequency: omentum, colon, stomach, liver, and small intestine.
- Left foramen relates to heart; thus, most herniations are seen on right side.

INCIDENCE/PREVALENCE AND EPIDEMIOLOGY

- Morgagni (parasternal) hernia is uncommon.
- Hernias are more common in adults than children.
- They are often associated with obesity or other situations involving increased intra-abdominal pressure such as severe effort or trauma.

WHAT THE REFERRING PHYSICIAN NEEDS TO KNOW
- This uncommon hernia is associated with obesity or trauma and usually asymptomatic.
- Some patients may complain of epigastric or lower sternal pressure and discomfort and sometimes cardiorespiratory and gastrointestinal symptoms.
- Occasionally stomach or colon may become incarcerated or strangulated, resulting in pain and vomiting.
- Diagnosis can be readily confirmed on CT.

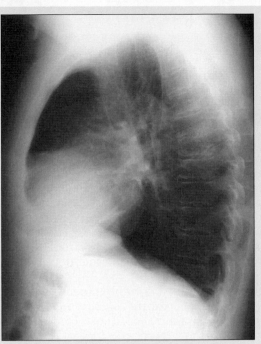

Figure 1. Morgagni hernia. Posteroanterior chest radiograph demonstrates a mass in the right costophrenic sulcus. The mass has a density lower than that of soft tissue, consistent with fat. The patient was a 49-year-old man.

Figure 2. Morgagni hernia. In the same patient as Figure 1, lateral chest radiograph demonstrates a mass in the right costophrenic sulcus. The mass has a density lower than that of soft tissue, consistent with fat. The patient was a 49-year-old man.

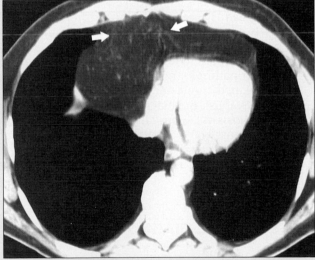

Figure 3. Morgagni hernia. In the same patient as Figure 1, CT image demonstrates omentum and omental vessels (*arrows*) herniating through the right lower parasternal region diagnostic of Morgagni hernia. The patient was a 49-year-old man.

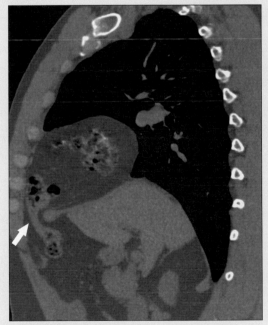

Figure 4. Morgagni hernia. Sagittal reformatted image demonstrates anterior herniation (*arrow*) of omentum and large bowel into the chest. The findings are characteristic of Morgagni hernia. The patient was a 54-year-old man.

Suggested Readings

Eren S, Ciris F: Diaphragmatic hernia: Diagnostic approaches with review of the literature. *Eur J Radiol* 54:448-459, 2005.

Loong TP, Kocher HM: Clinical presentation and operative repair of hernia of Morgagni. *Postgrad Med J* 81(951):41-44, 2005.

Mirvis SE: Imaging of acute thoracic injury: The advent of MDCT screening. *Semin Ultrasound CT MR* 26:305-331, 2005.

Sliker CW: Imaging of diaphragm injuries. *Radiol Clin North Am* 44:199-211, 2006.

Deformities of Chest Wall

DEFINITION: Congenital and developmental anomalies may affect the chest wall.

IMAGING

Radiography
Findings
- Poland syndrome: unilateral hyperlucency with absent axillary fold on the affected side, sometimes associated with rib deformities
- Pectus excavatum: obscured right-sided heart border, heart displaced to left and rotated, and spurious cardiomegaly
- Pectus excavatum: depression and deformity in lower portion of sternum
- Pectus carinatum: anterior prominence of sternum
- Kyphoscoliosis: curvature usually convex to the right
- Congenital rib anomalies (most commonly cervical rib)
- Rib notching: most commonly due to neurogenic tumor or coarctation of aorta

Utility
- In severe kyphoscoliosis, chest radiograph is difficult to evaluate because of rotation of the thorax and heart.

CT
Findings
- Poland syndrome: absence/hypoplasia of pectoral girdle musculature, with absent sternocostal head of pectoralis major and chest wall defects
- Pectus excavatum: depression and deformity of the lower sternum, with associated compression of lungs

Utility
- Best quantifies severity of pectus excavatum

MRI
Findings
- Poland syndrome: absence/hypoplasia of pectoral girdle musculature, with absent sternocostal head of pectoralis major and chest wall defects

Utility
- Modality of choice for assessment of chest wall soft tissue abnormalities

DIAGNOSTIC PEARLS

- Poland syndrome: unilateral hyperlucency with absent axillary fold on the affected side and sometimes associated with rib deformities
- Pectus excavatum: obscured right-sided heart border, heart displaced to left and rotated, and spurious cardiomegaly
- Pectus excavatum: lower portion of sternum shows depression and deformity
- Pectus carinatum: anterior prominence of sternum
- Kyphoscoliosis: abnormal posterior and lateral thoracic curvature

CLINICAL PRESENTATION

- Poland syndrome is associated with increased incidence of leukemia, non-Hodgkin lymphoma, lung cancer, and breast cancer; majority of patients present with cosmetic complaints, but in other cases the presentation varies according to the type of defect.
- Pectus excavatum is usually asymptomatic or presents as chest/back pain; it is associated with increased frequency of other congenital anomalies.
- Pectus carinatum is usually asymptomatic although may have arrhythmias or dyspnea; physical examination can establish the diagnosis.
- Kyphoscoliosis is abnormal posterior and lateral thoracic curvature, 80% of which is idiopathic, or with associated congenital causes.
- Cervical ribs cause thoracic outlet syndrome in less than 10% of patients.

DIFFERENTIAL DIAGNOSIS

- Poland syndrome
- Pectus excavatum
- Pectus carinatum

WHAT THE REFERRING PHYSICIAN NEEDS TO KNOW

- Cross-sectional imaging techniques enable precise localization of chest wall lesions and, in some cases, definitive diagnosis.
- Most common chest wall deformity is pectus excavatum (90%), followed by pectus carinatum (5%-7%).
- MRI is the imaging modality of choice for assessment of chest wall soft tissue abnormalities.

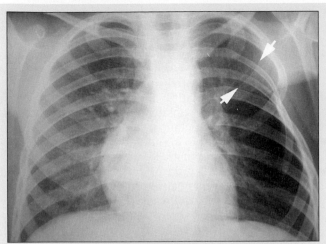

Figure 1. Poland syndrome. Anteroposterior chest radiograph shows hyperlucency of the left hemithorax compared with contralateral side. Two hypoplastic ribs are present in the ipsilateral hemithorax (*arrows*). (*Courtesy of Dr. Tomás Franquet, Barcelona, Spain*)

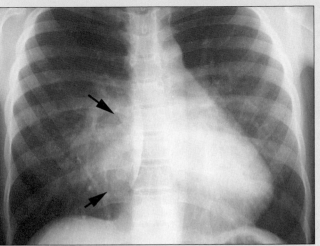

Figure 2. Pectus excavatum in a 22-year-old woman. Posteroanterior chest radiograph shows obscuration of the right-sided heart border (*arrows*) and displacement of the heart to the left. (*Courtesy of Dr. Tomás Franquet, Barcelona, Spain*)

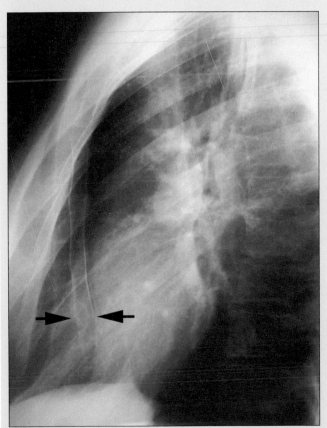

Figure 3. Pectus excavatum in a 22-year-old woman. In the same patient as Figure 2, lateral chest radiograph shows posterior displacement of the sternum (*arrows*). (*Courtesy of Dr. Tomás Franquet, Barcelona, Spain*)

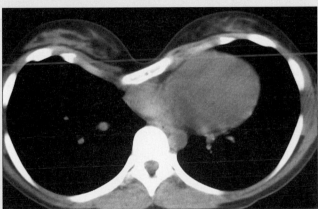

Figure 4. Pectus excavatum in a 22-year-old woman. In the same patient as Figure 2, CT scan demonstrates severe pectus excavatum with compression of the lungs and displacement of the heart to the left. (*Courtesy of Dr. Tomás Franquet, Barcelona, Spain*)

- Kyphoscoliosis
- Right middle lobe atelectasis
- Cardiomegaly
- Trauma

PATHOLOGY

- Poland syndrome is absence/hypoplasia of pectoral girdle musculature, with absent sternocostal head of pectoralis major and chest wall defects.
- Pectus excavatum generally present at birth and is progressive with increasing depth of sternal depression as the patient grows.
- Kyphoscoliosis, when severe, causes decreased compliance of lung and chest wall, with resultant restrictive lung disease.
- Rib notching results from rib erosion by dilated intercostal arteries taking part in collateral arterial flow such as in aortic coarctation and affects the lower margin of one or more ribs.

INCIDENCE/PREVALENCE AND EPIDEMIOLOGY

- Poland syndrome: three times more common in males than in females and involves the right side in 75% of patients

- Pectus excavatum: most common disorder of chest wall formation (1 case/300-400 live births), with 3:1 male-to-female ratio
- Pectus carinatum: less frequent than pectus excavatum (5%-7% vs. 90%), with 4:1 male-to-female ratio and positive familial predisposition
- Congenital rib anomalies: found in 1%-2% of chest radiographs and are isolated findings occurring sporadically and lacking clinical significance
- Cervical rib: present in about 0.5% of the general population and bilateral in 45%-70% of cases
- Rib notching: coarctation of aorta most common and important cause; other causes: intercostal nerve tumors (neurilemoma, neurofibroma), subclavian artery obstruction, arteriovenous malformation involving intercostal artery and vein, and hyperparathyroidism

Suggested Readings

Fefferman NR, Pinkney LP: Imaging evaluation of chest wall disorders in children. *Radiol Clin North Am* 43:355-370, 2005.

Glass RB, Norton KI, Mitre SA, Kang E: Pediatric ribs: A spectrum of abnormalities. *RadioGraphics* 22:87-104, 2002.

Goretsky MJ, Kelly RE Jr, Croitoru D, Nuss D: Chest wall anomalies: Pectus excavatum and pectus carinatum. *Adolesc Med Clin* 15:455-471, 2004.

Jeung MY, Gangi A, Gasser B, et al: Imaging of chest wall disorders. *RadioGraphics* 19:617-637, 1999.

Kuhlman JE, Bouchardy L, Fishman EK, Zerhouni EA: CT and MR imaging evaluation of chest wall disorders. *RadioGraphics* 14:571-595, 1994.

Tumors of Chest Wall

DEFINITION: Metastases to the chest wall and direct extension by pulmonary carcinoma are common, but primary chest wall tumors are uncommon.

IMAGING

Radiography

Findings

- Fibrous dysplasia: osteolytic lesion with homogeneous "ground-glass" matrix and endosteal scalloping, with or without bone expansion
- Osteochondroma: focal deformity or expansion of the rib with calcification of the cartilaginous cap
- Chondrosarcoma: large mineralized mass with characteristic rings and arches pattern of calcification, mainly arising from anterior rib or costochondral junction
- Osteosarcoma: mixed sclerotic and lucent areas within the medullary cavity; cortical disruption, aggressive periosteal reaction; and associated soft tissue mass.
- Ewing sarcoma/PNET: osteolytic lesions with cortical destruction, periosteal reaction, and associated soft tissue masses
- Multiple myeloma: multifocal osteolytic lesions with a "motheaten" appearance
- Metastases: lytic destructive process in the medullary cavity with ill-defined margins, cortical erosion, and frequent soft tissue extension
- Intercostal nerve tumor: may result in rib erosion

Utility

- Usually first imaging modality performed in these patients

CT

Findings

- Fibrous dysplasia: osteolytic lesion with homogeneous "ground-glass" matrix and endosteal scalloping, with or without bone expansion
- Osteochondroma; focal expansion of the rib with calcification of the cartilaginous cap
- Chondrosarcoma: large mineralized mass with characteristic rings and arches pattern of calcification, mainly arising from anterior rib or costochondral junction; soft tissue component evident on CT
- Lipoma: mass with homogeneous density similar to subcutaneous fat
- Elastofibroma: lenticular, unencapsulated, soft tissue mass with skeletal muscle attenuation interspersed with strands of fat attenuation

DIAGNOSTIC PEARLS

- Most common chest wall bone tumors: metastases and multiple myeloma
- Most common primary malignant chest wall bone tumor: chondrosarcoma
- Most common benign rib lesion: fibrous dysplasia
- Most common benign soft tissue tumor: lipoma
- Most common soft tissue malignant tumor: malignant fibrous histiocytoma

- Intercostal nerve sheath tumor (neurilemoma, neurofibroma): well-marginated, smooth mass along course of intercostal nerve; soft tissue or low attenuation with variable contrast enhancement
- Multiple myeloma: multifocal osteolytic lesions with a "motheaten" appearance
- Metastases: lytic destructive process in the medullary cavity with ill-defined margins, cortical erosion, and frequent soft tissue extension

Utility

- Fibrous dysplasia: CT enables more accurate assessment of lesion morphology, location, and extent over radiographs.
- Osteochondroma: CT is particularly helpful if lesions are in the ribs, shoulder, or spine.

MRI

Findings

- Chondrosarcoma: destructive lesion with large soft tissue mass having characteristic peripheral and septal enhancement after contrast agent administration
- Ewing sarcoma/PNET: large mixed-signal mass, disproportionately large compared with bone involvement
- Lipoma: mass with signal characteristics similar to subcutaneous fat
- Elastofibroma: lenticular, unencapsulated, soft tissue mass with skeletal muscle signal intensity interspersed with strands of fat signal intensity

Utility

- Fibrous dysplasia: MRI enables more accurate assessment of lesion morphology, location, and extent over radiographs

---

WHAT THE REFERRING PHYSICIAN NEEDS TO KNOW

- Benign bone tumors of the chest wall are uncommon, the most common being osteochondroma.
- Most common chest wall benign soft tissue tumor is lipoma.
- Most common primary malignant soft tissue tumor is malignant fibrous histiocytoma.
- MRI is the best method to assess the extent of malignant chest wall tumors.

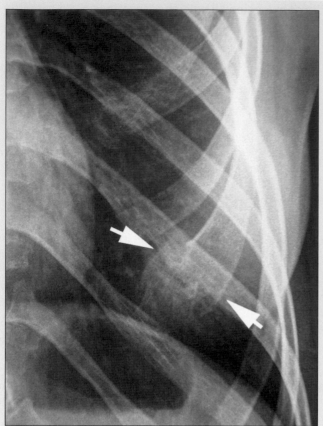

Figure 1. Fibrous dysplasia in a 16-year-old girl with chest pain. Close-up view from chest radiograph shows an expanding, osteolytic lesion in the anterior aspect of the sixth rib (*arrows*). (*Courtesy of Dr. Tomás Franquet, Barcelona, Spain*)

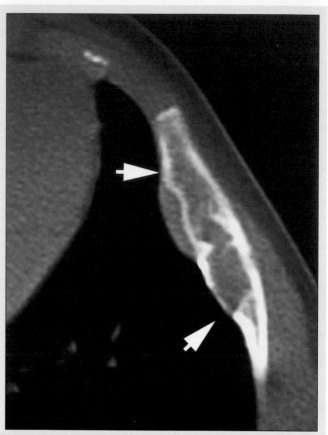

Figure 2. Fibrous dysplasia in a 16-year-old girl with chest pain. CT scan shows a large lytic lesion in the rib. The lesion has caused cortical thinning and expansile remodeling of the rib (*arrows*). (*Courtesy of Dr. Tomás Franquet, Barcelona, Spain*)

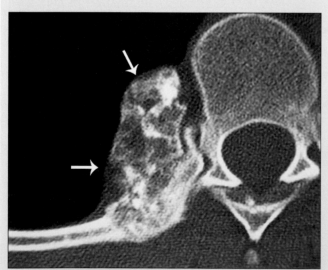

Figure 3. Osteochondroma of the rib in a 28-year-old man with an incidental finding on chest radiograph. CT scan at level of the costovertebral junction shows a mineralized mass arising from the rib (*arrows*). (*Courtesy of Dr. Tomás Franquet, Barcelona, Spain*)

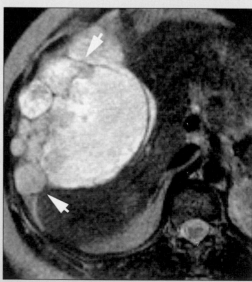

Figure 4. Chondrosarcoma of chest wall in a 45-year-old man with a painless, slowly growing mass in the lower chest wall. T2-weighted MR image shows a high signal intensity heterogenous mass, with lobulated appearance and low signal intensity septa between cartilaginous lobules (*arrows*). (*Courtesy of Dr. Tomás Franquet, Barcelona, Spain*)

- MRI is the best method to assess the extent of malignant chest wall tumors.

CLINICAL PRESENTATION

- Fibrous dysplasia: virtually affects any bone and may be monostotic or polyostotic
- Multiple myeloma: associated with presence of increased monoclonal immunoglobulin and light chain proteins in the blood and urine
- Metastases: pain, pathologic fractures, and hypercalcemia most common clinical manifestations
- Benign soft tissue tumors: typically manifest as painless, slow-growing, palpable masses
- Soft tissue sarcomas and primary malignant fibrous histiocytoma: manifest as painful and rapidly growing masses

DIFFERENTIAL DIAGNOSIS

- Metastases
- Multiple myeloma
- Chondrosarcoma
- Osteosarcoma
- Malignant fibrous histiocytoma
- Fibrous dysplasia
- Lipoma

PATHOLOGY

- Chest wall tumors are uncommon neoplasms that may arise from any of the chest wall tissues.
- Benign tumors are lipoma, osteochondroma, and fibrous dysplasia, whereas malignant tumor are chondrosarcoma, plasmacytoma, lymphoma, malignant fibrous histiocytoma, and osteosarcoma.
- Fibrous dysplasia is a skeletal developmental anomaly in which medullary bone is replaced by fibrous tissue with either monostotic or polyostotic involvement.
- Osteochondroma is characterized by cartilage-capped bony growth that projects from affected bone surface.
- Lipomas are composed of mature fat cells and are usually encapsulated.

- Osteosarcoma has malignant mesenchymal cells that produce osteoid or immature bone and has an aggressive pathologic behavior with mixed sclerosis/lucency within the medullary cavity.
- In children, primary malignancies are small round cell tumors, PNET, Askin tumors, rhabdomyosarcoma, and Ewing sarcoma.

INCIDENCE/PREVALENCE AND EPIDEMIOLOGY

- Most common benign rib lesion is fibrous dysplasia, followed by osteochondroma.
- Chondrosarcoma is most common adult malignant chest wall primary bone tumor, with 90% arising from the ribs.
- Ewing sarcoma/PNET is most common primary chest wall tumor in children.
- Metastases are most common malignant tumors involving the skeleton; the osteolytic type is encountered most frequently, although sclerotic or mixed types occur.
- Vast majority of primary chest wall soft tissue tumors are benign, the most common one being lipoma.
- Elastofibroma is a relatively common fibroelastic pseudotumor that in almost 99% of the cases occurs in the subscapular region.
- Soft tissue sarcomas and primary malignant fibrous histiocytoma of the chest wall are rare.

Suggested Readings

Jeung MY, Gangi A, Gasser B, et al: Imaging of chest wall disorders. *RadioGraphics* 19:617-637, 1999.

O'Sullivan P, O'Dwyer H, Flint J, et al: Malignant chest wall neoplasms of bone and cartilage: A pictorial review of CT and MR findings. *Br J Radiol* 80:678-684, 2007.

O'Sullivan P, O'Dwyer H, Flint J, et al: Soft tissue tumours and mass-like lesions of the chest wall: A pictorial review of CT and MR findings. *Br J Radiol* 80:574-580, 2007.

Tateishi U, Gladish GW, Kusumoto M, et al: Chest wall tumors: Radiologic findings and pathologic correlation: I. Benign tumors. *RadioGraphics* 23:1477-1490, 2003.

Tateishi U, Gladish GW, Kusumoto M, et al: Chest wall tumors: Radiologic findings and pathologic correlation: II. Malignant tumors. *RadioGraphics* 23:1491-1508, 2003.

Infection of Chest Wall

DEFINITION: A variety of inflammatory and infectious diseases may occur in the chest wall, ranging from inflammatory conditions of uncertain etiology to acute and chronic infections involving bone, joints, or soft tissues.

IMAGING

Radiography
Findings
- Soft tissue swelling

Utility
- Of limited value in the diagnosis

CT
Findings
- Soft tissue swelling, abscess formation
- Sternal osteomyelitis: suspected when soft tissue abnormalities are associated with bone destruction, dehiscence, or severe demineralization
- Necrotizing fasciitis: spontaneous necrosis and gas formation
- Actinomycosis: lung infection may result in empyema and extend into chest wall
- Tuberculosis: may result in chondritis, osteomyelitis, spondylitis, abscess formation, and empyema necessitatis

Utility
- CT is used to assess extent and depth of infection and can be useful for surgical planning.

CLINICAL PRESENTATION

- Chest pain, fever
- Necrotizing fasciitis: high fever; red, painful swelling that spreads rapidly

DIFFERENTIAL DIAGNOSIS

- Post-surgical hematoma or seroma
- Post-traumatic hematoma or seroma
- Chest wall abscess
- Sternal osteomyelitis
- Actinomycosis
- Tuberculosis

PATHOLOGY

- Lesions range from inflammatory conditions of uncertain etiology to acute or chronic infections involving bone, joints, or soft tissues.

DIAGNOSTIC PEARLS

- Sternal osteomyelitis: soft tissue abnormalities associated with bone destruction, dehiscence, or severe demineralization
- Tuberculosis: may result in chondritis, osteomyelitis, spondylitis, abscess formation, and empyema necessitatis
- Majority of chest wall infections follow surgery (particularly median sternotomy) or trauma

---

- Soft tissue infections may be classified into necrotizing fasciitis (subcutaneous fat and superficial fascia) and pyomyositis (muscles).
- Actinomycosis is a chronic granulomatous infection characterized by suppuration, sulfur granules, abscess formation, and sinus tracts; pulmonary infection may progress to empyema and extend into chest wall.
- Tuberculosis may result in chondritis, osteomyelitis, spondylitis, abscess formation, and empyema necessitatis.
- Empyema necessitatis is leakage of empyema through parietal pleura with discharge of its contents into subcutaneous tissues of chest wall.

INCIDENCE/PREVALENCE AND EPIDEMIOLOGY

- Majority of chest wall infections follow surgery (particularly median sternotomy) or trauma.
- Other causes include necrotizing fasciitis, intravenous drug use (abscess, osteomyelitis, diskitis), tuberculosis, and extension of intrathoracic infections (actinomycosis, tuberculosis, empyema necessitatis).

Suggested Readings

Kwong JS, Müller NL, Godwin JD, et al: Thoracic actinomycosis: CT findings in eight patients. *Radiology* 183:189-192, 1992.
Morris BS, Maheshwari M, Chalwa A: Chest wall tuberculosis: A review of CT appearances. *Br J Radiol* 77:449-457, 2004.
Templeton PA, Fishman EK: CT evaluation of poststernotomy complications. *AJR Am J Roentgenol* 159:45-50, 1992.

WHAT THE REFERRING PHYSICIAN NEEDS TO KNOW
- Contrast-enhanced CT is the imaging modality of choice for the diagnosis of presence and extent of chest wall infection.

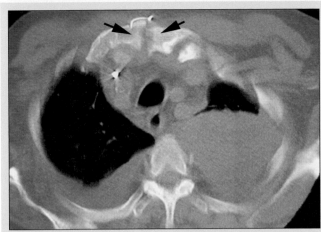

Figure 1. **Sternal dehiscence and infection from** ***Staphylococcus aureus*** **in a 65-year-old man after coronary artery bypass graft.** CT scan photographed at bone window settings shows sternal dehiscence (*arrows*). Also noted are bilateral pleural effusions. (*Courtesy of Dr. Tomás Franquet, Barcelona, Spain*)

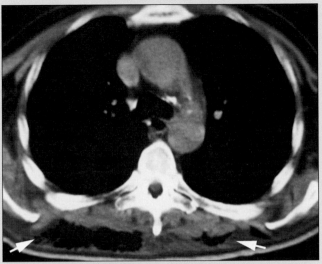

Figure 2. **Necrotizing fasciitis in a 66-year-old woman.** CT image photographed at lung window settings shows large gas collections dissecting the fascial planes of the posterior upper chest wall (*arrows*). (*Courtesy of Dr. Tomás Franquet, Barcelona, Spain*)

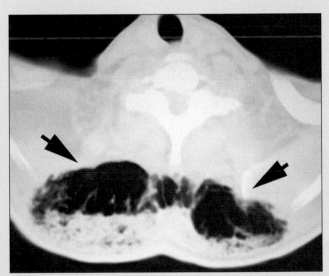

Figure 3. **Necrotizing fasciitis in a 66-year-old woman.** CT image photographed at soft window settings shows large gas collections dissecting the fascial planes of the posterior upper chest wall (*arrows*). (*Courtesy of Dr. Tomás Franquet, Barcelona, Spain*)

Index

Note: Page numbers followed by *f* indicate figures.